2011
YEAR BOOK OF
CARDIOLOGY®

The 2011 Year Book Series

Year Book of Anesthesiology and Pain Management™: Drs Chestnut, Abram, Black, Gravlee, Lien, Mathru, and Roizen

Year Book of Cardiology®: Drs Gersh, Cheitlin, Elliott, Gold, Graham, and Thourani

Year Book of Critical Care Medicine®: Drs Dellinger, Parrillo, Balk, Dorman, Dries, and Zanotti-Cavazzoni

Year Book of Dermatology and Dermatologic Surgery™: Dr Del Rosso

Year Book of Diagnostic Radiology®: Drs Osborn, Abbara, Elster, Manaster, Oestreich, Offiah, Rosado de Christenson, Stephens, and Walker

Year Book of Emergency Medicine®: Drs Hamilton, Bruno, Handly, Mullin, Quintana, and Ramoska

Year Book of Endocrinology®: Drs Schott, Apovian, Clarke, Eugster, Ludlam, Meikle, Ovalle, Schinner, Schteingart, and Toth

Year Book of Gastroenterology™: Drs Talley, DeVault, Harnois, Pearson, Picco, Scolapio, Smith, and Vege

Year Book of Hand and Upper Limb Surgery®: Drs Yao and Steinmann

Year Book of Medicine®: Drs Barker, Garrick, Gersh, Khardori, LeRoith, Seo, Talley, and Thigpen

Year Book of Neonatal and Perinatal Medicine®: Drs Fanaroff, Benitz, Donn, Neu, Papile, Polin, and van Marter

Year Book of Neurology and Neurosurgery®: Drs Klimo and Rabinstein

Year Book of Obstetrics, Gynecology, and Women's Health®: Drs Dungan and Shulman

Year Book of Oncology®: Drs Arceci, Bauer, Gordon, Lawton, and Thigpen

Year Book of Ophthalmology®: Drs Rapuano, Cohen, Flanders, Hammersmith, Milman, Myers, Nelson, Penne, Pyfer, Sergott, Shields, and Vander

Year Book of Orthopedics®: Drs Morrey, Beauchamp, Huddleston, Swiontkowski, and Trigg

Year Book of Otolaryngology-Head and Neck Surgery®: Drs Sindwani, Balough, Franco, Gapany, and Mitchell

Year Book of Pathology and Laboratory Medicine®: Drs Raab, Parwani, Bejarano, and Bissell

Year Book of Pediatrics®: Dr Stockman

Year Book of Plastic and Aesthetic Surgery™: Drs Miller, Gosain, Gurtner, Gutowski, Ruberg, Salisbury, and Smith

Year Book of Psychiatry and Applied Mental Health®: Drs Talbott, Ballenger, Buckley, Frances, Krupnick, and Mack

Year Book of Pulmonary Disease®: Drs Barker, Jones, Maurer, Raza, Tanoue, and Willsie

Year Book of Sports Medicine®: Drs Shephard, Cantu, Feldman, Jankowski, Khan, Lebrun, Nieman, Pierrynowski, and Rowland

Year Book of Surgery®: Drs Copeland, Behrns, Daly, Eberlein, Fahey, Huber, Klodell, Mozingo, and Pruett

Year Book of Urology®: Drs Andriole and Coplen

Year Book of Vascular Surgery®: Drs Moneta, Gillespie, Starnes, and Watkins

2011

The Year Book of CARDIOLOGY®

Editor in Chief

Bernard J. Gersh, MB, ChB, DPhil, FRCP

Professor of Medicine, Mayo Clinic College of Medicine; Consultant, Division of Cardiovascular Diseases, Mayo Clinic, Rochester, Minnesota

Editors

Melvin D. Cheitlin, MD, MACC

Emeritus Professor of Medicine, University of California, San Francisco; Former Chief of Cardiology, San Francisco General Hospital, San Francisco, California

William J. Elliott, MD, PhD

Professor of Preventive Medicine, Internal Medicine, and Pharmacology, Head, Division of Pharmacology, Pacific Northwest University of Health Sciences, Yakima, Washington

Michael R. Gold, MD, PhD

Michael E. Assey Professor of Medicine; Director of Cardiology, Medical University of South Carolina, Charleston, South Carolina

Thomas P. Graham, MD

Professor Emeritus of Pediatrics, Vanderbilt University School of Medicine; Division of Cardiology, Vanderbilt Children's Hospital, Nashville, Tennessee

Vinod H. Thourani, MD

Associate Professor of Cardiothoracic Surgery, Associate Director, Structural Heart Center, Associate Director, CT Surgery Clinical Research Unit, Associate Director, Residency Program, Emory University Hospital Midtown, Cardiac Surgery, Atlanta, Georgia

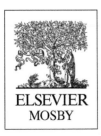

ELSEVIER
MOSBY

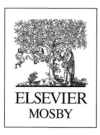

ELSEVIER
MOSBY

Vice President, Continuity: Kimberly Murphy
Developmental Editor: Katie Hartner
Production Supervisor, Electronic Year Books: Donna M. Skelton
Electronic Article Manager: Emily Ogle
Illustrations and Permissions Coordinator: Dawn A. Vohsen

2011 EDITION

Composition by TNQ Books and Journals Pvt Ltd, India

Editorial Office:
Elsevier
1600 John F. Kennedy Blvd.
Suite 1800
Philadelphia, PA 19103-2899

International Standard Serial Number: 0145-4145
International Standard Book Number: 978-0-323-08408-6

Printed and bound by CPI Group (UK) Ltd, Croydon, CR0 4YY

Transferred to Digital Print 2011

Contributing Editors

Michael L. Bernard, MD, PhD
Fellow, Division of Cardiology, Medical University of South Carolina, Charleston, South Carolina

William W. Brabham, MD
Fellow, Division of Cardiology, Medical University of South Carolina, Charleston, South Carolina

Frank A. Cuoco, Jr, MD, MBA
Assistant Professor, Department of Medicine, Medical University of South Carolina, Charleston, South Carolina

Jason Goebel, MD
Fellow, Division of Cardiology, Medical University of South Carolina, Charleston, South Carolina

W. Brent Keeling, MD
Chief Resident in Cardiothoracic Surgery, Emory University School of Medicine, Atlanta, Georgia

Robert B. Leman, MD, FACC, FACP
Professor of Medicine, Medical University of South Carolina, Charleston, South Carolina

Peter Netzler, MD
Fellow, Division of Cardiology, Medical University of South Carolina, Charleston, South Carolina

Christopher P. Rowley, MD
Fellow, Division of Cardiology, Medical University of South Carolina, Charleston, South Carolina

Darren S. Sidney, MD
Fellow, Division of Cardiology, Medical University of South Carolina, Charleston, South Carolina

J. Lacy Sturdivant, MD
Assistant Professor, Department of Medicine, Medical University of South Carolina, Charleston, South Carolina

Richard Norris Vest III, MD
Fellow, Division of Cardiology, Medical University of South Carolina, Charleston, South Carolina

J. Marcus Wharton, MD
Frank Tourville Professor of Medicine, Chief of Electrophysiology, Medical University of South Carolina, Charleston, South Carolina

William M. Yarbrough, MD
Assistant Professor, Cardiothoracic Surgery, Department of Surgery, Medical University of South Carolina, Charleston, South Carolina

Table of Contents

Journals Represented

STANDARD ABBREVIATIONS

The following terms are abbreviated in this edition: acquired immunodeficiency syndrome (AIDS), cardiopulmonary resuscitation (CPR), central nervous system

(CNS), cerebrospinal fluid (CSF), computed tomography (CT), deoxyribonucleic acid (DNA), electrocardiography (ECG), health maintenance organization (HMO), human immunodeficiency virus (HIV), intensive care unit (ICU), intramuscular (IM), intravenous (IV), magnetic resonance (MR) imaging (MRI), ribonucleic acid (RNA), and ultrasound (US).

NOTE

The YEAR BOOK OF CARDIOLOGY is a literature survey service providing abstracts of articles published in the professional literature. Every effort is made to assure the accuracy of the information presented in these pages. Neither the editors nor the publisher of the YEAR BOOK OF CARDIOLOGY can be responsible for errors in the original materials. The editors' comments are their own opinions. Mention of specific products within this publication does not constitute endorsement.

To facilitate the use of the YEAR BOOK OF CARDIOLOGY as a reference tool, all illustrations and tables included in this publication are now identified as they appear in the original article. This change is meant to help the reader recognize that any illustration or table appearing in the YEAR BOOK OF CARDIOLOGY may be only one of many in the original article. For this reason, figure and table numbers will often appear to be out of sequence within the YEAR BOOK OF CARDIOLOGY.

1 Hypertension

Introduction

Overall, the field of hypertension had a very "slow" year in 2010. The initial and final release dates for the Eighth Report of the Joint National Committee on Prevention, Detection, Evaluation, and Treatment of High Blood Pressure (JNC 8) were pushed back again (now March and June of 2011). The International Society on Hypertension in Blacks released an "update" of their 2003 treatment guidelines, which presented many recommendations that were not very "evidence-based." Perhaps the most impressive event was the simultaneous publication of 4 (!) papers from Professor Peter Rothwell and his group at Oxford, which suggested that much of the variability of the effects of antihypertensive drugs on stroke end points in clinical trials can be attributed to visit-to-visit blood pressure variability. Additional data, primarily from the Hypertension in the Very Elderly Trial (HYVET), allowed an updated meta-analysis to conclude that antihypertensive drug treatment significantly reduces stroke and heart failure in octogenarians, with only a nonsignificant 6% increase in mortality. An excellent review of preeclampsia reminded us that there are many unanswered questions in this disease. A review of recent clinical trials in hypertension suggested that such studies should move away from pharmaceutical marketing. Meta-analyses also suggested that the cough associated with angiotensin-converting enzyme (ACE) inhibitors is far more common than indicated in the manufacturers' product information, that diuretics are the most effective antihypertensive drug class for preventing heart failure, and that catheter-based interventions for renovascular hypertension due to fibromuscular dysplasia are not quite as uniformly curative as once thought. A meta-analysis also concluded that biofeedback doesn't lower blood pressure very much (if at all), despite a subsequent publication that suggested a very slight hypotensive effect of behavioral neurocardiac training (which involves biofeedback, among other potential modalities). Two meta-analyses of the blood pressure-lowering effects of cocoa were published, along with a randomized trial suggesting that the effect is not likely due to theobromine. Perhaps the most widely publicized meta-analysis about hypertension and its therapy claimed that angiotensin receptor blockers are associated with a significantly increased risk of cancer, which was hotly debated thereafter.

Surely the most important epidemiological study published in 2010 indicated that the target for blood pressure control in the United States, advocated by both Healthy People 2000 and 2010, has been achieved: Just over 50% of Americans with hypertension now have a blood pressure lower than 140/90 mm Hg. This feat can be interpreted as late by 7 to 8 years or early by 2 to 3 years. Two cohort studies suggested that angiotensin receptor blockers may have some special protective effects for stroke or Alzheimer disease, echoing previous mechanistic studies and some clinical trial data. Another cohort study suggested that visit-to-visit blood pressure variability contributes to white matter hyperintensities seen on MRI, consistent with the conclusions of Rothwell et al. Two publications of the long-term effects of the Antihypertensive and Lipid Lowering treatment to prevent Heart Attack Trial (ALLHAT) Dissemination Project and of the African American Study of Kidney disease and hypertension (AASK) were somewhat pessimistic: compared to what one might have hoped, fewer patients filled prescriptions for thiazide diuretics after ALLHAT, and more AASK patients ended up on dialysis. A cohort study of Canadian physicians indicated that prelicensure testing of their communication and management skills predicted their future patients' adherence to antihypertensive drug therapy. Analysis of data from US national surveys from 1999-2006 suggested that chronic kidney disease was quite prevalent in American adults with undiagnosed hypertension (23%) and prehypertension (17%). Data from a large United Kingdom pharmacy database indicated that angiotensin receptor blockers, ACE-inhibitors, and beta-blockers may prevent atrial fibrillation in treated patients with hypertension. Lastly, data from nearly 9000 Australian people who underwent ambulatory blood pressure monitoring allowed correlation of office and daytime average blood pressures, and the findings intimated that physicians probably should not measure blood pressures in the office, as their results are significantly higher and do not correlate well with 24-hour ambulatory averages.

There were fewer papers published in 2010 than usual correlating hypertension and cardiovascular risk (excluding reviews and clinical trials). A California cohort study with 37 years of follow-up correlated preeclampsia with cardiovascular death, validating the concept of pregnancy as a "cardiovascular stress test." Post-hoc analyses of the patients with diabetes enrolled in the INternational VErapamil-Sustained release/ Trandolapril (INVEST) trial suggested no benefit of a lower-than-usual blood pressure target. A case-control study from the Group Health Cooperative in Seattle (the investigative group that became famous in 1995 for a study with similar design and conclusions) of calcium antagonists after an initial diuretic showed a higher risk of myocardial infarction than with other second-line therapies. And lastly, a post-hoc analysis of the pilot study of antihypertensive therapy for patients with intracerebral hemorrhage suggested that patients who achieved the lowest blood pressures in the first 24 hours had the least short-term increase in hemorrhage volume. Although this doesn't change current recommendations for not treating such patients' blood pressure, it calls for completion of the larger trial to show that such treatment is indeed beneficial in the long term.

Four publications highlighted new information about the "causes" of hypertension. Two high-profile cost-effectiveness analyses of population-wide reduction in dietary sodium in the United States agreed that such programs would be likely to save many lives, myocardial infarctions, strokes, and a **great deal** of money. A post-hoc analysis of a large Italian clinical trial suggests that pravastatin does not significantly lower blood pressure (contrary to recent data from other sources). Despite better blood pressure control and improved renal function in those who received angioplasty, the incidence of renal artery stenosis during "drive-by renal angiograms" (after cardiac catheterization) was much lower in a Swiss cohort than reported by American sites.

Many clinical trials added to our understanding of hypertension and its treatment. Probably the most important was the blood pressure-lowering arm of Action to Control Cardiovascular Risk in Diabetes (ACCORD-BP), which showed a nonsignificant benefit on cardiovascular risk of a systolic blood pressure goal lower than 120 mm Hg, compared to lower than 140 mm Hg, despite a lower risk of stroke; this is expected to help shape the JNC 8 recommendation for the blood pressure target in diabetics. A large, international, placebo-controlled, 2 × 2 factorial design trial of valsartan ± nateglinide in patients with impaired fasting glucose showed a significant effect of the former (but not the latter) on incident diabetes, and no effects of either on cardiovascular events. Two Japanese trials involving valsartan were probably underpowered to detect significant differences in cardiovascular outcomes, either compared to amlodipine, or when used as initial therapy comparing 2 systolic blood pressure targets (<140 vs <150 mm Hg) in patients with isolated systolic hypertension. Two subgroup analyses from the Avoiding Cardiovascular COMplications in Patients LIving with Systolic Hypertension (ACCOMPLISH) trial confirmed the conclusions of the main trial: the combination of amlodipine + benazepril was more effective than hydrochlorothiazide + benazepril in preventing either the primary end point in diabetics (as well as nondiabetics), or doubling of serum creatinine or end-stage renal disease. Whether to continue or stop antihypertensive drug therapy for acute stroke victims was addressed by an English clinical trial, but enrollment was slow and funding was cut, allowing no definitive conclusion to be drawn; but continuing therapy was not associated with adverse outcomes. Home blood pressure telemonitoring and self-management of medication adjustments led to better blood pressure control than office-management in one trial, but home blood pressure monitoring (without telemonitoring) did not improve medication adherence in another (in which adherence was very good in both randomized groups). Two trials in resistant hypertensives showed the blood pressure-lowering effects of spironolactone and continuous positive airway pressure, setting the stage for their comparison. Involving either pharmacists or barbers in management of hypertension improved blood pressure control in 2 cluster-randomized trials. Adding exercise and weight loss to the Dietary Approaches to Stop Hypertension diet lowered blood pressure significantly, but only about 5/3 mm Hg more than the diet alone, after 4 months of careful supervision. Giving placebo or supplemental vitamins C and E to more than 10 000 unselected nulliparous women during weeks 9-16 of pregnancy did not reduce preeclampsia or its complications. And lastly, a 3.4-year placebo-controlled trial of sibutramine for weight loss in 9804 patients with preexisting cardiovascular conditions observed a slightly higher blood pressure (by 1.2/1.4 mm Hg) and a significant increase in nonfatal myocardial infarction and nonfatal stroke, leading to the removal of the drug from the worldwide marketplace. These important results show the power of carefully designed and well-executed clinical trials, even when the blood pressure differences across randomized groups are too small to measure in any given patient at a single visit.

William J. Elliott, MD, PhD

Guidelines and Overviews

Limitations of the usual blood-pressure hypothesis and importance of variability, instability, and episodic hypertension

Rothwell PM (John Radcliffe Hosp, Headington, Oxford, UK)
Lancet 375:938-948, 2010

Although hypertension is the most prevalent treatable vascular risk factor, how it causes end-organ damage and vascular events is poorly understood. Yet, a widespread belief exists that underlying usual blood pressure can alone account for all blood-pressure-related risk of vascular events and for the benefits of antihypertensive drugs, and this notion has come to underpin all major clinical guidelines on diagnosis and treatment of hypertension. Other potentially informative measures, such as variability in clinic blood pressure or maximum blood pressure reached, have been neglected, and effects of antihypertensive drugs on such measures are largely unknown. Clinical guidelines recommend that episodic hypertension is not treated, and the potential risks of residual variability in blood pressure in treated hypertensive patients have been ignored. This Review discusses shortcomings of the usual blood-pressure hypothesis, provides background to accompanying reports on the importance of blood-pressure variability in prediction of risk of vascular events and in accounting for benefits of antihypertensive drugs, and draws attention to clinical implications and directions for future research.

▶ This review adds definitions, epidemiological perspective, and rationale to the other new evidence published simultaneously in *The Lancet* with 2 more articles by Professor Rothwell and colleagues,[1,2] along with an accompanying editorial,[3] and simultaneously, with another study on a similar topic in *Lancet Neurology*[4] (with its own editorial[5]). Because this article provides the background for the other analytical articles, it is probably best for most people to read this review first.[6]

This report clearly defines the measures of blood pressure that are discussed in this and the accompanying articles. While, for example, blood pressure variability can be noted in 24-hour ambulatory blood pressure monitoring sessions, these articles deal with the visit-to-visit variability in blood pressure in clinical trials (or day-to-day variability in home readings). The authors extrapolate their results to blood pressure instability (transient fluctuations in blood pressure associated with changing position, emotional stress, or pain). They believe that these phenomena lead to similar increases in risk of stroke as do visit-to-visit blood pressure variability seen in their studies and meta-analyses.

These considerations lead to a host of potential applications in clinical medicine. Perhaps the most interesting is that blood pressure variability may play a role in vascular dementia. At least one meta-analysis has already suggested that calcium antagonists (which seem to reduce blood pressure variability the best) may be protective in both stroke and vascular dementia because of their propensity to reduce carotid intima-medial thickness.[7] This review provides a different potential explanation for this phenomenon. More controversial is the suggestion that future research may show that people with normal blood pressures but high degrees of blood pressure variability may benefit from drug treatment that reduces the variability (without changing the blood pressure). Lastly, there is the hope that specific drugs might be developed that reduce blood pressure variability, without affecting the mean blood pressure very much; statins and other drugs that reduce biomarkers of inflammation (eg, C-reactive protein) might be examples of such drugs.

W. J. Elliott, MD, PhD

References

1. Rothwell PM, Howard SC, Dolan E, et al. Prognostic significance of visit-to-visit variability, maximum systolic blood pressure, and episodic hypertension. *Lancet.* 2010;375:895-905.
2. Webb AJS, Fischer U, Mehta Z, Rothwell PM. Effects of antihypertensive-drug class on interindividual variation in blood pressure and risk of stroke: a systematic review and meta-analysis. *Lancet.* 2010;375:906-915.
3. Carlberg B, Lindholm LH. Stroke and blood-pressure variation: new permutations on an old theme. *Lancet.* 2010;375:867-869.
4. Rothwell PM, Howard SC, Dolan E, et al. Effects of beta blockers and calcium-channel blockers on within-individual variability in blood pressure and risk of stroke. *Lancet Neurol.* 2010;9:469-480.
5. Gorelick PM. Reducing blood pressure variability to prevent stroke? *Lancet Neurol.* 2010;9:448-449.
6. Donlan E, O'Brien E. Blood pressure variability: clarity for clinical practice. *Hypertension.* 2010;56:179-181.
7. Wang J-G, Staessen JA, Li Y, et al. Carotid intima-media thickness and antihypertensive treatment: a meta-analysis of randomized controlled trials. *Stroke.* 2006; 37:1933-1940.

Prognostic significance of visit-to-visit variability, maximum systolic blood pressure, and episodic hypertension

Rothwell PM, Howard SC, Dolan E, et al (John Radcliffe Hosp, Headington, Oxford, UK; Connolly Hosp, Dublin, Ireland; et al)
Lancet 375:895-905, 2010

Background.—The mechanisms by which hypertension causes vascular events are unclear. Guidelines for diagnosis and treatment focus only on underlying mean blood pressure. We aimed to reliably establish the prognostic significance of visit-to-visit variability in blood pressure, maximum blood pressure reached, untreated episodic hypertension, and residual variability in treated patients.

Methods.—We determined the risk of stroke in relation to visit-to-visit variability in blood pressure (expressed as standard deviation [SD] and parameters independent of mean blood pressure) and maximum blood pressure in patients with previous transient ischaemic attack (TIA; UK-TIA trial and three validation cohorts) and in patients with treated hypertension (Anglo-Scandinavian Cardiac Outcomes Trial Blood Pressure Lowering Arm [ASCOT-BPLA]). In ASCOT-BPLA, 24-h ambulatory blood-pressure monitoring (ABPM) was also studied.

Findings.—In each TIA cohort, visit-to-visit variability in systolic blood pressure (SBP) was a strong predictor of subsequent stroke (eg, top-decile hazard ratio [HR] for SD SBP over seven visits in UK-TIA trial: 6·22, 95% CI 4·16—9·29, p<0·0001), independent of mean SBP, but dependent on precision of measurement (top-decile HR over ten visits: 12·08, 7·40—19·72, p<0·0001). Maximum SBP reached was also a strong predictor of stroke (HR for top-decile over seven visits: 15·01, 6·56—34·38, p<0·0001, after adjustment for mean SBP). In ASCOT-BPLA, residual visit-to-visit variability in SBP on treatment was also a strong predictor of stroke and coronary events (eg, top-decile HR for stroke: 3·25, 2·32—4·54, p<0·0001), independent of mean SBP in clinic or on ABPM. Variability on ABPM was a weaker predictor, but all measures of variability were most predictive in younger patients and at lower (<median) values of mean SBP in every cohort.

Interpretation.—Visit-to-visit variability in SBP and maximum SBP are strong predictors of stroke, independent of mean SBP. Increased residual variability in SBP in patients with treated hypertension is associated with a high risk of vascular events.

▶ This report, published in the same issue with 2 others[1,2] (an essentially unprecedented feat), with an accompanying editorial,[3] and simultaneously with another study on a similar topic in *Lancet Neurology*[4] (with its own editorial[5]) probably is the most important scientific contribution to hypertension in 2010, if not many years or even the new millennium. It should force us to rethink the usual blood pressure paradigm, which traditionally placed emphasis on the average level of blood pressure over a defined time period.

The use of sophisticated statistical analyses and the plethora of graphs from such analyses have probably deterred many from giving this article the study it deserves. Most practicing clinicians are aware of the greater risk of a high degree of within-individual variability in heart rate (eg, sick sinus syndrome) or plasma glucose levels (hypoglycemic coma vs hyperosmolar coma), but a similar degree of variability in blood pressure has not previously been cause for much concern. Professor Rothwell is trying to change that.

The efforts of the investigative team in this article are remarkable. They gathered patient-specific blood pressure from every visit and outcomes data from 5 clinical trials (data from the Anglo-Scandinavian Cardiac Outcomes Trial [ASCOT][5] included 1.12 million measurements), characterized their standard deviation and coefficient of variation (standard deviation/mean), and then, created a third statistical variable (variation independent of the mean, VID) related to the coefficient of variation, but dividing the standard deviation by the mean, raised to the x power, where x is derived from curve fitting of the standard deviation of systolic blood pressure (y-axis) versus mean systolic blood pressure (x-axis). This parameter has no significant correlation with mean blood pressure (as do both the standard deviation and the coefficient of variation). It turned out that all of these factors were more predictive of stroke than the mean level of blood pressure; the most predictive was visit-to-visit variability in blood pressure. They had consistent findings from each of the 4 trials that were used to develop the analytical techniques and discovered similar significant relationships in each randomized arm of the main ASCOT trial data.

They took their concept a giant step further by performing similar analyses on the 24-hour ambulatory blood pressure monitoring (ABPM) data from 1905 patients in ASCOT. Perhaps because of limited power (because of the smaller number of outcome events; the coefficients of variability were more precise because of the greater number of blood pressure measurements per session), the results were not quite as strong. However, the daytime coefficient of variation of systolic blood pressure on the ABPMs done during the 6th to 30th months of follow-up was still a significant predictor of cardiovascular events.

These results have important implications for clinical practice and future research. The first is that we need not "toss out the baby with the bathwater," and reject the importance of control of (mean) blood pressure. Recall that these analyses all adjust for mean blood pressure, so these are second-order effects, even if they account for a great deal of the residual variance of cardiovascular event prevention with drug therapy. The authors suggest that episodic hypertension is intrinsically risky and should not be an exclusion criterion for clinical trials. Similarly, stabilization of blood pressures may be a useful target for treatment and drug development. It is difficult to predict whether these concepts will be accepted by regulatory authorities, but the recent approval of single-pill combinations containing different agents with multiple dosing options is consistent with the authors' interpretations.[6]

W. J. Elliott, MD, PhD

References

1. Webb AJS, Fischer U, Mehta Z, Rothwell PM. Effects of antihypertensive-drug class on interindividual variation in blood pressure and risk of stroke: a systematic review and meta-analysis. *Lancet.* 2010;375:906-915.
2. Rothwell PM. Limitations of the usual blood-pressure hypothesis and importance of variability, instability, and episodic hypertension. *Lancet.* 2010;375:938-948.
3. Carlberg B, Lindholm LH. Stroke and blood-pressure variation: new permutations on an old theme. *Lancet.* 2010;375:867-869.
4. Rothwell PM, Howard SC, Dolan E, et al. Effects of beta blockers and calcium-channel blockers on within-individual variability in blood pressure and risk of stroke. *Lancet Neurol.* 2010;9:469-480.
5. Gorelick PB. Reducing blood pressure variability to prevent stroke? *Lancet Neurol.* 2010;9:448-449.
6. Donlan E, O'Brien E. Blood pressure variability: clarity for clinical practice. *Hypertension.* 2010;56:179-181.

Effects of antihypertensive-drug class on interindividual variation in blood pressure and risk of stroke: a systematic review and meta-analysis
Webb AJS, Fischer U, Mehta Z, et al (John Radcliffe Hosp, Oxford, UK)
Lancet 375:906-915, 2010

Introduction.—Unexplained differences between classes of antihypertensive drugs in their effectiveness in preventing stroke might be due to class effects on intraindividual variability in blood pressure. We did a systematic review to assess any such effects in randomised controlled trials.

Methods.—Baseline and follow-up data for mean (SD) of systolic blood pressure (SBP) were extracted from trial reports. Effect of treatment on interindividual variance (SD^2) in blood pressure (a surrogate for within-individual variability), expressed as the ratio of the variances (VR), was related to effects on clinical outcomes. Pooled estimates were derived by use of random-effects meta-analysis.

Findings.—Mean (SD) SBP at follow-up was reported in 389 (28%) of 1372 eligible trials. There was substantial heterogeneity between trials in VR ($p<1\times10^{-40}$), 68% of which was attributable to allocated drug class. Compared with other drugs, interindividual variation in SBP was reduced by calcium-channel blockers (VR 0·81, 95% CI 0·76−0·86, p<0·0001) and non-loop diuretic drugs (0·87, 0·79−0·96, p=0·007), and increased by angiotensin-converting enzyme (ACE) inhibitors (1·08, 1·02−1·15, p=0·008), angiotensin-receptor blockers (1·16, 1·07−1·25, p=0·0002), and β blockers (1·17, 1·07−1·28, p=0·0007). Compared with placebo only, interindividual variation in SBP was reduced the most by calcium-channel blockers (0·76, 0·67−0·85, p<0·0001). Effects were consistent in parallel group and crossover design trials, and in analyses of dose-response. Across all trials, effects of treatment on VR of SBP ($r^2=0·372$, p=0·0006) and on mean SBP ($r^2=0·328$, p=0·0015) accounted for effects on stroke risk (eg, odds ratio 0·79, 0·71−0·87, p<0·0001, for VR≤0·80), and both remained significant in a combined model.

Interpretation.—Drug-class effects on interindividual variation in blood pressure can account for differences in effects of antihypertensive drugs on risk of stroke independently of effects on mean SBP.

▶ This report adds to other new evidence, published in 2 articles by Professor Rothwell and colleagues[1,2] in the same issue, with an accompanying editorial,[3] and simultaneously with another study on a similar topic in *Lancet Neurology*[4] (with its own editorial[5]) in favor of the object of reducing not only the blood pressure level but also the blood pressure variability, to reduce the risk of stroke.

This report differs from many other meta-analyses in that it used other meta-analyses as the source for its data search strategy. The authors included not only outcomes-based studies of antihypertensive drugs but also registration studies, comparative short-term efficacy studies, and found 389 studies that reported the standard deviation of the systolic blood pressure at both baseline and follow-up (typically at 1 year after randomization). These were meta-analyzed and resulted in the conclusion that both subclasses of calcium antagonists decreased the change in the pooled variance ratio (a surrogate for blood pressure variability).

They then performed a second set of meta-analyses using data from the 21 clinical trials that reported both on blood pressure variability and the risk of stroke. Unlike myocardial infarction or heart failure, there was an independent effect of their measure of blood pressure variability on stroke, which was confirmed in several meta-regression analyses, plotting the variance ratio of the compared drugs against the odds ratio from stroke.

The authors have agreed to work with the Blood Pressure Lowering Trialists Collaboration (who have gathered much data from nearly all recent clinical trials in hypertension) in an effort to extend their observations using patient-level blood pressures and long-term changes in blood pressure (and variability thereof).[6,7] Presuming those analyses result in similar, but probably even stronger, conclusions, we may begin to see reports of clinical trials that contain specific analyses of blood pressure variability. Whether such parameters will prove useful as a type of quality control measure for individual physicians or collaborative group practices remains to be seen.

W. J. Elliott, MD, PhD

References

1. Rothwell PM, Howard SC, Dolan E, et al. Prognostic significance of visit-to-visit variability, maximum systolic blood pressure, and episodic hypertension. *Lancet.* 2010;375:895-905.
2. Rothwell PM. Limitations of the usual blood-pressure hypothesis and importance of variability, instability, and episodic hypertension. *Lancet.* 2010;375:938-948.
3. Carlberg B, Lindholm LH. Stroke and blood-pressure variation: new permutations on an old theme. *Lancet.* 2010;375:867-869.
4. Rothwell PM, Howard SC, Dolan E, et al. Effects of beta-blockers and calcium-channel blockers on within-individual variability in blood pressure and risk of stroke. *Lancet Neurol.* 2010;9:469-480.
5. Gorelick PB. Reducing blood pressure variability to prevent stroke? *Lancet Neurol.* 2010;9:448-449.

6. Donlan E, O'Brien E. Blood pressure variability: clarity for clinical practice. *Hypertension*. 2010;56:179-181.
7. Turnbull F, Neal B, Ninomiya T, et al. Blood Pressure Lowering Treatment Trialists' Collaboration. Effects of different regimens to lower blood pressure on major cardiovascular events in older and younger adults: meta-analysis of randomised trials. *BMJ*. 2008;336:1121-1123.

Effects of β blockers and calcium-channel blockers on within-individual variability in blood pressure and risk of stroke

Rothwell PM, on behalf of the ASCOT-BPLA and MRC Trial Investigators (John Radcliffe Hosp, Oxford, UK; et al)
Lancet Neurol 9:469-480, 2010

Background.—Analyses of some randomised trials show that calcium-channel blockers reduce the risk of stroke more than expected on the basis of mean blood pressure alone and that β blockers are less effective than expected. We aimed to investigate whether the effects of these drugs on variability in blood pressure might explain these disparities in effect on stroke risk.

Methods.—The Anglo-Scandinavian Cardiac Outcomes Trial Blood Pressure Lowering Arm (ASCOT-BPLA) compared amlodipine-based regimens with atenolol-based regimens in 19 257 patients with hypertension and other vascular risk factors and the Medical Research Council (MRC) trial compared atenolol-based and diuretic-based regimens versus placebo in 4396 hypertensive patients aged 65–74 years. We expressed visit-to-visit variability of blood pressure during follow-up in the two trials as standard deviation (SD) and as transformations uncorrelated with mean blood pressure. For ASCOT-BPLA, we also studied within-visit variability and variability on 24 h ambulatory blood-pressure monitoring (ABPM).

Results.—In ASCOT-BPLA, group systolic blood pressure (SBP) SD was lower in the amlodipine group than in the atenolol group at all follow-up visits (p<0.0001), mainly because of lower within-individual visit-to-visit variability. Within-visit and ABPM variability in SBP were also lower in the amlodipine group than in the atenolol group (all p<0.0001). Analysis of changes from baseline showed that variability decreased over time in the amlodipine group and increased in the atenolol group. The lower risk of stroke in the amlodipine group (hazard ratio 0.78, 95% CI 0.67–0.90) was partly attenuated by adjusting for mean SBP during follow-up (0.84, 0.72–0.98), but was abolished by also adjusting for within-individual SD of clinic SBP (0.99, 0.85–1.16). Findings were similar for coronary events. In the ABPM substudy, reduced variability in daytime SBP in the amlodipine group (p<0.0001) partly accounted for the reduced risk of vascular events, but reduced visit-to-visit variability in clinic SBP had a greater effect. In the MRC trial, group SD SBP and all measures of within-individual visit-to-visit variability in SBP were increased in the atenolol group compared with both the placebo group and the diuretic group during initial follow-up (all p<0.0001). Subsequent temporal trends in variability in blood pressure during follow-up in the atenolol group correlated with trends in stroke risk.

Interpretation.—The opposite effects of calcium-channel blockers and beta blockers on variability of blood pressure account for the disparity in observed effects on risk of stroke and expected effects based on mean blood pressure. To prevent stroke most effectively, blood-pressure-lowering drugs should reduce mean blood pressure without increasing variability; ideally they should reduce both.

▶ This is perhaps the most detailed analysis of the "blood pressure variability hypothesis" papers, 3 of which were published simultaneously by Professor Rothwell and colleagues[1-3] in *The Lancet* (with an editorial),[4] along with this one (with its own accompanying editorial) in *Lancet Neurology*.[5] Although the analyses of the Medical Research Council trial in older hypertensive patients[6] and the Anglo-Scandinavian Cardiac Outcomes Trial-Blood Pressure Lowering Arm (ASCOT-BPLA)[7] come to similar conclusions about the role of blood pressure variability in predicting stroke, the latter included a 24-hour ambulatory blood pressure monitoring (ABPM) substudy. This data set provides much more information about variability (both circadian and ultradian), even if the much smaller number of subjects (and subjects with cardiovascular events) limits statistical power for showing the relationship of variability and stroke risk. The investigators were able, however, to discern a significant relationship in the ASCOT ABPM substudy population, between blood pressure variability and "all cardiovascular events and procedures," an end point specified and favored by the ASCOT investigators because it had the highest incidence of all their end points.[8]

The authors make much of the fact that their "visit-to-visit variability accounts for the previously unexplained treatment effects in ASCOT-BLPA and other trials" leaves the reader without an accounting of the proportion of the risk attributed to this new variable. In their meta-analysis,[3] they attribute 68% of the previously unexplained variation in blood pressure to different antihypertensive drug classes.

It is likely that this work, along with its companion papers,[1-3] will provide much impetus for investigators in other hypertension treatment trials to reanalyze their data, much as the focus on pulse pressure (rather than diastolic blood pressure) in the 1990s did. It is critically important that this be done for calcium antagonists, which these data (and the accompanying meta-analysis[3]) suggest have the greatest potential for reducing visit-to-visit blood pressure variability, since the authors' conclusions about the risk of cardiovascular outcomes associated with it are based solely on ASCOT.[2] It is likely, however, that more detailed reporting of follow-up blood pressure in trials should now become more common, even if outcome-based hypertension treatment trials are not as common as they were in the last 20 years.

W. J. Elliott, MD, PhD

References

1. Rothwell PM. Limitations of the usual blood-pressure hypothesis and importance of variability, instability, and episodic hypertension. *Lancet.* 2010;375:938-948.

2. Rothwell PM, Howard SC, Dolan E, et al. Prognostic significance of visit-to-visit variability, maximum systolic blood pressure, and episodic hypertension. *Lancet.* 2010;375:895-905.
3. Webb AJS, Fischer U, Mehta Z, Rothwell PM. Effects of antihypertensive-drug class on interindividual variation in blood pressure and risk of stroke: a systematic review and meta-analysis. *Lancet.* 2010;375:906-915.
4. Carlberg B, Lindholm LH. Stroke and blood-pressure variation: new permutations on an old theme. *Lancet.* 2010;375:867-869.
5. Gorelick PM. Reducing blood pressure variability to prevent stroke? *Lancet Neurol.* 2010;9:448-449.
6. Medical Research Council trial of treatment of hypertension in older adults: principal results. MRC Working Party. *BMJ.* 1992;304:405-412.
7. Dahlöf B, Sever PS, Poulter NR, et al. Prevention of cardiovascular events with an antihypertensive regimen of amlodipine adding perindopril as required versus atenolol adding bendroflumethiazide as required, in the Anglo-Scandinavian Cardiac Outcomes Trial-Blood Pressure Lowering Arm (ASCOT-BPLA): a multicentre randomised controlled trial. *Lancet.* 2005;366:895-906.
8. Poulter NR, Wedel H, Dahlöf B, et al. Role of blood pressure and other variables in the differential cardiovascular event rates noted in the Anglo-Scandinavian Cardiac Outcomes Trial-Blood Pressure Lowering Arm (ASCOT-BPLA). *Lancet.* 2005;366:907-913.

Management of High Blood Pressure in Blacks: An Update of the International Society on Hypertension in Blacks Consensus Statement

Flack JM, on behalf of the International Society on Hypertension in Blacks (Wayne State Univ, Detroit, MI; et al)

Hypertension 56:780-800, 2010

Since the first International Society on Hypertension in Blacks consensus statement on the "Management of High Blood Pressure in African Americans" in 2003, data from additional clinical trials have become available. We reviewed hypertension and cardiovascular disease prevention and treatment guidelines, pharmacological hypertension clinical end point trials, and blood pressure—lowering trials in blacks. Selected trials without significant black representation were considered. In this update, blacks with hypertension are divided into 2 risk strata, primary prevention, where elevated blood pressure without target organ damage, preclinical cardiovascular disease, or overt cardiovascular disease for whom blood pressure consistently <135/85 mm Hg is recommended, and secondary prevention, where elevated blood pressure with target organ damage, preclinical cardiovascular disease, and/or a history of cardiovascular disease, for whom blood pressure consistently <130/80 mm Hg is recommended. If blood pressure is ≤10 mm Hg above target levels, monotherapy with a diuretic or calcium channel blocker is preferred. When blood pressure is >15/10 mm Hg above target, 2-drug therapy is recommended, with either a calcium channel blocker plus a renin-angiotensin system blocker or, alternatively, in edematous and/or volume-overload states, with a thiazide diuretic plus a renin-angiotensin system blocker. Effective multidrug therapeutic combinations through 4 drugs are described. Comprehensive lifestyle modifications should be initiated in blacks when blood pressure is ≥115/75 mm Hg. The updated International Society on Hypertension in Blacks consensus statement on hypertension management in blacks lowers the minimum target blood pressure level for the lowest-risk blacks, emphasizes effective multidrug regimens, and de-emphasizes monotherapy.

▶ This report updates the consensus guidelines from the International Society on Hypertension in Blacks (ISHIB) from the original,[1] published before the Seventh Report of the Joint National Committee (JNC 7) on Prevention, Detection, Evaluation, and Treatment of High Blood Pressure in 2003.[2] Those who felt that the original recommendations were too aggressive (and not very evidence based) will likely have a similar opinion of this statement, which the editorialists, prominent authorities in hypertension, have characterized as "unsupported by randomized clinical trial evidence, and moreover, are inconsistent with the most recent results of large randomized clinical outcome trials in black hypertensive patients."[3] They take issue with the recommendation of the universal blood pressure (BP) target of < 135/85 mm Hg (for primary prevention) and < 130/80 mm Hg for all blacks with what the American Society of Hypertension's Writing Group called Stage 2 hypertension.[4] This includes all blacks with target organ damage, preclinical cardiovascular disease (including albuminuria, chronic kidney disease, or impaired fasting glucose), or a history of cardiovascular disease. The complex proposed sequence of drug addition (Fig 2 in the original article) for those requiring multidrug therapy eventually has all patients taking a diuretic, a calcium antagonist, and an inhibitor of the renin-angiotensin system (which includes angiotensin-converting enzyme inhibitors, angiotensin II receptor blockers, or a direct renin inhibitor).

The authors of this consensus statement avoid calling their document a set of guidelines, as these may be forthcoming soon in the JNC 8. Nonetheless, many feel that the ISHIB statements represent the definitive state of the art in managing hypertension in blacks, particularly African Americans.

The editorialists for this article recommend its review of the epidemiology, prevention, and diagnosis of hypertension in blacks but disagree with the target BPs recommended (< 135/85 mm Hg for primary prevention in low-risk blacks and < 130/80 mm Hg for high-risk blacks) and the proposed drug treatment algorithm. We shall see how JNC 8 resolves these issues.

W. J. Elliott, MD, PhD

References

1. Douglas JG, Bakris GL, Epstein M, et al. Hypertension in African Americans Working Group of the International Society on Hypertension in Blacks. Management of high blood pressure in African Americans: consensus statement of the Hypertension in African Americans Working Group of the International Society on Hypertension in Blacks. *Arch Intern Med.* 2003;163:525-541.
2. Chobanian AV, Bakris GL, Black HR, et al. National High Blood Pressure Education Program Coordinating Committee. Seventh report of the Joint National Committee on Prevention, Detection, Evaluation and Treatment of High Blood Pressure. *Hypertension.* 2003;42:1206-1252.

3. Wright JT Jr, Agodoa LY, Appel L, et al. New recommendations for treating hypertension in black patients: evidence and/or consensus? *Hypertension.* 2010;56: 801-803 [editorial].
4. Giles TD, Berk BC, Black HR, et al. on behalf of the Hypertension Writing Group. Expanding the definition and classification of hypertension. *J Clin Hypertens (Greenwich).* 2005;7:505-512.

Implications of Recently Published Trials of Blood Pressure–Lowering Drugs in Hypertensive or High-Risk Patients

Staessen JA, Richart T, Wang Z, et al (Univ of Leuven, Belgium; Peking Union Med College and Chinese Academy of Med Sciences, Beijing, China)

Hypertension 55:819-831, 2010

We reviewed 6 recent outcome trials of blood pressure (BP)–lowering drugs in 74 524 randomized hypertensive or high-risk patients. Over interpretation of nonsignificant or marginal probability values in large trials with overlapping end points, exclusion of patients not tolerating or not adhering to experimental treatments, labeling nonsignificant treatment effects as modest, and insufficient information on the quality of the BP measurements or on the BP changes early after randomization raise concern. From a clinical viewpoint, results should not be extrapolated to patients with characteristics dissimilar from those randomized. The benefit beyond BP lowering in cardiovascular prevention is tiny. Dual inhibition of the renin system should only be used in patients at high risk, in whom all drug combinations have been tried and who cannot be controlled by a single renin system inhibitor. Current evidence does not support BP lowering in normotensive patients or the use of renin system inhibitors for prevention of stroke recurrence. Because angiotensin-receptor blockers might offer less protection against myocardial infarction than angiotensin-converting enzyme inhibitors, the latter should remain the preferred renin system inhibitor for cardiovascular prevention in angiotensin-converting enzyme inhibitor-tolerant patients. In 2 trials, in which new-onset diabetes was a predefined end point, 1000 patients had to be treated for 1 year with an angiotensin-receptor blocker instead of placebo to prevent just 2 cases. From a design viewpoint, the time has come to revise the concept of large simple trials and to pursue research questions that serve patient interests more than showing noninferiority or highlight the ancillary qualities of marketable antihypertensive drugs.

▶ This article is a version of the authors' summary of the "State of the Art" in hypertension trials, presented as a plenary lecture at the 2009 American Society of Hypertension meeting. The authors point out that most recent clinical trials in hypertension are industry funded and intended to show benefits (typically either in composite cardiovascular outcomes or in ancillary properties) of expensive, branded, antihypertensive drugs. The authors criticize the many shortcomings of these trials and propose that the time has come to move beyond such myopic perspectives and to design and execute studies that are more relevant to, and primarily serve, patient care rather than the manufacturer or sponsor.

The editorialist for this article,[1] who was the primary principal investigator of several of the recent trials that came under criticism (Heart Outcomes Prevention Evaluation,[2] Ongoing Telmisartan Alone and in Combination with Ramipril Global Endpoint Trial,[3] Telmisartan Randomised AssessmeNt Study in ACE iNtolerant subjects with cardiovascular Disease,[4] and The Prevention Regimen for Effectively Avoiding Second Strokes Trial[5]), understandably and predictably disagrees with some of the arguments presented.

W. J. Elliott, MD, PhD

References

1. Yusuf S. Unresolved issues in the management of hypertension. *Hypertension.* 2010;55:832-834 [Editorial].
2. Yusuf S, Sleight P, Pogue J, Bosch J, Davies R, Dagenais G. Effects of an angiotensin-converting-enzyme inhibitor, ramipril, on death from cardiovascular events in high-risk patients. The Heart Outcomes Prevention Evaluation (HOPE) Study Investigators. *N Engl J Med.* 2000;342:145-153.
3. The ONTARGET Investigators. Telmisartan, ramipril or both in patients at high risk for vascular events. *N Engl J Med.* 2008;358:1547-1549.
4. Yusuf S, Teo K, Anderson C, et al. for the Telmisartan Randomised AssessmeNt Study in ACE iNtolerant subjects with cardiovascular Disease (TRANSCEND) Investigators. Effects of the angiotensin-receptor blocker telmisartan on cardiovascular events in high-risk patients intolerant to angiotensin-converting enzyme inhibitors: a randomised controlled trial. *Lancet.* 2008;372:1174-1183.
5. Yusuf S, Diener H-C, Sacco R, et al. Telmisartan to prevent recurrent stroke and cardiovascular events. *N Engl J Med.* 2008;359:1225-1237.

Treatment of hypertension in patients 80 years and older: the lower the better? A meta-analysis of randomized controlled trials

Bejan-Angoulvant T, Saadatian-Elahi M, Wright JM, et al (Hospices Civils de Lyon, France; Univ of British Columbia, Vancouver, Canada; et al)
J Hypertens 28:1366-1372, 2010

Background.—Results of randomized controlled trials are consistent in showing reduced rates of stroke, heart failure and cardiovascular events in very old patients treated with antihypertensive drugs. However, inconsistencies exist with regard to the effect of these drugs on total mortality.

Methods.—We performed a meta-analysis of available data on hypertensive patients 80 years and older by selecting total mortality as the main outcome. Secondary outcomes were coronary events, stroke, cardiovascular events, heart failure and cause-specific mortality. The common relative risk (RR) of active treatment versus placebo or no treatment was assessed using a random-effect model. Linear metaregression was performed to explore the relationship between intensity of antihypertensive therapy and blood pressure (BP) reduction and the log-transformed value of total mortality odds ratios (ORs).

Results.—The overall RR for total mortality was 1.06 (95% confidence interval 0.89–1.25), with significant heterogeneity between hypertension in the very elderly trial (HYVET) and the other trials. This heterogeneity was not explained by differences in the follow-up duration between trials. The meta-regression suggested that a reduction in mortality was achieved in trials with the least BP reductions and the lowest intensity of therapy. Antihypertensive therapy significantly reduced ($P<0.001$) the risk of stroke (35%), cardiovascular events (27%) and heart failure (50%). Cause-specific mortality was not different between treated and untreated patients.

Conclusion.—Treating hypertension in very old patients reduces stroke and heart failure with no effect on total mortality. The most reasonable strategy is the one associated with significant mortality reduction; thiazides as first-line drugs with a maximum of two drugs.

▶ These results depend heavily on both the Hypertension in the Very Elderly Trial (HYVET)[1] and the pioneering work of the last author, who organized the Individual Data ANalysis of Antihypertensive drug intervention trials (INDANA) group, the meta-analysis of which provoked many anxious questions when it was published in 1999.[2] This group gathered all the then-existing data about subjects older than 80 years of age enrolled in hypertension clinical trials involving placebo or no treatment and came to the conclusion that stroke and heart failure were significantly prevented by antihypertensive drug therapy but mortality was increased by 14%. Although this was not statistically significant, it gave pause to many geriatricians and others, who claimed that octogenarians ought not to be given antihypertensive medications, as the first duty of the physician is to do no harm.

The HYVET data account for 48% of the deaths (and 57% of the subjects) in this meta-analysis, so this single study obviously influences all the results. However, the overall trend is still a nonsignificant 6% increase in mortality. The authors also limited their trials to those that used placebo or no treatment as initial therapy, thus excluding trials such as the Kyoto Heart Study[3] and the Heart Institute of Japan—Candesartan Randomized Trial for Evaluation in Coronary Artery Disease,[4] both of which enrolled only hypertensive patients but used other background antihypertensive agents in addition to the randomized placebo or angiotensin receptor blocker. The authors performed a number of other important calculations, for example, showing that cardiovascular events are now significantly prevented (by 27%) and heart failure prevention jumps up to 50% (primarily again influenced by the HYVET data). Because HYVET was stopped prematurely because of a mortality benefit, the cumulative hazard ratios for all trials over time still show a disturbing trend past 2 years. The authors also performed meta-regression analyses for mortality risk and the maximum intensity of treatment and achieved systolic blood pressure reductions. Both suggest (but do not prove) that lower intensity of treatment and a smaller drop in achieved systolic blood pressure were associated with lower mortality. This is the rationale for the authors' conclusions to use only 2 drugs at low doses and to lower the systolic blood pressure to < 150 mm Hg, both of which are familiar to readers of HYVET but also likely to be controversial, and the impetus for much discussion. The editorialists for this article question the authors' heavy weighting of HYVET, reporting the results of a fixed-effects model with significant inhomogeneity ($P = .07$, which was higher than the prespecified $P < .10$) for mortality (which was no longer observed using a random-effects model), use of a fixed-effects meta-regression analysis for only 7 studies (to dissect the effects of intensity of treatment and the change in systolic blood pressure) and their recommendation of a thiazide diuretic as initial therapy.[5]

W. J. Elliott, MD, PhD

References

1. Beckett NS, Peters R, Fletcher AE, et al. Treatment of hypertension in patients 80 years of age or older. *N Engl J Med.* 2008;358:1887-1898.
2. Gueyffier F, Bulpitt C, Boissel JP, et al. Antihypertensive drugs in very old people: a subgroup meta-analysis of randomised controlled trials. INDANA Group. *Lancet.* 1999;353:793-796.
3. Sawada T, Yamada H, Dahlöf B, Matsubara H, KYOTO HEART Study Group. Effects of valsartan on morbidity and mortality in uncontrolled hypertensive patients with high cardiovascular risks: KYOTO HEART Study. *Eur Heart J.* 2009;30:2461-2469.
4. Kasanuki H, Hagiwara N, Hosoda S, et al. for the HIJ-CREATE Investigators. Angiotensin II receptor blocker-based vs. non-angiotensin II receptor blocker-based therapy in patients with angiographically documented coronary artery disease and hypertension: the Heart Institute of Japan Candesartan Randomized Trial for Evaluation in Coronary Artery Disease (HIJ-CREATE). *Eur Heart J.* 2009;30:1203-1212.
5. Reboldi G, Gentile G, Angeli F, Verdecchia P. Blood pressure lowering in the oldest old. *J Hypertens.* 2010;28:1373-1376 [Editorial].

Pre-eclampsia

Steegers EAP, von Dadelszen P, Duvekot JJ, et al (Univ Med Centre Rotterdam, Netherlands; Univ of British Columbia, Vancouver, Canada; et al)
Lancet 376:631-644, 2010

Pre-eclampsia remains a leading cause of maternal and perinatal mortality and morbidity. It is a pregnancy-specific disease characterised by de-novo development of concurrent hypertension and proteinuria, sometimes progressing into a multiorgan cluster of varying clinical features. Poor early placentation is especially associated with early onset disease. Predisposing cardiovascular or metabolic risks for endothelial dysfunction, as part of an exaggerated systemic inflammatory response, might dominate in the origins of late onset pre-eclampsia. Because the multifactorial pathogenesis of different pre-eclampsia phenotypes has not been fully elucidated, prevention and prediction are still not possible, and symptomatic clinical management should be mainly directed to prevent maternal morbidity (eg, eclampsia) and mortality. Expectant management of women with early onset disease to improve perinatal outcome should not preclude timely delivery—the only definitive cure. Pre-eclampsia foretells raised rates of cardiovascular and metabolic disease in later life, which could be reason for subsequent lifestyle education and intervention.

▶ Despite the short summary, this article concisely presents most of what we know, and more importantly, much of what is not known (and especially what is controversial) about this condition. The 10 pages of well-written text are followed by 10 more pages containing 149 small print references, which should allow intent readers to learn the details of recent research into the pathophysiology, risk factors, management, and sequelae of this challenging medical problem. Sad to say, it appears that there are still large gaps in our understanding of most, if not all, of these issues. But this multifaceted review is the closest we have to a setting out of the research agenda that might attempt to answer some of the questions that still remain.

Like many phenomena in hypertension, there are disagreements between US and international guideline committees,[1,2] even on such basic issues as the nomenclature of terms useful in defining pre-eclampsia, for example, the systolic blood pressure threshold of 160 or 170 mm Hg. Particularly because these guidelines are now somewhat old, it is likely that they will soon be revisited and revised; perhaps that is why so many other groups[3] have felt the need to publish their own sets of recommendations. It will be interesting to see how these inconsistencies are resolved in upcoming guideline statements.

W. J. Elliott, MD, PhD

References

1. ACOG Committee on Obstetric Practice. ACOG practice bulletin. Diagnosis and management of preeclampsia and eclampsia. Number 33, January 2002. American College of Obstetricians and Gynecologists. *Int J Gynaecol Obstet.* 2002;77: 67-75.
2. Brown MA, Lindheimer MD, de Swiet M, Van Assche A, Moutquin JM. The classification and diagnosis of the hypertensive disorders of pregnancy: statement from the International Society for the Study of Hypertension in Pregnancy (ISSHP). *Hypertens Pregnancy.* 2001;20:IX-XIV.
3. Chobanian AV, Bakris GL, Black HR, et al. National High Blood Pressure Education Program Coordinating Committee. Seventh report of the Joint National Committee on Prevention, Detection, Evaluation and Treatment of High Blood Pressure. *Hypertension.* 2003;42:1206-1252.

Antihypertensive Treatment and Development of Heart Failure in Hypertension: A Bayesian Network Meta-analysis of Studies in Patients With Hypertension and High Cardiovascular Risk

Sciarretta S, Palano F, Tocci G, et al (Univ of Rome "Sapienza," Italy)
Arch Intern Med 171:384-394, 2011

Background.—It is still debated whether there are differences among the various antihypertensive strategies in heart failure prevention. We performed a network meta-analysis of recent trials in hypertension aimed at investigating this issue.

Methods.—Randomized, controlled trials published from 1997 through 2009 in peer-reviewed journals indexed in the PubMed and EMBASE databases were selected. Selected trials included patients with hypertension or a high-risk population with a predominance of patients with hypertension.

Results.—A total of 223 313 patients were enrolled in the selected studies. Network meta-analysis showed that diuretics (odds ratio [OR], 0.59; 95% credibility interval [CrI], 0.47-0.73), angiotensin-converting enzyme (ACE) inhibitors (OR, 0.71; 95% CrI, 0.59-0.85) and angiotensin II receptor blockers (ARBs) (OR, 0.76; 95% CrI, 0.62-0.90) represented the most efficient classes of drugs to reduce the heart failure onset compared with placebo. On the one hand, a diuretic-based therapy represented the best treatment because it was significantly more efficient than that based on ACE inhibitors (OR, 0.83; 95% CrI, 0.69-0.99) and ARBs (OR, 0.78; 95% CrI, 0.63-0.97). On the other hand, diuretics (OR, 0.71; 95% CrI, 0.60-0.86), ARBs (OR, 0.91; 95% CrI, 0.78-1.07), and ACE inhibitors (OR, 0.86; 95% CrI, 0.75-1.00) were superior to calcium channel blockers, which were among the least effective first-line agents in heart failure prevention, together with β-blockers and α-blockers.

Conclusions.—Diuretics represented the most effective class of drugs in preventing heart failure, followed by renin-angiotensin system inhibitors. Thus, our findings support the use of these agents as first-line antihypertensive strategy to prevent heart failure in patients with hypertension at risk to develop heart failure. Calcium channel blockers and β-blockers were found to be less effective in heart failure prevention.

▶ These results are not surprisingly little different from those of previous reports of network meta-analyses of heart failure end points in clinical trials in hypertension: Psaty et al[1] reported the superiority of diuretics in preventing heart failure in 42 trials of initial therapy in 2003; we reported preliminary data from 47 to 53 trials of initial randomized antihypertensive drug therapy in 2007 and 2008[2,3]; Bangalore et al[4] reported the results of 12 trials using beta-blockers as initial therapy for hypertension; Verdecchia et al[5] performed many meta-analyses of 31 recent trials; and Wright and Musini[6] meta-analyzed 57 trials of initial therapy and concluded that low-dose diuretics were the best first-line choice for hypertension. The methodology used here is different from many previous reports, in that the Markov chain Monte Carlo Bayesian meta-analytic method was used to compare drug classes, based on prior probabilities derived from the clinical trial results. This method, however, does not overcome the challenges associated with attributing the trial results to a drug that is used very late in the therapeutic sequence (eg, the Heart Outcomes Prevention Evaluation Study and studies with a similar design,[7] in which the test agent or placebo was layered onto other antihypertensive medications).

The authors' conclusions are based on but a small subset of recent clinical trials, and do not include older classic hypertension trials, in which diuretics were very effective in preventing stroke, myocardial infarction, and heart failure.[8] Why the authors did not include the Kyoto Heart Study,[9] the Candesartan Antihypertensive Survival Evaluation in Japan,[10] and more recent trials is uncertain. The authors' conclusions are heavily influenced by the controversial heart failure results of the Antihypertensive and Lipid-Lowering to prevent Heart Attack Trial,[11] which accounts for more than 88% of the diuretic-associated heart failure end points. One wonders if their conclusion should single out chlorthalidone, based on its overwhelmingly large numbers (> 90% of the diuretic-associated heart failure cases) in their meta-analysis.[2,3]

W. J. Elliott, MD, PhD

References

1. Psaty BM, Lumley T, Furberg CD, et al. Health outcomes associated with various antihypertensive therapies used as first-line agents: a network meta-analysis. *JAMA*. 2003;289:2534-2544.
2. Elliott WJ, Meyer PM. Antihypertensive drug therapy and incident heart failure in clinical trials in hypertension: an updated network meta-analysis. *J Clin Hypertens (Greenwich)*. 2007;9:A210.
3. Elliott WJ, Basu S, Meyer PM. Initial antihypertensive drugs for heart failure prevention: network and Bayesian meta-analyses of clinical trial data. *Circulation*. 2008;118:S886.
4. Bangalore S, Wild D, Parkar S, Kukin M, Messerli FH. Beta-blockers for primary prevention of heart failure in patients with hypertension: insights from a meta-analysis. *J Am Coll Cardiol*. 2008;52:1062-1072.
5. Verdecchia P, Angeli F, Cavallini C, et al. Blood pressure reduction and renin-angiotensin system inhibition for prevention of congestive heart failure: a meta-analysis. *Eur Heart J*. 2009;30:679-688.
6. Wright JM, Musini VM. First-line drugs for hypertension. *Cochrane Database Syst Rev*. 2009; 10.1002/14651858. CD001841.
7. Effects of an angiotensin-converting-enzyme inhibitor, ramipril, on death from cardiovascular causes, myocardial infarction, and stroke in high-risk patients. The Heart Outcomes Prevention Evaluation (HOPE) Study Investigators. *N Engl J Med*. 2000;342:145-153.
8. Collins R, Peto R, MacMahon S, et al. Blood pressure, stroke, and coronary heart disease: Part 2, Short-term reductions in blood pressure: overview of randomised drug trials in their epidemiological context. *Lancet*. 1990;335:827-838.
9. Sawada T, Yamada H, Dahlöf B, Matsubara H, Kyoto Heart Study Group. Effects of valsartan on morbidity and mortality in uncontrolled hypertensive patients with high cardiovascular risks: Kyoto Heart Study. *Eur Heart J*. 2009; 30:2461-2469.
10. Ogihara T, Nakao K, Fukui T, et al. Candesartan Antihypertensive Survival Evaluation in Japan Trial Group. Effects of candesartan compared with amlodipine in hypertensive patients with high cardiovascular risks: candesartan antihypertensive survival evaluation in Japan trial. *Hypertension*. 2008;51:393-398.
11. The ALLHAT Officers and Coordinators for the ALLHAT Collaborative Research Group. Major outcomes in high-risk hypertensive patients randomized to angiotensin-converting enzyme inhibitor or calcium channel blocker vs. diuretic: the Antihypertensive and Lipid-Lowering Treatment to Prevent Heart Attack Trial (ALLHAT). *JAMA*. 2002;288:2981-2997.

Angiotensin-Converting Enzyme Inhibitor Associated Cough: Deceptive Information from the *Physicians' Desk Reference*
Bangalore S, Kumar S, Messerli FH (Harvard Med School, Boston, MA; Columbia Univ College of Physicians & Surgeons, NY)
Am J Med 123:1016-1030, 2010

Background.—Dry cough is a common, annoying adverse effect of all angiotensin-converting enzyme (ACE) inhibitors. The present study was designed to compare the rate of coughs reported in the literature with reported rates in the *Physicians' Desk Reference (PDR)*/drug label.

Methods.—We searched MEDLINE/EMBASE/CENTRAL for articles published from 1990 to the present about randomized clinical trials (RCTs) of ACE inhibitors with a sample size of at least 100 patients in the ACE inhibitors arm with follow-up for at least 3 months and reporting the incidence or withdrawal rates due to cough. Baseline characteristics, cohort enrolled, metrics used to assess cough, incidence, and withdrawal rates due to cough were abstracted.

Results.—One hundred twenty-five studies that satisfied our inclusion criteria enrolled 198,130 patients. The pooled weighted incidence of cough for enalapril was 11.48% (95% confidence interval [CI], 9.54% to 13.41%), which was ninefold greater compared to the reported rate in the *PDR*/drug label (1.3%). The pooled weighted withdrawal rate due to cough for enalapril was 2.57% (95% CI, 2.40-2.74), which was 31-fold greater compared to the reported rate in the *PDR*/drug label (0.1%). The incidence of cough has increased progressively over the last 2 decades with accumulating data, but it has been reported consistently several-fold less in the *PDR* compared to the RCTs. The results were similar for most other ACE inhibitors.

Conclusion.—The incidence of ACE inhibitor-associated cough and the withdrawal rate (the more objective metric) due to cough is significantly greater in the literature than reported in the *PDR*/drug label and is likely to be even greater in the real world when compared with the data from RCTs. There exists a gap between the data available from the literature and that which is presented to the consumers (prescribing physicians and patients).

▶ The authors' conclusion that the real incidence of cough associated with angiotensin-converting enzyme (ACE) inhibitor therapy is much higher than reported in the Food and Drug Administration (FDA)-approved package insert information is not a big surprise because the data that comprise the latter are typically drawn from the placebo-controlled randomized trials that supported the New Drug Application. In the case of the ACE inhibitors, it is not surprising that cough was not reported (either spontaneously or in response to the usual question, "Have you had any changes in your health status since your last visit?"), as there were no drugs that were recognized as causing cough at the time. Cough was first reported to be associated with ACE inhibitors in the English literature in 1985,[1] about 6 to 7 years after they were first given to hypertensive patients in clinical trials. It is a good reminder of the old saying, "You won't find a fever if you don't take a temperature."

The authors have compiled an impressive body of data from clinical trials in which cough was reported as a secondary (or lower) and/or safety end point and did not include some trials that compared an ACE inhibitor and an angiotensin receptor blocker for which cough was the prespecified primary end point.[2-9] They also excluded some studies that enrolled patients who had previously reported a cough with an ACE inhibitor, which is a very strong predictor of a second episode of coughing with another ACE inhibitor.[10]

The authors and editorialist[11] recommend that the FDA-approved prescription be updated periodically to reflect gathered information. The drug's registration trials would break new ground; however, updates would likely strain the already overburdened agency with contentious discussions with the drug's sponsors. These sponsors would wish to severely limit both the perception of hazards and the amount of printing required in order to disseminate the updated information.

W. J. Elliott, MD, PhD

References

1. Sesoko S, Kaneko Y. Cough associated with the use of captopril. *Arch Intern Med.* 1985;145:1524-1525.
2. Maillion JM, Goldberg AL. Global efficacy and tolerability of losartan, an angiotensin II subtype 1-receptor antagonist, in the treatment of hypertension. *Blood Press Suppl.* 1996;2:82-86.
3. Larochelle P, Flack JM, Marbury TC, Sareli P, Krieger EM, Reeves RA. Effects and tolerability of irbesartan versus enalapril in patients with severe hypertension. irbesartan Multicenter investigators. *Am J Cardiol.* 1997;80:1613-1615.
4. Malmqvist K, Kahan T, Dahl M. Angiotensin II type 1 (AT1) receptor blockade in hypertensive women: benefits of candesartan cilexetil versus enalapril or hydrochlorothiazide. *Am J Hypertens.* 2000;13:504-511.
5. McInnes GT, O'Kane KP, Istad H, Keinänen-Kiukaanniemi S, Van Mierlo HF. Comparison of the AT1-receptor blocker, candesartan cilexetil, and the ACE-inhibitor, lisinopril, in fixed combination with low dose hydrochlorothiazide in hypertensive patients. *J Hum Hypertens.* 2000;14:263-269.
6. Ogihara T, Arakawa K. Clinical efficacy and tolerability of candesartan cilexetil. Candesartan Study Groups in Japan. *J Hum Hypertens.* 1999;13:S27-S31.
7. Karlberg BE, Lins L-E, Hermansson K. Efficacy and safety of telmisartan, a selective AT1 receptor antagonist, compared with enalapril in elderly patients with primary hypertension. TEES Study Group. *J Hypertens.* 1999;17:293-302.
8. Lacourcière Y. A multicenter, randomized, double-blind study of the antihypertensive efficacy and tolerability of irbesartan in patients aged ≥ 65 years with mild-to-moderate hypertension. *Clin Ther.* 2000;22:1213-1224.
9. Ogihara T, Yoshinaga K. The clinical efficacy and tolerability of the angiotensin II-receptor antagonist losartan in Japanese patients with hypertension. *Blood Press Suppl.* 1996;2:78-81.
10. Elliott WJ. Cough with ACE-inhibitors or angiotensin II receptor blockers: Meta-analysis of randomized hypertension studies. *J Hypertens.* 2002;20:S161.
11. Serebruany VL. Realistic assessment of drug-induced adverse events: a double-edged sword. *Am J Med.* 2010;123:971.

Efficacy of Revascularization For Renal Artery Stenosis Caused by Fibromuscular Dysplasia: A Systematic Review and Meta-Analysis

Trinquart L, Mounier-Vehier C, Sapoval M, et al (Institut National de la Santé et de la Recherche Médicale Centre d'Investigation Clinique et Epidémiologie Clinique 4, Paris, France; Université Lille 2, France; Université Paris Descartes, France)
Hypertension 56:525-532, 2010

In patients with fibromuscular dysplasia and renal artery stenosis, renal artery revascularization has been used to cure hypertension or to improve blood pressure control. To provide an up-to-date assessment of the benefits and risks associated with revascularization in this condition, we performed a systematic review of studies in which hypertensive patients with fibromuscular dysplasia renal artery stenosis underwent percutaneous transluminal renal angioplasty or surgical reconstruction. We assessed how often periprocedural complications and hypertension cure and improvement occurred. We selected 47 angioplasty studies (1616 patients) and 23 surgery studies (1014 patients). Combined rates of hypertension cure, defined according to the criteria in each study, after angioplasty or surgery were estimated to be 46% (95% CI: 40% to 52%) and 58% (95% CI: 53% to 62%), respectively, with substantial variations across studies. The probability of being cured was negatively associated with patient age and time of publication. Cure rates using current definitions of hypertension cure (blood pressure <140/90 mm Hg without treatment) were only 36% and 54% after angioplasty and surgery, respectively. The combined risks of periprocedural complications were 12% and 17% after angioplasty and surgery, respectively, with less major complications after angioplasty than surgery (6% versus 15%). In conclusion, angioplasty or surgical revascularization yielded moderate benefits in patients with fibromuscular dysplasia renal artery stenosis, with substantial variation across studies. The blood pressure outcome was strongly influenced by patient age.

▶ The diagnosis and treatment of renovascular hypertension has become something of a nonissue since the recent reports of no benefit of renal angioplasty stenting in large groups of patients.[1-4] These reports, however, largely dealt with atherosclerotic renal artery stenosis; the consensus for many years has been that patients with fibromuscular dysplasia (who are typically much younger and have few systemic manifestations of atherosclerotic vascular disease) have a much better response to angioplasty and a much better prognosis.[5]

The authors of this report challenge conventional wisdom by compiling all the data they could find about outcomes after angioplasty or surgical procedures for fibromuscular dysplasia of the renal arteries. Perhaps not surprisingly, they found that the data are not nearly as compelling as is commonly taught. Strict definition of normotension (blood pressure < 140/90 mm Hg without antihypertensive medication) was probably the stumbling block for most of the studies included, although the teaching has long been that about 40% to 50% of patients subjected to revascularization procedures are able to reduce either the dose or the number of antihypertensive drugs (which was not taken into account by the authors). As usual, initial (and smaller) studies were very positive about improved outcomes after the procedure, but more recent (and larger) reports are more realistic and have lower success rates. The complication rates after angioplasty averaged about 12% (95% confidence interval [CI]: 8.2%-15.9%) compared with about 17% (95% CI: 10.3%-24.7%) with surgery. The authors found that, like nearly all procedures, younger patients fared better; it is also likely that those who have the procedure soon after hypertension is diagnosed also do better, as is the case for many animal studies of renovascular disease.

Perhaps most interesting is the recommendation at the conclusion of their article that a randomized trial needs to be done to show that revascularization procedures are actually better than maximal medical therapy for fibromuscular renal artery stenosis. Whether any center that does angioplasty would allow any of their patients to be randomized to medical therapy, or (more likely) would have a very low threshold for angioplasty (even a few months after randomization) in patients assigned to medical therapy, is uncertain.

W. J. Elliott, MD, PhD

References

1. Dworkin LD, Cooper CJ. Clinical practice. Renal-artery stenosis. *N Engl J Med.* 2009;361:1972-1978.
2. van Jaarsveld BC, Krijnen P, Pieterman H, et al. The effect of balloon angioplasty on hypertension in atherosclerotic renal-artery stenosis. Dutch Renal Artery Stenosis Intervention Cooperative Study Group. *N Engl J Med.* 2000;342: 1007-1014.
3. Bax L, Woittiez AJ, Kouwenberg HJ, et al. Stent placement in patients with atherosclerotic renal artery stenosis and impaired renal function: a randomized trial. *Ann Intern Med.* 2009;150:840-848.
4. Wheatley K, Ives N, Kalra PA, et al. On behalf of the Angioplasty and Stenting for Renal Artery Lesions (ASTRAL) Investigators. Revascularization versus Medical Therapy for Renal-Artery Stenosis. *N Engl J Med.* 2009;361:1953-1962.
5. Slovut DP, Olin JW. Fibromuscular dysplasia. *N Engl J Med.* 2004;350:1862-1871.

Biofeedback for hypertension: a systematic review
Greenhalgh J, Dickson R, Dundar Y (Univ of Liverpool, Brownlow Hill, UK)
J Hypertens 28:644-652, 2010

Objective.—To assess the evidence for the long-term effectiveness of biofeedback for the treatment of essential hypertension in adults.

Methods.—A systematic review following accepted international guidelines was conducted. Randomized controlled trials that compared biofeedback procedures with antihypertensive medication, placebo (sham biofeedback treatment), no intervention or other behavioural treatments were included. The outcome measure was change in blood pressure.

Results.—The inclusion criteria were fulfilled by 36 trials. Twenty-one trials employed biofeedback treatment with no adjunctive therapy, whereas 15 others used biofeedback treatment alongside another treatment. The majority of trials were small with no posttreatment follow-up or follow-up of less than 6 months. Qualitative heterogeneity of the included studies (e.g. poor quality of the trials, differences in interventions and inconsistencies in the measurement of outcomes) meant that it was inappropriate to pool data in the form of a meta-analysis. A narrative summary of the data based on trial authors' conclusions is presented. No studies reported long-term (>12 months) follow-up of patients. Data were grouped first by treatment type and then by comparator. Trial results were variable and conflicting, demonstrating no clear benefits of biofeedback in relation to moderation of hypertension.

Conclusion.—Although there may be other reported life benefits to its use, we found no convincing evidence that consistently demonstrates the effectiveness of the use of any particular biofeedback treatment in the control of essential hypertension when compared with pharmacotherapy, placebo, no intervention or other behavioural therapies. Any future research needs to be conducted using accepted quality standards and given current guidelines for the treatment of hypertension is likely to be considered only as an adjunct to pharmacological treatment.

▶ The authors apparently wanted to reassess the relatively old meta-analyses suggesting that there was a slight, but significant, effect of biofeedback on blood pressure,[1,2] but after collecting the published data, they concluded that there was too much heterogeneity to attempt even a random effects model (which typically does not report a *P*-value for homogeneity). They therefore provide a narrative summary of their findings, which suggests that overall, there is little, if any, effect of biofeedback on blood pressure. The authors are relatively careful about defining what (to their eyes and understanding) constitutes biofeedback because some either recent[3] or older[4] studies, including some that included device- or music-guided[5] breathing (as a type of biofeedback), have shown a significant blood pressure—lowering effect.

The authors make a number of recommendations for researchers who wish to study the phenomenon further. These include enrollment of a large number of research subjects, differences in baseline blood pressure levels (as any intervention is more likely to show a significant fall in blood pressure if the initial values are very high), a long duration of biofeedback treatment (as hypertension is usually a life-long condition), simple versus complex biofeedback equipment necessary for initial training and continuous use during biofeedback sessions, and high-quality measures of blood pressure (eg, ambulatory blood pressure monitoring) with appropriate statistical measures for detecting clinically important differences in blood pressure. The authors opine that this situation is analogous to that of the early 1950s, when pharmacological therapy was still experimental and most trials were small and did not include cardiovascular outcomes.

The authors believe that biofeedback may have its true efficacy assessed if it were used as an adjunct to antihypertensive drug therapy. This has been done in more recent studies[3,5,6] and no longer is an impediment to interpretation of most studies. The more challenging question is how many people, once taught the techniques, will continue to use them to maintain the initial blood pressure reduction. The issue of adherence is as important to biobehavioral techniques as it is to pharmacological treatments.

W. J. Elliott, MD, PhD

References

1. Nakao M, Yano E, Nomura S, Kuboki T. Blood pressure-lowering effects of biofeedback treatment in hypertension: A meta-analysis of randomized clinical trials. *Hypertens Res.* 2003;26:37-46.
2. Yucha CB, Clark L, Smith M, Uris P, LaFleur B, Duval S. The effect of biofeedback in hypertension. *Appl Nurs Res.* 2001;14:29-35.
3. Nolan RP, Floras JS, Harvey PJ, et al. Behavioral neurocardiac training in hypertension: a randomized, controlled trial. *Hypertension.* 2010;55:1033-1039.
4. Patel C. 12-month follow-up of yoga and biofeedback in the management of hypertension. *Lancet.* 1975;305:62-64.
5. Modesti PA, Ferrari A, Bazzini C, et al. Psychological predictors of the antihypertensive effects of music-guided slow breathing. *J Hypertens.* 2010;28:1097-1103.
6. Gavish B. Device-guided breathing in the home setting: Technology, performance and clinical outcomes. *Biol Psychol.* 2010;84:150-156.

Does chocolate reduce blood pressure? A meta-analysis

Ried K, Sullivan T, Fakler P, et al (The Univ of Adelaide, South Australia, Australia)

BMC Med 8:39, 2010

Background.—Dark chocolate and flavanol-rich cocoa products have attracted interest as an alternative treatment option for hypertension, a known risk factor for cardiovascular disease. Previous meta-analyses concluded that cocoa-rich foods may reduce blood pressure. Recently, several additional trials have been conducted with conflicting results. Our study summarises current evidence on the effect of flavanol-rich cocoa products on blood pressure in hypertensive and normotensive individuals.

Methods.—We searched Medline, Cochrane and international trial registries between 1955 and 2009 for randomised controlled trials investigating the effect of cocoa as food or drink compared with placebo on systolic and diastolic blood pressure (SBP/DBP) for a minimum duration of 2 weeks. We conducted random effects meta-analysis of all studies fitting the inclusion criteria, as well as subgroup analysis by baseline blood pressure (hypertensive/normotensive). Meta-regression analysis explored the association between type of treatment, dosage, duration or baseline blood pressure and blood pressure outcome. Statistical significance was set at $P < 0.05$.

Results.—Fifteen trial arms of 13 assessed studies met the inclusion criteria. Pooled meta-analysis of all trials revealed a significant blood pressure-reducing effect of cocoa-chocolate compared with control (mean BP change ± SE: SBP: -3.2 ± 1.9 mmHg, $P = 0.001$; DBP: -2.0 ± 1.3 mmHg, $P = 0.003$). However, subgroup meta-analysis was significant only for the hypertensive or prehypertensive subgroups (SBP: -5.0 ± 3.0 mmHg; $P = 0.0009$; DBP: -2.7 ± 2.2 mmHg, $P = 0.01$), while BP was not significantly reduced in the normotensive subgroups (SBP: -1.6 ± 2.3 mmHg, $P = 0.17$; DBP: -1.3 ± 1.6 mmHg, $P = 0.12$). Nine trials used chocolate containing 50% to 70% cocoa compared with white chocolate or other cocoa-free controls, while six trials compared high- with low-flavanol cocoa products. Daily flavanol dosages ranged from 30 mg to 1000 mg in the active treatment groups, and interventions ran for 2 to 18 weeks. Meta-regression analysis found study design and type of control to be borderline significant but possibly indirect predictors for blood pressure outcome.

Conclusion.—Our meta-analysis suggests that dark chocolate is superior to placebo in reducing systolic hypertension or diastolic prehypertension. Flavanol-rich chocolate did not significantly reduce mean blood pressure below 140 mmHg systolic or 80 mmHg diastolic.

▶ The potential antihypertensive effects of cocoa have now been studied by many investigators, possibly in response to epidemiological studies that purport to show a benefit of cocoa consumption on hard cardiovascular end points.[1,2] This meta-analysis is 1 of 2 published in a 6-month period that come to the same conclusion: dark (but not white) chocolate seems to lower blood pressure in prehypertensive and hypertensive individuals, but not by very much.[3] A group that includes a prominent hypertension expert has recently cast doubt on the clinical significance of these data[4] but leaves open the possibility that dark chocolate might eventually prove useful to selected people in the distant future, if ongoing research continues to find a significant lowering of blood pressure in better-designed studies.

The mechanism by which dark chocolate lowers blood pressure is still uncertain, despite several well-designed and executed studies.[5,6] Five very probing unanswered questions about the potential blood pressure—lowering effects of dark chocolate are posed by Egan et al.[4] Only further research is likely to be able to evaluate whether the caloric intake, saturated fat, and salt content of some dark chocolate preparations will outweigh its statistically significant (but clinically small) blood pressure—lowering effect. This is one area of research in hypertension in which it will presumably not be very challenging to recruit subjects for clinical trials!

W. J. Elliott, MD, PhD

References

1. Corti R, Flammer AJ, Hollenberg NK, Lüscher TF. Cocoa and cardiovascular health. *Circulation.* 2009;119:1433-1441.
2. Buijsse B, Feskens EJ, Kok FJ, Kromhout D. Cocoa intake, blood pressure and cardiovascular mortality: the Zutphen Elderly Study. *Arch Intern Med.* 2006; 166:411-417.
3. Desch S, Schmidt J, Kobler D, et al. Effect of cocoa products on blood pressure: systematic review and meta-analysis. *Am J Hypertens.* 2010;23:97-103.

4. Egan BM, Laken MA, Donovan JL, Woolson RF. Does dark chocolate have a role in the prevention and management of hypertension? Commentary on the evidence. *Hypertension.* 2010;55:1289-1295.
5. Taubert D, Roesen R, Lehmann C, Jung N, Schömig E. Effects of low habitual cocoa intake on blood pressure and bioactive nitric oxide: a randomized controlled trial. *JAMA.* 2007;298:49-60.
6. van den Bogaard B, Draijer R, Westerhof BE, van den Meiracker AH, van Montfrans GA, van den Born BJ. Effects on peripheral and central blood pressure of cocoa with natural or high-dose theobromine: a randomized, double-blind crossover trial. *Hypertension.* 2010;56:839-846.

Angiotensin-receptor blockade and risk of cancer: meta-analysis of randomised controlled trials

Sipahi I, Debanne SM, Rowland DY, et al (Case Western Reserve Univ School of Medicine, Cleveland, OH)
Lancet Oncol 11:627-636, 2010

Background.—Angiotensin-receptor blockers (ARBs) are a widely used drug class approved for treatment of hypertension, heart failure, diabetic nephropathy, and, recently, for cardiovascular risk reduction. Experimental studies implicate the renin-angiotensin system, particularly angiotensin II type-1 and type-2 receptors, in the regulation of cell proliferation, angiogenesis, and tumour progression. We assessed whether ARBs affect cancer occurrence with a meta-analysis of randomised controlled trials of these drugs.

Methods.—We searched Medline, Scopus (including Embase), Cochrane Central Register of Controlled Trials, Cochrane Database of Systematic Reviews, and the US Food and Drug Administration website for studies published before November, 2009, that included any of the seven currently available ARBs. Randomised controlled trials with an ARB given in at least one group, with a follow-up of at least 1 year, and that enrolled at least 100 patients were included. New cancer data were available for 61 590 patients from five trials. Data on common types of solid organ cancers were available for 68 402 patients from five trials, and data on cancer deaths were available for 93 515 patients from eight trials.

Findings.—Telmisartan was the study drug in 30 014 (85·7%) patients who received ARBs as part of the trials with new cancer data. Patients randomly assigned to receive ARBs had a significantly increased risk of new cancer occurrence compared with patients in control groups (7·2% *vs* 6·0%, risk ratio [RR] 1·08, 95% CI 1·01−1·15; p=0·016). When analysis was limited to trials where cancer was a prespecified endpoint, the RR was 1·11 (95% CI 1·04−1·18, p=0·001). Among specific solid organ cancers examined, only new lung-cancer occurrence was significantly higher in patients randomly assigned to receive ARBs than in those assigned to receive control (0·9% *vs* 0·7%, RR 1·25, 1·05−1·49; p=0·01). No statistically significant difference in cancer deaths was observed (1·8% *vs* 1·6%, RR 1·07, 0·97−1·18; p=0·183).

Interpretation.—This meta-analysis of randomised controlled trials suggests that ARBs are associated with a modestly increased risk of new cancer diagnosis. Given the limited data, it is not possible to draw conclusions about the exact risk of cancer associated with each particular drug. These findings warrant further investigation.

▶ This was certainly the most widely covered research article in hypertension in 2010. The first author and the editorialist for this article[1] were heavily featured and quoted in nearly all daily newspapers, blogs, and health-related internet sites. They uniformly recommended that United States and European regulatory authorities should immediately launch a formal investigation into (1) when the manufacturers (and the US Food and Drug Administration [FDA]) either knew or should have known of this significantly increased risk of cancer, (2) why the manufacturers of angiotensin receptor blockers (ARBs) and the US FDA did not disclose this fact as soon as it became known, and (3) why these drugs were not immediately removed from the US market. The FDA was targeted for criticism because some of the data included in this meta-analysis were available only in FDA briefing documents rather than in the published medical literature.

Rebuttal to these requests came in several forms.[2-5] Some criticized the authors' methodology, as data from some ARB trials were apparently not included (notably the Valsartan Antihypertensive Long-term Use Evaluation [VALUE]).[4,6] One of the leaders of the VALUE trial commented soon after this study's publication that when the VALUE data were added to those in this meta-analysis, the summary odds ratio was nearly exact unity. Subsequent letters to the editor did not resolve the issue of why the VALUE data were not included.[5] Others were concerned about the authors' explanation of biological plausibility: while cultured cells exposed to stimuli of the angiotensin II type 2 receptor experience a decrease in apoptosis and an increase in both angiogenesis and cytokines associated with tumorigenesis, the relevance of these models to intact humans is uncertain.[2,3] The median follow-up of patients in the trials was about 2.5 years, which some correspondents felt was not long enough to observe the de novo growth of a clinically detectable cancer.[3,4] Lastly, some commentators noted that the editorialist chosen for this article was formerly a research colleague and mentor of the first author, suggesting a less than independent appraisal of the article. Since ~83% of the cancers in the meta-analysis involved telmisartan, many were most concerned about this specific agent, despite the fact that the highest risk of incident cancer was seen when telmisartan was combined with ramipril in the Ongoing Telmisartan Alone and in Combination with Ramipril Global Endpoint Trial.[7]

By the time these issues came to light, however, many patients panicked and either discarded their ARBs or requested a different kind of antihypertensive medication from their physicians. The situation is vaguely reminiscent of the calcium channel blocker scare of 5:32 PM ET of March 11, 1995,[8] which launched a great deal of subsequent research, including "the largest and most important clinical trial in hypertension ever in the USA,"[9] which showed on December 17, 2002, that the alleged significant 60% increase in risk of myocardial infarction was actually a nonsignificant 2% decrease, compared with a diuretic.[10] As it is unlikely that the National Institutes of Health will fund another large study in hypertension comparing specific drug classes,[11] the open question of whether ARBs cause cancer will likely be solved only after all the available data can be gathered and analyzed. This may take a while, although the European Medicines Agency announced soon after this article's publication that they will start such a project.

W. J. Elliott, MD, PhD

References

1. Nissen SE. Angiotensin-receptor blockers and cancer: urgent regulatory review needed. *Lancet Oncol.* 2010;11:605-606.
2. Goldstein MR, Mascatelli L, Pezzetta F, et al. Angiotensin-receptor blockade, cancer and concerns. *Lancet Oncol.* 2010;11:817-821.
3. Meredith PA, McInnes GT. Angiotensin-receptor blockade, cancer and concerns. *Lancet Oncol.* 2010;11:819.
4. Barrios V, Escobar C. Angiotensin-receptor blockade, cancer and concerns. *Lancet Oncol.* 2010;11:819-820.
5. Julius S, Kjeldsen SE, Weber MA. Angiotensin-receptor blockade, cancer and concerns. *Lancet Oncol.* 2010;11:820-821.
6. Julius S, Kjeldsen S, Weber M, et al. Outcomes in hypertensive patients at high cardiovascular risk treated with regimens based on valsartan or amlodipine: the VALUE randomised trial. *Lancet.* 2004;363:2022-2031.
7. Yusuf S, Teo KK, Pogue J, et al. ONTARGET Investigators. Telmisartan, ramipril or both in patients at high risk for vascular events. *N Engl J Med.* 2008;358: 1547-1549.
8. Psaty BM, Heckbert SR, Koepsell TD, et al. The risk of myocardial infarction associated with antihypertensive drug therapies. *JAMA.* 1995;274:620-625.
9. Elliott WJ. ALLHAT: the largest and most important clinical trial in hypertension ever done in the USA. Antihypertensive and Lipid Lowering Treatment to Prevent Heart Attack Trial. *Am J Hypertens.* 1996;9:409-411.
10. The ALLHAT Officers and Coordinators for the ALLHAT Collaborative Research Group. Major outcomes in high-risk hypertensive patients randomized to angiotensin-converting enzyme inhibitor or calcium channel blocker vs diuretic: the Antihypertensive and Lipid-Lowering Treatment to Prevent Heart Attack Trial (ALLHAT). *JAMA.* 2002;288:2981-2997.
11. The National Heart Lung and Blood Institute Working Group on Future Directions in Hypertension Treatment Trials. Major clinical trials of hypertension: what should be done next? *Hypertension.* 2005;46:1-6.

Epidemiological Studies

US Trends in Prevalence, Awareness, Treatment, and Control of Hypertension, 1988-2008

Egan BM, Zhao Y, Axon RN (Med Univ of South Carolina, Charleston)
JAMA 303:2043-2050, 2010

Context.—Hypertension is a major risk factor for cardiovascular disease and treatment and control of hypertension reduces risk. The Healthy People 2010 goal was to achieve blood pressure (BP) control in 50% of the US population.

Objective.—To assess progress in treating and controlling hypertension in the United States from 1988-2008.

Design, Setting, and Participants.—The National Health and Nutrition Examination Survey (NHANES) 1988-1994 and 1999-2008 in five 2-year blocks included 42 856 adults aged older than 18 years, representing a probability sample of the US civilian population.

Main Outcome Measures.—Hypertension was defined as systolic BP of at least 140 mm Hg and diastolic BP of at least 90 mm Hg, self-reported use of antihypertensive medications, or both. Hypertension control was defined as systolic BP values of less than 140 mm Hg and diastolic BP values of less than 90 mm Hg. All survey periods were age-adjusted to the year 2000 US population.

Results.—Rates of hypertension increased from 23.9% (95% confidence interval [CI], 22.7%-25.2%) in 1988-1994 to 28.5% (95% CI, 25.9%-31.3%; $P<.001$) in 1999-2000, but did not change between 1999-2000 and 2007-2008 (29.0%; 95% CI, 27.6%-30.5%; $P=.24$). Hypertension control increased from 27.3% (95% CI, 25.6%-29.1%) in 1988-1994 to 50.1% (95% CI, 46.8%-53.5%; $P=.006$) in 2007-2008, and BP among patients with hypertension decreased from 143.0/80.4 mm Hg (95% CI, 141.9-144.2/79.6-81.1 mm Hg) to 135.2/74.1 mm Hg (95% CI, 134.2-136.2/73.2-75.0 mm Hg; $P=.02/P<.001$). Blood pressure control improved significantly more in absolute percentages between 1999-2000 and 2007-2008 vs 1988-1994 and 1999-2000 (18.6%; 95% CI, 13.3%-23.9%; vs 4.1%; 95% CI, −0.5% to 8.8%; $P<.001$). Better BP control reflected improvements in awareness (69.1%; 95% CI, 67.1%-71.1%; vs 80.7%; 95% CI, 78.1%-83.0%; P for trend=.03), treatment (54.0%; 95% CI, 52.0%-56.1%; vs 72.5%; 95% CI, 70.1%-74.8%; $P=.004$), and proportion of patients who were treated and had controlled hypertension (50.6%; 95% CI, 48.0%-53.2%; vs 69.1%; 95% CI, 65.7%-72.3%; $P=.006$). Hypertension control improved significantly between 1988-1994 and 2007-2008, across age, race, and sex groups, but was lower among individuals aged 18 to 39 years vs 40 to 59 years ($P<.001$) and 60 years or older ($P<.001$), and in Hispanic vs white individuals ($P=.004$).

Conclusions.—Blood pressure was controlled in an estimated 50.1% of all patients with hypertension in NHANES 2007-2008, with most of the improvement since 1988 occurring after 1999-2000. Hypertension control was significantly lower among younger than middle-aged individuals and older adults, and Hispanic vs white individuals.

▶ American public health authorities, including the Chair of the Seventh Report of the Joint National Committee (JNC 7[1]) on Prevention, Detection, Evaluation, and Treatment of High Blood Pressure, have much to be happy about since this nationwide survey about hypertension was reported.[2] One of the major messages of JNC 7 was the poor progress that had been made in the United States in the war on hypertension, which started in 1973 with the formation of the National High Blood Pressure Education Program. Earlier *National Health and Nutrition Examination Survey* (NHANES) data had shown some mild but continuous improvements in the proportion of American hypertensives achieving the target blood pressure of < 140/90 mm Hg.[3-6] Unfortunately, these reports were discomforting because they always fell short of the Healthy People 2000 (and then the updated but unchanged Healthy People 2010) goal of 50% of the hypertensive population being controlled.

Many other data, including those from the US National Ambulatory Care Survey and the Healthcare Employer Data Information Set (collected by the National Committee on Quality Assurance), have suggested that more Americans are achieving goal blood pressure than ever before, but these conclusions are based on data from office visits and do not include or sample individuals who do not seek health care.

These data from the most recent NHANES report show significant improvements in the overall control of hypertension, despite relatively constant prevalence, which is a little surprising, given the aging and growth (in body mass index) of the US population, both of which would be expected to increase the overall prevalence. There is lesser focus in this report on racial/ethnic disparities, but it seems clear that the much higher prevalence of uncontrolled hypertension in the non-Hispanic blacks seen in earlier reports[7,8] has continued to improve. These data suggest that Mexican Americans now are the group with the highest proportion of unaware, untreated, and uncontrolled hypertension, which may be due to limited access to care.

These data are important from a historical perspective but do not reflect the current standard of care, which has moved the target blood pressure for individuals, with diabetes, chronic kidney disease, and, more recently, heart disease, to less than 130/80 mm Hg. Perhaps in the next report from this database, investigators may determine the proportion of American adults who meet their individual current blood pressure targets. There is little doubt that the proportion will be smaller than the overall 50.1% success rate reported here.

W. J. Elliott, MD, PhD

References

1. Chobanian AV, Bakris GL, Black HR, et al. The seventh report of the Joint National Committee on Prevention, Detection, Evaluation, and Treatment of High Blood Pressure: the JNC 7 report. *JAMA*. 2003;289:2560-2572.
2. Chobanian AV. Improved hypertension control: cause for some celebration. *JAMA*. 2010;303:2082-2083.
3. Ostchega Y, Yoon SS, Hughes J, Louis T. Hypertension awareness, treatment and control—Continued disparities in adults: United States, 2005−2006. *NCHS Data Brief*. 2008;3:1-8.
4. Ong KL, Cheung BMY, Man YB, Lau CP, Lam KSL. Prevalence, awareness, treatment, and control of hypertension among United States adults 1999−2004. *Hypertension*. 2007;49:69-75.
5. Hajjar I, Kotchen TA. Trends in prevalence, awareness, treatment, and control of hypertension in the United States, 1988−2000. *JAMA*. 2003;290:199-206.
6. Burt VL, Cutler JA, Higgins M, et al. Trends in the prevalence, awareness, treatment, and control of hypertension in the adult US population. Data from the health examination surveys, 1960 to 1991. *Hypertension*. 1995;26:60-69.
7. Glover MJ, Greenlund KJ, Ayala C, Croft JB. Racial/ethnic disparities in prevalence, treatment and control of hypertension—United States, 1999−2002. *MMWR Morb Mortal Wkly Rep*. 2005;54:7-9.
8. Hertz RP, Unger AN, Cornell JA, Saunders E. Racial disparities in hypertension prevalence, awareness and management. *Arch Intern Med*. 2005;165:2098-2104.

Use of angiotensin receptor blockers and risk of dementia in a predominantly male population: prospective cohort analysis

Li N-C, Lee A, Whitmer RA, et al (Boston Univ School of Public Health, MA; Veteran Affairs Med Ctr, Bedford, MA; Kaiser Permanente, Oakland, CA; et al)

BMJ 340:b5465, 2010

Objective.—To investigate whether angiotensin receptor blockers protect against Alzheimer's disease and dementia or reduce the progression of both diseases.

Design.—Prospective cohort analysis.

Setting.—Administrative database of the US Veteran Affairs, 2002-6.

Population.—819 491 predominantly male participants (98%) aged 65 or more with cardiovascular disease.

Main Outcome Measures.—Time to incident Alzheimer's disease or dementia in three cohorts (angiotensin receptor blockers, lisinopril, and other cardiovascular drugs, the "cardiovascular comparator") over a four year period (fiscal years 2003-6) using Cox proportional hazard models with adjustments for age, diabetes, stroke, and cardiovascular disease. Disease progression was the time to admission to a nursing home or death among participants with pre-existing Alzheimer's disease or dementia.

Results.—Hazard rates for incident dementia in the angiotensin receptor blocker group were 0.76 (95% confidence interval 0.69 to 0.84) compared with the cardiovascular comparator and 0.81 (0.73 to 0.90) compared with the lisinopril group. Compared with the cardiovascular comparator, angiotensin receptor blockers in patients with pre-existing Alzheimer's disease were associated with a significantly lower risk of admission to a nursing home (0.51, 0.36 to 0.72) and death (0.83, 0.71 to 0.97). Angiotensin receptor blockers exhibited a dose-response as well as additive effects in combination with angiotensin converting enzyme inhibitors. This combination compared with angiotensin converting enzyme inhibitors alone was associated with a reduced risk of incident dementia (0.54, 0.51 to 0.57) and admission to a nursing home (0.33, 0.22 to 0.49). Minor differences were shown in mean systolic and diastolic blood pressures between the groups. Similar results were observed for Alzheimer's disease.

Conclusions.—Angiotensin receptor blockers are associated with a significant reduction in the incidence and progression of Alzheimer's disease and dementia compared with angiotensin converting enzyme inhibitors or other cardiovascular drugs in a predominantly male population.

▶ This very interesting report has many strengths. The authors carefully framed their hypothesis, developed 2 concomitant control groups, and examined a large, presumably representative cohort of older men in the Veteran Affairs Healthcare system, not only for incident dementia (including Alzheimer disease) but also for the most-feared sequelae of these problems: nursing home placement and death. They examined their data in many ways (eg, including the dose-response relationship: higher doses of angiotensin receptor blockers [ARBs] were associated with an even greater protective effect against Alzheimer disease than lower doses as well as the very complex issue of switchers from ARB therapy to angiotensin converting enzyme [ACE]-inhibitor therapy and back) and found nothing that contradicted their primary conclusion: the higher the dose and the greater the duration of ARB therapy, the greater was the protection from Alzheimer disease, all-cause dementia, nursing home placement, or death.

Suggestions that antihypertensive therapy (and ARB therapy in particular) may protect from Alzheimer disease have been made before, in meta-analyses,[1] some (but not all[2]) clinical trials,[3,4] and other reports.[5] This may be the largest, well-designed, cohort study to see the same phenomenon.

The authors' choice of lisinopril as the positive control may have occurred because it is the most popular of the ACE inhibitors (in their database and in the United States in general) and therefore afforded the largest possible numbers of subjects within the database taking a specific ACE inhibitor. They do mention that lisinopril is not a brain penetrant. In fact, lisinopril was synthesized and developed precisely because it was enalapril with an extra epsilon-amino group and when protonated, was unlikely to cross the blood-brain barrier. From the perspective of preventing diseases that involve the central nervous system (CNS), lisinopril may have been a suboptimal choice, particularly because candesartan, perhaps the ARB with the greatest CNS penetration, appears to be the most active of the ARBs in preventing Alzheimer disease (based on the authors' data and analyses).

It is a pity that these data have come to light only shortly before the first ARB loses its patent protection, as developing an ARB for this indication might have proved very useful for the public health. Because we have so many ARBs now, it seems unlikely that a new research program involving long-term clinical trials could be done quickly enough to result in a profitable endeavor for a pharmaceutical company. Perhaps governmental funding could be procured to test the hypothesis that an ARB can prevent Alzheimer disease in a large, randomized, clinical trial. The size of the cohorts used in this study was not impossibly huge (11 703 received an ARB in the incident Alzheimer disease analysis, and only 476 received an ARB in the progression to nursing home placement or death analysis), compared with other recent clinical trials involving ARBs.

W. J. Elliott, MD, PhD

References

1. Feigin V, Ratnasabapathy Y, Anderson C. Does blood pressure lowering treatment prevents dementia or cognitive decline in patients with cardiovascular and cerebrovascular disease? *J Neurol Sci.* 2005;229-230:151-155.
2. Lithell H, Hansson L, Skoog I, et al. The study on Cognition and Prognosis in the Elderly (SCOPE): principal results of a randomized double-blind intervention trial. *J Hypertens.* 2003;21:875-886.
3. Forette F, Seux ML, Staessen JA, et al. Prevention of dementia in randomised double-blind placebo-controlled Systolic Hypertension in Europe (Syst-Eur) trial. *Lancet.* 1998;352:1347-1351.
4. PROGRESS Collaborative Group. Randomised trial of a perindopril-based blood-pressure-lowering regimen among 6,105 individuals with previous stroke or transient ischaemic attack. *Lancet.* 2001;358:1033-1041.

5. Li G, Rhew IC, Shofer JB, et al. Age-varying association between blood pressure and risk of dementia in those aged 65 and older: a community-based prospective cohort study. *J Am Geriatr Soc.* 2007;55:1161-1167.

Treatment with angiotensin receptor blockers before stroke could exert a favourable effect in acute cerebral infarction

Fuentes B, Fernández-Domínguez J, Ortega-Casarrubios MÁ, et al (La Paz Univ Hosp, Madrid, Spain)

J Hypertens 28:575-581, 2010

Introduction.—Evidence from experimental and clinical studies is accumulating about the possible cerebral protective properties of antihypertensive drugs, mainly angiotensin receptor blockers (ARB) or angiotensin-converting enzyme inhibitors (ACEI). Our aim was to analyse the impact of prestroke use of antihypertensive drugs on stroke severity and outcome.

Methods.—We analysed 1968 consecutive patients with first-ever acute cerebral infarction admitted to an acute stroke unit. Stroke severity was evaluated using the Canadian Neurological Scale and the modified Rankin Score (mRS) was used to evaluate the outcome at discharge.

Results.—Previous diagnosis of arterial hypertension was reported in 1212 patients and 73% were on antihypertensive treatment. No significant differences in stroke severity were found between patients with or without previous arterial hypertension, either in patients with or without antihypertensive treatment. Patients taking antihypertensive drugs at stroke onset had lower rates of poor outcome than those not on antihypertensive treatment (47 vs. 53%; $P = 0.047$) and those taking ARB had better outcomes than those without ARB (mRS $\leq$ 2: 75 vs. 65.8%; $P = 0.029$), with no differences in the analysis of other antihypertensive drugs. The multivariable logistic regression analysis showed that previous treatment with ARB was independently associated with reduced stroke severity (OR: 0.40; 95%CI 0.24–0.65; $P < 0.001$) and against poor outcome (OR: 0.41; 95%CI 0.23–0.78; $P = 0.003$).

Conclusion.—Our study suggests that prestroke treatment with ARB may be associated with reduced stroke severity and also with better outcome. This finding agrees with experimental data that suggest a cerebral protective effect.

▶ This article is very reminiscent of one 20 years ago in the *BMJ*, reporting that patients in Perth, Australia, who took a beta-blocker before their first myocardial infarction had an impressive 50% lower 28-day mortality rate, after adjustment for age and other predictors of cardiac death.[1] There was, however, no difference in the unadjusted rates. Although the authors attributed this to a lower mean peak creatine kinase activity (and smaller infarcts), subsequent clinical trials and meta-analyses have suggested that (except when administered soon after an acute myocardial infarction)[2] beta-blockers do not protect against death or myocardial infarction in hypertensive patients.[2,3] These authors at least have a consistent data set: their unadjusted data show a lower stroke severity and a better stroke outcome in the small subset of patients who were given an angiotensin receptor blocker (ARB); these conclusions were changed only a little after statistical adjustment. They also found that patients who were taking antihypertensive drugs had better outcomes than those who were untreated at the time of the stroke. Whether this reflects a lower prestroke blood pressure, closer follow-up, or better medical care before the event is unclear.

The authors bolster their case by citing conclusions from animal studies and some early clinical trials that suggest that ARBs seem to have some special neuroprotective benefit.[4,5] Sadly, the most direct test of telmisartan in poststroke patients did not show significant benefits,[6] although some recent meta-analyses continue to show better prevention of stroke than myocardial infarction with an ARB for hypertension.[2,7-10]

The editorialist for this article also points out that only 7.2% of the patients in the study were taking an ARB prior to the stroke, which opens the conclusions to many forms of bias and confounding.[11]

W. J. Elliott, MD, PhD

References

1. Nidorf SM, Parsons RW, Thompson PL, Jamrozik KD, Hobbs MS. Reduced risk of death at 28 days in patients taking a beta-blocker before admission to hospital with myocardial infarction. *BMJ.* 1990;300:71-74.
2. Law MR, Morris JK, Wald NJ. Use of blood pressure lowering drugs in the prevention of cardiovascular disease: meta-analysis of 147 randomised trials in the context of expectations from prospective epidemiological studies. *BMJ.* 2009;338:b1665.
3. Lindholm LH, Carlberg B, Samuelsson O. Should β-blockers remain first choice in the treatment of primary hypertension? A meta-analysis. *Lancet.* 2005;366: 1545-1553.
4. Schrader J, Lüders S, Kulschewski A, et al. The ACCESS Study: evaluation of Acute Candesartan Cilexetil Therapy in Stroke Survivors. *Stroke.* 2003;34: 1699-1703.
5. Schrader J, Lüders S, Kulschewski A, et al. Morbidity and Mortality After Stroke, Eprosartan Compared with Nitrendipine for Secondary Prevention: principal results of a prospective randomized controlled study (MOSES). *Stroke.* 2005; 36:1218-1226.
6. Yusuf S, Diener H-C, Sacco RL, et al. PRoFESS Study Group. Telmisartan to prevent recurrent stroke and cardiovascular events. *N Engl J Med.* 2008;359: 1225-1237.
7. Turnbull F, Neal B, Ninomiya T, et al. Blood Pressure Lowering Treatment Trialists' Collaboration. Effects of different regimens to lower blood pressure on major cardiovascular events in older and younger adults: meta-analysis of randomised trials. *BMJ.* 2008;336:1121-1123.
8. Wright JM, Musini VM. First-line drugs for hypertension. *Cochrane Database Syst Rev.* 2009;(3) 10.1002/14651858. CD001841.
9. Elliott WJ, Basu S, Meyer PM. Initial drugs for stroke prevention in hypertensive patients: Network and Bayesian meta-analyses of clinical trial data. *J Clin Hypertens (Greenwich).* 2009;11:A7.
10. Elliott WJ, Basu S, Meyer PM. Initial drugs for coronary heart disease prevention in hypertensive patients: Network and Bayesian meta-analyses of clinical trial data [abstract]. *J Clin Hypertens (Greenwich).* 2009;11:A7.
11. Anderson C. More indirect evidence of potential neuroprotective benefits of angiotensin receptor blockers. *J Hypertens.* 2010;28:429.

Long-term Blood Pressure Fluctuation and Cerebrovascular Disease in an Elderly Cohort

Brickman AM, Reitz C, Luchsinger JA, et al (Columbia Univ, NY; et al)
Arch Neurol 67:564-569, 2010

Background.—The importance of subclinical cerebrovascular disease in the elderly is increasingly recognized, but its determinants have not been fully explicated. Elevated blood pressure (BP) and fluctuation in BP may lead to cerebrovascular disease through ischemic changes and compromised cerebral autoregulation.

Objective.—To determine the association of BP and long-term fluctuation in BP with cerebrovascular disease.

Design.—A community-based epidemiological study of older adults from northern Manhattan.

Setting.—The Washington Heights—Inwood Columbia Aging Project.

Participants.—A total of 686 nondemented older adults who had BP measurements during 3 study visits at 24-month intervals and underwent structural magnetic resonance imaging (corresponding temporally with the third assessment). We derived the mean (SD) of the mean BP for each participant during the 3 intervals and divided the participants into 4 groups defined as below or above the group median ($\leq$96.48 or >96.48 mm Hg) and further subdivided them as below or above the median SD ($\leq$7.21 or >7.21 mm Hg). This scheme yielded 4 groups representing the full range of BPs and fluctuations in BP.

Main Outcome Measures.—Differences in white matter hyperintensity (WMH) volume and presence of brain infarctions across groups.

Results.—White matter hyperintensity volume increased across the 4 groups in a linear manner, with the lowest WMH volume in the lowest mean/lowest SD group and the highest WMH volume in the highest mean/highest SD group ($F_{3,610} = 3.52$, $P = .02$). Frequency of infarction also increased monotonically across groups (from 22% to 41%, P for trend = .004).

Conclusions.—Compared with individuals with low BP and low fluctuations in BP, the risk of cerebrovascular disease increased with higher BP and BP fluctuations. Given that cerebrovascular disease is associated with disability, these findings suggest that interventions should focus on long-term fluctuating BP and elevated BP.

▶ This article was written and accepted well before the series of blood pressure variability hypothesis articles were published by Professor Rothwell and colleagues,[1-4] but it comes to similar conclusions, using a totally different research design. It is likely that these authors will wish to reanalyze their data, using the statistical methodology of the Oxford group, but it is likely that they will reach the same conclusion as that derived here from a traditional cohort study.

These authors took their cohort of 686 older individuals, examined each on 3 occasions over 6 years, and then performed a structural magnetic resonance imaging study of the brain at the last visit, to determine the volume of white matter hyperintensity volume (which corresponds pathologically to areas of lacunes and infarcts). They divided their cohort into 4 groups, based on the variability of, and mean blood pressure across the 3 biennial time periods. As with the Rothwell data set, the subjects with the most variability had the highest blood pressures; unlike the Rothwell data set, these authors did not adjust statistically in a single linear model for the different blood pressure levels in the 4 groups, which they now presumably will do, using one of the statistical parameters recommended by the Oxford group that is independent of mean blood pressure.[1,2] The results showed a significant trend for more white matter hyperintensity volume as the blood pressure (and its variability) increased. This suggests that at least one of Rothwell's hypotheses[1] may be correct: the brain does not easily tolerate fluctuations in blood pressure, particularly in this older cohort of patients.

The authors' conclusion that blood pressure variability (or fluctuation, as they call it) is associated with significantly more white matter lesions is based on comparison of groups 1 versus 2 and then groups 3 versus 4. The mean blood pressures in these 2 pairs were close (130/68 vs 131/68 and 152/80 vs 156/81 mm Hg, respectively), and there were numerically more white matter lesions in groups 2 and 4, compared with groups 1 and 3. Yet the authors didn't test specifically for a difference in white matter lesions between these 2 paired groups but instead performed only comparisons across the 4 groups. It is likely that they will perform such analyses now since their observation is a direct test of the usual blood pressure hypothesis.

W. J. Elliott, MD, PhD

References

1. Rothwell PM. Limitations of the usual blood-pressure hypothesis and importance of variability, instability, and episodic hypertension. *Lancet.* 2010;375:938-948.
2. Rothwell PM, Howard SC, Dolan E, et al. Prognostic significance of visit-to-visit variability, maximum systolic blood pressure, and episodic hypertension. *Lancet.* 2010;375:895-905.
3. Webb AJS, Fischer U, Mehta Z, Rothwell PM. Effects of antihypertensive-drug class on interindividual variation in blood pressure and risk of stroke: a systematic review and meta-analysis. *Lancet.* 2010;375:906-915.
4. Rothwell PM, Howard SC, Dolan E, et al. Effects of beta blockers and calcium-channel blockers on within-individual variability in blood pressure and risk of stroke. *Lancet Neurol.* 2010;9:469-480.

Impact of the ALLHAT/JNC7 Dissemination Project on Thiazide-Type Diuretic Use

Stafford RS, for the ALLHAT Collaborative Research Group (Stanford Univ, CA; et al)
Arch Intern Med 170:851-858, 2010

Background.—Strategies are needed to improve the translation of clinical trial results into practice. We assessed the impact of the ALLHAT/JNC7 Dissemination Project's academic detailing component on thiazide-type diuretic prescribing (ALLHAT indicates Antihypertensive and Lipid-Lowering Treatment to Prevent Heart Attack Trial; JNC7 indicates the Seventh Report of the Joint National Committee on Detection, Evaluation, and Treatment of High Blood Pressure).

Methods.—We used 2 national databases available from IMS Health: a physician survey of medications reported for hypertension and a pharmacy dispensing database on antihypertensive medications. At a county level, we correlated medication data with Dissemination Project intensity. Practices before the Dissemination Project in 2004 were compared with those after its completion in 2007. We also examined 2000-2008 national trends.

Results.—Academic detailing reached 18 524 physicians in 1698 venues via 147 investigator-educators. We noted an association between ALLHAT/JNC7 academic detailing activities and increased prescribing of thiazide-type diuretics. Physician survey data showed that the percentage of hypertension visits where the physician recorded a thiazide-type diuretic increased the most in counties where academic detailing activity was the highest (an increase of 8.6%, from 37.9% to 46.5%) compared with counties where activity was moderate (an increase of 2%) or low (a decrease of 2%), or where there was none (an increase of 2%; P value for trend, <.05). Pharmacy dispensing data showed that thiazide-type diuretic prescribing increased by 8.7% in counties with Dissemination Project activities compared with 3.9% in those without activities (P<.001). Nationally, thiazide-type diuretic use did not increase between 2004 and 2008.

Conclusions.—The ALLHAT/JNC7 Dissemination Project was associated with a small effect on thiazide-type diuretic use consistent with its small dose and the potential of external factors to diminish its impact. Academic detailing may increase physicians' implementation of clinical trial results, thereby making prescribing more consistent with evidence.

▶ This fascinating article describes the results of a National Institutes of Health—funded effort to make the results and conclusions[1] of the largest and most important clinical trial in hypertension ever done in the United States,[2] the Antihypertensive and Lipid-Lowering treatment to prevent Heart Attack Trial (ALLHAT), more widely known to practicing physicians. Perhaps more importantly, the authors compared the numbers of prescription diuretics before and after the intervention in specific counties that received more or less of the intervention, reflecting a change in prescribing habits. Because so many of the ALLHAT officers, investigators, and coordinators were part of the many writing groups of the Seventh Report of the Joint National Committee (JNC 7) on Prevention, Detection, Evaluation, and Treatment of High Blood Pressure[3] and the recommendations of JNC 7 so closely paralleled those of ALLHAT, the results of this dissemination project could be seen as translating both the clinical trial results and the concordant national guidelines into general medical practice.

Ironically, the real experts at changing prescription-writing behaviors in the United States are pharmaceutical industry employees, who are generally well rewarded for their efforts when successful, but they are often fired when not as successful as their marketing departments had projected. The designers of this dissemination project were presumably less experienced in their mission than their industry-sponsored competition, had to rely on volunteer physicians, trained once on a general theme (rather than well-motivated, continuously trained, and highly paid pharmaceutical sales representatives, formerly detail men, clearly focused on a single product), and had fewer resources to influence physician prescribing habits than the competing pharmaceutical industry (which was heavily promoting angiotensin receptor blockers) simultaneously. Unlike the pharmaceutical industry, the authors did not focus on new starts or new Rxs, but instead counted only total dispensings, which (based on prior information[4,5]) should have yielded more impressive results, given the large installed base of diuretic users.

Despite these disadvantages, the authors were able to discern a positive impact of their intervention, particularly in high-intensity counties. Similar nationwide trends had been noted immediately after the initial publications of ALLHAT results[6,7] and in other national databases.[8,9] The editorialist for this article (and the inventor of the term, academic detailing) makes some interesting reflections on how the efforts of academic detailing might have been diluted and some interesting suggestions[10] of how such efforts might be improved in the future.[7] But it is likely that the federal government and its agents will not soon be more effective than the pharmaceutical industry, given the latter's experience, much larger budget, and legions of trained, targeted, and loaded sales representatives. Recent restrictions on their unfettered access to physicians, negative publicity regarding sales incentives, formulary additions, and prohibition against participation in continuing medical education activities seem to have had little recent impact on pharmaceutical sales.

W. J. Elliott, MD, PhD

References

1. The ALLHAT Officers and Coordinators for the ALLHAT Collaborative Research Group. Major outcomes in high-risk hypertensive patients randomized to angiotensin-converting enzyme inhibitor or calcium channel blocker vs diuretic: The Antihypertensive and Lipid-Lowering Treatment to Prevent Heart Attack Trial (ALLHAT). *JAMA.* 2002;288:2981-2997.
2. Elliott WJ. ALLHAT: The largest and most important clinical trial in hypertension ever done in the U.S.A. Antihypertensive and Lipid Lowering Treatment to Prevent Heart Attack Trial. *Am J Hypertens.* 1996;9:409-411.
3. Chobanian AV, Bakris GL, Black HR, et al. National High Blood Pressure Education Program Coordinating Committee. Seventh report of the Joint National Committee on Prevention, Detection, Evaluation and Treatment of High Blood Pressure. *Hypertension.* 2003;42:1206-1252.
4. Muntner P, Krousel-Wood M, Hyre AD, et al. Antihypertensive prescriptions for newly treated patients before and after the main antihypertensive and lipid-lowering treatment to prevent heart attack trial and seventh report of the joint national committee on prevention, detection, evaluation, and treatment of high blood pressure. *Hypertension.* 2009;53:617-623.
5. Ho PM, Zeng C, Tavel HM, et al. Trends in first-line therapy for hypertension in the Cardiovascular Research Network Hypertension Registry, 2002–2007. *Arch Intern Med.* 2010;170:912-913.

6. Stafford RS, Furberg CD, Finkelstein SN, Cockburn IM, Alehegn T, Ma J. Impact of clinical trial results on national trends in alpha-blocker prescribing, 1996–2002. *JAMA.* 2004;291:54-62.
7. Player MS, Gill JM, Fagan HB, Mainous AG III. Antihypertensive prescribing practices: impact of the Antihypertensive and Lipid-Lowering treatment to prevent Heart Attack Trial. *J Clin Hypertens (Greenwich).* 2006;8:860-864.
8. Xie F, Petitti DB, Chen W. Prescribing patterns for antihypertensive drugs after the Antihypertensive and Lipid-Lowering treatment to prevent Heart Attack Trial: report of experience in a health maintenance organization. *Am J Hypertens.* 2005;18:464-469.
9. Stafford RS, Monti V, Furberg CD, Ma J. Long-term and short-term changes in antihypertensive prescribing by office-based physicians in the United States. *Hypertension.* 2006;48:213-218.
10. Avorn J. Transforming trial results into practice change: The final translational hurdle: Comment on "Impact of the ALLHAT/JNC7 Dissemination Project on thiazide-type diuretic use." *Arch Intern Med.* 2010;170:858-860.

Intensive Blood-Pressure Control in Hypertensive Chronic Kidney Disease

Appel LJ, for the AASK Collaborative Research Group (Johns Hopkins Med Institutions, Baltimore, MD; et al)

N Engl J Med 363:918-929, 2010

Background.—In observational studies, the relationship between blood pressure and end-stage renal disease (ESRD) is direct and progressive. The burden of hypertension-related chronic kidney disease and ESRD is especially high among black patients. Yet few trials have tested whether intensive blood-pressure control retards the progression of chronic kidney disease among black patients.

Methods.—We randomly assigned 1094 black patients with hypertensive chronic kidney disease to receive either intensive or standard blood-pressure control. After completing the trial phase, patients were invited to enroll in a cohort phase in which the blood pressure target was less than 130/80 mm Hg. The primary clinical outcome in the cohort phase was the progression of chronic kidney disease, which was defined as a doubling of the serum creatinine level, a diagnosis of ESRD, or death. Follow-up ranged from 8.8 to 12.2 years.

Results.—During the trial phase, the mean blood pressure was 130/78 mm Hg in the intensive-control group and 141/86 mm Hg in the standard-control group. During the cohort phase, corresponding mean blood pressures were 131/78 mm Hg and 134/78 mm Hg. In both phases, there was no significant between-group difference in the risk of the primary outcome (hazard ratio in the intensive-control group, 0.91; $P = 0.27$). However, the effects differed according to the baseline level of proteinuria ($P = 0.02$ for interaction), with a potential benefit in patients with a protein-to-creatinine ratio of more than 0.22 (hazard ratio, 0.73; $P = 0.01$).

Conclusions.—In overall analyses, intensive blood-pressure control had no effect on kidney disease progression. However, there may be differential effects of intensive blood-pressure control in patients with and those without baseline proteinuria. (Funded by the National Institute of Diabetes and Digestive and Kidney Diseases, the National Center on Minority Health and Health Disparities, and others.)

▶ This report may have the longest follow-up of any clinical trial in chronic kidney disease that compared 2 different blood pressure targets in patients who were at high risk of end-stage renal disease. This is important because the traditional surrogate end point (doubling of serum creatinine, end-stage renal disease, or death) used in the Irbesartan Diabetic Nephropathy Trial[1] and the Reduction of Endpoints in NIDDM with the Angiotensin II Antagonist Losartan[2] trial is not as definitive (or as costly) as the harder end point of dialysis.

The good news from this report is that there is great similarity between the conclusions of the original clinical trial, the African American Study of Kidney Disease and Hypertension,[3] and those derived from this long-term follow-up of the cohort drawn from the clinical trial. In both, there is a hint that prognosis may be slightly better in individuals with baseline proteinuria (here defined as a 24-hour protein/creatinine ratio of 0.22) who were assigned to the lower blood pressure goal. A similar observation was made, post hoc, in the Modification of Diet in Renal Disease study,[4] but there were several potential confounders in that report (particularly during long-term follow-up).[5]

It is likely that these data, and those from other shorter trials in renal disease, may help shape the next set of guidelines, from both the Eighth Report of the Joint National Committee on Prevention, Detection, Evaluation, and Treatment of High Blood Pressure and the National Kidney Foundation. Some have argued that the blood pressure target of < 140/90 mm Hg is acceptable for patients with or without chronic kidney disease, except if proteinuria is present, in which case < 125/75 mm Hg may be somewhat better, but < 130/80 mm Hg is a reasonable compromise and easier to achieve.

W. J. Elliott, MD, PhD

References

1. Lewis EJ, Hunsicker LG, Clarke WR, et al. Renoprotective effect of the angiotensin-receptor antagonist irbesartan in patients with nephropathy due to type 2 diabetes. *N Engl J Med*. 2001;345:851-860.
2. Brenner BM, Cooper ME, de Zeeuw D, et al. Effects of losartan on renal and cardiovascular outcomes in patients with type 2 diabetes and nephropathy. *N Engl J Med*. 2001;345:861-869.
3. Wright JT Jr, Bakris GL, Greene T, et al. Effect of blood pressure lowering and antihypertensive drug class on progression of hypertensive kidney disease: results from the AASK trial. *JAMA*. 2002;288:2421-2431.
4. Peterson JC, Adler S, Burkart JM, et al. Blood pressure control, proteinuria, and the progression of renal disease: The Modification of Diet in Renal Disease Study. *Ann Intern Med*. 1995;123:754-762.
5. Sarnak MJ, Greene T, Wang X, et al. The effect of a lower target blood pressure on the progression of kidney disease: long-term follow-up of the Modification of Diet in Renal Disease Study. *Ann Intern Med*. 2005;142:342-351.

Influence of Physicians' Management and Communication Ability on Patients' Persistence With Antihypertensive Medication

Tamblyn R, Abrahamowicz M, Dauphinee D, et al (McGill Univ, Montreal, Quebec, Canada; et al)
Arch Intern Med 170:1064-1072, 2010

Background.—Less than 75% of people prescribed antihypertensive medication are still using treatment after 6 months. Physicians determine treatment, educate patients, manage side effects, and influence patient knowledge and motivation. Although physician communication ability likely influences persistence, little is known about the importance of medical management skills, even though these abilities can be enhanced through educational and practice interventions. The purpose of this study was to determine whether a physician's medical management and communication ability influence persistence with antihypertensive treatment.

Methods.—This was a population-based study of 13 205 hypertensive patients who started antihypertensive medication prescribed by a cohort of 645 physicians entering practice in Quebec, Canada, between 1993 and 2007. Medical Council of Canada licensing examination scores were used to assess medical management and communication ability. Population-based prescription and medical services databases were used to assess starting therapy, treatment changes, comorbidity, and persistence with antihypertensive treatment in the first 6 months.

Results.—Within 6 months after starting treatment, 2926 patients (22.2%) had discontinued all antihypertensive medication. The risk of nonpersistence was reduced for patients who were treated by physicians with better medical management (odds ratio per 2-SD increase in score, 0.74; 95% confidence interval, 0.63-0.87) and communication (0.88; 0.78-1.00) ability and with early therapy changes (odds ratio, 0.45; 95% confidence interval, 0.37-0.54), more follow-up visits, and nondiuretics as the initial choice of therapy. Medical management ability was responsible for preventing 15.8% (95% confidence interval, 7.5%-23.3%) of nonpersistence.

Conclusion.—Better clinical decision-making and data collection skills and early modifications in therapy improve persistence with antihypertensive therapy.

▶ Although persistence with antihypertensive drug therapy has many risk factors, most people typically blame the patient for not being willing to continue to take the prescribed medication. These authors use some novel techniques to assess physician behaviors that might be predictors of patients' persistence with prescribed pharmaceuticals.

The authors have previously capitalized on the Canadian requirement, beginning in 1992, for physicians who wish to be licensed to take and pass a standardized clinical skills examination, consisting of 18 to 20 standardized patient cases that can provide an objective assessment of the person's communication, physical examination, and clinical management skills. Scores on these examinations have previously been shown by this research team to correlate inversely with patient complaints about care, peer review proceedings,[1,2] and adjudicated quality-of-care scores in future practice.[3]

The hypothesis tested in this work was that, for the first time, objective measures of a physician's communication and/or management skills (represented by the clinical skills examination scores in 1993-1996) would predict patients' 6-month adherence to initial antihypertensive medications (in 1993-2007). Not only was the hypothesis successfully supported but also the authors estimated that better medical management skills prevented about 16% (95% confidence interval: 8%-23%) of their patients' nonpersistence with antihypertensive therapy. They also identified (as have others) early therapy changes, more follow-up visits, and nondiuretic initial therapy as independent predictors of better persistence.

The authors admit to a number of possible confounders of their described association. One hopes that physicians who had low scores on their first licensure examination improved their skills during their several subsequent years of practice. The authors suggest that a physician's ability to incorporate patient preferences into the treatment plan may be an important characteristic of physicians and may predict better patient persistence, which is a question worthy of further research.

W. J. Elliott, MD, PhD

References

1. Tamblyn R, Abrahamowicz M, Dauphinee D, et al. Physician scores on a national clinical skills examination as predictors of complaints to medical regulatory authorities. *JAMA.* 2007;298:993-1001.
2. Tamblyn R, Abrahamowicz M, Dauphinee D, et al. Association between licensure examination scores and practice in primary care. *JAMA.* 2002;288:3019-3026.
3. Wenghofer E, Klass D, Abrahamowicz M, et al. Doctor scores on national qualifying examinations predict quality of care in future practice. *Med Educ.* 2009;43:1166-1173.

Prevalence of Chronic Kidney Disease in Persons With Undiagnosed or Prehypertension in the United States
Crews DC, for the Centers for Disease Control and Prevention Chronic Kidney Disease Surveillance Team (Johns Hopkins Univ, Baltimore, MD; et al)
Hypertension 55:1102-1109, 2010

Hypertension is both a cause and a consequence of chronic kidney disease, but the prevalence of chronic kidney disease throughout the diagnostic spectrum of blood pressure has not been established. We determined the prevalence of chronic kidney disease within blood pressure categories in 17 794 adults surveyed by the National Health and Nutrition Examination Survey during 1999–2006. Diagnosed hypertension was defined as self-reported provider diagnosis (n = 5832); undiagnosed hypertension was defined as systolic blood pressure ≥140 mm Hg or diastolic blood pressure ≥90 mm Hg, without report of provider diagnosis (n = 3046); prehypertension was defined as systolic blood pressure ≥120 and <140 mm Hg or diastolic blood pressure ≥80 and <90 mm Hg (n = 3719); and normal was defined as systolic blood pressure <120 mm Hg and diastolic blood pressure <80 mm Hg (n = 5197). Chronic kidney disease was defined as estimated glomerular filtration rate <60 mL/min per 1.73 m² or urinary albumin:creatinine ratio >30 mg/g. Prevalences of chronic kidney disease among those with prehypertension and undiagnosed hypertension were 17.3% and 22.0%, respectively, compared with 27.5% with diagnosed hypertension and 13.4% with normal blood pressure, after adjustment for age, sex, and race in multivariable logistic regression. This pattern persisted with varying definitions of kidney disease; macroalbuminuria (urinary albumin:creatinine ratio >300 mg/g) had the strongest association with increasing blood pressure category (odds ratio: 2.37 [95% CI: 2.00 to 2.81]). Chronic kidney disease is prevalent in undiagnosed and prehypertension. Earlier identification and treatment of both these conditions may prevent or delay morbidity and mortality from chronic kidney disease.

▶ This is probably the first report of the prevalence of chronic kidney disease (CKD) in a population-based sample of either normotensive (blood pressure <120/80 mm Hg[1]) or prehypertensive (120/80 mm Hg < blood pressure <139/89 mm Hg[1]) US adults. The implications for policymakers are clear: even if only a very small percent of those with CKD go on to very expensive dialysis, the opportunity to prevent CKD progression will be missed if such individuals are not screened, identified, and treated.

This conclusion is based on the idea that there are appropriate and cost-effective treatments to postpone end-stage renal disease in patients with stage 1 or 2 CKD. Furthermore, the definition of CKD is age independent, whereas renal function normally declines with increasing age.[2] This puts everyone older than 75 years with a serum creatinine >1.5 mg/dL into at least stage 3 CKD, even though their renal function is exactly what is predicted for people their age.

The editorialist for this article also is concerned that the estimates of CKD in the nonhypertensive population depend strictly on the definitions used for CKD.[3] He quite correctly points out that if one uses a more specific (or more conservative) definition (eg, estimated glomerular filtration rate <45 mL/min/1.73 m²), the prevalence decreases dramatically, whereas using a more sensitive (or more liberal) definition (eg, one abnormal albumin/creatinine ratio), it increases up to 26-fold. These considerations also depend somewhat on the blood pressure level, which for patients with CKD is considered treatable and not at target unless it is <130/80 mm Hg (prehypertension by current US guidelines[1]). These considerations suggest that there are many US adults, particularly in the older age groups, with mild CKD and fortunately, not so many with severe CKD who are likely soon to require dialysis. He makes the case that greater awareness of CKD in the population at risk would probably be helpful, as would more widespread use of home blood pressure measurements. Neither of these is likely to be very costly to the already-strained US health care budget.

W. J. Elliott, MD, PhD

References

1. Chobanian AV, Bakris GL, Black HR, et al. National High Blood Pressure Education Program Coordinating Committee. Seventh Report of the Joint National Committee on Prevention, Detection, Evaluation and Treatment of High Blood Pressure. *Hypertension.* 2003;42:1206-1252.
2. Kidney Disease Outcomes Quality Initiative (K/DOQI). K/DOQI clinical practice guidelines on hypertension and antihypertensive agents in chronic kidney disease. *Am J Kidney Dis.* 2004;43:S1-S290.
3. Agarwal R. Epidemiology of chronic kidney disease among normotensives: but what is chronic kidney disease? *Hypertension.* 2010;55:1097-1099.

Risk for Incident Atrial Fibrillation in Patients Who Receive Antihypertensive Drugs: A Nested Case–Control Study

Schaer BA, Schneider C, Jick SS, et al (Univ Hosp, Basel, Switzerland; Boston Univ Med Ctr, Lexington, MA)
Ann Intern Med 152:78-84, 2010

Background.—Different antihypertensive drug classes may alter risk for atrial fibrillation. Some studies suggest that drugs that interfere with the renin–angiotensin system may be favorable because of their effect on atrial remodeling.

Objective.—To assess and compare the relative risk for incident atrial fibrillation among hypertensive patients who receive antihypertensive drugs from different classes.

Design.—Nested case–control analysis.

Setting.—The United Kingdom–based General Practice Research Database, a well-validated primary care database comprising approximately 5 million patient records.

Patients.—4661 patients with atrial fibrillation and 18 642 matched control participants from a population of 682 993 patients treated for hypertension.

Measurements.—A comparison of the risk for atrial fibrillation among hypertensive users of angiotensin-converting enzyme (ACE) inhibitors, angiotensin II–receptor blockers (ARBs), or β-blockers with the reference group of users of calcium-channel blockers. Patients with clinical risk factors for atrial fibrillation were excluded.

Results.—Current exclusive long-term therapy with ACE inhibitors (odds ratio [OR], 0.75 [95% CI, 0.65 to 0.87]), ARBs (OR, 0.71 [CI, 0.57 to 0.89]), or β-blockers (OR, 0.78 [CI, 0.67 to 0.92]) was associated with a lower risk for atrial fibrillation than current exclusive therapy with calcium-channel blockers.

Limitation.—Blood pressure changes during treatment courses could not be evaluated, and risk for bias by indication cannot be fully excluded in an observational study.

Conclusion.—In hypertensive patients, long-term receipt of ACE inhibitors, ARBs, or β-blockers reduces the risk for atrial fibrillation compared with receipt of calcium-channel blockers.

▶ Atrial fibrillation has the highest odds ratio for incident stroke of all risk factors, although the population prevalence is low. Antihypertensive drugs that lower heart rate (beta-blockers and nondihydropyridine calcium antagonists) are used to treat acute atrial fibrillation (presumably by controlling rate, but perhaps not the risk of recurrent atrial fibrillation). It came therefore as something of a surprise that either angiotensin-converting enzyme (ACE) inhibitors or angiotensin II receptor blockers (ARBs) were associated with a lower risk of incident atrial fibrillation in several recent large clinical trials in heart failure[1-4] or hypertension, respectively.[5,6] Subsequent studies in cardiac surgery patients and those undergoing direct-current cardioversion for acute atrial fibrillation also showed the effect.[5,6] These authors therefore examined their large database, covering about 5 million people in the United Kingdom, to see if these associations were also present.

Perhaps the most difficult issue in addressing the question is what drug to use as the referent agent. Perhaps because dihydropyridine calcium antagonists are more widely prescribed than nondihydropyridine agents, and the former had not been associated with a reduced risk for atrial fibrillation, calcium antagonists were selected as the referent agent. The authors make no clear distinction between the calcium antagonist subclasses, except to mention that cases needed to have an antidysrhythmic agent (eg, verapamil and diltiazem) or an anticoagulant and a cardiological evaluation for a rhythm disturbance. One presumes that patients taking a nondihydropyridine calcium antagonist were excluded from the study. For simplicity, the authors selected only patients who received antihypertensive drug monotherapy (except that concomitant coadministration of a low-dose diuretic in a single-pill combination was allowed).

The results basically corroborate previous retrospective analyses of clinical trials: either ACE inhibitors or ARBs appear to prevent atrial fibrillation if used in the long-term.[7] Those who received less than 12 months of therapy with any of the 3 effective drug classes had no significant reduction in atrial fibrillation risk. There are major strengths to the study design and execution, typical of this research group's efforts with their large database in many pharmacoepidemiological evaluations. But the possibility of confounding by indication (physicians preferentially prescribing drugs based on an estimated risk of future atrial fibrillation) cannot easily be ruled out. Such estimations, however, are not yet easily codified, and this possibility seems rather remote. It is likely, from the preponderance of the evidence, that both ACE inhibitors and ARBs reduce the risk of future atrial fibrillation, which may perhaps be important in stroke prevention. Evidence to the contrary comes from meta-analyses of clinical trials in hypertension, which suggest that ARBs appear to be rather effective in preventing stroke, whereas ACE inhibitors are more effective for prevention of coronary heart disease than stroke.[8-10]

W. J. Elliott, MD, PhD

References

1. Vermes E, Tardif JC, Bourassa MG, et al. Enalapril decreases the incidence of atrial fibrillation in patients with left ventricular dysfunction: insight from the Studies of Left Ventricular Dysfunction (SOLVD) trials. *Circulation.* 2003;107: 2926-2931.
2. Alsheikh-Ali AA, Wang PJ, Rand W, et al. Enalapril treatment and hospitalization with atrial tachyarrhythmias in patients with left ventricular dysfunction. *Am Heart J.* 2004;147:1061-1065.
3. Maggioni AP, Latini R, Carson PE, et al. for the Val-HeFT Investigators. Valsartan reduces the incidence of atrial fibrillation in patients with heart failure: results from the Valsartan Heart Failure Trial (Val-HeFT). *Am Heart J.* 2005;149: 548-557.
4. Ducharme A, Swedberg K, Pfeffer MA, et al. for the CHARM Investigators. Prevention of atrial fibrillation in patients with symptomatic chronic heart failure by candesartan in the Candesartan in Heart failure: Assessment of Reduction of Mortality and morbidity (CHARM) program. *Am Heart J.* 2006;152:86-92.
5. Wachtell K, Lehto M, Gerdts E, et al. Angiotensin II receptor blockade reduces new-onset atrial fibrillation and subsequent stroke compared to atenolol: the Losartan Intervention for End Point Reduction in Hypertension (LIFE) study. *J Am Coll Cardiol.* 2005;45:712-719.
6. Schmieder RE, Kjeldsen SE, Julius S, McInnes GT, Zanchetti A, Hua TA, for the VALUE Trial Group. Reduced incidence of new-onset atrial fibrillation with angiotensin II receptor blockade: the VALUE trial. *J Hypertens.* 2008;26: 403-411.
7. Aksnes TA, Flaa A, Strand A, Kjeldsen SE. Prevention of new-onset atrial fibrillation and its predictors with angiotensin II-receptor blockers in the treatment of hypertension and heart failure. *J Hypertens.* 2007;25:15-23.
8. Elliott WJ, Basu S, Meyer PM. Initial drugs for coronary heart disease prevention in hypertensive patients: Network and Bayesian meta-analyses of clinical trial data. *J Clin Hypertens (Greenwich).* 2009;11:A7.
9. Elliott WJ, Basu S, Meyer PM. Initial drugs for stroke prevention in hypertensive patients: Network and Bayesian meta-analyses of clinical trial data. *J Clin Hypertens (Greenwich).* 2009;11:A7.
10. Verdecchia P, Reboldi G, Angeli F, et al. Angiotensin-converting enzyme inhibitors and calcium channel blockers for coronary heart disease and stroke prevention. *Hypertension.* 2005;46:386-392.

Definition of ambulatory blood pressure targets for diagnosis and treatment of hypertension in relation to clinic blood pressure: prospective cohort study

Head GA, for the Ambulatory Blood Pressure Working Group of the High Blood Pressure Research Council of Australia (Baker IDI Heart and Diabetes Inst, Melbourne, Victoria, Australia; et al)
BMJ 340:c1104, 2010

Background.—Twenty-four hour ambulatory blood pressure thresholds have been defined for the diagnosis of mild hypertension but not for its treatment or for other blood pressure thresholds used in the diagnosis of moderate to severe hypertension. We aimed to derive age and sex related ambulatory blood pressure equivalents to clinic blood pressure thresholds for diagnosis and treatment of hypertension.

Methods.—We collated 24 hour ambulatory blood pressure data, recorded with validated devices, from 11 centres across six Australian states (n=8575). We used least product regression to assess the relation between these measurements and clinic blood pressure measured by trained staff and in a smaller cohort by doctors (n=1693).

Results.—Mean age of participants was 56 years (SD 15) with mean body mass index 28.9 (5.5) and mean clinic systolic/diastolic blood pressure 142/82 mm Hg (19/12); 4626 (54%) were women. Average clinic measurements by trained staff were 6/3 mm Hg higher than daytime ambulatory blood pressure and 10/5 mm Hg higher than 24 hour blood pressure, but 9/7 mm Hg lower than clinic values measured by doctors. Daytime ambulatory equivalents derived from trained staff clinic measurements were 4/3 mm Hg less than the 140/90 mm Hg clinic threshold (lower limit of grade 1 hypertension), 2/2 mm Hg less than the 130/80 mm Hg threshold (target upper limit for patients with associated conditions), and 1/1 mm Hg less than the 125/75 mm Hg threshold. Equivalents were 1/2 mm Hg lower for women and 3/1 mm Hg lower in older people compared with the combined group.

Conclusions.—Our study provides daytime ambulatory blood pressure thresholds that are slightly lower than equivalent clinic values. Clinic blood pressure measurements taken by doctors were considerably higher than those taken by trained staff and therefore gave inappropriate estimates of ambulatory thresholds. These results provide a framework for the diagnosis and management of hypertension using ambulatory blood pressure values.

▶ The results of this large Australian undertaking suggest 2 major conclusions. The first is that the daytime average of a 24-hour ambulatory blood pressure monitoring (ABPM) is lower than the corresponding office reading for important thresholds of blood pressure, with the difference mainly depending on the absolute level of blood pressure (eg, for clinic thresholds of 130/80 or 180/110 mm Hg, the corresponding daytime ABPM readings are 128/78 and 168/105 mm Hg, respectively). Second, like many other investigators, more than 25 years ago[1] and since,[2] they found that doctors' office blood pressures are higher than 24-hour ABPM daytime averages, whereas other trained health care providers' measurements are very similar to the ABPM daytime averages. The implication is that physicians ought not to be taking office readings to minimize the white-coat effect.

As might be expected, there was some inconsistency in the way the readings were obtained. Different ABPM machines were used at different sites, which probably is inconsequential. Doctors' readings were reported only for a small subset of the patients studied; those more than 2 weeks in time away from the ABPM session were excluded. The routine assignment of sleep and wake times for data analysis can be inaccurate for patients who do not work the usual 9AM to 5PM shift. The differences observed between genders are not well explained in the article but could result from differences in physical activity, which is known to influence daytime ABPM averages.

It is likely that these results are generalizable to non-Australian populations, as the overall averages for comparable situations are quite similar to those from other national and international databases.[3,4] Whether Australians have a larger white-coat effect than Americans is uncertain, but other studies have suggested that it is more common in Italians, Spaniards, and perhaps Mexicans. Because of the many problems inherent in office measurements of blood pressure, a prominent Canadian physician has recently recommended that automated sphygmomanometers can be used for all in-office readings, with the health care provider out of the examination room.[5]

W. J. Elliott, MD, PhD

References

1. Mancia G, Bertinieri G, Grassi G, et al. Effects of blood-pressure measurement by the doctor on patient's blood pressure and heart rate. *Lancet.* 1983;2:695-698.
2. Mancia G, Parati G, Pomidossi G, Grassi G, Casadei R, Zanchetti A. Alerting reaction and rise in blood pressure during measurement by physician and nurse. *Hypertension.* 1987;9:209-215.
3. Pickering TG, Hall JE, Appel LJ, et al. Recommendations for blood pressure measurement in humans and experimental animals: Part 1: blood pressure measurement in humans: a statement for professionals from the Subcommittee of Professional and Public Education of the American Heart Association Council on High Blood Pressure Research. *Hypertension.* 2005;45:142-161.
4. Staessen JA, O'Brien ET, Atkins N, Amery AK. Short report: ambulatory blood pressure in normotensive compared with hypertensive subjects. The Ad-Hoc Working Group. *J Hypertension.* 1993;11:1289-1297.
5. Myers MG. A proposed algorithm for diagnosing hypertension using automated office blood pressure measurement. *J Hypertens.* 2010;28:703-708.

Hypertension and Cardiovascular Risk

Tight Blood Pressure Control and Cardiovascular Outcomes Among Hypertensive Patients With Diabetes and Coronary Artery Disease

Cooper-DeHoff RM, Gong Y, Handberg EM, et al (Univ of Florida, Gainesville; et al)

JAMA 304:61-68, 2010

Context.—Hypertension guidelines advocate treating systolic blood pressure (BP) to less than 130 mm Hg for patients with diabetes mellitus; however, data are lacking for the growing population who also have coronary artery disease (CAD).

Objective.—To determine the association of systolic BP control achieved and adverse cardiovascular outcomes in a cohort of patients with diabetes and CAD.

Design, Setting, and Patients.—Observational subgroup analysis of 6400 of the 22 576 participants in the International Verapamil SR-Trandolapril Study (INVEST). For this analysis, participants were at least 50 years old and had diabetes and CAD. Participants were recruited between September 1997 and December 2000 from 862 sites in 14 countries and were followed up through March 2003 with an extended follow-up through August 2008 through the National Death Index for US participants.

Intervention.—Patients received first-line treatment of either a calcium antagonist or β-blocker followed by angiotensin-converting enzyme inhibitor, a diuretic, or both to achieve systolic BP of less than 130 and diastolic BP of less than 85 mm Hg. Patients were categorized as having tight control if they could maintain their systolic BP at less than 130 mm Hg; usual control if it ranged from 130 mm Hg to less than 140 mm Hg; and uncontrolled if it was 140 mm Hg or higher.

Main Outcome Measures.—Adverse cardiovascular outcomes, including the primary outcomes which was the first occurrence of all-cause death, nonfatal myocardial infarction, or nonfatal stroke.

Results.—During 16 893 patient-years of follow-up, 286 patients (12.7%) who maintained tight control, 249 (12.6%) who had usual control, and 431 (19.8%) who had uncontrolled systolic BP experienced a primary outcome event. Patients in the usual-control group had a cardiovascular event rate of 12.6% vs a 19.8% event rate for those in the uncontrolled group (adjusted hazard ratio [HR], 1.46; 95% confidence interval [CI], 1.25-1.71; $P<.001$). However, little difference existed between those with usual control and those with tight control. Their respective event rates were 12.6% vs 12.7% (adjusted HR, 1.11; 95% CI, 0.93-1.32; $P=.24$). The all-cause mortality rate was 11.0% in the tight-control group vs 10.2% in the usual-control group (adjusted HR, 1.20; 95% CI, 0.99-1.45; $P=.06$); however, when extended follow-up was included, risk of all-cause mortality was 22.8% in the tight control vs 21.8% in the usual control group (adjusted HR, 1.15; 95% CI, 1.01-1.32; $P=.04$).

Conclusion.—Tight control of systolic BP among patients with diabetes and CAD was not associated with improved cardiovascular outcomes compared with usual control.

Trial Registration.—clinicaltrials.gov Identifier: NCT00133692.

▶ Like a recent meta-analysis,[1] this report questions the long-held belief that patients with diabetes ought to have lower blood pressures than the nondiabetic hypertensive population. The authors point out that in previous clinical trials in hypertensive patients with diabetes, systolic blood pressure was seldom, if ever, reduced to < 130 mm Hg, as current guidelines recommend.[2,3] These data suggest that there is no benefit on cardiovascular end points associated with achieving systolic blood pressure < 130 mm Hg. The authors performed many sensitivity analyses to consider multiple variations on their data sets, including a 5-year extension of follow-up for mortality in patients enrolled at centers in the United States.

This report also addresses some of the controversy arising from the American Heart Association's Scientific Statement in 2007 that recommended a blood pressure target of < 130/80 mm Hg for hypertensive patients with established heart disease,[4] based primarily on a post hoc subgroup analysis of the intravascular ultrasound substudy of the Comparison of Amlodipine versus Enalapril to Limit Occurrences of Thrombosis trial,[5] and the general impression that high-risk patients should benefit from a lower blood pressure target.[2]

There are some challenges in accepting these conclusions as public health policy, however. These data are derived from a randomized clinical trial, but the analyses constituted a post hoc cohort study and performed many statistical adjustments for baseline variables, which may or may not lead to proper conclusions. For example, patients were trichotomized into those whose systolic blood pressures were, on average, < 130 mm Hg, between 130 and 139 mm Hg, or ≥140 mm Hg. This enriches the tight control group with those who were known to have an increased risk of myocardial infarction in the entire International Verapamil SR-Trandolapril Study data set.[6] Recent data have suggested that in addition to the average office blood pressure, its inter-visit variability may be an important determinant of cardiovascular outcomes.[7] There are also concerns about interpreting the results of this study too broadly, as it included subjects with both diabetes and coronary heart disease. Lastly, it may be dangerous to form policy based on potentially confounded observational studies; most would prefer clinical trials that randomized and successfully treated at-risk individuals to different blood pressure targets, as was recently done in the Avoiding Cardiovascular Complications in Diabetes trial.[8]

W. J. Elliott, MD, PhD

References

1. Arguedas JA, Perez MI, Wright JM. Treatment blood pressure targets for hypertension. *Cochrane Database Syst Rev.* 2009;(3):CD004349. 10.1002/14651858. CD004349.pub2, mrw.interscience.wiley.com/cochrane/clsysrev/articles/CD004349/frame.htm; 2009. Accessed July 10, 2009.
2. Chobanian AV, Bakris GL, Black HR, et al. National High Blood Pressure Education Program Coordinating Committee. Seventh report of the Joint National Committee on Prevention, Detection, Evaluation and Treatment of High Blood Pressure. *Hypertension.* 2003;42:1206-1252.
3. American Diabetes Association. Standards of medical care in diabetes—2010. *Diabetes Care.* 2010;33:S11-S61.
4. Rosendorff C, Black HR, Cannon CP, et al. Treatment of hypertension in the prevention and management of ischemic heart disease: a scientific statement from the American Heart Association Council for High Blood Pressure Research and the Councils on Clinical Cardiology and Epidemiology and Prevention. *Circulation.* 2007;115:2761-2788.
5. Sipahi I, Tuzcu EM, Schoenhagen P, et al. Effects of normal, pre-hypertensive, and hypertensive blood pressure levels on progression of coronary atherosclerosis. *J Am Coll Cardiol.* 2006;48:833-838.
6. Messerli FH, Mancia G, Conti CR, et al. for the International Verapamil-Trandolapril Study Investigators. Dogma disputed: can aggressively lowering blood pressure in hypertensive patients with coronary artery disease be dangerous? *Ann Intern Med.* 2006;144:884-893.
7. Rothwell PM. Limitations of the usual blood-pressure hypothesis and importance of variability, instability, and episodic hypertension. *Lancet.* 2010;375:938-948.
8. Cushman WC, Evans GW, Byington RP, et al. ACCORD Study Group. Effects of intensive blood-pressure control in type 2 diabetes mellitus. *N Engl J Med.* 2010; 362:1575-1585.

Myocardial infarction and stroke associated with diuretic based two drug antihypertensive regimens: population based case-control study

Boger-Megiddo I, Heckbert SR, Weiss NS, et al (Univ of Washington, Seattle; et al)
BMJ 340:c103, 2010

Objective.—To examine the association of myocardial infarction and stroke incidence with several commonly used two drug antihypertensive treatment regimens.

Design.—Population based case-control study.

Setting.—Group Health Cooperative, Seattle, WA, USA.

Participants.—Cases (n=353) were aged 30-79 years, had pharmacologically treated hypertension, and were diagnosed with a first fatal or non-fatal myocardial infarction or stroke between 1989 and 2005. Controls (n=952) were a random sample of Group Health members who had pharmacologically treated hypertension. We excluded individuals with heart failure, evidence of coronary heart disease, diabetes, or chronic kidney disease.

Exposures.—One of three common two drug combinations: diuretics plus β blockers; diuretics plus calcium channel blockers; and diuretics plus angiotensin converting enzyme inhibitors or angiotensin receptor blockers.

Main Outcome Measures.—Myocardial infarction or stroke.

Results.—Compared with users of diuretics plus β blockers, users of diuretics plus calcium channel blockers had an increased risk of myocardial infarction (adjusted odds ratio (OR) 1.98, 95% confidence interval 1.37 to 2.87) but not of stroke (OR 1.02, 95% CI 0.63 to 1.64). The risks of myocardial infarction and stroke in users of diuretics plus angiotensin converting enzyme inhibitors or angiotensin receptor blockers were slightly but not significantly lower than in users of diuretics plus β blockers (myocardial infarction: OR 0.76, 95% CI 0.52 to 1.11; stroke: OR 0.71, 95% CI 0.46 to 1.10).

Conclusions.—In patients with hypertension, diuretics plus calcium channel blockers were associated with a higher risk of myocardial infarction than other common two drug treatment regimens. A large trial of second line antihypertensive treatments in patients already on low dose diuretics is required to provide a solid basis for treatment recommendations.

▶ This report is similar to 2 others: a prospective cohort study from the Women's Health Initiative (by many of the same authors)[1] and the infamous case-control study (by many of the same authors)[2] that launched the calcium channel blocker scare of 1995 and (many believe) may have been the impetus for National Institutes of Health to fund the Antihypertensive and Lipid-Lowering treatment to prevent Heart Attack Trial.[3] One of the major challenges to these case-control studies is the possibility of indication bias, which has been well described by one of this article's senior authors, who has suggested measures that make it less likely.[4] This type of bias is notoriously difficult to detect, either by the researchers or by readers of their reports.[5] Some have suggested that this was the major reason that these authors' 1995 study suggested a significant 60% increased risk of myocardial infarction with calcium antagonists (compared with a diuretic),[2] whereas the prospective, randomized, double-blinded, clinical trial showed a nonsignificant 2% reduction in said risk.[3] In the penultimate paragraph of the methods section, the authors discuss the steps they took to minimize indication bias in this report.

The authors interpret their findings of higher risk of diuretic + calcium antagonist to be consistent with the renin hypothesis[6] and the British National Institute for Health and Clinical Excellence guidelines.[7] In their discussion of trials of second-line antihypertensive therapy, they do not mention either the Study on Cognition and Prognosis in the Elderly (which added candesartan or other agents to hydrochlorothiazide 12.5 mg/d)[8] or the Felodipine Event Reduction trial, which showed significant benefit over placebo on stroke in Chinese patients whose blood pressures were not controlled with hydrochlorothiazide 12.5 mg/d.[9] They concluded by extolling the virtues of the recent National Institutes of Health (NIH) Consensus Conference,[10] which called for a large randomized trial of different second-line antihypertensive therapies and mentioned Systolic blood Pressure Intervention Trial (SPRINT) as a trial currently in planning that could address this important topic. An NIH meeting in 2007 concluded that the issue of the optimal second drug for hypertensive patients was not as important as determination of an optimal blood pressure target.[11] The current description of the SPRINT protocol on the ClinicalTrials.gov Web site makes no mention of a second randomization to different classes of antihypertensive agents but instead only to systolic blood pressure targets of < 120 or < 140 mm Hg.[12]

W. J. Elliott, MD, PhD

References

1. Wassertheil-Smoller S, Psaty BM, Greenland P, et al. Association between cardiovascular outcomes and antihypertensive drug treatment in older women. *JAMA.* 2004;292:2849-2859.
2. Psaty BM, Heckbert SR, Koepsell TD, et al. The risk of myocardial infarction associated with antihypertensive drug therapies. *JAMA.* 1995;274:620-625.
3. The ALLHAT Officers and Coordinators for the ALLHAT Collaborative Research Group. Major outcomes in high-risk hypertensive patients randomized to angiotensin-converting enzyme inhibitor or calcium channel blocker vs. diuretic: The Antihypertensive and Lipid-Lowering Treatment to Prevent Heart Attack Trial (ALLHAT). *JAMA.* 2002;288:2981-2997.
4. Psaty BM, Siscovick DS. Minimizing bias due to confounding by indication in comparative effectiveness research: the importance of restriction. *JAMA.* 2010; 304:897-898.
5. Joffe MM. Confounding by indication: the case of calcium channel blockers. *Pharmacoepidemiol Drug Saf.* 2000;9:37-41.
6. Laragh JH. Laragh's lessons in pathophysiology and clinical pearls for treating hypertension. Lesson XVI: how to choose the correct drug treatment for each hypertensive patient using a plasma renin-based method and the volume-vasoconstriction analysis. *Am J Hypertens.* 2001;14:491-503.
7. Littlejohns P, Ranson P, Sealey C, et al, for the National Collaborating Centre for Chronic Conditions. Hypertension: Management of hypertension in adults in

primary care (partial update of NICE Clinical Guideline 18). National Institute for Health and Clinical Excellence, http://www.nice.org.uk/page.aspx?o=278167. Accessed June 25, 2006.

8. Lithell H, Hansson L, Skoog I, et al. SCOPE Study Group. The Study on Cognition and Prognosis in the Elderly (SCOPE): principal results of a randomized double-blind intervention trial. *J Hypertens.* 2003;21:875-886.

9. Liu L, Zhang Y, Liu G, Li W, Zhang X, Zanchetti A, FEVER Study Group. The Felodipine Event Reduction (FEVER) study: a randomized long-term placebo-controlled trial in Chinese hypertensive patients. *J Hypertens.* 2005;23: 2157-2172.

10. National Heart, Lung, and Blood Institute Working Group on Future Directions in Hypertension Treatment Trials. Major clinical trials of hypertension: what should be done next? *Hypertension.* 2005;46:1-6.

11. Working Group Report: Expert Panel on a Hypertension Treatment Trial Initiative Meeting Summary, http://www.nhlbi.nih.gov/meetings/workshops/hypertsnsion-full.pdf. Accessed November 01, 2010.

12. Systolic Blood Pressure Intervention Trial (SPRINT), http://www.clinicaltrials. gov/ct2/show/NCT01206062. Accessed November 01, 2010.

Preeclampsia and Cardiovascular Disease Death: Prospective Evidence From the Child Health and Development Studies Cohort

Mongraw-Chaffin ML, Cirillo PM, Cohn BA (Public Health Inst, Berkeley, CA)
Hypertension 56:166-171, 2010

This study prospectively investigates the contribution of pregnancy complications and other reproductive age risk factors on the risk of subsequent cardiovascular disease death. Participants were 14 403 women in the Child Health and Development Studies pregnancy cohort drawn from the Kaiser Permanente Health Plan in California. Only women with nonmissing parity and no previously diagnosed heart conditions were included. A total of 481 had observed preeclampsia, and 266 died from cardiovascular disease. The median age at enrollment was 26 years, and the median follow-up time was 37 years. Cardiovascular disease death was determined by linkage with the California Department of Vital Statistics. Observed preeclampsia was independently associated with cardiovascular disease death (mutually adjusted hazard ratio: 2.14 [95% CI: 1.29 to 3.57]). The risk of subsequent cardiovascular disease death was notably higher among women with onset of preeclampsia by 34 weeks of gestation (hazard ratio: 9.54 [95% CI: 4.50 to 20.26]). At 30 years of follow-up and a median age of 56 years, the cumulative cardiovascular disease death survival for women with early preeclampsia was 85.9% compared with 98.3% for women with late preeclampsia and 99.3% for women without preeclampsia. Women with preeclampsia had an increased risk of cardiovascular disease death later in life, independent of other measured risk factors. These findings reinforce previously reported recommendations that a history of preeclampsia should be used to target women at risk for cardiovascular disease. Additionally, women with preeclampsia earlier in pregnancy may be particularly at risk for cardiovascular disease death and could be targeted for early and intensive screening and intervention.

▶ The emerging concept of pregnancy being a stress test for future cardiovascular disease, with pre-eclampsia indicating a flunking grade, is supported by 2 recent meta-analyses[1,2] and several retrospective cohort studies. This report is one (of 2[3]) of the prospective cohort studies of the association of pre-eclampsia and cardiovascular disease death, has the longest follow-up period, and uses standardized definitions of both terms. As such, it may be the most persuasive evidence for the link and may bolster the efforts of those who advocate using a history of pre-eclampsia as a method of targeting and motivating such women to have more intensive treatment of cardiovascular risk factors.

There are many intriguing aspects to this report. Of the 14 403 women in the original database (enrollment from 1957-1968), 481 developed pre-eclampsia and 226 (or 47%) died from a cardiovascular cause over 37 years of average follow-up, allowing the authors to calculate the proper incidence rates of cardiovascular death. More importantly, they calculated and compared Kaplan-Meier survival curves for women without pre-eclampsia and women who developed it before and after 34 weeks of pregnancy. These were strikingly different, with nearly 10-fold increase in the risk of death for women who developed pre-eclampsia at or before 34 weeks of pregnancy. Similarly, they identified risk factors for cardiovascular death, which included pre-eclampsia, pre-existing hypertension before pregnancy, prior birth of a child with intrauterine growth retardation, smoking, higher body mass index at enrollment, and age.

With the advent of the Health Information Portability and Accountability Act restrictions on retention of health information in place since April 14, 2003, similar data are unlikely to ever be collected or seen again in the United States. Despite the fact that the pathophysiology of pre-eclampsia is complex and poorly understood currently,[4] these data serve as a reminder that epidemiological investigations can inform current theories and practices, even when the data were collected during the last millennium.

W. J. Elliott, MD, PhD

References

1. Bellamy L, Casas JP, Hingorani AD, Williams DJ. Pre-eclampsia and risk of cardiovascular disease and cancer in later life: systematic review and meta-analysis. *BMJ.* 2007;335:974-986.
2. McDonald SD, Malinowski A, Zhou Q, Yusuf S, Devereaux PJ. Cardiovascular sequelae of preeclampsia/eclampsia: a systematic review and meta-analyses. *Am Heart J.* 2008;156:918-930.
3. Hannaford P, Ferry S, Hirsch S. Cardiovascular sequelae of toxaemia of pregnancy. *Heart.* 1997;77:154-158.
4. Steegers EAP, von Dadelszen P, Duvekot JJ, Pijnenborg R. Pre-eclampsia. *Lancet.* 2010;376:631-644.

Lower Treatment Blood Pressure Is Associated With Greatest Reduction in Hematoma Growth After Acute Intracerebral Hemorrhage
Arima H, for the Intensive Blood Pressure Reduction in Acute Cerebral Haemorrhage Trial Investigators (Royal Prince Alfred Hosp and the Univ of Sydney, New South Wales, Australia; et al)
Hypertension 56:852-858, 2010

The pilot phase of the Intensive Blood Pressure Reduction in Acute Cerebral Haemorrhage Trial (INTERACT) showed that rapid blood pressure (BP) lowering can attenuate hematoma growth in acute intracerebral hemorrhage. We sought to define the systolic BP level associated with greatest attenuation of hematoma growth. INTERACT included 404 patients with computed tomographic—confirmed intracerebral hemorrhage, elevated systolic BP (150 to 220 mm Hg), and capacity to commence BP lowering treatment within 6 hours of onset. Computed tomography was done at baseline and at 24 hours using standardized techniques, with digital images analyzed centrally, blinded to clinical data. Associations of baseline and achieved on-treatment (mean during the first 24 hours) systolic BP levels with the primary outcome of increase in hematoma volume were explored. There were 346 patients with duplicate computed tomographic scans. There was no significant association between baseline systolic BP levels and either the absolute or proportional growth in hematoma volume (P trend=0.26 and 0.12, respectively). By contrast, achieved on-treatment systolic BP levels in the first 24 hours were clearly associated with both absolute and proportional hematoma growth (both P trend=0.03). Maximum reduction in hematoma growth occurred in the one third of participants with the lowest on-treatment systolic BP levels (median: 135 mm Hg). Intensive BP reduction to systolic levels between 130 and 140 mm Hg is likely to provide the maximum protection against hematoma growth after intracerebral hemorrhage.

▶ The Intensive Blood Pressure Reduction in Acute Cerebral Haemorrhage Trial (INTERACT) was a pilot feasibility study carried out in Australasia that intended to lower blood pressure to < 140 mm Hg within an hour of randomization (intensive treatment group) or < 180 mm Hg (control group). Not powered to assess long-term outcomes, the primary end point was the proportional change in hematoma volume at 24 hours.[1] This end point significantly favored the intensively treated group, despite having baseline and 24-hour computed tomographic scans available for only 346 of their 404 randomized patients. This report is a post hoc analysis of the paired scans that identified predictors of hematoma growth in their patients. Perhaps not surprisingly, given the overall trial results, lowered blood pressure was associated with barely significant lower absolute and proportional growth rates of the hematomas ($P = .03$ for trend in both cases). Their data suggest, but cannot prove, that lowering systolic blood pressure to between 130 and 140 mm Hg may be associated with the slowest hematoma progression rate in hemorrhagic stroke.

These results challenge, but do not refute, current US guidelines for allowing blood pressure to remain elevated and untreated in acute stroke victims.[2,3] Exceptions are generally made if the blood pressure is very high (typically > 200/120 mm Hg) or, only in ischemic stroke, as a prelude to thrombolytic therapy (which is contraindicated in very hypertensive stroke victims). Perhaps because hemorrhagic stroke is far less common than ischemic stroke in the United States, these results of INTERACT will solidify the authors' conviction that the larger outcome-based trial should proceed in Australasia but may not be very pertinent to most US stroke victims. Research seems to be chipping away at prohibitions for using antihypertensive medications in acute stroke,[4,5] but so far no trial has shown clear and convincing evidence that such treatment is beneficial. Practitioners of evidence-based medicine are therefore more likely to support the need for continued research in this area[6] but are probably not yet ready to recommend acute blood pressure lowering in the stroke survivors under their care. As in pediatrics and stroke rehabilitation, many small steps are necessary before everyone can run.

W. J. Elliott, MD, PhD

References

1. Anderson CS, Huang Y, Wang JG, et al. INTERACT Investigators. Intensive blood pressure reduction in acute cerebral hemorrhage trial (INTERACT): a randomized pilot trial. *Lancet Neurol*. 2008;7:391-399.
2. Adams HP, del Zoppa G, Alberts MJ, et al. Guidelines for the early management of adults with ischemic stroke: a guideline from the American Heart Association/American Stroke Association Stroke Council, Clinical Cardiology Council, Cardiovascular Radiology and Intervention Council, and the Atherosclerotic Peripheral Vascular Disease and Quality of Care Outcomes in Research Interdisciplinary Working Groups: the American Academy of Neurology affirms the value of this guideline as an educational tool for neurologists. *Stroke*. 2007;38: 1655-1711.
3. Sacco RL, Adams R, Albers G, et al. Guidelines for prevention of stroke in patients with ischemic stroke or transient ischemic attack: a statement for healthcare professionals from the American Heart Association/American Stroke Association Council on Stroke: co-sponsored by the Council on Cardiovascular Radiology and Intervention: the American Academy of Neurology affirms the value of this guideline. *Stroke*. 2006;37:577-617.
4. Schrader J, Luders S, Kulschewski A, et al. Acute Candesartan Cilexitil Therapy in Stroke Survivors Study Group. The ACCESS Study: evaluation of Acute Candesartan Cilexetil Therapy in Stroke Survivors. *Stroke*. 2003;34:1699-1703.
5. Potter JF, Robinson TJ, Ford GA, et al. Controlling hypertension and hypotension immediately post-stroke (CHHIPS): a randomised, placebo-controlled, double-blind pilot trial. *Lancet Neurol*. 2009;8:48-56.
6. Elijovich F, Laffer CL. Acute stroke: lower blood pressure looks better and better. *Hypertension*. 2010;56:808-810 [editorial].

"Causes" of Hypertension

Projected Effect of Dietary Salt Reductions on Future Cardiovascular Disease
Bibbins-Domingo K, Chertow GM, Coxson PG, et al (Univ of California, San Francisco; Stanford Univ, Palo Alto, CA; et al)
N Engl J Med 362:590-599, 2010

Background.—The U.S. diet is high in salt, with the majority coming from processed foods. Reducing dietary salt is a potentially important target for the improvement of public health.

Methods.—We used the Coronary Heart Disease (CHD) Policy Model to quantify the benefits of potentially achievable, population-wide reductions in dietary salt of up to 3 g per day (1200 mg of sodium per day). We estimated the rates and costs of cardiovascular disease in subgroups defined by age, sex, and race; compared the effects of salt reduction with those of other interventions intended to reduce the risk of cardiovascular disease; and determined the cost-effectiveness of salt reduction as compared with the treatment of hypertension with medications.

Results.—Reducing dietary salt by 3 g per day is projected to reduce the annual number of new cases of CHD by 60,000 to 120,000, stroke by 32,000 to 66,000, and myocardial infarction by 54,000 to 99,000 and to reduce the annual number of deaths from any cause by 44,000 to 92,000. All segments of the population would benefit, with blacks benefiting proportionately more, women benefiting particularly from stroke reduction, older adults from reductions in CHD events, and younger adults from lower mortality rates. The cardiovascular benefits of reduced salt intake are on par with the benefits of population-wide reductions in tobacco use, obesity, and cholesterol levels. A regulatory intervention designed to achieve a reduction in salt intake of 3 g per day would save 194,000 to 392,000 quality-adjusted life-years and $10 billion to $24 billion in health care costs annually. Such an intervention would be cost-saving even if only a modest reduction of 1 g per day were achieved gradually between 2010 and 2019 and would be more cost-effective than using medications to lower blood pressure in all persons with hypertension.

Conclusions.—Modest reductions in dietary salt could substantially reduce cardiovascular events and medical costs and should be a public health target.

▶ This fascinating gedanken experiment uses a computer model to predict outcomes in the entire US population (and important subpopulations) if it were somehow possible to reduce salt intake from the 2005 to 2006 average of 10.4 g/d (=4124 mEq/d in men) and 7.3 g/d (=2895 mEq/d in women) by 3 g/d (=1200 mEq/d).[1] The current recommendation from the US Departments of Agriculture and Health and Human Services is 5.8 g/d (=2300 mEq/d) for all Americans and 3.7 g/d (=1467 mEq/d) for high-risk individuals (eg, hypertensives, African Americans, and those older than 40 years of age).[2] The results of their computer simulation are overwhelmingly positive; such an intervention saves strokes, myocardial infarctions, lives, and money overall. The authors calculate that such an intervention would overall be more cost-effective than drug treatment of hypertension, which most people see as a relative health care bargain, compared with many other interventions in clinical practice.

The authors cite similar national programs to gradually reduce the sodium content of prepared foods, which contain about 70% to 80% of the salt in most people's diets.[3] Such programs have been quite successful in the United Kingdom, Japan, Finland, Portugal, and are now being implemented in certain provinces of China that have an excessively high stroke and stroke mortality rate. Probably the most impressive data come from England, where a law was passed to implement a progressive 10% decrease in sodium added to processed foods over a 4-year period, which saw no reduction in sales of such food items.[4] Carefully collected data from the last millennium suggest that taste buds adjust only slowly to decreased dietary sodium but in the long term, most prefer the taste of low-sodium foods.[5]

Editorialists for this article point out many assumptions, estimations, projections, and other uncertainties in the methodologies used by the authors but conclude that their estimates of the benefits of population-wide salt restriction (to be spearheaded by laws and governmental regulation) may well be underestimated.[6] Whether the American people will permit their elected representative to force the food industry to provide healthier menu items, probably at an increased price, in this politically charged debate, remains to be seen. A recent survey of purchased lunches in New York City showed a very high proportion of meals from various fast food emporia that contained more than 2300 mEq of sodium.[7] It will take more than just advertising campaigns to reverse this challenge.

W. J. Elliott, MD, PhD

References

1. Application of lower sodium intake recommendations for adults—United States 1999–2006. *MMWR Morb Mortal Wkly Rep.* 2009;58:281-283.
2. Henney JE, Taylor CL, Boon CS, eds.. Institute of Medicine: Strategies to Reduce Sodium Intake in the United States. Washington, DC: National Academies Press; 2010, http://www.nap.edu/catalog/php?record_id=12818#description. Accessed October 23, 2010.
3. Mattes RD, Donnelly D. Relative contributions of dietary sodium sources. *J Am Coll Nutr.* 1991;10:383-393.
4. *Dietary Sodium Level Surveys.* Aberdeen, UK: Food Standards Agency; 2008, http://www.food.gov.uk/science/dietarysurveys/urinary. Accessed October 23, 2010.
5. Blais CA, Pangborn RM, Borhani NO, Ferrell MF, Prineas RJ, Laing B. Effect of dietary sodium restriction on taste responses to sodium chloride: a longitudinal study. *Am J Clin Nutr.* 1986;44:232-243.
6. Appel LJ, Anderson CAM. Compelling evidence for public health action to reduce salt intake. *N Engl J Med.* 2010;362:650-652.
7. Johnson CM, Angel SY, Lederer A, et al. Sodium content of lunchtime fast food purchases at major US chains. *Arch Intern Med.* 2010;170:732-734.

Population Strategies to Decrease Sodium Intake and the Burden of Cardiovascular Disease: A Cost-Effectiveness Analysis
Smith-Spangler CM, Juusola JL, Enns EA, et al (Veterans Affairs Palo Alto Healthcare System, CA; Stanford Univ, CA)
Ann Intern Med 152:481-487, 2010

Background.—Sodium consumption raises blood pressure, increasing the risk for heart attack and stroke. Several countries, including the United States, are considering strategies to decrease population sodium intake.

Objective.—To assess the cost-effectiveness of 2 population strategies to reduce sodium intake: government collaboration with food manufacturers to voluntarily cut sodium in processed foods, modeled on the United Kingdom experience, and a sodium tax.

Design.—A Markov model was constructed with 4 health states: well, acute myocardial infarction (MI), acute stroke, and history of MI or stroke.

Data Sources.—Medical Panel Expenditure Survey (2006), Framingham Heart Study (1980 to 2003), Dietary Approaches to Stop Hypertension trial, and other published data.

Target Population.—U.S. adults aged 40 to 85 years.

Time Horizon.—Lifetime.

Perspective.—Societal.

Outcome Measures.—Incremental costs (2008 U.S. dollars), quality-adjusted life-years (QALYs), and MIs and strokes averted.

Results of Base-Case Analysis.—Collaboration with industry that decreases mean population sodium intake by 9.5% averts 513 885 strokes and 480 358 MIs over the lifetime of adults aged 40 to 85 years who are alive today compared with the status quo, increasing QALYs by 2.1 million and saving $32.1 billion in medical costs. A tax on sodium that decreases population sodium intake by 6% increases QALYs by 1.3 million and saves $22.4 billion over the same period.

Results of Sensitivity Analysis.—Results are sensitive to the assumption that consumers have no disutility with modest reductions in sodium intake.

Limitation.—Efforts to reduce population sodium intake could result in other dietary changes that are difficult to predict.

Conclusion.—Strategies to reduce sodium intake on a population level in the United States are likely to substantially reduce stroke and MI incidence, which would save billions of dollars in medical expenses.

▶ This is a slightly different approach to the population-based consequences of getting Americans to consume a low-sodium diet, compared with a similar recent gedanken experiment of somehow reducing salt intake from the 2005-06 average of 10.4 gm/d (=4124 mEq/d in men) and 7.3 gm/d (=2895 mEq/d in women) by 3 gm/d (=1200 mEq/d).[1] These authors compare the results of 2 interventions: the governmentally facilitated voluntary reduction in hidden salt in prepared foods that worked so well in the United Kingdom and elsewhere[2,3] and a more draconian tax that would force Americans to pay higher prices for high-sodium food items.

The results of the authors' calculations are overwhelmingly positive: both interventions save strokes, myocardial infarctions, lives, and billions of dollars overall. These conclusions are quite similar to those of a different cost-effectiveness analysis that did not prespecify the method of sodium restriction.[1] As usual, examination of the base-case assumptions and the many sensitivity analyses provides an interesting look into how the conclusions change because of wide variance in the initial conditions. As an example, the authors claim that an acute myocardial infarction costs $9000, which is close to the cost of a single dose of one thrombolytic drug in some centers in the United States. The range of costs modeled is $7000 to $19 000, which is much lower than current estimates from the American Heart Association.[4]

Editorialists for this article (from the US Centers for Disease Control and Prevention, which has been tasked by Congress to provide a road map for nationwide sodium restriction) point out that the voluntary gradual reduction in sodium added to prepared foods is much more likely to be successful (even at 9% reduction) than the proposed salt tax, which faces many philosophical and practical challenges.[5] This may be the reason the authors chose to model only a 6% reduction in sodium consumption for this intervention as their base case. It is no surprise that the less effective intervention results in a lower overall savings of morbid/mortal events and money. Exactly how the nationwide reduction in salt intake will be implemented may turn out to be a political issue, and hotly debated, even though both sides agree that it may well be worthwhile.[6] Whatever program is chosen, one hopes that it will be more successful than the halt the salt campaign of the early 1980s.

W. J. Elliott, MD, PhD

References

1. Bibbins-Domingo K, Chertow GM, Coxson PG, et al. Projected effect of dietary salt reductions on future cardiovascular disease. *N Engl J Med.* 2010;362:590-599.
2. He FJ, MacGregor GA. A comprehensive review on salt and health and current experience of worldwide salt reduction programmes. *J Hum Hypertens.* 2009;23:363-384.
3. *Dietary Sodium Level Surveys.* Aberdeen, UK: Food Standards Agency; 2008, http://www.food.gov.uk/science/dietarysurveys/urinary; 2008.
4. Lloyd-Jones DM, Adams RJ, Brown TM, et al. Heart disease and stroke statistics—2010 update: a report from the American Heart Association. *Circulation.* 2010;121:e46-e215.
5. Frieden TR, Briss PA. We can reduce dietary sodium, save money and save lives. *Ann Intern Med.* 2010;152:526-528.
6. Henney JE, Taylor CL, Boon CS, eds.. Institute of Medicine: Strategies to reduce sodium intake in the United States. Washington, DC: National Academies Press; 2010, http://www.nap.edu/catalog/php?record_id=12818#description.

Statins, antihypertensive treatment, and blood pressure control in clinic and over 24 hours: evidence from PHYLLIS randomised double blind trial
Mancia G, Parati G, Revera M, et al (Univ of Milano-Bicocca, Milan, Italy; et al)
BMJ 340:c1197, 2010

Objective.—To investigate the possibility that statins reduce blood pressure as well as cholesterol concentrations through clinic and 24 hour ambulatory blood pressure monitoring.
Design.—Randomised placebo controlled double blind trial.
Setting.—13 hospitals in Italy.
Participants.—508 patients with mild hypertension and hypercholesterolaemia, aged 45 to 70 years.
Intervention.—Participants were randomised to antihypertensive treatment (hydrochlorothiazide 25 mg once daily or fosinopril 20 mg once daily) with or without the addition of a statin (pravastatin 40 mg once daily).
Main Outcome Measures.—Clinic and ambulatory blood pressure measured every year throughout an average 2.6 year treatment period.
Results.—Both the group receiving antihypertensive treatment without pravastatin (n=254) (with little change in total cholesterol) and the group receiving antihypertensive treatment with pravastatin (n=253) (with marked and sustained reduction in total cholesterol and low density lipoprotein cholesterol) had a clear cut sustained reduction in clinic measured systolic and diastolic blood pressure as well as in 24 hour, and day and night, systolic and diastolic blood pressure. Pravastatin performed slightly worse than placebo, and between group differences did not exceed 1.9 (95% confidence interval −0.6 to 4.3, P=0.13) mm Hg throughout the treatment period. This was also the case when participants who remained on monotherapy with hydrochlorothiazide or fosinopril throughout the study were considered separately.
Conclusions.—Administration of a statin in hypertensive patients in whom blood pressure is effectively reduced by concomitant antihypertensive treatment does not have an additional blood pressure lowering effect.
Trial Registration.—BRISQUI_*IV_2004_001 (registered at Osservatorio Nazionale sulla Sperimentazione Clinica dei Medicinali—National Monitoring Centre on Clinical Research with Medicines).

▶ Statins (or 3-hydroxy-3-methylglutaryl coenzyme A reductase inhibitors) have many benefits, seemingly beyond the changes in circulating lipid levels that they were primarily designed to achieve. Controversy still exists as to whether these drugs lower blood pressure as well as serum low-density lipoprotein-cholesterol levels.[1-3]

The authors hypothesized that some of the studies reporting a blood pressure reduction might have been confounded because of an accommodation effect (blood pressure decreases on repeated visits to the clinical site, as patients become used to the personnel, procedures, and surroundings). They therefore dusted off some of their old data from a randomized clinical trial[4] that used, as one of the efficacy measures, 24-hour ambulatory blood pressure monitoring (ABPM), which typically has very little, if any, accommodation or placebo effect.

Their results indicate that pravastatin, at doses used in Plaque Hypertension Lipid-Lowering Italian Study (PHYLLIS), had no significant effect on either clinic monitoring or 24-hour ABPM, whereas the antihypertensive drug regimens (fosinopril, hydrochlorothiazide, or their combination) had a major significant blood pressure reduction. The authors point out that the most recent meta-analysis that suggested a blood pressure-lowering effect included clinic measurements from 563 patients,[2] whereas their study included 508 patients; if one counts the number of blood pressure determinations, the ABPM data overwhelm the clinic measurements. They also cite data from the Anglo-Scandinavian Cardiac Outcomes Trial (ASCOT),[5] the Conduit Artery Function Evaluation (CAFE) substudy of ASCOT,[6] and the Cholesterol and Recurrent Events (CARE) trial,[7] none of which used ABPM to evaluate blood pressures, that support their contention that neither pravastatin (in PHYLLIS and CARE) nor atorvastatin (in ASCOT and CAFE) significantly lowered blood pressure, and the beneficial effects of these drugs (and presumably other statins) are therefore more likely because of alterations in lipid levels.

W. J. Elliott, MD, PhD

References

1. Wierzbicki AS. Lipid lowering: another method of reducing blood pressure? *J Hum Hypertens*. 2002;16:753-760.
2. Strazzullo P, Kerry SM, Barbato A, Versiero M, D'Elia L, Cappuccio FP. Do statins reduce blood pressure?: a meta-analysis of randomized, controlled trials. *Hypertension*. 2007;49:792-798.
3. Golomb BA, Dimsdale JE, White HL, Ritchie JB, Criqui MH. Reduction in blood pressure with statins: results from the UCSD Statin Study, a randomized trial. *Arch Intern Med*. 2008;168:721-727.
4. Zanchetti A, Crepaldi G, Bond G, et al. Different effects of antihypertensive regimens based on fosinopril or hydrochlorothiazide, with or without lipid lowering by pravastatin on progression of asymptomatic carotid atherosclerosis: principal results of PHYLLIS—a randomized double-blind trial. *Stroke*. 2004;35:2807-2812.
5. Sever PS, Dahlöf B, Poulter NR, et al. for the ASCOT Investigators. Prevention of coronary and stroke events with atorvastatin in hypertensive patients who have average or lower-than-average cholesterol concentrations, in the Anglo-Scandinavian Cardiac Outcomes Trial—Lipid Lowering Arm (ASCOT-LLA): a multicentre randomized controlled trial. *Lancet*. 2003;361:1149-1158.
6. Tonelli M, Sacks F, Pfeffer M, Lopez-Jimenez F, Jhangri GS, Curhan G. Effect of pravastatin on blood pressure in people with cardiovascular disease. *J Hum Hypertens*. 2006;20:560-565.
7. Williams B, Lacy PS, Cruickshank JK, et al. Impact of statin therapy on central aortic pressures and hemodynamics: principal results of the Conduit Artery Functional Evaluation-Lipid-Lowering Arm (CAFE-LLA) Study. *Circulation*. 2009;119:53-61.

Screening renal artery angiography in hypertensive patients undergoing coronary angiography and 6-month follow-up after ad hoc percutaneous revascularization

Rimoldi SF, de Marchi SF, Windecker S, et al (Univ Hosp Bern, Switzerland)
J Hypertens 28:842-847, 2010

Objective.—To determine the prevalence and independent predictors of significant atherosclerotic renal artery stenosis (RAS) in unselected hypertensive patients undergoing coronary angiography and to assess the 6-month outcome of those patients with a significant RAS.

Methods.—One thousand, four hundred and three consecutive hypertensive patients undergoing drive-by renal arteriography were analyzed retrospectively. Univariate and multivariate logistic regression analyses were performed to identify independent predictors of RAS. In patients with significant RAS ($\geq 50\%$ luminal narrowing), 6-month follow-up was assessed and outcome was compared between patients with or without renal revascularization.

Results.—The prevalence of significant RAS was 8%. After multivariate analysis, coronary [odds ratio 5.3; 95% confidence interval (CI) 2.7—10.3; $P < 0.0001$], peripheral (odds ratio 3.3; 95% CI 2.0—5.5; $P < 0.0001$), and cerebral artery (odds ratio 2.8; 95% CI 1.5-5.3; $P = 0.001$) diseases, and impaired renal function (odds ratio 2.9; 95% CI 1.8—4.5; $P < 0.0001$) were found as independent predictors. At least one of these predictors was present in 96% of patients with RAS. In 74 patients (66%) with significant RAS, an ad hoc revascularization was performed. At follow-up, creatinine clearance was significantly higher in revascularized than in nonrevascularized patients (69.2 vs. 55.5 ml/min per 1.73 m, $P = 0.029$). By contrast, blood pressure was comparable between both groups, but nonrevascularized patients were taking significantly more antihypertensive drugs as compared with baseline (2.7 vs. 2.1, follow-up vs. baseline; $P = 0.0066$).

Conclusion.—The prevalence of atherosclerotic RAS in unselected hypertensive patients undergoing coronary angiography was low. Coronary, peripheral, and cerebral artery diseases, and impaired renal function were independent predictors of RAS. Ad hoc renal revascularization was associated with better renal function and fewer intake of antihypertensive drugs at follow-up.

▶ This article rather strongly contradicts much other information in the literature. Several series of American patients put the prevalence of significant renal artery stenosis at 11% to 39% among patients undergoing cardiac catheterization,[1] which would be a much larger clinical burden of disease than this group sees in Switzerland. The American Heart Association had to publish guidelines for appropriate investigation of renal artery stenosis during cardiac catheterization[2] because so many angiographers were performing drive-by renal angiograms. Because renal artery stenosis is more common in older patients, patients with obstructive atherosclerotic disease in other vascular beds, and patients with increasing degrees of renal impairment,[3] it would be interesting to know if the authors' cohort was much different than many American series with regard to these parameters; the descriptive data provided by the authors in Table 1 would suggest any such differences were minor.

The other area in which these authors' conclusions differ from those of other investigators is the improved outcomes in patients who received renal angioplasty. At least 3 large clinical trials have now shown no benefit of such therapy in intention-to-treat analyses, compared with maximal medical therapy alone.[4-6] One wonders about the possibility of indication bias that might account for the authors' observation that the patients they selected for angioplasty were different from those that they chose not to intervene. This may be another instance in which case series and cohort studies come to different conclusions than randomized clinical trials about the efficacy of a given therapy.

It is unlikely that angiographers in the United States will soon have a chance to repeat these findings because it took more than 3 years of work to accumulate 1043 subjects in Switzerland. Most health care financing authorities in the United States now routinely deny prior authorization requests for angiography and renal artery angioplasty, with or without stenting, unless very specific criteria are met and maximal medical therapy has been unsuccessful in lowering blood pressure over a defined (and relatively long) time period.

W. J. Elliott, MD, PhD

References

1. de Mast Q, Beutler JJ. The prevalence of atherosclerotic renal artery stenosis in risk groups: a systematic literature review. *J Hypertens.* 2009;27:1333-1340.
2. White CJ, Jaff MR, Haskal ZJ, et al. Indications for renal arteriography at the time of coronary arteriography: A science advisory from the American Heart Association Committee on Diagnostic and Interventional Cardiac Catheterization, Council on Clinical Cardiology, and the Councils on Cardiovascular Radiology and Intervention and on Kidney in Cardiovascular Disease. *Circulation.* 2006; 114:1892-1895.
3. Buller CE, Nogareda JG, Ramanathan K, et al. The profile of cardiac patients with renal artery stenosis. *J Am Coll Cardiol.* 2003;43:1606-1613.
4. van Jaarsveld BC, Krijnen P, Pieterman H, et al. The effect of balloon angioplasty on hypertension in atherosclerotic renal-artery stenosis. Dutch Renal Artery Stenosis Intervention Cooperative Study Group. *N Engl J Med.* 2000;342:1007-1014.
5. Bax L, Woittiez A-J, Kouwenberg HJ, et al. Stent placement in patients with atherosclerotic renal artery stenosis and impaired renal function: a randomized trial. *Ann Intern Med.* 2009;150:840-848.
6. Wheatley K, Ives N, Kalra PA, et al. on behalf of the Angioplasty and Stenting for Renal Artery Lesions (ASTRAL) Investigators. Revascularization versus medical therapy for renal-artery stenosis. *N Engl J Med.* 2009;361:1953-1962.

Clinical Trials

Effects of Intensive Blood-Pressure Control in Type 2 Diabetes Mellitus

The ACCORD Study Group (Memphis Veterans Affairs (VA) Med Ctr; Wake Forest Univ School of Medicine, Winston-Salem, NC; et al)

N Engl J Med 362:1575-1585, 2010

Background.—There is no evidence from randomized trials to support a strategy of lowering systolic blood pressure below 135 to 140 mm Hg in persons with type 2 diabetes mellitus. We investigated whether therapy targeting normal systolic pressure (i.e., <120 mm Hg) reduces major cardiovascular events in participants with type 2 diabetes at high risk for cardiovascular events.

Methods.—A total of 4733 participants with type 2 diabetes were randomly assigned to intensive therapy, targeting a systolic pressure of less than 120 mm Hg, or standard therapy, targeting a systolic pressure of less than 140 mm Hg. The primary composite outcome was nonfatal myocardial infarction, nonfatal stroke, or death from cardiovascular causes. The mean follow-up was 4.7 years.

Results.—After 1 year, the mean systolic blood pressure was 119.3 mm Hg in the intensive-therapy group and 133.5 mm Hg in the standard-therapy group. The annual rate of the primary outcome was 1.87% in the intensive-therapy group and 2.09% in the standard-therapy group (hazard ratio with intensive therapy, 0.88; 95% confidence interval [CI], 0.73 to 1.06; P = 0.20). The annual rates of death from any cause were 1.28% and 1.19% in the two groups, respectively (hazard ratio, 1.07; 95% CI, 0.85 to 1.35; P = 0.55). The annual rates of stroke, a prespecified secondary outcome, were 0.32% and 0.53% in the two groups, respectively (hazard ratio, 0.59; 95% CI, 0.39 to 0.89; P = 0.01). Serious adverse events attributed to antihypertensive treatment occurred in 77 of the 2362 participants in the intensive-therapy group (3.3%) and 30 of the 2371 participants in the standard-therapy group (1.3%) (P<0.001).

Conclusions.—In patients with type 2 diabetes at high risk for cardiovascular events, targeting a systolic blood pressure of less than 120 mm Hg, as compared with less than 140 mm Hg, did not reduce the rate of a composite outcome of fatal and nonfatal major cardiovascular events. (ClinicalTrials.gov number, NCT00000620.)

▶ This report raises many questions. Perhaps the most interesting of these is why the designers of the Action to Control Cardiovascular Risk in Diabetes (ACCORD) trial chose a target systolic blood pressure (BP) of < 140 mm Hg for their standard therapy group when, since at least 1997,[1] American patients with diabetes have been recommended to achieve and maintain a systolic BP of < 130 mm Hg. Some would argue that this recommendation has never been properly evidence based,[2] and others would point to the controversy surrounding the J-shaped curve[3] as requiring a definitive answer. Unkind individuals might assert that the US federal government has focused its clinical trial funding on studies designed to show that more expensive therapies are not better (eg, chlorthalidone was superior to more expensive antihypertensive drugs, and pravastatin was not significantly better than usual care in the Antihypertensive and Lipid-Lowering treatment to prevent Heart Attack Trial).[4,5] Some would argue that the same theme runs through all 3 components of ACCORD.[6,7]

The fact that stroke was significantly reduced in the group with the low target BP is perhaps not surprising, as stroke is the cardiovascular end point that is most sensitive to BP lowering. The question of whether this was an important lesson from ACCORD-BP is controversial, as many public health authorities have reminded us that one should be reticent to accept a secondary end point as public health policy, when the overall results of the trial (as expressed in the primary end point) did not achieve statistical significance.

It will be most interesting to see how the results of ACCORD-BP are integrated into clinical guidelines, both in the Eighth Report of the Joint National Committee on Prevention, Detection, Evaluation, and Treatment of High Blood Pressure and by the guidelines committees of the American Diabetes Association. If, as might be expected, these results dampen the enthusiasm for a lower BP goal for patients with diabetes, fewer prescriptions for antihypertensive drugs and fewer office visits to control the BPs of patients with diabetes will be needed. These savings may be offset, however, to some degree, by higher pay for performance revenues to physicians, if more patients with diabetes achieve their (higher) office BP targets.

These data indicate that it is possible to treat many patients with diabetes to a very low systolic BP (< 120 mm Hg), but there seems to be little reason to do so (except possibly to reduce stroke rates). The higher cost, higher frequency of severe adverse effects, and the lack of a significant overall cardiovascular benefit, all make it unlikely that this target can be generally recommended. Whether the same can be said for the systolic BP target of < 130 mm Hg is still an open question.

W. J. Elliott, MD, PhD

References

1. The Sixth Report of the Joint National Committee on Prevention, Detection, Evaluation, and Treatment of High Blood Pressure (JNC VI). *Arch Intern Med.* 1997; 157:2413-2446.
2. Arguedas JA, Perez MI, Wright JM. Treatment blood pressure targets for hypertension. *Cochrane Database Syst Rev.* 2009;(4) 10.1002/14651858.CD004349.pub2, mrw.interscience.wiley.com/cochrane/clsysrev/articles/CD004349/frame.htm. Accessed July 10, 2010.
3. Messerli FH, Panjrath GS. The J-curve between blood pressure and coronary artery disease or essential hypertension: exactly how essential? *J Am Coll Cardiol.* 2009;54:1827-1834.
4. The ALLHAT Officers and Coordinators for the ALLHAT Collaborative Research Group. Major outcomes in high-risk hypertensive patients randomized to angiotensin-converting enzyme inhibitor or calcium channel blocker vs. diuretic: The Antihypertensive and Lipid Lowering Treatment to Prevent Heart Attack Trial (ALLHAT). *JAMA.* 2002;288:2981-2997.

5. The ALLHAT Officers and Coordinators for the ALLHAT Collaborative Research Group. Major outcomes in moderately hypercholesterolemic, hypertensive patients randomized to pravastatin vs. usual care: The Antihypertensive and Lipid-Lowering Treatment to Prevent Heart Attack Trial (ALLHAT-LLT). *JAMA.* 2002;288:2998-3007.
6. Gerstein HC, Miller ME, Byington RP, et al. The Action to Control Cardiovascular Risk in Diabetes Study Group. Effects of intensive glucose lowering in type 2 diabetes. *N Engl J Med.* 2008;358:2545-2559.
7. Ginsberg HN, Elam MB, Lovato LC, et al. The Action to Control Cardiovascular Risk in Diabetes(ACCORD) Study Group. Effects of combination lipid therapy in type 2 diabetes mellitus. *N Engl J Med.* 2010;362:1563-1574.

Effect of Valsartan on the Incidence of Diabetes and Cardiovascular Events

The NAVIGATOR Study Group (Univ of Glasgow, UK; Univ of Oxford, UK; Univ of Texas Health Science Ctr, San Antonio; et al)
N Engl J Med 362:1477-1490, 2010

Background.—It is not known whether drugs that block the renin–angiotensin system reduce the risk of diabetes and cardiovascular events in patients with impaired glucose tolerance.

Methods.—In this double-blind, randomized clinical trial with a 2-by-2 factorial design, we assigned 9306 patients with impaired glucose tolerance and established cardiovascular disease or cardiovascular risk factors to receive valsartan (up to 160 mg daily) or placebo (and nateglinide or placebo) in addition to lifestyle modification. We then followed the patients for a median of 5.0 years for the development of diabetes (6.5 years for vital status). We studied the effects of valsartan on the occurrence of three coprimary outcomes: the development of diabetes; an extended composite outcome of death from cardiovascular causes, nonfatal myocardial infarction, nonfatal stroke, hospitalization for heart failure, arterial revascularization, or hospitalization for unstable angina; and a core composite outcome that excluded unstable angina and revascularization.

Results.—The cumulative incidence of diabetes was 33.1% in the valsartan group, as compared with 36.8% in the placebo group (hazard ratio in the valsartan group, 0.86; 95% confidence interval [CI], 0.80 to 0.92; P<0.001). Valsartan, as compared with placebo, did not significantly reduce the incidence of either the extended cardiovascular outcome (14.5% vs. 14.8%; hazard ratio, 0.96; 95% CI, 0.86 to 1.07; P=0.43) or the core cardiovascular outcome (8.1% vs. 8.1%; hazard ratio, 0.99; 95% CI, 0.86 to 1.14; P=0.85).

Conclusions.—Among patients with impaired glucose tolerance and cardiovascular disease or risk factors, the use of valsartan for 5 years, along with lifestyle modification, led to a relative reduction of 14% in the incidence of diabetes but did not reduce the rate of cardiovascular events. (ClinicalTrials.gov number, NCT00097786.)

▶ This report is somewhat reminiscent of the Diabetes Reduction Assessment with ramipril and rosiglitazone Medications (DREAM) trial.[1] Both were 2 × 2 factorial design studies of a renin-angiotensin system blocker and a hypoglycemic agent, each compared simultaneously with placebo, on the prevention of type 2 diabetes. This trial sets a record by having 2 additional coprimary end points, as these drugs' effects on cardiovascular events were simultaneously monitored but without any significant differences being noted.

In DREAM, rosiglitazone was much more effective than placebo in preventing diabetes, which left less diabetes to be prevented by ramipril (and may have been the reason for its 9% reduction but nonsignificant difference from placebo). In this trial, no significant benefit of nateglinide was noted, perhaps leaving more diabetes to be prevented by valsartan.

These data are consistent with a prior network meta-analysis that included all data up to and including DREAM,[2] in which an angiotensin converting enzyme (ACE)inhibitor was slightly (but not significantly) inferior to an angiotensin receptor blocker (ARB) in preventing diabetes. A subsequent network metaanalysis, updated with all trials through (and including) Nateglinide and Valsartan in Impaired Glucose Tolerance Outcomes Research (NAVIGATOR), still shows a slight (but nonsignificant) advantage for the ARB.[3]

The more challenging question is why valsartan did not reduce the rates of cardiovascular events in this large group of prediabetic individuals, who had many other cardiovascular risk factors. Although just over half were women, more than 77% of the participants were hypertensive, nearly 25% had a previous cardiovascular event, more than half had some form of dyslipidemia, and about 11% smoked. Perhaps because their blood pressures were already reasonably well controlled (139.7/82.5 mm Hg on average at baseline), and they received (either at randomization or later during follow-up) effective preventive treatments for cardiovascular events (including antiplatelet drugs in 45%, lipidlowering drugs in 50%, β-blockers in 41%, and calcium antagonists in 36%, all at the last follow-up visit), there were fewer cardiovascular events than the study designers anticipated. This research group originally chose the ONgoing Telmisartan Alone and in combination with Ramipril Global Endpoint Trial (ONTARGET)[4] and Telmisartan Randomised AssessmeNt Study in ACE iNtolerant subjects with cardiovascular Disease (TRANSCEND)[5] primary end point as their first secondary end point, but it was promoted to the third coprimary end point for NAVIGATOR early during follow-up, with the appropriate downward adjustment in the acceptable P-value for multiple comparisons. Interestingly, the authors report that the observed rate of their core cardiovascular outcomes was 14.0/1000 patient-years, whereas those for the ARBtreated patients in ONTARGET and TRANSCEND were about 35.7 and 33.8 per 1000 patient-years, respectively. These comparisons give some credence to the suggestion that NAVIGATOR may have been underpowered to see a difference in cardiovascular outcomes, perhaps because the primary enrollment criterion was the presence of impaired glucose tolerance, and patients with diabetes were actively excluded.

These data add to our knowledge about the relative efficacy of ARBs in preventing diabetes (for which the 5-year number needed to treat was about 27) as well as the relative ineffectiveness of ARBs (when added to other effective therapies) in preventing rare cardiovascular events in what were probably lower-risk patients than in other recent ARB trials.[4-8]

W. J. Elliott, MD, PhD

References

1. Bosch J, Yusuf S, Gerstein HC, et al. for the DREAM Trial Investigators. Effect of ramipril on the incidence of diabetes. *N Engl J Med.* 2006;355:1551-1562.
2. Elliott WJ, Meyer PM. Incident diabetes in clinical trials of antihypertensive drugs: a network meta-analysis. *Lancet.* 2007;369:201-207.
3. Elliott WJ, Basu S, Meyer PM. Incident diabetes with antihypertensive drugs: Updated network and Bayesian meta-analyses of clinical trial data. *J Clin Hypertens (Greenwich).* 2010;12:A20 [abstract].
4. Yusuf S, Teo KK, Pogue J, et al. ONTARGET Investigators. Telmisartan, ramipril or both in patients at high risk for vascular events. *N Engl J Med.* 2008;358: 1547-1549.
5. Yusuf S, Teo K, Anderson C, et al. for the Telmisartan Randomised AssessmeNt Study in ACE iNtolerant subjects with cardiovascular Disease (TRANSCEND) Investigators. Effects of the angiotensin-receptor blocker telmisartan on cardiovascular events in high-risk patients intolerant to angiotensin-converting enzyme inhibitors: a randomised controlled trial. *Lancet.* 2008;372:1174-1183.
6. Mochizuki S, Dahlöf B, Shimizu M, et al. Valsartan in a Japanese population with hypertension and other cardiovascular disease (Jikei Heart Study): a randomised, open-label, blinded endpoint morbidity-mortality study. *Lancet.* 2007;369: 1431-1439.
7. Kasanuki H, Hagiwara N, Hosoda S, et al. for the HIJ-CREATE Investigators. Angiotensin II receptor blocker-based vs. non-angiotensin II receptor blocker-based therapy in patients with angiographically documented coronary artery disease and hypertension: the Heart Institute of Japan Candesartan Randomized Trial for Evaluation in Coronary Artery Disease (HIJ-CREATE). *Eur Heart J.* 2009;30:1203-1212.
8. Sawada T, Yamada H, Dahlöf B, Matsubara H, for the Kyoto Heart Study Group. Effects of valsartan on morbidity and mortality in uncontrolled hypertensive patients with high cardiovascular risks: Kyoto Heart Study. *Eur Heart J.* 2009; 30:2461-2469.

Target Blood Pressure for Treatment of Isolated Systolic Hypertension in the Elderly: Valsartan in Elderly Isolated Systolic Hypertension Study
Ogihara T, for the Valsartan in Elderly Isolated Systolic Hypertension Study Group (Osaka Univ Graduate School of Medicine, Japan; et al)
Hypertension 56:196-202, 2010

In this prospective, randomized, open-label, blinded end point study, we aimed to establish whether strict blood pressure control (<140 mm Hg) is superior to moderate blood pressure control (≥140 mm Hg to <150 mm Hg) in reducing cardiovascular mortality and morbidity in elderly patients with isolated systolic hypertension. We divided 3260 patients aged 70 to 84 years with isolated systolic hypertension (sitting blood pressure 160 to 199 mm Hg) into 2 groups, according to strict or moderate blood pressure treatment. A composite of cardiovascular events was evaluated for ≥2 years. The strict control (1545 patients) and moderate control (1534 patients) groups were well matched (mean age: 76.1 years; mean blood pressure: 169.5/81.5 mm Hg). Median follow-up was 3.07 years. At 3 years, blood pressure reached 136.6/74.8 mm Hg and 142.0/76.5 mm Hg, respectively. The blood pressure difference between the 2 groups was 5.4/1.7 mm Hg. The overall rate of the primary composite end point was 10.6 per 1000 patient-years in the strict control group and 12.0 per 1000 patient-years in the moderate control group (hazard ratio: 0.89; [95% CI: 0.60 to 1.34]; P=0.38). In summary, blood pressure targets of <140 mm Hg are safely achievable in relatively healthy patients ≥70 years of age with isolated systolic hypertension, although our trial was underpowered to definitively determine whether strict control was superior to less stringent blood pressure targets.

▶ The optimal target blood pressure for older patients with isolated systolic hypertension is debatable. The landmark clinical trial, the Systolic Hypertension in the Elderly Program, found a highly significant benefit on stroke (and other cardiovascular end points, notably heart failure) with a chlorthalidone-based anti-hypertensive regimen, compared with placebo, but the target systolic blood pressure was <160 mm Hg and/or a drop in systolic blood pressure by ≥20 mm Hg.[1] A post hoc analysis of the data showed significant benefits on stroke with achieved systolic blood pressures of <160 mm Hg and <150 mm Hg, but not <140 mm Hg, presumably because so few patients achieved that level of systolic blood pressure with the antihypertensive drug regimens used in the late 1980s.[2] Similarly, the Systolic Hypertension in Europe and China trials showed significant prevention of stroke, but other end points were less impressive (perhaps again because the primary end point was so well prevented).[3,4] The most recent clinical trial, Hypertension in the Very Elderly Trial, had a target systolic blood pressure of <150 mm Hg, but did not show a significant benefit on stroke, perhaps because the Data Safety and Monitoring Board recommended stopping the study early because of a significant mortality benefit of active treatment.[5] Disciples of evidence-based medicine thus assert that the clinical trial evidence favors a systolic blood pressure target of <150 mm Hg, but not lower, in patients with isolated systolic hypertension. They discount the results of the Cardio-Sis trial because it included younger patients, without isolated systolic hypertension, and it was a secondary end point that showed a benefit of the lower target (<130/80 mm Hg) on cardiovascular events.[6]

Unfortunately, the results of this Prospective, Randomized, Open-label Blinded Endpoints clinical trial failed to show a significant difference between blood pressure targets. One could argue that the trial itself was underpowered, should have used stroke as the primary end point (rather than a veritable hodge-podge of cardiovascular and renal events), might have done better with a diuretic as initial therapy,[1,5] or had many other potential criticisms. For reasons that are not clear, the trial's designers did not use the evidence-based target of <150 mm Hg in their referent group, somewhat reminiscent of the Action to Control Cardiovascular Risk in Diabetes-Blood Pressure trial, which ignored the currently recommended target of <130/80 mm Hg in patients with diabetes in favor of comparing the systolic targets of <120 and <140 mm Hg.[7]

These data add to the point of view espoused by recent Cochrane Collaboration meta-analysts, who claim that there are no good data to support any blood pressure targets < 140/90 mm Hg.[8] Whether guideline committees will agree with them remains to be seen.

W. J. Elliott, MD, PhD

References

1. Prevention of stroke by antihypertensive drug treatment in older persons with isolated systolic hypertension. Final results of the Systolic Hypertension in the Elderly Program (SHEP). SHEP Cooperative Study Group. *JAMA.* 1991;265:3255-3264.
2. Perry HM Jr, Davis BR, Price TR, et al. Effect of treating isolated systolic hypertension on the risk of developing various types and subtypes of stroke. the Systolic Hypertension in the Elderly Program (SHEP). *JAMA.* 2000;284:465-471.
3. Staessen JA, Fagard R, Thijs L, et al. for the Systolic Hypertension—Europe (Syst-EUR) Trial Investigators. Morbidity and mortality in the placebo-controlled European Trial on Isolated Systolic Hypertension in the Elderly. *Lancet.* 1997; 350:757-764.
4. Wang JG, Staessen JA, Gong L, Liu L. Chinese trial on isolated systolic hypertension in the elderly. Systolic Hypertension in China (Syst-China) Collaborative Group. *Arch Intern Med.* 2000;160:211-220.
5. Beckett NS, Peters R, Fletcher AE, et al. Treatment of hypertension in patients 80 years of age or older. *N Engl J Med.* 2008;358:1887-1898.
6. Verdecchia P, Staessen JA, Angeli F, et al. for the Cardio-Sis Investigators. Usual versus tight control of systolic blood pressure in non-diabetic patients with hypertension (Cardio-Sis): an open-label randomised trial. *Lancet.* 2009;374:525-533.
7. Cushman WC, Evans GW, Byington RP, et al, on behalf of The Action to Control Cardiovascular Risk in Diabetes (ACCORD) Study Group. Effects of intensive blood-pressure control in type 2 diabetes mellitus. *N Engl J Med.* 2010;362: 1575-1585.
8. Arguedas JA, Perez MI, Wright JM. Treatment blood pressure targets for hypertension. *Cochrane Database Syst Rev.* 2009;(4) 10.1002/14651858.CD004349.pub2, mrw.interscience.wiley.com/cochrane/clsysrev/articles/CD004349/frame.htm. Accessed October 10, 2010.

Renal outcomes with different fixed-dose combination therapies in patients with hypertension at high risk for cardiovascular events (ACCOMPLISH): a prespecified secondary analysis of a randomised controlled trial
Bakris GL, for the ACCOMPLISH Trial investigators (Univ of Chicago-Pritzker School of Medicine, IL; et al)
Lancet 375:1173-1181, 2010

Background.—The Avoiding Cardiovascular Events through Combination Therapy in Patients Living with Systolic Hypertension (ACCOMPLISH) trial showed that initial antihypertensive therapy with benazepril plus amlodipine was superior to benazepril plus hydrochlorothiazide in reducing cardiovascular morbidity and mortality. We assessed the effects of these drug combinations on progression of chronic kidney disease.

Methods.—ACCOMPLISH was a double-blind, randomised trial undertaken in five countries (USA, Sweden, Norway, Denmark, and Finland). 11 506 patients with hypertension who were at high risk for cardiovascular events were randomly assigned via a central, telephone-based interactive voice response system in a 1:1 ratio to receive benazepril (20 mg) plus amlodipine (5 mg; n=5744) or benazepril (20 mg) plus hydrochlorothiazide (12.5 mg; n=5762), orally once daily. Drug doses were force-titrated for patients to attain recommended blood pressure goals. Progression of chronic kidney disease, a prespecified endpoint, was defined as doubling of serum creatinine concentration or end-stage renal disease (estimated glomerular filtration rate <15 mL/min/1.73 m^2 or need for dialysis). Analysis was by intention to treat (ITT). This trial is registered with ClinicalTrials.gov, number NCT00170950.

Findings.—The trial was terminated early (mean follow-up 2.9 years [SD 0.4]) because of superior efficacy of benazepril plus amlodipine compared with benazepril plus hydrochlorothiazide. At trial completion, vital status was not known for 143 (1%) patients who were lost to follow-up (benazepril plus amlodipine, n=70; benazepril plus hydrochlorothiazide, n=73). All randomised patients were included in the ITT analysis. There were 113 (2.0%) events of chronic kidney disease progression in the benazepril plus amlodipine group compared with 215 (3.7%) in the benazepril plus hydrochlorothiazide group (HR 0.52, 0.41–0.65, p<0.0001). The most frequent adverse event in patients with chronic kidney disease was peripheral oedema (benazepril plus amlodipine, 189 of 561, 33.7%; benazepril plus hydrochlorothiazide, 85 of 532, 16.0%). In patients with chronic kidney disease, angio-oedema was more frequent in the benazepril plus amlodipine group than in the benazepril plus hydrochlorothiazide group. In patients without chronic kidney disease, dizziness, hypokalaemia, and hypotension were more frequent in the benazepril plus hydrochlorothiazide group than in the benazepril plus amlodipine group.

Interpretation.—Initial antihypertensive treatment with benazepril plus amlodipine should be considered in preference to benazepril plus hydrochlorothiazide since it slows progression of nephropathy to a greater extent.

▶ This article presents the results of the prespecified secondary end point pertaining to renal function in the Avoiding Cardiovascular Events Through Combination Therapy in Patients Living with Systolic Hypertension (ACCOMPLISH) trial.[1] This study was terminated earlier than expected because of a significant reduction in the composite cardiovascular end point (cardiovascular death, myocardial infarction, stroke, hospitalization for angina, resuscitated arrest, or coronary revascularization) in the group randomized to amlodipine + benazepril, compared with those initially given hydrochlorothiazide and benazepril.

In addition to the usual issues of chlorthalidone versus hydrochlorothiazide, the editorialists for this article describe 3 major challenges to interpret these data.[2] First, there is the fact that the amlodipine + benazepril–treated group had lower blood pressure than the comparator group, which is consistent with a benefit attributed to a lower blood pressure target for people with chronic kidney disease, which is now recommended by some guideline committees[3-5] but has recently been challenged.[6] Second is the concern about overinterpretation of differences in secondary end points when the trial did not run to completion. But third is the concern that the entire conclusion is driven by a difference in doubling of serum creatinine (compared with baseline), which may have either a hemodynamic or structural basis. Calcium antagonists often initially decrease serum creatinine, whereas diuretics typically increase it in the first few weeks or months of therapy. This significant difference at 12 weeks between the 2 randomized treatment groups was seen (and reported) in the ACCOMPLISH trial cohort in 2009.[7] Because there were so few patients who ended up on dialysis (20 of 11 506) and the progression to an estimated glomerular filtration rate of < 15 mL/min/1.73 m^2 was actually slightly more common in the group randomized to amlodipine + benazepril, the editorialists believe that the significant difference seen across the entire trial is because of an acute hemodynamic effect, not a real long-term effect on kidney function. The African American Study of Kidney disease and hypertension trial was designed to take this difference into account; it used as its primary end point the long-term slopes of the decline in renal function, ignoring the first 90 days of therapy.[8] The accompanying figure in the editorial suggests that the long-term slopes of the decline in renal function do not differ in ACCOMPLISH.

As might be expected, in this trial, albuminuria was more likely to be reduced by the combination of hydrochlorothiazide + benazepril than amlodipine + benazepril, but this did not correlate with either renal or cardiovascular outcomes (both of which were said to be better with the latter regimen). This is presumably one of the major reasons why albuminuria is not currently accepted by the US Food and Drug Administration as a surrogate for progressive renal disease. It will be interesting to see how Eighth Report of the Joint National Committee on Prevention, Detection, Evaluation, and Treatment of High Blood Pressure and other kidney-focused guidelines will use these data in making recommendations about lowering blood pressure to prevent progression of kidney disease.

W. J. Elliott, MD, PhD

References

1. Jamerson K, Weber MA, Bakris GL, et al. for the ACCOMPLISH Trial Investigators. Benazepril plus amlodipine or hydrochlorothiazide for hypertension in high-risk patients. *N Engl J Med.* 2008;359:2417-2428.
2. Heerspink HL, de Zeeuw D. Composite renal endpoints: was ACCOMPLISH accomplished? *Lancet.* 2010;375:1440-1442.
3. Chobanian AV, Bakris GL, Black HR, et al. National High Blood Pressure Education Program Coordinating Committee. Seventh report of the Joint National Committee on Prevention, Detection, Evaluation and Treatment of High Blood Pressure. *Hypertension.* 2003;42:1206-1252.
4. Kidney Disease Outcomes Quality Initiative (K/DOQI). K/DOQI clinical practice guidelines on hypertension and antihypertensive agents in chronic kidney disease. *Am J Kidney Dis.* 2004;43:S1-S290.
5. Mancia G, Laurent S, Agabiti-Rosei E, et al. Reappraisal of European guidelines on hypertension management: a European Society of Hypertension Task Force document. *J Hypertens.* 2009;27:2121-2158.

6. Arguedas JA, Perez MI, Wright JM. Treatment blood pressure targets for hypertension. *Cochrane Database Syst Rev.* 2009;(4) 10.1002/14651858.CD004349.pub2.
7. Sarafidis PA, Bakris GL, Weber MA, et al. *Changes in Glomerular Filtration Rate with Benazepril Plus Amlodipine or Benazepril Plus Hydrochlorothiazide Treatment in Hypertensive Patients at High Risk: An Analysis of the ACCOMPLISH Trial.* Milan, Italy: World Congress of Nephrology; 2009. http://www. abstracts2view.com/wcn/view.php?nu=WCN09L_455.
8. Wright JT Jr, Bakris GL, Greene T, et al. Effect of blood pressure lowering and antihypertensive drug class on progression of hypertensive kidney disease: results from the AASK trial. *JAMA.* 2002;288:2421-2431.

Cardiovascular Events During Differing Hypertension Therapies in Patients With Diabetes

Weber MA, for the ACCOMPLISH Investigators (SUNY Downstate College of Medicine, Brooklyn, NY; et al)
J Am Coll Cardiol 56:77-85, 2010

Objectives.—The aim of this study was to determine which combination therapy in patients with hypertension and diabetes most effectively decreases cardiovascular events.

Background.—The ACCOMPLISH (Avoiding Cardiovascular Events Through COMbination Therapy in Patients Living With Systolic Hypertension) trial compared the outcomes effects of a renin-angiotensin system blocker, benazepril, combined with amlodipine (B+A) or hydrochlorothiazide (B+H). A separate analysis in diabetic patients was pre-specified.

Methods.—A total of 6,946 patients with diabetes were randomized to treatment with B+A or B+H. A subgroup of 2,842 diabetic patients at very high risk (previous cardiovascular or stroke events) was also analyzed, as were 4,559 patients without diabetes. The primary end point was a composite of cardiovascular death, myocardial infarction, stroke, hospitalization for angina, resuscitated arrest, and coronary revascularization.

Results.—In the full diabetes group, the mean achieved blood pressures in the B+A and B+H groups were 131.5/72.6 and 132.7/73.7 mm Hg; during 30 months, there were 307 (8.8%) and 383 (11.0%) primary events (hazard ratio [HR]: 0.79, 95% confidence interval [CI]: 0.68 to 0.92, p = 0.003). For the diabetic patients at very high risk, there were 195 (13.6%) and 244 (17.3%) primary events (HR: 0.77, 95% CI: 0.64 to 0.93, p = 0.007). In the nondiabetic patients, there were 245 (10.8%) and 296 (12.9%) primary events (HR: 0.82, 95% CI: 0.69 to 0.97, p = 0.020). In the diabetic patients, there were clear coronary benefits with B+A, including both acute clinical events (p = 0.013) and revascularizations (p = 0.024). There were no unexpected adverse events.

Conclusions.—In patients with diabetes and hypertension, combining a renin-angiotensin system blocker with amlodipine, compared with hydrochlorothiazide, was superior in reducing cardiovascular events and could influence future management of hypertension in patients with diabetes.

(Avoiding Cardiovascular Events Through COMbination Therapy in Patients Living With Systolic Hypertension [ACCOMPLISH]; NCT00170950).

▶ On the face of it, this prespecified subgroup analysis of the Avoiding Cardiovascular Events Through COMbination Therapy in Patients Living With Systolic Hypertension (ACCOMPLISH) trial comes to a similar conclusion as the analyses of the originally reported, full cohort: the primary composite outcome was significantly lower in the group randomized to the combination of amlodipine + benazepril, compared with that given hydrochlorothiazide + benazepril.[1] However, in patients with diabetes, the restricted end point of cardiovascular death, myocardial infarction, or stroke (the Heart Outcomes Prevention Evaluation primary endpoint[2]) was not significantly different (hazard ratio: 0.84, 95% confidence interval: 0.69-1.03). This suggests that major benefit was experienced regarding the nontraditional or softer end points of the composite primary outcome, which included hospitalization for unstable angina, coronary revascularization, or (less likely, given the overall results[1]) resuscitated cardiac arrest. Some say this subgroup comparison, by definition, was underpowered in the first place, and the situation may have been made worse by the early termination of the trial.[1] Whether the results might have been different if the blood pressures had been assessed by 24-hour ambulatory blood pressure monitoring[3] in the entire diabetic cohort (rather than in the subgroup of 353 reported here) or if chlorthalidone had been used instead of hydrochlorothiazide[4] (as in the Antihypertensive and Lipid-Lowering to prevent Heart Attack Trial)[5] remains an unsolved mystery.

Although 60.3% of the participants in ACCOMPLISH were diabetic, a further analysis was done of those who had a prior cardiovascular event (so-called high-risk diabetics) that constituted only ~25% of the enrolled subjects. For the composite primary end point, there was a significant 23% reduction noted in the group receiving amlodipine + benazepril, compared with those assigned to hydrochlorothiazide + benazepril. None of the individual components of the composite primary end point achieved statistical significance, although the amlodipine + benazepril group had significantly fewer nonrevascularization coronary events (myocardial infarction, unstable angina pectoris, or sudden cardiac death) and ≥50% increase in serum creatinine (and above the normal range). Whether the latter had anything to do with intravascular volume depletion and hemoconcentration is uncertain.

With the recent publication of the Action to Control Cardiovascular Risk in Diabetes trial,[5] there is much interest in the proper blood pressure target for patients with diabetes. The average office blood pressures in patients with diabetes in the ACCOMPLISH trial after dose titration were ~132/73 and ~133/74 mm Hg, with 46% and 44% achieving the blood pressure target of < 130/80 mm Hg, in the amlodipine + benazepril and hydrochlorothiazide + benazepril groups, respectively. It is likely that the authors will soon do a post hoc analysis to determine whether those who achieved blood pressures < 130/80 mm Hg had a better prognosis than those who did not.[6]

W. J. Elliott, MD, PhD

References

1. Jamerson K, Weber MA, Bakris GL, et al. for the ACCOMPLISH Trial Investigators. Benazepril plus amlodipine or hydrochlorothiazide for hypertension in high-risk patients. *N Engl J Med.* 2008;359:2417-2428.
2. Yusuf S, Sleight P, Pogue J, Bosch J, Davies R, Dagenais G. Effects of an angiotensin converting enzyme inhibitor, ramipril, on cardiovascular events in high-risk patients. The Heart Outcomes Prevention Evaluation (HOPE) Investigators. *N Engl J Med.* 2000;342:145-153.
3. Jamerson KA, Bakris GL, Weber MA. 24-hour ambulatory blood pressure in the ACCOMPLISH trial. *N Engl J Med.* 2010;363:98 [letter].
4. Ernst ME, Carter BL, Goerdt CJ, et al. Comparative antihypertensive effects of hydrochlorothiazide and chlorthalidone on ambulatory and office blood pressure. *Hypertension.* 2006;47:352-358.
5. The ALLHAT Officers and Coordinators for the ALLHAT Collaborative Research Group. Major outcomes in high-risk hypertensive patients randomized to angiotensin-converting enzyme inhibitor or calcium channel blocker vs. diuretic: The Antihypertensive and Lipid Lowering Treatment to Prevent Heart Attack Trial (ALLHAT). *JAMA.* 2002;288:2981-2997.
6. Cushman WC, Evans GW, Byington RP, et al. on behalf of The Action to Control Cardiovascular Risk in Diabetes (ACCORD) Study Group. Effects of intensive blood-pressure control in type 2 diabetes mellitus. *N Engl J Med.* 2010;362: 1575-1585.

Effects of antihypertensive treatment after acute stroke in the Continue Or Stop post-Stroke Antihypertensives Collaborative Study (COSSACS): a prospective, randomised, open, blinded-endpoint trial

Robinson TG, on behalf of the COSSACS Investigators (Univ of Leicester, UK; et al)
Lancet Neurol 9:767-775, 2010

Background.—Up to 50% of patients with acute stroke are taking antihypertensive drugs on hospital admission. However, whether such treatment should be continued during the immediate post-stroke period is unclear. We therefore aimed to assess the efficacy and safety of continuing or stopping pre-existing antihypertensive drugs in patients who had recently had a stroke.

Methods.—The Continue Or Stop post-Stroke Antihypertensives Collaborative Study (COSSACS) was a UK multicentre, prospective, randomised, open, blinded-endpoint trial. Patients were recruited at 49 UK National Institute for Health Research Stroke Research Network centres from January 1, 2003, to March 31, 2009. Patients aged over 18 years who were taking antihypertensive drugs were enrolled within 48 h of stroke and the last dose of antihypertensive drug. Patients were randomly assigned (1:1) by secure internet central randomisation to either continue or stop pre-existing antihypertensive drugs for 2 weeks. Patients and clinicians who randomly assigned patients were unmasked to group allocation. Clinicians who assessed 2-week outcomes and 6-month outcomes were masked to group allocation. The primary endpoint was death or dependency at 2 weeks, with dependency defined as a modified Rankin scale score greater than 3 points. Analysis was by intention to treat. This trial is registered with the International Standard Randomised Controlled Trial Register, number ISRCTN89712435.

Findings.—763 patients were assigned to continue (n=379) or stop (n=384) pre-existing antihypertensive drugs. 72 of 379 patients in the continue group and 82 of 384 patients in the stop group reached the primary endpoint (relative risk 0·86, 95% CI 0·65—1·14; p=0·3). The difference in systolic blood pressure at 2 weeks between the continue group and the stop group was 13 mm Hg (95% CI 10—17) and the difference in diastolic blood pressure was 8 mm Hg (6—10; difference between groups p<0·0001). No substantial differences were observed between groups in rates of serious adverse events, 6-month mortality, or major cardiovascular events.

Interpretation.—Continuation of antihypertensive drugs did not reduce 2-week death or dependency, cardiovascular event rate, or mortality at 6 months. Lower blood pressure levels in those who continued antihypertensive treatment after acute mild stroke were not associated with an increase in adverse events. These neutral results might be because COSSACS was underpowered owing to early termination of the trial, and support the continuation of ongoing research trials.

▶ In the United States, lowering blood pressure in patients with an acute stroke in evolution is still thought to be dangerous and likely to cause more harm than good.[1,2] Most, if not the vast majority, of stroke victims have a spontaneous fall in blood pressure, without treatment, over the first few days of hospitalization.[3] For this reason, most stroke neurologists recommend discontinuing, or at least holding, antihypertensive medications for the first day or two after a stroke in order to maintain blood flow to watershed areas of the ischemic penumbrum. Exceptions are generally made if the blood pressure is very high (typically > 200/120 mm Hg) or as a prelude to thrombolytic therapy (which is contraindicated in very hypertensive stroke victims). Suggestions to the contrary come from Germany (overall benefit of candesartan vs placebo, given 24 hours after stroke onset),[4] from this group in the United Kingdom (significant reduction in 3-month mortality after labetalol or lisinopril, compared with placebo),[5] and from Australia (smaller hematoma formation in hemorrhagic stroke if treated acutely with antihypertensive drugs).[6] Note that only the underenrolled German trial showed a significant difference in hard endpoints, and even that was unexpected.[4]

In the Continue Or Stop post-Stroke Antihypertensives Collaborative Study, the investigators attempted to answer the simple question of whether continuing or stopping previously prescribed antihypertensive agents would lead to better outcomes in acute stroke survivors. They were ultimately unable to gather enough data, however, because trial enrollment was slow and funding for the trial was discontinued. There were, however, no suggestions that continuing antihypertensive drug therapy was unsafe. Even the editorialist for this article (the principal investigator of the Australian trial on intracerebral hemorrhage, who might be expected to have a positive opinion about acute blood pressure lowering) says we must await the results of further trials before adopting such a strategy for most acute stroke victims.[7]

W. J. Elliott, MD, PhD

References

1. Adams HP Jr, del Zoppa G, Alberts MJ, et al. Guidelines for the early management of adults with ischemic stroke: a guideline from the American Heart Association/American Stroke Association Stroke Council, Clinical Cardiology Council, Cardiovascular Radiology and Intervention Council, and the Atherosclerotic Peripheral Vascular Disease and Quality of Care Outcomes in Research Interdisciplinary Working Groups: the American Academy of Neurology affirms the value of this guideline as an educational tool for neurologists. *Stroke.* 2007;38: 1655-1711.
2. Sacco RL, Adams R, Albers G, et al. Guidelines for prevention of stroke in patients with ischemic stroke or transient ischemic attack: a statement for healthcare professionals from the American Heart Association/American Stroke Association Council on Stroke: co-sponsored by the Council on Cardiovascular Radiology and Intervention: the American Academy of Neurology affirms the value of this guideline. *Stroke.* 2006;37:577-617.
3. Qureshi AI. Acute hypertensive response in patients with stroke: pathophysiology and management. *Circulation.* 2008;118:176-187.
4. Schrader J, Lüders S, Kulschewski A, et al. For the Acute Candesartan Cilexitil Therapy in Stroke Survivors Study Group. The ACCESS study: evaluation of Acute Candesartan Cilexetil Therapy in Stroke Survivors. *Stroke.* 2003;34: 1699-1703.
5. Potter JF, Robinson TG, Ford GA, et al. Controlling hypertension and hypotension immediately post-stroke (CHHIPS): a randomised, placebo-controlled, double-blind pilot trial. *Lancet Neurol.* 2009;8:48-56.
6. Anderson CS, Huang Y, Wang JG, et al. For the INTERACT Investigators. Intensive blood pressure reduction in acute cerebral haemorrhage trial (INTERACT): a randomized pilot trial. *Lancet Neurol.* 2008;7:391-399.
7. Anderson CS. A step forward in resolving uncertainties over blood-pressure management in acute stroke. *Lancet Neurol.* 2010;9:752-753.

Telemonitoring and self-management in the control of hypertension (TASMINH2): a randomised controlled trial
McManus RJ, Mant J, Bray EP, et al (Univ of Birmingham and Natl Inst for Health Res (NIHR) Natl School for Primary Care Res, UK; Univ of Cambridge, UK; et al)
Lancet 376:163-172, 2010

Background.—Control of blood pressure is a key component of cardiovascular disease prevention, but is difficult to achieve and until recently has been the sole preserve of health professionals. This study assessed whether self-management by people with poorly controlled hypertension resulted in better blood pressure control compared with usual care.

Methods.—This randomised controlled trial was undertaken in 24 general practices in the UK. Patients aged 35−85 years were eligible for enrolment if they had blood pressure more than 140/90 mm Hg despite antihypertensive treatment and were willing to self-manage their hypertension. Participants were randomly assigned in a 1:1 ratio to self-management, consisting of self-monitoring of blood pressure and self-titration of antihypertensive drugs, combined with telemonitoring of home blood pressure measurements or to usual care. Randomisation was done by use of a central web-based system and was stratified by general practice with minimisation for sex, baseline systolic blood pressure, and presence or absence of diabetes or chronic kidney disease. Neither participants nor investigators were masked to group assignment. The primary endpoint was change in mean systolic blood pressure between baseline and each follow-up point (6 months and 12 months). All randomised patients who attended follow-up visits at 6 months and 12 months and had complete data for the primary outcome were included in the analysis, without imputation for missing data. This study is registered as an International Standard Randomised Controlled Trial, number ISRCTN17585681.

Findings.—527 participants were randomly assigned to self-management (n=263) or control (n=264), of whom 480 (91%; self-management, n=234; control, n=246) were included in the primary analysis. Mean systolic blood pressure decreased by 12·9 mm Hg (95% CI 10·4−15·5) from baseline to 6 months in the self-management group and by 9·2 mm Hg (6·7−11·8) in the control group (difference between groups 3·7 mm Hg, 0·8−6·6; p=0·013). From baseline to 12 months, systolic blood pressure decreased by 17·6 mm Hg (14·9−20·3) in the self-management group and by 12·2 mm Hg (9·5−14·9) in the control group (difference between groups 5·4 mm Hg, 2·4−8·5; p=0·0004). Frequency of most side-effects did not differ between groups, apart from leg swelling (self-management, 74 patients [32%]; control, 55 patients [22%]; p=0·022).

Interpretation.—Self-management of hypertension in combination with telemonitoring of blood pressure measurements represents an important new addition to control of hypertension in primary care.

▶ This trial combines 2 interventions that have been previously shown to improve blood pressure control rates: self-titration of antihypertensive drugs, based on home blood pressure measurements[1-3] and remote monitoring of home blood pressure measurements by health care professionals (done here primarily to ensure patient safety, instead of forming a basis for medication titration).[3-5] Some would say that since these 2 techniques work well in patients with diabetes mellitus, asthma, and need for chronic anticoagulation, it is only fitting that they be tried in hypertensive patients.

There are many groundbreaking assumptions in the authors' choices for their study. They chose home blood pressure thresholds of 130/85 or 130/75 mm Hg for titration of antihypertensive drugs for patients without diabetes or with diabetes, respectively; these are lower than current US recommendations[6] but may be appropriate now, given the results of the Action to Control Cardiovascular Risk in Diabetes trial.[7] They restricted enrollment to patients with uncontrolled hypertension taking less than 3 medications, to minimize the probability of resistant hypertension. Their patients were told to monitor home blood pressures only 1 week of the month; many patients develop a habit of daily home measurements. And the primary outcome was not ambulatory blood pressure (as in previous studies[1]) but instead an office blood pressure measurement taken by an automated device (with which the intervention participants were likely to be more familiar). The number of patients in the control group who used home blood pressure monitoring on their own is not stated. It is interesting that 20% of patients in the intervention group did not follow the study plan (8% didn't attend the initial training and 12% discontinued home readings before the year-end), yet the results of the intervention were significant.

Whether these results are generalizable to routine medical care is uncertain, as discussed by the authors and the editorialist.[8] It is likely that more corroborative studies, the planned cost-effectiveness analysis, and decisions of health care financing authorities[9] (particularly large health maintenance organizations) will all have to be positive before self-titration of antihypertensive medications based on home blood pressure readings will become widespread.

W. J. Elliott, MD, PhD

References

1. Zarnke KB, Feagan BG, Mahon JL, Feldman RD. A randomized study comparing a patient-directed hypertension management strategy with usual office-based care. *Am J Hypertens.* 1997;10:58-67.
2. Bobrie G, Postel-Vinay N, Delonca J, Corvol P. Self-measurement and self-titration in hypertension: a pilot telemedicine study. *Am J Hypertens.* 2007;20:1314-1320.
3. Pickering TG, Gerin W, Holland JK. Home blood pressure teletransmission for better diagnosis and treatment. *Curr Hypertens Rep.* 1999;1:489-494.
4. Rogers MA, Small D, Buchan DA, et al. Home monitoring service improves mean arterial pressure in patients with essential hypertension. A randomized, controlled trial. *Ann Intern Med.* 2001;134:1024-1032.
5. Green BB, Cook AJ, Ralston JD, et al. Effectiveness of home blood pressure monitoring, Web communication, and pharmacist care on hypertension control: a randomized controlled trial. *JAMA.* 2008;299:2857-2867.
6. Pickering TG, Hall JE, Appel LJ, et al. Recommendations for blood pressure measurement in humans and experimental animals: Part 1: blood pressure measurement in humans: a statement for professionals from the Subcommittee of Professional and Public Education of the American Heart Association Council on High Blood Pressure Research. *Hypertension.* 2005;45:142-161.
7. Cushman WC, Evans GW, Byington RP, et al. ACCORD Study Group. Effects of intensive blood-pressure control in type 2 diabetes mellitus. *N Engl J Med.* 2010; 362:1575-1585.
8. Ogedegbe G. Self-titration for treatment of uncomplicated hypertension [editorial]. *Lancet.* 2010;376:144-146.
9. Pickering TG, Miller NH, Ogedegbe G, Krakoff LR, Artinian NT, Goff D, American Heart Association, American Society of Hypertension, Preventive Cardiovascular Nurses Association. Call to action on use and reimbursement for home blood pressure monitoring: executive summary: a joint scientific statement from the American Heart Association, American Society of Hypertension, and Preventive Cardiovascular Nurses Association. *Hypertension.* 2008;52:1-9.

Effect of self-measurement of blood pressure on adherence to treatment in patients with mild-to-moderate hypertension

van Onzenoort HAW, Verberk WJ, Kroon AA, et al (Univ Med Ctr St Radboud, Nijmegen, The Netherlands; Microlife Corporation, Taipei, Taiwan; Maastricht Univ, The Netherlands; et al)
J Hypertens 28:622-627, 2010

Background.—Poor adherence to treatment is one of the major problems in the treatment of hypertension. Self blood pressure measurement may help patients to improve their adherence to treatment.

Method.—In this prospective, randomized, controlled study coordinated by a university hospital, a total of 228 mild-to-moderate hypertensive patients were randomized to either a group that performed self-measurements at home in addition to office blood pressure measurements [the self-pressure group ($n = 114$)] or a group that only underwent office blood pressure measurement [the office pressure group ($n = 114$)]. Patients were followed for 1 year in which treatment was adjusted, if necessary, at each visit to the physician's office according to the achieved blood pressure. Adherence to treatment was assessed by means of medication event monitoring system TrackCaps.

Results.—Median adherence was slightly greater in patients from the self-pressure group than in those from the office pressure group (92.3 vs. 90.9%; $P = 0.043$). Although identical among both groups, in the week directly after each visit to the physician's office, adherence [71.4% (interquartile range 71−79%)] was significantly lower ($P<0.001$) than that at the last 7 days prior to each visit [100% (interquartile range 90−100%)]. On the remaining days between the visits, patients from the self-pressure group displayed a modestly better adherence than patients from the office pressure group (97.6 vs. 97.0%; $P = 0.024$).

Conclusion.—Although self-blood pressure measurement as an adjunct to office blood pressure measurement led to somewhat better adherence to treatment in this study, the difference was only small and not clinically significant. The time relative to a visit to the doctor seems to be a more important predictor of adherence.

▶ This article, derived from the randomized trial Home versus Office Measurements: Reduction of Unnecessary Treatment Study,[1] contradicts the conventional wisdom (now going back 35 years)[2] that self- (or home) monitoring of blood pressure is associated with better adherence to medication and thereafter to better blood pressure control.[3-5] The authors have a great deal of experience with the electronic medication monitoring system used in this study as the gold standard, and there is little reason to suspect that it didn't work as it usually does. A more likely explanation of why the extra home monitoring group did not have better adherence than the standard office blood pressure measurement group is that both groups were very well motivated to take their pills, being in a clinical trial that involved informed consent and a pill counter that tracked their adherence. This is most easily seen in the mean levels of adherence:

92.3% versus 90.9%, which is much higher than rates seen in routine clinical practice.

These authors have also redescribed in this article what is often called the toothbrush effect: adherence improves for the week or so prior to an office visit, as compared with the week afterward.[6] Dentists were among the first to show that the frequency of toothbrushing increases in the week or so prior to a dental appointment and that phenomenon has previously been seen in adherence with antihypertensive pills, especially when the electronic pill-cap monitoring system was used.

There are many reasons to recommend that many patients obtain home blood pressure readings, regardless of the conclusions of this work. The challenge for the health care system is how to have these readings interpreted and feedback given by the health care provider and paid for in the current reimbursement schemes.[7]

W. J. Elliott, MD, PhD

References

1. Verberk WJ, Kroon AA, Lenders JW, et al. for the Home Versus Office Measurement, Reduction of Unnecessary Treatment Study Investigators. Self-measurement of blood pressure at home reduces the need for antihypertensive drugs: a randomized, controlled trial. *Hypertension.* 2007;50:1019-1025.
2. Carnahan JE, Nugent CA. The effects of self-monitoring by patients on the control of hypertension. *Am J Med Sci.* 1975;269:69-73.
3. Vrijens B, Goetghebeur E. Comparing compliance patterns between randomized treatments. *Control Clin Trials.* 1997;18:187-203.
4. Márquez-Contreras E, Martell-Claros N, Gil-Guillén V, et al. Efficacy of a home blood pressure monitoring programme on therapeutic compliance in hypertension: The EAPACUM-HTA study. *J Hypertens.* 2006;24:169-175.
5. Ashida T, Sugiyama T, Okuno S, Ebihara A, Fujii J. Relationship between home blood pressure measurement and medication compliance and name recognition of antihypertensive drugs. *Hypertens Res.* 2000;23:21-24.
6. Waeber B, Burnier M, Brunner HR. How to improve adherence with prescribed treatment in hypertensive patients? *J Cardiovasc Pharmacol.* 2000;35:S23-S26.
7. Pickering TG, Miller NH, Ogedegbe G, Krakoff LR, Artinian NT, Goff D. Call to action on use and reimbursement for home blood pressure monitoring: executive summary: a joint scientific statement from the American Heart Association, American Society Of Hypertension, and Preventive Cardiovascular Nurses Association. *Hypertension.* 2008;52:1-9.

Continuous positive airway pressure treatment in sleep apnea patients with resistant hypertension: a randomized, controlled trial
Lozano L, Tovar JL, Sampol G, et al (Universitat Autònoma de Barcelona, Spain)
J Hypertens 28:2161-2168, 2010

Objectives.—This controlled trial assessed the effect of continuous positive airway pressure (CPAP) on blood pressure (BP) in patients with obstructive sleep apnea (OSA) and resistant hypertension (RH).

Methods.—We evaluated 96 patients with resistant hypertension, defined as clinic BP at least 140/90 mmHg despite treatment with at least three drugs at adequate doses, including a diuretic. Patients underwent a polysomnography and a 24-h ambulatory BP monitoring (ABPM). They were classified as consulting room or ABPM-confirmed resistant hypertension, according to 24-h BP lower or higher than 125/80 mmHg. Patients with an apnea-hypopnea index at least 15 events/h ($n = 75$) were randomized to receive either CPAP added to conventional treatment ($n = 38$) or conventional medical treatment alone ($n = 37$). ABPM was repeated at 3 months. The main outcome was the change in systolic and diastolic BP.

Results.—Sixty-four patients completed the follow-up. Patients with ABPM-confirmed resistant hypertension treated with CPAP ($n = 20$), unlike those treated with conventional treatment ($n = 21$), showed a decrease in 24-h diastolic BP (-4.9 ± 6.4 vs. 0.1 ± 7.3 mmHg, $P = 0.027$). Patients who used CPAP > 5.8 h showed a greater reduction in daytime diastolic BP {-6.12 mmHg [confidence interval (CI) -1.45; -10.82], $P = 0.004$}, 24-h diastolic BP (-6.98 mmHg [CI -1.86; -12.1], $P = 0.009$) and 24-h systolic BP (-9.71 mmHg [CI -0.20; -19.22], $P = 0.046$). The number of patients with a dipping pattern significantly increased in the CPAP group (51.7% vs. 24.1%, $P = 0.008$).

Conclusion.—In patients with resistant hypertension and OSA, CPAP treatment for 3 months achieves reductions in 24-h BP. This effect is seen in patients with ABPM-confirmed resistant hypertension who use CPAP more than 5.8 h.

▶ Most authorities agree that sleep apnea is an important cause of hypertension and appears to be even more common in patients with resistant hypertension.[1] Many previous observational studies have shown that patients with sleep apnea benefit from continuous positive airway pressure (CPAP), both in terms of blood pressure lowering[2] and in mortality,[3] but proper long-term randomized trials could typically not be done in this patient population because some would be randomized to not receive the standard-of-care therapy, CPAP.

These authors have now some short-term data from a randomized clinical trial (although only 64 of their 96 patients completed follow-up), showing a 3-month lowering in blood pressure (using the very sensitive technique of ambulatory blood pressure monitoring) as well as a restoration of the normal dipping pattern of blood pressure at night.

It now seems timely to organize the large clinical trial comparing CPAP and a selective aldosterone antagonist in a large number of hypertensive patients with obstructive sleep apnea, using both blood pressure and cardiovascular events as outcomes.[4,5] As both spironolactone and eplerenone are now generically available, such a study would likely require governmental funding and would require so many patients to be enrolled that its cost would likely be very high.

W. J. Elliott, MD, PhD

References

1. Calhoun DA, Jones D, Textor S, et al. Resistant hypertension: diagnosis, evaluation, and treatment. A scientific statement from the American Heart Association Professional Education Committee of the Council for High Blood Pressure Research. *Hypertension.* 2008;51:1403-1419.
2. Haentjens P, Van Meerhaeghe A, Moscariello A, et al. The impact of continuous positive airway pressure on blood pressure in patients with obstructive sleep apnea syndrome: evidence from a meta-analysis of placebo-controlled randomized trials. *Arch Intern Med.* 2007;167:757-764.
3. Marin JM, Carrizo SJ, Vicente E, Agusti AG. Long-term cardiovascular outcomes in men with obstructive sleep apnoea-hypopnoea with or without treatment with continuous positive airway pressure: an observational study. *Lancet.* 2005;365: 1046-1053.
4. Nishizaka MK, Zaman MA, Calhoun DA. Efficacy of low-dose spironolactone in subjects with resistant hypertension. *Am J Hypertens.* 2003;16:925-930.
5. Ouzan J, Pérault C, Lincoff AM, Carré E, Mertes M. The role of spironolactone in the treatment of patients with refractory hypertension. *Am J Hypertens.* 2002;15: 333-339.

Efficacy of Spironolactone Therapy in Patients With True Resistant Hypertension

de Souza F, Muxfeldt E, Fiszman R, et al (Federal Univ of Rio de Janeiro, Brazil)
Hypertension 55:147-152, 2010

The role of spironolactone in resistant hypertension management is unclear. The aim of this prospective trial was to evaluate the antihypertensive effect of spironolactone in patients with true resistant hypertension diagnosed by ambulatory blood pressure monitoring. A total of 175 patients had clinical and complementary exams obtained at baseline and received spironolactone in doses of 25 to 100 mg/d. A second ambulatory blood pressure monitoring was performed after a median interval of 7 months. Paired Student t test was used to assess differences in blood pressure before and during spironolactone administration, and multivariate analysis adjusted for age, sex, and number of antihypertensive drugs to assess the predictors of blood pressure fall. There were mean reductions of 16 and 9 mm Hg, respectively, in 24-hour systolic and diastolic blood pressures (95% CIs: 13 to 18 and 7 to 10 mm Hg; $P<0.001$). Office systolic blood pressure and diastolic blood pressure also decreased (14 and 7 mm Hg). Controlled ambulatory blood pressure was reached in 48% of patients. Factors associated with better response were higher waist circumference, lower aortic pulse wave velocity, and lower serum potassium. No association with plasma aldosterone or aldosterone:renin ratio was found. Adverse effects were observed in 13 patients (7.4%). A third ambulatory blood pressure monitoring performed in 78 patients after a median of 15 months confirmed the persistence of the spironolactone effect. In conclusion, spironolactone administration to true resistant hypertensive patients is safe and effective in decreasing blood pressure, especially in those with abdominal obesity and lower arterial stiffness.

Its addition to an antihypertensive regimen as the fourth or fifth drug is recommended.

▶ Several earlier reports of the efficacy of spironolactone for resistant hypertension had greater scientific rigor than this uncontrolled, nonrandomized, open-label cohort study.[1,2] The Anglo-Scandinavian Cardiac Outcomes Trial (ASCOT) used spironolactone as a fourth-line antihypertensive therapy in 1411 patients,[3] but one could argue that not all had true resistant hypertension, if one uses the now-current definition from the American Heart Association's Scientific Statement on Resistant Hypertension.[4] One could argue that obstructive sleep apnea was not systematically evaluated in their patients, but the efficacy of spironolactone in sleep apnea is now well established.[5,6]

Like the ASCOT investigators, these authors tried to tease out factors that might predict a better-than-expected blood pressure response to spironolactone, but the only one that is shared between the 2 studies is a low baseline serum potassium (which is hardly surprising). Compared with the most recent previous placebo-controlled clinical trial with spironolactone,[7] or the ASCOT experience,[3] the ~1% rate of hyperkalemia (> 5.5 mEq/L) and the 4% rate of gynecomastia (requiring discontinuation in 3%) observed by the authors appear low. These authors do not report any deterioration in glucose tolerance with spironolactone that was seen in ASCOT.[3] They also do not mention many of the situations in which spironolactone is at least relatively contraindicated: hyperkalemia, impaired renal function, pregnancy, and lactation. Prior experience with widespread use of spironolactone in patients with heart failure who were not carefully monitored has been troublesome.[8]

It is likely that for most hypertensive patients who are not achieving goal blood pressure with 3 well-chosen antihypertensive drugs, a therapeutic trial of this inexpensive, generically available drug that has a proven safety record going back at least 20 years will be widely recommended, rather than a long, expensive, and involved evaluation for secondary causes of hypertension. This approach is consistent with, but not yet recommended by, recent reviews and guidelines.[9,10]

W. J. Elliott, MD, PhD

References

1. Nishizaka MK, Zaman MA, Calhoun DA. Efficacy of low-dose spironolactone in subjects with resistant hypertension. *Am J Hypertens.* 2003;16:925-930.
2. Ouzan J, Pérault C, Lincoff AM, Carré E, Mertes M. The role of spironolactone in the treatment of patients with refractory hypertension. *Am J Hypertens.* 2002; 15:333-339.
3. Chapman N, Dobson J, Wilson S, et al. Anglo-Scandinavian Cardiac Outcomes Trial Investigators. Effect of spironolactone on blood pressure in subjects with resistant hypertension. *Hypertension.* 2007;49:839-845.
4. Calhoun DA, Jones D, Textor S, et al. Resistant hypertension: diagnosis, evaluation, and treatment. A scientific statement from the American Heart Association Professional Education Committee of the Council for High Blood Pressure Research. *Hypertension.* 2008;51:1403-1419.
5. Calhoun DA, Nishizaka MK, Zaman MA, Thakkar RB, Weissmann P. Hyperaldosteronism among black and white subjects with resistant hypertension. *Hypertension.* 2002;40:892-896.

6. Goodfriend TL, Calhoun DA. Resistant hypertension, obesity, sleep apnea and aldosterone: theory and therapy. *Hypertension.* 2004;43:518-524.
7. Pitt B, Zannad F, Remme WJ, et al. The effect of spironolactone on morbidity and mortality in patients with severe heart failure. Randomized Aldactone Evaluation Study Investigators. *N Engl J Med.* 1999;341:709-717.
8. Juurlink DN, Mamgami MM, Lee DS, et al. Rates of hyperkalemia after publication of the Randomized Aldactone Evaluation Study. *N Engl J Med.* 2004; 351:543-551.
9. Moser M, Setaro JF. Clinical practice. Resistant or difficult-to-control hypertension. *N Engl J Med.* 2006;355:385-392.
10. Garg JP, Elliott WJ, Folker A, Izhar M, Black HR. Resistant hypertension revisited: a comparison of two university-based cohorts. *Am J Hypertens.* 2005;18:619-626.

Effects on Peripheral and Central Blood Pressure of Cocoa With Natural or High-Dose Theobromine: A Randomized, Double-Blind Crossover Trial

van den Bogaard B, Draijer R, Westerhof BE, et al (Univ of Amsterdam, The Netherlands; Unilever Res and Development, Vlaardingen, The Netherlands; BMEYE BV, Amsterdam, The Netherlands; et al)
Hypertension 56:839-846, 2010

Flavanol-rich cocoa products have been reported to lower blood pressure. It has been suggested that theobromine is partially responsible for this effect. We tested whether consumption of flavanol-rich cocoa drinks with natural or added theobromine could lower peripheral and central blood pressure. In a double-blind, placebo-controlled 3-period crossover trial we assigned 42 healthy individuals (age 62 ± 4.5 years; 32 men) with office blood pressure of 130 to 159 mm Hg/85 to 99 mm Hg and low added cardiovascular risk to a random treatment sequence of dairy drinks containing placebo, flavanol-rich cocoa with natural dose consisting of 106 mg of theobromine, or theobromine-enriched flavanol-rich cocoa with 979 mg of theobromine. Treatment duration was 3 weeks with a 2-week washout. The primary outcome was the difference in 24-hour ambulatory systolic blood pressure between placebo and active treatment after 3 weeks. The difference in central systolic blood pressure between placebo and active treatment was a secondary outcome. Treatment with theobromine-enriched cocoa resulted in a mean $\pm$ SE of 3.2 ± 1.1 mm Hg higher 24-hour ambulatory systolic blood pressure compared with placebo ($P<0.01$). In contrast, 2 hours after theobromine-enriched cocoa, laboratory peripheral systolic blood pressure was not different from placebo, whereas central systolic blood pressure was 4.3 ± 1.4 mm Hg lower ($P=0.001$). Natural dose theobromine cocoa did not significantly change either 24-hour ambulatory or central systolic blood pressure compared with placebo. In conclusion, theobromine-enriched cocoa significantly increased 24-hour ambulatory systolic blood pressure while lowering central systolic blood pressure.

▶ The blood pressure—lowering (and other health-promoting) effects of chocolate remain controversial,[1-5] particularly because the mechanism of the process is not well understood. Some propose that flavanols, which are more common in dark chocolate, are the active compounds. Others suggest that theobromine (a methylxanthine), which is also found in high concentrations in chocolate, is responsible for the vasodilating action of chocolate by inhibition of phosphodiesterase.[6] The results of this fairly straightforward 3-period crossover study are somewhat difficult to interpret. In this study, cocoa containing the usual and customary dose of theobromine had no significant effect on either 24-hour ambulatory blood pressure or hemodynamic measurements 2 hours after a dose, compared with placebo (which allegedly tasted identical to cocoa). One wonders if the tested dose of cocoa (1200 mL cup/day) was therefore similar to that of other studies that report a significant blood pressure—lowering effect of cocoa. The results with theobromine-enriched cocoa are even more complex: there was a significant blood pressure—raising effect on 24-hour ambulatory blood pressures, compared with placebo but a lowering of estimated central aortic pressures 2 hours after consumption. Although other interpretations are possible, this may mean that theobromine is likely not the substance responsible for the peripheral blood pressure—lowering properties of cocoa.

W. J. Elliott, MD, PhD

References

1. Desch S, Schmidt J, Kobler D, et al. Effect of cocoa products on blood pressure: systematic review and meta-analysis. *Am J Hypertens.* 2010;23:97-103.
2. Ried K, Sullivan T, Fakler P, Frank OR, Stocks NP. Does chocolate reduce blood pressure? A meta-analysis. *BMC Med.* 2010;8:39.
3. Taubert D, Roesen R, Lehmann C, Jung N, Schömig E. Effects of low habitual cocoa intake on blood pressure and bioactive nitric oxide: a randomized controlled trial. *JAMA.* 2007;298:49-60.
4. Buijsse B, Feskens EJ, Kok FJ, Kromhout D. Cocoa intake, blood pressure and cardiovascular mortality: the Zutphen Elderly Study. *Arch Intern Med.* 2006; 166:411-417.
5. Egan BM, Laken MA, Donovan JL, Woolson RF. Does dark chocolate have a role in the prevention and management of hypertension? commentary on the evidence. *Hypertension.* 2010;55:1289-1295.
6. Kelly CJ. Effects of theobromine should be considered in future studies. *Am J Clin Nutr.* 2005;82:486-487.

Pharmacist-Physician Comanagement of Hypertension and Reduction in 24-Hour Ambulatory Blood Pressures
Weber CA, Ernst ME, Sezate GS, et al (The Univ of Iowa)
Arch Intern Med 170:1634-1639, 2010

Background.—Pharmacist-physician comanagement of hypertension has been shown to improve office blood pressures (BPs). We sought to describe the effect of such a model on 24-hour ambulatory BPs.

Methods.—We performed a prospective, cluster-randomized, controlled clinical trial, enrolling 179 patients with uncontrolled hypertension from 5 primary care clinics in Iowa City, Iowa. Patients were randomized by clinic to receive pharmacist-physician collaborative management of hypertension (intervention) or usual care (control) for a 9-month period. In the intervention group, pharmacists helped patients to identify barriers to BP control, counseled on lifestyle and dietary modifications, and adjusted antihypertensive therapy in collaboration with the patients' primary care providers. Patients were seen by pharmacists a minimum of every 2 months. Ambulatory BP was measured at baseline and at study end.

Results.—Baseline and end-of-study ambulatory BP profiles were evaluated for 175 patients. Mean (SD) ambulatory systolic BPs (SBPs), reported in millimeters of mercury, were reduced more in the intervention group than in the control group: daytime change in (delta) SBP, 15.2 (11.5) vs 5.5 (13.5) ($P < .001$); nighttime deltaSBP, 12.2 (14.8) vs 3.4 (13.3) ($P < .001$); and 24-hour deltaSBP, 14.1 (11.3) vs 5.5 (12.5) ($P < .001$). More patients in the intervention group than in the control group had their BP controlled at the end of the study (75.0% vs 50.7%) ($P < .001$), as defined by overall 24-hour ambulatory BP monitoring.

Conclusion.—Pharmacist-physician collaborative management of hypertension achieved consistent and significantly greater reduction in 24-hour BP and a high rate of BP control.

Trial Registration.—clinicaltrials.gov Identifier: NCT00201045.

▶ Many have decried the suboptimal rates of blood pressure control in the United States and elsewhere.[1] Some believe that this occurs because physicians are too busy or too inattentive to address patients' needs in the short time span of an office visit.[2] In many studies, antihypertensive therapy was more often intensified (and blood pressure better controlled) when pharmacists or other health care professionals managed the patient's medications.[3] Some believe that pharmacists are better prepared to address patient concerns about medications, as they have at least 5 years of training, specifically regarding medications, whereas most physicians have only a 1-year course in pharmacology and little (if any) formal training in therapeutics. Pharmacists have been incorporated into many practices for these reasons; in many Department of Veterans Affairs Medical Centers, the Hypertension Clinic is run by pharmacists, sometimes in collaboration with a physician.[4] This article builds on these ideas to broaden the role of community pharmacists in the management of antihypertensive pharmacotherapy[5] compared with the usual care model in which pharmacists' role was the more traditional filling of physicians' prescriptions.

The results of this study are sure to please pharmacists interested in billing for cognitive services under the *Current Procedural Terminology* codes (99605, 99606, 99607), approved on January 1, 2008, strictly for pharmacists to use for medication management services.[6] They are also likely to appeal to the Center for Medicare and Medicaid Services and all those interested in decreasing health care costs because these codes reimburse less (per visit) than an office-based physician visit. Whether this type of pharmacist-physician collaboration can be implemented in many more communities remains to be seen.

W. J. Elliott, MD, PhD

References

1. Chobanian AV, Bakris GL, Black HR, et al. National High Blood Pressure Education Program Coordinating Committee. Seventh Report of the Joint National Committee on Prevention, Detection, Evaluation and Treatment of High Blood Pressure. *Hypertension*. 2003;42:1206-1252.
2. Berlowitz DR, Ash AS, Hickey EC, et al. Inadequate management of blood pressure in a hypertensive population. *N Engl J Med*. 1998;339:1957-1963.
3. Walsh JM, McDonald KM, Shojania KG, et al. Quality improvement strategies for hypertension management: a systematic review. *Med Care*. 2006;44:646-657.
4. Carter BL, Malone BC, Ellis SL, Dombrowski RC. Antihypertensive drug utilization in hypertensive veterans with complex medication profiles. *J Clin Hypertens (Greenwich)*. 2000;2:172-180.
5. Carter BL, Rogers M, Daly J, Zheng S, James PA. The potency of team-based care interventions for hypertension: a meta-analysis. *Arch Intern Med*. 2009;169:1748-1755.
6. Thompson CA. Pharmacists' CPT codes become permanent: next step is to set valuation for each code. *Am J Health Syst Pharm*. 2007;64:2410-2412.

Behavioral Neurocardiac Training in Hypertension: A Randomized, Controlled Trial

Nolan RP, Floras JS, Harvey PJ, et al (Univ of Toronto, Ontario, Canada; et al)
Hypertension 55:1033-1039, 2010

It is not established whether behavioral interventions add benefit to pharmacological therapy for hypertension. We hypothesized that behavioral neurocardiac training (BNT) with heart rate variability biofeedback would reduce blood pressure further by modifying vagal heart rate modulation during reactivity and recovery from standardized cognitive tasks ("mental stress"). This randomized, controlled trial enrolled 65 patients with uncomplicated hypertension to BNT or active control (autogenic relaxation), with six 1-hour sessions over 2 months with home practice. Outcomes were analyzed with linear mixed models that adjusted for antihypertensive drugs. BNT reduced daytime and 24-hour systolic blood pressures (-2.4 ± 0.9 mm Hg, $P=0.009$, and -2.1 ± 0.9 mm Hg, $P=0.03$, respectively) and pulse pressures (-1.7 ± 0.6 mm Hg, $P=0.004$, and -1.4 ± 0.6 mm Hg, $P=0.02$, respectively). No effect was observed for controls ($P>0.10$ for all indices). BNT also increased RR-high-frequency power (0.15 to 0.40 Hz; $P=0.01$) and RR interval ($P<0.001$) during cognitive tasks. Among controls, high-frequency power was unchanged ($P=0.29$), and RR interval decreased ($P=0.03$). Neither intervention altered spontaneous baroreflex sensitivity ($P>0.10$). In contrast to relaxation therapy, BNT with heart rate variability biofeedback modestly lowers ambulatory blood pressure during wakefulness, and it augments tonic vagal heart rate modulation. It is unknown whether efficacy of this treatment can be improved with biofeedback of baroreflex gain. BNT, alone or as an adjunct to drug therapy, may represent a promising new intervention for hypertension.

▶ This article builds on the pioneering work of Chandra Patel,[1] who showed a significant lowering of blood pressure after yoga training,[2] presumably mediated by the relaxation response. Similar reductions in autonomic cardiovascular rhythms have been seen using other relaxation techniques (eg, mantra recitation and rosary prayer)[3]; some studies included subjects with pharmacologically treated hypertension.[4] Some believe that blood pressure lowering (in either treated or untreated hypertensives) with device-guided breathing also involves the relaxation response, at least in part.[5,6]

These authors interpret the existing literature as showing little to no effect of relaxation therapy or stress management, either in medicated hypertensives or compared with an active biobehavioral control. They therefore designed this trial to see if behavioral neurocardiac training with heart rate variability biofeedback would lower blood pressure more than passive relaxation training. The primary outcome was daytime and 24-hour ambulatory blood pressure measurements (ABPMs), done before randomization and 1 week after the final training session (which is probably sufficient time to have the acute effects dissipate). Several other outcome variables were also analyzed, primarily having to do with heart rate variability in response to psychological testing, which presumably assured that the relaxation response was having the desired effect on vagal tone and other physiological parameters.

All subjects were educated with 4 weekly and then 2 biweekly sessions. Each began with a 10-minute review of cognitive behavioral techniques to manage stress, supplemented by a 20-minute audiotape that reviewed these procedures (meant for daily home use, but its use was not quantified). The hour-long neurocardiac training sessions included exercises to induce the relaxation response and achieve a respiratory rate of ~6 breaths/minute, guided by continuous biofeedback from a monitor that displayed measures of heart rate variability and respiratory rate. Control subjects received a 30-minute audio-taped self-initiated relaxation procedure intended to promote relaxation of major muscle groups.

The results are interesting in that the absolute lowering of awake systolic blood (and pulse) pressure (and corresponding 24-hour ABPM averages) are small, yet significant, for those receiving neurocardiac training. No significant change was seen in diastolic blood pressures for those receiving neurocardiac training nor was any change seen for any blood pressures in the control groups. The authors conclude that their training program may have a role in biobehavioral treatment for hypertension. No comments are made about the magnitude of the effect nor comparisons to other biofeedback techniques (eg, device-guided breathing) or antihypertensive drug therapy, which might be important issues.

W. J. Elliott, MD, PhD

References

1. Patel CH. Yoga and bio-feedback in management of hypertension. *Lancet.* 1973;2: 1053-1055.

2. Patel C. 12-month follow-up of yoga and biofeedback in the management of hypertension. *Lancet.* 1975;305:62-64.

3. Bernardi L, Sleight P, Bandinelli G, et al. Effect of rosary prayer and yoga mantras on autonomic cardiovascular rhythms: comparative study. *BMJ.* 2001;323: 1446-1449.

4. Benson H, Rosner BA, Marzetta BR, Klemchuk HM. Decreased blood-pressure in pharmacologically treated hypertensive patients who regularly elicited the relaxation response. *Lancet.* 1974;303:289-291.

5. Elliott WJ, Izzo JL Jr, White WB, et al. Graded blood pressure reduction in hypertensive outpatients associated with use of a device to assist with slow breathing. *J Clin Hypertens (Greenwich).* 2004;6:553-561.

6. Gavish B. Device-guided breathing in the home setting: Technology, performance and clinical outcomes. *Biol Psychol.* 2010;84:150-156.

Effects of the DASH Diet Alone and in Combination With Exercise and Weight Loss on Blood Pressure and Cardiovascular Biomarkers in Men and Women With High Blood Pressure: The ENCORE Study

Blumenthal JA, Babyak MA, Hinderliter A, et al (Duke Univ Med Ctr, Durham, NC; Univ of North Carolina at Chapel Hill; et al)
Arch Intern Med 170:126-135, 2010

Background.—Although the DASH (Dietary Approaches to Stop Hypertension) diet has been shown to lower blood pressure (BP) in short-term feeding studies, it has not been shown to lower BP among free-living individuals, nor has it been shown to alter cardiovascular biomarkers of risk.

Objective.—To compare the DASH diet alone or combined with a weight management program with usual diet controls among participants with prehypertension or stage 1 hypertension (systolic BP, 130-159 mm Hg; or diastolic BP, 85-99 mm Hg).

Design and Setting.—Randomized, controlled trial in a tertiary care medical center with assessments at baseline and 4 months. Enrollment began October 29, 2003, and ended July 28, 2008.

Participants.—Overweight or obese, unmedicated outpatients with high BP (N = 144).

Interventions.—Usual diet controls, DASH diet alone, and DASH diet plus weight management.

Outcome Measures.—The main outcome measure is BP measured in the clinic and by ambulatory BP monitoring. Secondary outcomes included pulse wave velocity, flow-mediated dilation of the brachial artery, baroreflex sensitivity, and left ventricular mass.

Results.—Clinic-measured BP was reduced by 16.1/9.9 mm Hg (DASH plus weight management); 11.2/7.5 mm (DASH alone); and 3.4/3.8 mm (usual diet controls) (*P* < .001). A similar pattern was observed for ambulatory BP (*P* < .05). Greater improvement was noted for DASH plus weight management compared with DASH alone for pulse wave velocity, baroreflex sensitivity, and left ventricular mass (all *P* < .05).

Conclusion.—For overweight or obese persons with above-normal BP, the addition of exercise and weight loss to the DASH diet resulted in even larger BP reductions, greater improvements in vascular and autonomic function, and reduced left ventricular mass.

Clinical Trial Registration.—clinicaltrials.gov Identifier: NCT00571844.

▶ The Dietary Approaches to Stop Hypertension (DASH) diet is now a cornerstone of lifestyle modifications for blood pressure control and has become the most common download from the National Institutes of Health's public website. Its efficacy in lowering blood pressure was first shown in short-term feeding studies,[1,2] but 6- and 18-month results were not significant in free-living individuals.[3] This research team therefore attempted to add an exercise and weight management program to the DASH diet and compare its results with the DASH diet alone and a usual-care control in improving blood pressure and other subclinical markers of cardiovascular disease. Perhaps as a homage to the DASH diet, they entitled their study, "Exercise and Nutritional interventions for CardiOvasculaR hEalth" (or ENCORE).

Despite much previous and successful work in their locale, they report that it took 1734 days to recruit 144 subjects (or < 5% of those originally contacted) for their study (average: 12 days per recruit). This may have been because of very strict enrollment criteria (unmedicated overweight people without cardiovascular disease and above-normal blood pressure) and the need to assure that recruits would be adherent to the program for at least the 4 months of follow-up. The efforts to provide appropriate instruction and counseling to these subjects must have been immense; the 10 authors thank 29 staff members of the trial and 3 members of the Data and Safety Monitoring Board for their contributions.

The good news is that the multifaceted intervention worked better than just the DASH diet alone, and both interventions worked better than usual care in reducing office blood pressures. Similar but less impressive differences were seen across groups in the ambulatory blood pressure monitoring data. The authors had to impute data for several subjects who withdrew prior to the completion of the 4-month study period: 2 in the DASH diet and exercise group and 1 in the usual control group (because the person was not happy with the result of randomization). Most of the results of testing for biomarkers and other subclinical cardiovascular disease end points favored the combined intervention.

Even the authors regard their results as another proof-of-concept study and recommend further follow-up of their cohort as well as larger clinical trials with "harder endpoints." Given the recent challenges of getting Americans to lose weight (and with few Food and Drug Administration—approved drugs for this purpose in the US market), there may be a larger opportunity for more outcomes research studying biobehavioral interventions for cardiovascular disease prevention, particularly in overweight subjects.

W. J. Elliott, MD, PhD

References

1. Appel L, Moore T, Obarzanek E, et al. A clinical trial of the effects of dietary patterns on blood pressure. DASH Collaborative Research Group. *N Engl J Med*. 1997;336:1117-1124.
2. Sacks FM, Svetkey LP, Vollmer WM, et al. Effects on blood pressure of reduced dietary sodium and the Dietary Approaches to Stop Hypertension (DASH) diet. DASH-Sodium Collaborative Research Group. *N Engl J Med*. 2001;344:3-10.
3. Appel LJ, Champagne CM, Harsha DW, et al. Writing Group of the PREMIER Collaborative Research Group. Effects of comprehensive lifestyle modification on blood pressure control: main results of the PREMIER clinical trial. *JAMA*. 2003;289:2083-2093.

Effectiveness of a Barber-Based Intervention for Improving Hypertension Control in Black Men: The BARBER-1 Study: A Cluster Randomized Trial
Victor RG, Ravenell JE, Freeman A, et al (Univ of Texas Southwestern Med Ctr, Dallas; et al)
Arch Intern Med 171:342-350, 2011

Background.—Barbershop-based hypertension (HTN) outreach programs for black men are becoming increasingly common, but whether they are an effective approach for improving HTN control remains uncertain.

Methods.—To evaluate whether a continuous high blood pressure (BP) monitoring and referral program conducted by barbers motivates male patrons with elevated BP to pursue physician follow-up, leading to improved HTN control, a cluster randomized trial (BARBER-1) of HTN control was conducted among black male patrons of 17 black-owned barbershops in Dallas County, Texas (March 2006—December 2008). Participants underwent 10-week baseline BP screening, and then study sites were randomized to a comparison group that received standard BP pamphlets (8 shops, 77 hypertensive patrons per shop) or an intervention group in which barbers continually offered BP checks with haircuts and promoted physician follow-up with sex-specific peer-based health messaging (9 shops, 75 hypertensive patrons per shop). After 10 months, follow-up data were obtained. The primary outcome measure was change in HTN control rate for each barbershop.

Results.—The HTN control rate increased more in intervention barbershops than in comparison barbershops (absolute group difference, 8.8% [95% confidence interval (CI), 0.8%-16.9%]) (*P* =.04); the intervention effect persisted after adjustment for covariates (*P* =.03). A marginal intervention effect was found for systolic BP change (absolute group difference, −2.5 mm Hg [95% CI, −5.3 to 0.3 mm Hg]) (*P* =.08).

Conclusions.—The effect of BP screening on HTN control among black male barbershop patrons was improved when barbers were enabled to become health educators, monitor BP, and promote physician follow-up. Further research is warranted.

Trial Registration.—clinicaltrials.gov Identifier: NCT00325533.

▶ The results of this fascinating cluster-randomized trial of blood pressure control rates in African American men who receive haircuts, social support, relevant community-based news, and other benefits from barbers in their local area should perhaps not be very surprising. In many African American communities, barbershops serve many roles, not just as a place to get a haircut. Because of the burden of early and often undetected hypertension in urban African American men, targeted screening and education efforts in social gathering places frequented by these often underdiagnosed and undertreated men have been attempted for many years. These programs, which date back to the early 1980s in Chicago, typically involved a partnership between local healthcare providers (who provided secondary screening and a source of clinical care), the American Heart Association (which provided the funding), and a local authority figure trusted by the community (pastor, church nurse, barber, coach/trainer for the local basketball team, barkeeper) and were moderately successful (using historical controls) in discovering new cases of hypertension and referring them to an appropriate source of clinical care. But these efforts did not involve a control group, were not randomized, and generally involved blood pressure measurements that were obtained by a licensed healthcare professional at the screening site. Now that accurate automated sphygmomanometers are available that can be used easily by laypeople, a trial such as this became feasible.

The design of the study is rather straightforward, although cluster-randomized trials are not very common in hypertension.[1] They are much more common in infectious diseases in which the unit of randomization is the source of care, but the unit of analysis is the patient cohort seen by each source of care.[2,3] Thus, each barber and barbershop could be randomized to receive the special intervention (education, automated blood pressure monitor, and focus on successful blood pressure management) or the control group (American Heart Association pamphlet about blood pressure in African Americans) and the patrons of each barbershop could be assessed for blood pressure control 10 months after starting the program. The results were promising, in that control rates increased from ∼34% to ∼54% in the patrons of barbershops that received the special intervention, but there was also an improvement in the patrons of control barbershops (∼40%–∼51%), consistent with recent secular trends.[4] Many other analyses of their data persistently showed barely significant differences in many parameters related to hypertension awareness, treatment, and control.

The editorialist, a famous African American cardiologist who has worked since 1982 (and frequented the same barber for 17 years) in Dallas, rhetorically wondered why such special efforts were needed to bring hypertension control to the attention of the African American men in the study.[5] Most were insured, had been screened for hypertension many times previously, and should have received proper instruction and opportunity for blood pressure control in their medical care homes. It is likely, however, that such community-based programs that target high-risk individuals for screening and nagging about their likely healthcare problems will be more successful than simply inviting these individuals to an off-site source of medical care that does not enjoy the level of trust, community support, and social networking commonly found in urban barbershops, churches, gymnasia, and taverns.

W. J. Elliott, MD, PhD

References

1. Feldman RD, Zou GY, Vandervoort MK, Wong CJ, Nelson SAE, Feagen BJ. A simplified approach to the treatment of uncomplicated hypertension: a cluster-randomized controlled trial. *Hypertension.* 2009;53:646-653.
2. Thiam S, LeFevre AM, Hane F, et al. Effectiveness of a strategy to improve adherence to tuberculosis treatment in a resource-poor setting: a cluster randomized controlled trial. *JAMA.* 2007;297:380-386.
3. Welliver R, Monto AS, Carewicz O, et al, for the Oseltamivir Post-Exposure Prophylaxis Investigator Group. Effectiveness of oseltamivir in preventing influenza in household contacts: a randomized controlled trial. *JAMA.* 2001;285:748-754.
4. Egan BM, Zhao Y, Axon RN. US trends in prevalence, awareness, treatment, and control of hypertension: 1998-2008. *JAMA.* 2010;303:2043-2050.
5. Yancy CW. A bald fade and a BP check: Comment on "Effectiveness of a barbershop-based intervention for improving hypertension control in black men". *Arch Intern Med.* 2010 Oct 25;170.

Vitamins C and E to Prevent Complications of Pregnancy-Associated Hypertension
Roberts JM, for the Eunice Kennedy Shriver National Institute of Child Health and Human Development Maternal—Fetal Medicine Units Network (Univ of Pittsburgh, PA; et al)
N Engl J Med 362:1282-1291, 2010

Background.—Oxidative stress has been proposed as a mechanism linking the poor placental perfusion characteristic of preeclampsia with the clinical manifestations of the disorder. We assessed the effects of antioxidant supplementation with vitamins C and E, initiated early in pregnancy, on the risk of serious adverse maternal, fetal, and neonatal outcomes related to pregnancy-associated hypertension.

Methods.—We conducted a multicenter, randomized, double-blind trial involving nulliparous women who were at low risk for preeclampsia. Women were randomly assigned to begin daily supplementation with 1000 mg of vitamin C and 400 IU of vitamin E or matching placebo between the 9th and 16th weeks of pregnancy. The primary outcome was severe pregnancy-associated hypertension alone or severe or mild hypertension with elevated liver-enzyme levels, thrombocytopenia, elevated serum creatinine levels, eclamptic seizure, medically indicated preterm birth, fetal-growth restriction, or perinatal death.

Results.—A total of 10,154 women underwent randomization. The two groups were similar with respect to baseline characteristics and adherence to the study drug. Outcome data were available for 9969 women. There was no significant difference between the vitamin and placebo groups in the rates of the primary outcome (6.1% and 5.7%, respectively; relative risk in the vitamin group, 1.07; 95% confidence interval [CI], 0.91 to 1.25) or in the rates of preeclampsia (7.2% and 6.7%, respectively; relative risk, 1.07; 95% CI, 0.93 to 1.24). Rates of adverse perinatal outcomes did not differ significantly between the groups.

Conclusions.—Vitamin C and E supplementation initiated in the 9th to 16th week of pregnancy in an unselected cohort of low-risk, nulliparous women did not reduce the rate of adverse maternal or perinatal outcomes related to pregnancy-associated hypertension (ClinicalTrials.gov number, NCT00135707).

▶ The pathophysiology of preeclampsia is not well understood[1]; perhaps because of this, potential therapies for it (including aspirin,[2] calcium supplements,[3] and other vitamins[4]) have not been effective in all populations for preventing the clinical syndrome. There is evidence, however, that in higher-risk populations, these therapies may be somewhat effective, whereas in lower-risk populations, no significant benefit is seen.[5] This may be the explanation for why an early study of antioxidants (including vitamins E and C) was positive in a relatively small number (n = 283) of carefully selected high-risk women.[6] The authors tried to build on this success by attempting a much larger trial in a broader spectrum of women, including some at relatively low risk of preeclampsia.

Unfortunately, the results of this well-performed clinical trial failed to show a significant benefit of these inexpensive and relatively innocuous vitamins. One could argue that the recruitment of primarily low-risk women into the trial worked against finding a benefit, but the overall relative risk estimates pointed in the direction of harm, not benefit. One could quibble with the over-inclusive primary end point, but the fact that the women were all at low risk for preeclampsia meant that a complex and broader composite end point was justified. The authors worry about the doses of vitamins used in the trial compared with those available in prenatal vitamins, which were routinely used in their study subjects, but it appears that this was not the explanation for why no significant benefit of vitamin supplements was seen. A more recent, smaller trial (n = 762) in patients with type 1 diabetes also showed no significant benefit, although the trend was at least positive (19% risk reduction, 95% confidence interval, −12%-41%).[7]

When the meta-analysis of vitamin C and E supplementation for prevention of preeclampsia is completed, it is likely that, like aspirin and calcium supplementation, no overall benefit will be evident. It seems that we are still searching for a better understanding of this complex problem's pathophysiology, which may perhaps eventually lead to effective preventive therapies.

W. J. Elliott, MD, PhD

References

1. Steegars EAP, von Dadelszen P, Duvekot JJ, Pijnenborg R. Pre-eclampsia. *Lancet.* 2010;376:631-642.

2. Askie LM, Duley L, Henderson-Smart DJ, et al. Antiplatelet agents for prevention of pre-eclampsia: a meta-analysis of individual patient data. *Lancet.* 2007;369: 1791-1798.

3. Hofmeyr GJ, Atallah AN, Duley L. Calcium supplementation during pregnancy for preventing hypertensive disorders and related problems. *Cochrane Database Syst Rev.* 2006;(3) 10.1002/14651858.CD001059.pub2. CD001059.

4. Villar J, Purwar M, Merialdi M, et al. World Health Organisation multicentre randomised trial of supplementation with Vitamins C and E among pregnant women at high risk for pre-eclampsia in populations of low nutritional status from developing countries. *BJOG.* 2009;116:780-788.

5. Elliott WJ, Black HR. Special situations in the management of hypertension. Chapter 12. In: Hollenberg NK, ed. *Atlas of Hypertension.* 6th ed. Philadelphia, PA: Current Medicine, Inc; 2009:274-299.

6. Chappell LC, Seed PT, Briley AL, et al. Effect of antioxidants on the occurrence of pre-eclampsia in women at increased risk: a randomised trial. *Lancet.* 1999;354: 810-816.

7. McCance DR, Holmes VA, Maresh MJ, et al. for the Diabetes and Pre-eclampsia Intervention Trial Study Group. Vitamins C and E for prevention of pre-eclampsia in women with type 1 diabetes (DAPIT): a randomised placebo-controlled trial. *Lancet.* 2010;376:259-266.

Effect of Sibutramine on Cardiovascular Outcomes in Overweight and Obese Subjects

James WPT, for the SCOUT Investigators (London School of Hygiene and Tropical Medicine, UK; et al)

N Engl J Med 363:905-917, 2010

Background.—The long-term effects of sibutramine treatment on the rates of cardiovascular events and cardiovascular death among subjects at high cardiovascular risk have not been established.

Methods.—We enrolled in our study 10,744 overweight or obese subjects, 55 years of age or older, with preexisting cardiovascular disease, type 2 diabetes mellitus, or both to assess the cardiovascular consequences of weight management with and without sibutramine in subjects at high risk for cardiovascular events. All the subjects received sibutramine in addition to participating in a weight-management program during a 6-week, single-blind, lead-in period, after which 9804 subjects underwent random assignment in a double-blind fashion to sibutramine (4906 subjects) or placebo (4898 subjects). The primary end point was the time from randomization to the first occurrence of a primary outcome event (nonfatal myocardial infarction, nonfatal stroke, resuscitation after cardiac arrest, or cardiovascular death).

Results.—The mean duration of treatment was 3.4 years. The mean weight loss during the lead-in period was 2.6 kg; after randomization, the subjects in the sibutramine group achieved and maintained further weight reduction (mean, 1.7 kg). The mean blood pressure decreased in both groups, with greater reductions in the placebo group than in the sibutramine group (mean difference, 1.2/1.4 mm Hg). The risk of a primary outcome event was 11.4% in the sibutramine group as compared with 10.0% in the placebo group (hazard ratio, 1.16; 95% confidence interval [CI], 1.03 to 1.31; P = 0.02). The rates of nonfatal myocardial infarction and nonfatal stroke were 4.1% and 2.6% in the sibutramine group and 3.2% and 1.9% in the placebo group, respectively (hazard ratio for nonfatal myocardial infarction, 1.28; 95% CI, 1.04 to 1.57; P = 0.02; hazard ratio for nonfatal stroke, 1.36; 95% CI, 1.04 to 1.77; P = 0.03). The rates of cardiovascular death and death from any cause were not increased.

Conclusions.—Subjects with preexisting cardiovascular conditions who were receiving long-term sibutramine treatment had an increased risk of nonfatal myocardial infarction and nonfatal stroke but not of cardiovascular death or death from any cause. (Funded by Abbott; ClinicalTrials. gov number, NCT00234832.)

▶ This report from the Sibutramine Cardiovascular Outcomes Trial (SCOUT) triggered the marketer of sibutramine to voluntarily withdraw it from the United States, although it had previously been withdrawn from Europe and other countries.[1] This leaves us with only orlistat as a Food and Drug Administration (FDA)-approved medication for weight loss in the United States, despite the huge current epidemic of obesity.[2] There had previously been some controversy about the clinical importance of the small amount of blood pressure and heart rate increase seen in registration trials with the drug, such that its FDA-approved product information contained a warning about its use in obese hypertensive patients.[3] There was, however, no contraindication for its use in patients with hypertension or pre-existing cardiovascular disease. But this report not only solidified the data about the excessive risk in obese populations, it also highlights the clinical importance of "a few mm Hg of blood pressure elevation." Many physicians believe that if they can't measure a 2-mm Hg increase in blood pressure with their sphygmomanometers, it cannot be a clinically important difference, even if it achieves traditional levels of statistical significance. Here, the difference in blood pressure was only 1.2/1.4 mm Hg in the sibutramine versus placebo groups, less than what can be measured in an individual patient at a single visit. Yet the cardiovascular event rate was 16% higher in the sibutramine-treated patients, a significant difference, with a 28% increase in risk of nonfatal myocardial infarction and an even higher 36% increase in risk of a nonfatal stroke (just as one would predict from the blood pressure differences alone). These increases in risk were primarily seen in patients with pre-existing cardiovascular disease, a group that might particularly benefit from weight loss.

Editorialists for this article decried the fact that it took 13 years to design and execute this long-term outcome study regarding the safety of this drug.[3] They also complain that in this long-term study, sibutramine was associated with only a 4.5-kg weight loss (compared with baseline) at 12 months,[4] when the FDA usually expects at least a 5.0 kg decline in weight for proof of efficacy.[5] Eventually, the authors of SCOUT should consider attempting to discern whether the increased cardiovascular risk could be more closely linked to the between-group differences in blood pressure or heart rate, but the fact that the marketer has withdrawn the compound makes it unlikely that such analyses will be funded and published.

W. J. Elliott, MD, PhD

References

1. *European Medicines Agency Recommends Suspension of Marketing Authorization for Sibutramine.* European Medicines Agency Press; 2010. http://www.ema. europa.eu/pdfs/human/referral/sibutramine/3940810en.pdf. Accessed October 22, 2010.
2. Hedley AA, Ogden CL, Johnson CL, Carroll MD, Curtin LR, Flegal KM. Prevalence of overweight and obesity among US children, adolescents, and adults, 1999-2002. *JAMA.* 2004;291:2847-2850.
3. *Sibutramine (Meridia®) Product Information (Package Insert).* North Chicago, IL: Abbott Laboratories; 2010. http://www.fda.gov/downloads/Drugs/Drugsafety/ PublicHealthAdvisories/UCM130745.pdf. Accessed October 22, 2010.
4. Curfman GD, Morrissey S, Drazen JM. Sibutramine—another flawed diet pill [editorial]. *N Engl J Med.* 2010;363:972-974.
5. *Guidance for Industry. Developing Products for Weight Management.* Rockville, MD: US Food and Drug Administration; 2007. http://www.fda.gov/downloads/ Drugs/GuidanceComplianceRegulatoryInformation/Guidances/ucm071612.pdf.

2 Pediatric Cardiovascular Disease

Tetralogy of Fallot

Arrhythmia Burden in Adults With Surgically Repaired Tetralogy of Fallot: A Multi-Institutional Study

Khairy P, for the Alliance for Adult Research in Congenital Cardiology (AARCC) (Univ of Montreal, Quebec, Canada; et al)
Circulation 122:868-875, 2010

Background.—The arrhythmia burden in tetralogy of Fallot, types of arrhythmias encountered, and risk profile may change as the population ages.

Methods and Results.—The Alliance for Adult Research in Congenital Cardiology (AARCC) conducted a multicenter cross-sectional study to quantify the arrhythmia burden in tetralogy of Fallot, to characterize age-related trends, and to identify associated factors. A total of 556 patients, 54.0% female, 36.8 ± 12.0 years of age were recruited from 11 centers. Overall, 43.3% had a sustained arrhythmia or arrhythmia intervention. Prevalence of atrial tachyarrhythmias was 20.1%. Factors associated with intraatrial reentrant tachycardia in multivariable analyses were right atrial enlargement (odds ratio [OR], 6.2; 95% confidence interval [CI], 2.8 to 13.6), hypertension (OR, 2.3; 95% CI, 1.1 to 4.6), and number of cardiac surgeries (OR, 1.4; 95% CI, 1.2 to 1.6). Older age (OR, 1.09 per year; 95% CI, 1.05 to 1.12), lower left ventricular ejection fraction (OR, 0.93 per unit; 95% CI, 0.89 to 0.96), left atrial dilation (OR, 3.2; 95% CI, 1.5 to 6.8), and number of cardiac surgeries (OR, 1.5; 95% CI, 1.2 to 1.9) were jointly associated with atrial fibrillation. Ventricular arrhythmias were prevalent in 14.6% and jointly associated with number of cardiac surgeries (OR, 1.3; 95% CI, 1.1 to 1.6), QRS duration (OR, 1.02 per 1 ms; 95% CI, 1.01 to 1.03), and left ventricular diastolic dysfunction (OR, 3.3; 95% CI, 1.5 to 7.1). Prevalence of atrial fibrillation and ventricular arrhythmias markedly increased after 45 years of age.

Conclusions.—The arrhythmia burden in adults with tetralogy of Fallot is considerable, with various subtypes characterized by different profiles. Atrial fibrillation and ventricular arrhythmias appear to be influenced more by left-than right-sided heart disease.

▶ This reasonably large multi-institutional study documents quite well the markedly increased prevalence of both atrial and ventricular tachyarrhythmias in postoperative tetralogy patients with increasing age. These patients require close follow-up and combined care by experts in adult congenital heart disease (ACHD) and electrophysiology to attempt to modify their course and decrease the incidence of premature morbidity and mortality. Hopefully the prevalence of these complications will decrease with those patients now entering their second and third decade who will benefit from earlier repair and improved hemodynamics.

T. P. Graham, Jr, MD

Can we use the end systolic volume index to monitor intrinsic right ventricular function after repair of tetralogy of Fallot?
Uebing A, Fischer G, Schlangen J, et al (Univ Hosp of Schleswig-Holstein, Kiel, Germany; et al)
Int J Cardiol 147:52-57, 2011

Background.—After tetralogy of Fallot (ToF) repair the right ventricle (RV) is commonly exposed to abnormal volume load resulting from pulmonary regurgitation (PR) leading to progressive RV dilatation. The objective of this study was to assess the relationship between RV volumes, especially the end systolic volume index (ESVi), and RV contractility in patients after ToF repair and significant PR and to determine whether RV dilatation reflects intrinsic RV dysfunction in these patients.

Methods.—Twenty-nine ToF patients were studied 11.6 (range: 1.9–30.1) years after repair with the pressure–volume conductance system. The patient cohort was divided into two groups according to the median ESVi (*group 1*: ESVi<34.7 ml/m$^{2\times1.18}$, $n = 14$; *group 2*: ESVi≥34.7 ml/m$^{2\times1.18}$, $n = 15$).

Results.—The slope of the end systolic pressure-volume relationship (end systolic elastance, Ees) was higher in *group 1* compared to *group 2* both at baseline and during dobutamine infusion (0.87 ± 0.36 vs. 0.46 ± 0.28 mm Hg/ml and 1.50 ± 0.77 vs. 0.92 ± 0.37 mm Hg/ml; $P<0.005$ and $P=0.02$, respectively).

Overall, *Ees* at baseline correlated significantly with ESVi and also with the end diastolic volume index ($r = -0.64$, and $P<0.001$ for both). Receiver operating characteristic curve analysis revealed that ESVi was superior to RV ejection fraction (EF) in predicting an *Ees* in the lowest quartile of the study group (area under curve ESVi vs. EF: 0.84 (0.64–0.95) vs. 0.68 (0.47–0.85); $P=0.015$).

Conclusion.—ESVi is a valid estimate of intrinsic RV function in repaired ToF patients with residual PR and in this respect seems superior to EF. These data underscore the importance of serial ventricular volume assessment in the follow-up of these patients.

▶ This is a sophisticated study using a conductance catheter to estimate right ventricular volumes in postoperative tetralogy of Fallot patients before and after dobutamine infusion. The data indicate that right ventricular end systolic volume indexed for body size yields a reasonably good estimate of contractility that could prove quite useful in improving timing of pulmonary valve replacement in this patient group.

T. P. Graham, Jr, MD

Determinants of outcome after surgical treatment of pulmonary atresia with ventricular septal defect and major aortopulmonary collateral arteries
Carotti A, Albanese SB, Filippelli S, et al (Bambino Gesù Children's Hosp, Rome, Italy)
J Thorac Cardiovasc Surg 140:1092-1103, 2010

Objectives.—Identification of variables influencing surgical outcome in patients treated for pulmonary atresia with ventricular septal defect and major aortopulmonary collateral arteries.

Methods.—A total of 90 consecutive patients (median age, 12 months; range, 20 days to 35 years), who had primarily undergone either 1-stage unifocalization (n = 69) or palliation to promote native pulmonary arterial development (n = 21), were studied. Chromosome 22q11 deletion had occurred in 37% of the cases. Ventricular septal defect closure was accomplished in 70 patients (78%), with a mean postoperative right/left ventricular pressure ratio of 0.48 ± 0.14.

Results.—The rate of 14-year survival, freedom from conduit reintervention, and freedom from percutaneous intervention on the pulmonary arteries was 75%, 46%, and 52%, respectively. At a median interval of 95 months (range, 1.5-164 months), the right/left ventricular pressure ratio did not differ significantly from early postoperatively. Univariate analysis showed that an absence of confluent intrapericardial pulmonary arteries favorably affected the postoperative right/left ventricular pressure ratio after ventricular septal defect closure ($P = .04$). Kaplan-Meier estimates showed age of 30 days or younger ($P = .0004$) and weight of 3 kg or less ($P = .0004$) at unifocalization and chromosome 22q11 deletion ($P = .001$) significantly affected survival. Chromosome 22q11 deletion was significantly associated with mortality, even in the Cox regression model (hazard ratio, 8.26; $P = .003$). Finally, ventricular septal defect closure during single-stage and single/multiple-stage procedures significantly correlated with both early ($P = .0013$ and $P < .00001$, respectively) and overall ($P = .013$ and $P = .0007$, respectively) survival.

Conclusions.—The results of surgery were satisfactory and durable, despite the need for repeated percutaneous or surgical reinterventions. The outcomes were negatively affected by neonatal age and low body weight and positively affected by simultaneous or staged ventricular septal defect closure. Finally, chromosome 22q11 deletion remained an independent variable affecting survival.

▶ This series adds to the literature regarding a generally positive outcome for aggressive treatment of the patients with unifocalization as an integral part of the process even when one only has major aortopulmonary collateral arteries or collateral arteries to use for the pulmonary arteries. The mean age at unifocalization was 15 months; this was due largely to later referrals. These authors favor doing the procedure at a body weight of 5 kg. The consensus from the 3 largest studies performing infant unifocalization as noted in the remarks following the article by Dr Hanley are that when unifocalization is performed aggressively and relatively early in life, midterm outcomes are improved. Second, these patients need aggressive follow-up with early postoperative catheterization and interventional studies to dilate and frequently stent small stenotic arteries in an attempt to maximize pulmonary perfusion and number of pulmonary segments that receive significant blood flow. Small infants with this condition and small to hypoplastic arteries remain among the most difficult and challenging patients. These results help us to be more committed to a long process with ultimately a much improved outlook for a good functional outcome.

T. P. Graham, Jr, MD

Transposition of the Great Arteries

Cardiac Outcomes in Young Adult Survivors of the Arterial Switch Operation for Transposition of the Great Arteries
Tobler D, Williams WG, Jegatheeswaran A, et al (Univ of Toronto, Ontario, Canada)
J Am Coll Cardiol 56:58-64, 2010

Objectives.—We sought to determine cardiac outcomes in young adults with complete transposition of the great arteries (TGA) after the arterial switch operation (ASO).

Background.—Although cardiac outcomes in the pediatric population with TGA after ASO have been well described, outcomes in the adult population have not to our knowledge been studied.

Methods.—We determined late survival in all operative survivors with TGA after ASO performed before 1991 at our local pediatric referring hospital. In the subset of adults (n = 65) followed in our adult congenital cardiac clinic, we examined cardiac outcomes in adulthood.

Results.—Survival of the 132 infants discharged from hospital after ASO was 97% (70% confidence interval [CI]: 95.0% to 98.1%) at 20 years. In the 65 patients (mean age 21 ± 3 years, 62% male) followed at our institution, 17% (11 of 65) had at least 1 clinically significant cardiac lesion, including ventricular dysfunction, valvular dysfunction, or arrhythmias. Residual lesions were more common in those who had had cardiac reinterventions in childhood (odds ratio: 10.7, 95% CI: 2.1 to 55). In adulthood, 5 patients (8%) had arrhythmia requiring treatment and 7 patients (11%) required reinterventions (5 reoperations and 2 pacemaker implantations). Intervention for aortic valve regurgitation and aortic root dilation were not observed. Exercise capacity was reduced in most adults (82%) after ASO.

Conclusions.—Although most adults after ASO are well, and few have residual defects, there are subgroups, particularly those who needed further cardiac intervention in childhood, who are at higher risk for ventricular and valve dysfunction and arrhythmias.

▶ This represents one of the first reports of adult survivors of the arterial switch operation (ASO) for transposition of the great arteries (TGA). Excellent survival is shown, and the numbers of reinterventions are mostly related to earlier operations before modifications were put in place that have almost eliminated right ventricular outflow obstruction. Aortic root dilation was common, but the degree of AR was not sufficient enough to warrant aortic valve replacement in any patient to date. Left ventricular systolic dysfunction was present in 14%, but none were reported to have symptomatic congestive heart failure. Exercise capacity was mildly depressed and questionably related to complex TGA and/or reoperations. The 4 deaths were related to myocardial infarction in 2, subacute bacterial endocarditis in 1, and with sudden unexplained death in 1. Perfusion defects were present in 5 of 23 who were tested; only 1 of these patients had coronary angiograms performed which were normal. This group of patients obviously is much improved from those who had arterial switch operations, but long-term follow-up is still very important, as coronary and aortic abnormalities are common. I feel that imaging of coronary anatomy by cardiac magnetic resonance would be useful in all patients before they get chest pain and appear in emergency departments, where they may get the standard referral to the chest pain center and where they will not have the usual anatomy or physiology.

T. P. Graham, Jr, MD

Coronary Diameter and Vasodilator Function in Children Following Arterial Switch Operation for Complete Transposition of the Great Arteries
Turner DR, Muzik O, Forbes TJ, et al (Wayne State Univ School of Medicine, Detroit, MI; et al)
Am J Cardiol 106:421-425, 2010

Coronary reimplantation during arterial switch operation (ASO) may affect coronary artery growth and function during childhood. The purpose of this study was to assess coronary artery diameter and regional myocardial blood flow (MBF) and myocardial flow reserve (MFR) in children after neonatal ASO. We measured proximal diameters of left anterior descending (LAD), left circumflex, and posterior descending coronary arteries on coronary angiogram in 12 children (median age 11 years, range 7.6 to 15.1) with a history of neonatal ASO. These children then underwent cardiac positron emission tomographic imaging using nitrogen-13 ammonia to assess MBF at baseline and during intravenous adenosine hyperemia in regions supplied by these 3 coronary arteries. Coronary artery z-scores were within normal range (-2.0 to 2.0) for 32 of 36 coronary arteries. MFR (ratio of hyperemic to basal MBF) was normal (>2.5) in all myocardial regions in 10 of 12 patients. The remaining 2 patients, 1 with a dual LAD and 1 with LAD origin from the right coronary artery, had generalized impairment of hyperemic MBF (<2.0 ml/g/min) and low MFR (<2.5). Coronary artery z-scores and MFR in corresponding myocardial territories were not correlated ($r = 0.15$, $p = 0.36$). In conclusion, coronary growth and function appear to be normal in most children after neonatal ASO. Children with anatomic LAD abnormalities may be at increased risk of impaired MFR.

▶ This is certainly good news for most children post arterial switch operation (ASO) for transposition of the great arteries. Hopefully a larger cohort will have similar findings. It does behoove the follow-up cardiologist to know the details of the ASO well so that those patients who had abnormal origins of the left anterior descending artery can get appropriate studies of their coronaries.

T. P. Graham, Jr, MD

Effects of Morphologic Left Ventricular Pressure on Right Ventricular Geometry and Tricuspid Valve Regurgitation in Patients With Congenitally Corrected Transposition of the Great Arteries

Kral Kollars CA, Gelehrter S, Bove EL, et al (Univ of Michigan Med School, Ann Arbor)
Am J Cardiol 105:735-739, 2010

Congenitally corrected transposition of the great arteries (CCTGA) is associated with tricuspid regurgitation (TR), which has been postulated to arise from the effect of ventricular septal position on the attachments of the tricuspid valve. This study was performed to determine the effect of left ventricular (LV) pressure on right ventricular (RV) and LV geometry and the degree of TR. Serial echocardiograms were reviewed from, 30 patients with CCTGA who underwent pulmonary artery banding to train the morphologic left ventricle ($n = 14$) or left ventricle–to–pulmonary artery conduit placement and ventricular septal defect closure in conjunction with physiologic repair ($n = 16$). The degree of TR, the LV/RV pressure ratio, RV and LV sphericity indexes, and tricuspid valve tethering distance and coaptation length were analyzed. After pulmonary artery banding, an increase in LV systolic pressure to $\geq 2/3$ systemic resulted in a decrease in TR from severe to moderate (p = 0.02). The percentage of patients with severe TR decreased from 64% to 18% (p = 0.06). The RV sphericity index decreased (p = 0.05), and the LV sphericity index increased (p = 0.02). After left ventricle—to—pulmonary artery conduit placement, a decrease in LV pressure to ≤1/2 systemic resulted in an increase in TR from none to mild (p = 0.003). In conclusion, these data indicate that LV pressure in patients with CCTGA affects the degree of TR and that septal shift caused by changes in LV and RV pressure is an important mechanism.

▶ Although the association of right ventricular/left ventricular pressure ratios and septal position with the severity of tricuspid regurgitation (TR) in patients with congenitally corrected transposition of the great arteries has been noted previously, this report solidifies that hypothesis. Occasionally, pulmonary artery banding in patients with severe TR and congestive heart failure (CHF) has resulted in such improvement in TR and CHF that nothing further is needed therapeutically for a considerable period of time.

T. P. Graham, Jr, MD

Outcomes of Biventricular Repair for Congenitally Corrected Transposition of the Great Arteries
Lim H-G, Lee JR, Kim YJ, et al (Seoul Natl Univ Children's Hosp, Korea; Seoul Natl Univ Hosp, Korea; Seoul Natl Univ, Korea; et al)
Ann Thorac Surg 89:159-167, 2010

Background.—This study was undertaken to evaluate long-term results of biventricular repairs for congenitally corrected transposition of the great arteries, and to analyze the risk factors that affect mortality and morbidity.

Methods.—Between 1983 and 2009, 167 patients with congenitally corrected transposition of the great arteries underwent biventricular repairs. The physiologic repairs were performed in 123 patients, and anatomic repairs in 44. Average follow-up was 9.3 ± 6.6 years.

Results.—Kaplan-Meier estimated survival was 83.3% ± 0.5% at 25 years in biventricular repair. In anatomic repair, left ventricular training and right ventricular dysfunction had negative impact on survival, but bidirectional cavopulmonary shunt had positive impact on survival. The reoperation-free ratio was 10.1% ± 7.8% at 22 years after physiologic repair, and 46.2% ± 12.4% at 15 years after anatomic repair (*p* = 0.885). Freedom from any arrhythmia was 49.6% ± 7.5% at 22 years after physiologic repair, and 60.8% ± 14.8% at 18 years after anatomic repair (*p* = 0.458). Freedom from systemic atrioventricular valve and ventricular dysfunction as well as tricuspid valve and right ventricular dysfunction was significantly higher in anatomic repair than in physiologic repair.

Conclusions.—Long-term results of biventricular repair were satisfactory. Patients presenting with right ventricular dysfunction or need for left ventricular training represent a high-risk group of anatomic repair for which selection criteria are particularly important. Late functional outcomes of anatomic repair were excellent compared with physiologic repair. Anatomic repair is the procedure of choice for those patients if both ventricles are adequate or if surgical technique is modified with the help of additional a bidirectional cavopulmonary shunt.

▶ This report from 4 institutions has a lot of data and affords midterm follow-up comparing anatomic and physiologic repair of patients with congenitally corrected transposition of the great arteries. They do show a superiority of the anatomic repair in terms of atrioventricular valve regurgitation and ventricular function, freedom from arrhythmia, and fewer reoperations. These authors reaffirm the difficulty in patient selection for left ventricle retraining and in successfully carrying out this process. They do recommend the use of a superior caval bidirectional shunt if there is any indication of compromise of the pulmonary ventricular size or function after either anatomic or physiologic repair.

T. P. Graham, Jr, MD

Fontan Operation

Arrhythmias in a Contemporary Fontan Cohort: Prevalence and Clinical Associations in a Multicenter Cross-Sectional Study
Stephenson EA, for the Pediatric Heart Network Investigators (The Hosp for Sick Children, Toronto, Ontario, Canada; et al)
J Am Coll Cardiol 56:890-896, 2010

Objectives.—Our aim was to examine the prevalence of arrhythmias and identify independent associations of time to arrhythmia development.
Background.—Since introduction of the Fontan operation in 1971, long-term results have steadily improved with newer modifications. However, atrial arrhythmias are frequent and contribute to ongoing morbidity and mortality. Data are lacking regarding the prevalence of arrhythmias and risk factors for their development in the current era.
Methods.—The Pediatric Heart Network Fontan Cross-Sectional study evaluated data from 7 centers, with 520 patients age 6 to 18 years (mean 8.6 ± 3.4 years after the Fontan operation), including echocardiograms, electrocardiograms, exercise testing, parent-reported Child Health Questionnaire (CHQ) results, and medical history.
Results.—Supraventricular tachycardias were present in 9.4% of patients. Intra-atrial re-entrant tachycardia (IART) was present in 7.3% (32 of 520). The hazard of IART decreased until 4 to 6 years post-Fontan, and then increased with age thereafter. Cardiac anatomy and resting heart rate (including marked bradycardia) were not associated with IART. We identified 3 independent associations of time to occurrence of IART: lower CHQ physical summary score ($p < 0.001$); predominant rhythm ($p = 0.002$; highest risk with paced rhythm), and type of Fontan operation ($p = 0.037$; highest risk with atriopulmonary connection).

Time to IART did not differ between patients with lateral tunnel and extracardiac conduit types of Fontan repair. Ventricular tachycardia was noted in 3.5% of patients.

Conclusions.—Overall prevalence of IART was lower in this cohort (7.3%) than previously reported. Lower functional status, an atriopulmonary connection, and paced rhythm were determined to be independently associated with development of IART after Fontan. (Relationship Between Functional Health Status and Ventricular Performance After Fontan—Pediatric Heart Network; NCT00132782).

▶ This study does show an improvement in prevalence of arrhythmias, post-Fontan with a contemporary cohort. It is of interest that this study did not show a decreased incidence of rhythm disturbance with an extracardiac conduit versus a lateral tunnel connection. In addition, I thought a paced rhythm might actually protect from atrial arrhythmia. Perhaps it does in individual patients, but when compared with others in this series who did not require pacing, those who were paced may have other characteristics, such as larger atria, more atrial suture lines, or more complex anatomy, that were not wholly accounted for by the statistical tests, which were possible to use.

T. P. Graham, Jr, MD

Exercise capacity, quality of life, and daily activity in the long-term follow-up of patients with univentricular heart and total cavopulmonary connection
Müller J, Christov F, Schreiber C, et al (Technische Universität München, Germany)
Eur Heart J 30:2915-2920, 2009

Aims.—Patients with congenital heart disease usually show diminished exercise capacity and quality of life. However, there is only little information about daily activity, a marker for lifestyle, exercise capacity, and the prevention of arteriosclerosis. This study investigated exercise capacity, quality of life, daily activity, and their interaction with univentricular heart physiology after total cavopulmonary connection (TCPC).

Methods and Results.—Fifty-seven patients (18 females, 39 males, age 8–52 years) after TCPC (lateral tunnel 28, extra-cardiac conduit 29) who underwent surgery during 1994–2001 were examined in our institution. They performed a symptom-limited cardiopulmonary exercise test. Those patients 14 years of age and older filled in the health-related quality-of-life questionnaire SF-36, and those who were 8–13 years of age, the CF-87. Daily activity parameters were obtained by using a triaxial accelerometer over the next three consecutive days. Exercise capacity was severely reduced after TCPC (25.0 mL/min/kg corresponding to 59.7% of age- and sex-related reference values). Daily activity was within the recommendations of the United Kingdom Expert Consensus Group (≥60 min, ≥3 metabolic equivalent, ≥5 days/week) in 72% of the investigated patients. It was reduced in older patients (Spearman $r = -0.506$, $P < 0.001$) and patients with a lower peak oxygen uptake (Spearman $r = 0.432$, $P = 0.001$). In children <14 years, mental health was related to daily activity.

Conclusion.—Despite their diminished exercise capacity, patients after TCPC show a fairly normal activity pattern. However, their activity depends not only on age, but also on exercise capacity, which, in contrast to healthy people, decreases already from early adolescence on.

▶ These Fontan patients are most likely the best of their peer group in that they were able to complete the testing and had a normal activity profile. Despite all of these provisions and the lack of atrial-pulmonary or atrial-ventricular connections in these patients, their exercise capacity was significantly reduced—similar to most, if not all, previous Fontan exercise studies. The Fontan operation has been a huge overall success and at its best has afforded wonderful mid- to long-term palliation and quality of life. These patients need lifelong follow-up to be sure that any new issues can be evaluated and treated quickly to try to prevent late complications.

T. P. Graham, Jr, MD

How Good Is a Good Fontan? Quality of Life and Exercise Capacity of Fontans Without Arrhythmias

d'Udekem Y, Cheung MMH, Setyapranata S, et al (Royal Children's Hosp, Victoria, Australia; Univ of Melbourne, Victoria, Australia, Royal Melbourne Hosp, Victoria, Australia)

Ann Thorac Surg 88:1961-1969, 2009

Background.—Poor long-term outcomes are expected after Fontan surgery, but these perspectives have been tainted by the poorly functioning Fontans suffering from arrhythmias. No predictions of outcome can be quoted to the increasing number of Fontan patients free from arrhythmic complications. The parameters determining improved exercise capacity and quality of life in this subgroup are yet unknown.

Methods.—Fontan survivors from our institution and living in Victoria were invited to participate in the study if they were more than 10 years of age, and free of arrhythmias. A mean of 17 ± 4 years after Fontan, 36 patients, 23 with a classical atriopulmonary connection (AP) and 13 with a lateral tunnel (LT) underwent transthoracic echocardiography, cycloergometer exercise study, neurohumoral screening, and assessment of quality of life.

Results.—The only factor predicting worse exercise capacity was the type of Fontan performed; patients with LT having better exercise capacity than those with AP (percentage of predicted anaerobic threshold: $88 \pm 14\%$ vs $72 \pm 14\%$, $p < 0.005$; percentage of predicted Vo_2max: $62 \pm 8\%$ vs $54 \pm 7\%$, $p < 0.005$). Endothelin-1 levels were elevated in all patients (2.9 pmol/L, 2.5 to 3.7). Responses from the quality of life measures placed our Fontan cohort mainly within the normal population range. None of the preoperative and postoperative variables adversely affected patients' quality of life.

Conclusions.—The anaerobic threshold of arrhythmia-free Fontan patients operated with the lateral tunnel technique was relatively preserved. Despite restricted exercise capacity, Fontan patients, provided that they are free of arrhythmias, have a normal quality of life reflected in their reports of psychiatric symptoms and family relationships.

▶ This well-studied group of Fontan patients without arrhythmias at midterm follow-up demonstrates similar findings in terms of depressed peak exercise performance as shown by virtually all previous studies. The lateral tunnel patients did show improved exercise capacity compared with a larger and older group of patients with atriopulmonary connections. The good news is that these patients' quality of life profiles were relatively well preserved. Is the presence or absence of arrhythmias a marker of poor hemodynamics, time since operation, surgical technique, atrial incisions/suture lines, or all of these? I am amazed that these investigators have such a relatively large group of atriopulmonary connection patients without arrhythmias. They do quote an 87 % freedom from arrhythmias using the lateral tunnel approach. Good results from a very active group in Melbourne. There must be something to the Aussie can-do positive approach to difficult problems.

T. P. Graham, Jr, MD

Improved management of systemic venous anomalies in a single ventricle: New rationale
Amodeo A, Grigioni M, Filippelli S, et al (Bambino Gesù Paediatric Hosp, Rome, Italy; Health of the ISS (Italian Natl Inst of Health), Rome, Italy; et al)
J Thorac Cardiovasc Surg 138:1154-1159, 2009

Objectives.—Two innovative surgical approaches addressing systemic venous anomalies in single-ventricle patients are evaluated.

Methods.—Between 2003 and 2007, 7 patients underwent a unifocal bilateral bidirectional cavopulmonary anastomosis, and 5 patients underwent a hepatoazygos venous connection associated with a previous (n = 4) or concomitant (n = 1) Kawashima operation. Computational fluid dynamics simulations allowed investigation of 2 sets of comparative models: (1) bifocal versus unifocal bilateral bidirectional cavopulmonary anastomosis and (2) classic hepatic vein—pulmonary artery channel versus hepatoazygos direct anastomosis for Fontan completion after or combined with the Kawashima operation.

Results.—There was 1 hospital death in the unifocal bilateral bidirectional cavopulmonary anastomosis group. At a mean follow-up of 15.6 ± 7.40 months after a unifocal bilateral bidirectional cavopulmonary anastomosis and of 38.7 ± 13.2 months after direct hepatoazygos venous connection, respectively, all 11 survivors are in New York Heart Association class I with functional anastomoses. Computational assessment of bifocal bilateral bidirectional cavopulmonary anastomosis demonstrated weak perfusion between caval veins against symmetric and steady bilateral flow fields in the unifocal arrangement. In the classic post-Kawashima Fontan completion model, the hepatic venous flow to the pulmonary artery was held back by means of preponderant opposite flow, whereas in the direct hepatoazygos venous connection model, the hepatic venous flow merged smoothly into the azygos vein. Power-loss calculation showed no significant difference between bifocal and unifocal bilateral bidirectional cavopulmonary anastomosis topology, whereas the hepatoazygos connection clearly had better energy preservation than the classical connection.

Conclusions.—This limited clinical and computational fluid dynamics assessment suggests the efficacy of this new rationale to reduce the additional thrombotic risks produced by systemic venous anomalies in single-ventricle patients.

▶ These innovative surgical techniques have definite theoretical advantages for avoiding colliding venous pathways with potential for stagnant flow and thrombosis. In the hepatoazygous connection, the improved flow dynamics were apparent, but no improved fluid dynamics were found in the unifocalized superior bicaval anastomosis. Any advantage to promoting pulmonary flow in patients undergoing Fontan operation is worthwhile if these variations can be performed without increasing surgical risk.

T. P. Graham, Jr, MD

Laboratory Measures of Exercise Capacity and Ventricular Characteristics and Function Are Weakly Associated With Functional Health Status After Fontan Procedure

McCrindle BW, for the Pediatric Heart Network Investigators (Univ of Toronto, Ontario, Canada; et al)
Circulation 121:34-42, 2010

Background.—Patients after the Fontan procedure are at risk for suboptimal functional health status, and associations with laboratory measures are important for planning interventions and outcome measures for clinical trials.

Methods and Results.—Parents completed the generic Child Health Questionnaire for 511 Fontan Cross-Sectional Study patients 6 to 18 years of age (61% male). Associations of Child Health Questionnaire Physical and Psychosocial Functioning Summary Scores (FSS) with standardized measurements from prospective exercise testing, echocardiography, magnetic resonance imaging, and measurement of brain natriuretic peptide were determined by regression analyses. For exercise variables for maximal effort patients only, the final model showed that higher Physical FSS was associated only with higher maximum work rate, accounting for 9% of variation in Physical FSS. For echocardiography, lower Tei index (particularly for patients with extracardiac lateral tunnel connections), lower indexed end-systolic volume, and the absence of atrioventricular valve regurgitation for patients having Fontan procedure at age <2 years were associated with higher Physical FSS, accounting for 14% of variation in Physical FSS. For magnetic resonance imaging, ratio of lower mass to end-diastolic volume and midquartiles of indexed end-systolic volume (nonlinear) were associated with higher Physical FSS, accounting for 11% of variation. Lower brain natriuretic peptide was significantly but weakly associated with higher Physical FSS (1% of variation). Significant associations for Psychosocial FSS with laboratory measures were fewer and weaker than for Physical FSS.

Conclusions.—In relatively healthy Fontan patients, laboratory measures account for a small proportion of the variation in functional health status and therefore may not be optimal surrogate end points for trials of therapeutic interventions.

▶ This study shows very weak correlations between functional health status as determined by a questionnaire completed by parents and exercise testing, ventricular function measurements, and BNP levels in a relatively large cohort of post-Fontan patients. Patients and parents tend to minimize symptoms because they clearly want to be as normal as possible and do not need further invasive procedures or surgery—a clearly universal human phenomenon. What does one do with these data? First, as the authors suggest, pay attention to and evaluate any psychosocial issues and consider rehabilitation programs for all. Second, continue to evaluate intermittently the objective measures of cardiopulmonary function and continue research to try to develop strategies to prevent late clinical deterioration of these patients.

T. P. Graham, Jr, MD

Hypoplastic Left Heart Syndrome

A contemporary comparison of the effect of shunt type in hypoplastic left heart syndrome on the hemodynamics and outcome at Fontan completion
Ballweg JA, Dominguez TE, Ravishankar C, et al (Children's Hosp of Philadelphia, PA; et al)
J Thorac Cardiovasc Surg 140:537-544, 2010

Objective.—We previously reported no difference in morbidity or mortality in a cohort of infants undergoing stage 1 and 2 reconstructions for hypoplastic left heart syndrome with either a modified Blalock—Taussig shunt or a right ventricular to pulmonary artery conduit. This article compares the hemodynamics and perioperative course at the time of the Fontan completion and reports longer-term survival for this cohort.

Methods.—We retrospectively reviewed the hospital records of all patients who underwent stage 1 reconstruction between January 2002 and May 2005 and subsequent surgical procedures, as well as cross-sectional analysis of hospital survivors.

Results.—A total of 176 patients with hypoplastic left heart syndrome or a variant underwent stage 1 reconstruction with either modified Blalock—Taussig shunt (n = 114) or right ventricular to pulmonary artery conduit (n = 62). Shunt selection was at the discretion of the surgeon. The median duration of follow-up was 58 months (range 1—87 months). By Kaplan—Meier analysis, shunt type did not influence survival or freedom from transplant at 5 years (right ventricular to pulmonary artery conduit 61%; 95% confidence limit, 47—72 vs modified Blalock—Taussig shunt 70%; 95% confidence limit, 60—77; $P = .55$). A total of 107 patients underwent Fontan (69 modified Blalock—Taussig shunts and 38 right ventricular to pulmonary artery conduits) with 98% (105/107) early survival. Patients with a right ventricular to pulmonary artery conduit shunt pre-Fontan had higher pulmonary artery (13 ± 8 mm Hg vs 11 ± 3 mm Hg, $P = .026$) and common atrial (8 ± 2.3 mm Hg vs 6.8 ± 2.7 mm Hg, $P = .039$) pressures. By echocardiography evaluation, there was more qualitative moderate to severe ventricular dysfunction (right ventricular to pulmonary artery conduit 31% [12/36] vs modified Blalock—Taussig shunt 17% [11/67], $P = .05$) and moderate to severe atrioventricular valve regurgitation (right ventricular to pulmonary artery conduit 40% [14/35] vs modified Blalock—Taussig shunt 16% [11/67], $P = .01$) in the right ventricular to pulmonary artery conduit group. Use of diuretic therapy, angiotensin-converting enzyme inhibition, reflux medications, and tube feedings were not different between groups. Overall, 5 patients underwent heart transplantation (right ventricular to pulmonary artery conduit 4 vs modified Blalock—Taussig shunt 1, $P = .1$) before Fontan. There was no difference in age or weight at Fontan, bypass time, intensive care unit or hospital length of stay, postoperative pleural effusions, or need for reoperation between groups.

Conclusions.—Interim analyses continue to suggest there is no survival advantage of one shunt type compared with the other. Longer-term follow-up of a randomized patient population remains of utmost importance.

▶ This comparison of right ventricle to pulmonary artery (RV-PA) connection versus Blalock-Taussig shunt for initial palliation of hypoplastic left heart syndrome provides another bit of data indicating the virtual equivalent early and mid-term survival of patients both for initial palliation and for Fontan completion. The data do show more qualitative RV dysfunction in the RV-PA group. I agree with the authors that a longer follow-up of a randomized large population of patients is needed to sort out any small differences in outcome.

T. P. Graham, Jr, MD

Surgical Therapy

Adults or Big Kids: What Is the Ideal Clinical Environment for Management of Grown-Up Patients With Congenital Heart Disease?

Karamlou T, Diggs BS, Ungerleider RM, et al (Oregon Health and Science Univ, Portland; Case Western Reserve Univ, Cleveland, OH; Mary Bridge Children's Hosp and Health Ctr, Tacoma, WA)
Ann Thorac Surg 90:573-579, 2010

Background.—Initiatives to develop Adult Congenital Centers for management of grown-up congenital heart disease (GUCH) patients (aged ≥18 years) have widened without evidence identifying the ideal clinical environment. To elucidate the optimum care paradigm, we investigated whether mortality for patients with GUCH was influenced by the type of hospital where they had surgery, children's specialty hospital (CH) versus general hospital (GH), and by the clinical focus of the surgeon, congenital heart surgery (CHS) or noncongenital (adult acquired) heart surgery (NCHS).

Methods.—In the Nationwide Inpatient Sample 1988–2003, we identified index procedures in patients 18 or more years of age within 12 congenital cardiac disease diagnostic groups. The CHS surgeons were defined as those whose annual practice volume consisted of more than 75% pediatric cardiac operations. Four clinical environment combinations were constructed: CH plus CHS, CH plus NCHS, GH plus CHS, and GH plus NCHS. Years were grouped into quartiles to identify trends in management over time.

Results.—In all, 29,070 operations occurred at GH and 10,971 occurred at CH. Unadjusted in-hospital mortality was lowest in the CH plus CHS environment (1.14%), and highest for in the GH plus CHS environment (9.93%; $p < 0.001$). After risk adjustment for patient factors, the CH plus CHS environment remained optimum, whereas the other three environments increased the risk of in-hospital death (GH plus NCHS: odds ratio 2.4 [95% confidence interval: 0.9 to 6.2]; CH plus NCHS: odds ratio 2.4 [95% confidence interval: 0.9 to 6.5]; GH plus CHS: odds ratio 9.1 [95% confidence interval: 3.0 to 27.6]). Over the study period, there was a dramatic rise in the number of GUCH patients treated in GH plus NCHS and CH plus NCHS, suggesting that the shift in clinical environment was provider specific rather than hospital-type specific.

Conclusions.—Case mix varies with the clinical environment, with more complex procedures performed at GH plus CHS. The optimal environment for complex GUCH surgery involved CHS operating within CH. Initiatives to develop adult congenital centers dedicated to the care of GUCH patients are warranted, and should include congenital heart surgeons operating in a setting mimicking children's hospitals.

▶ In this study, there is an attempt to determine the best setting and surgeon to minimize mortality for congenital heart surgery for the patient with adult congenital heart disease (ACHD). The study indicates that CHD surgeons in a children's hospital do the best but leaves some questions that will require clarification in the future. What are the results for similar high-risk patients in terms of complexity of CHD and/or comorbidities when operated on in children's hospitals versus adult hospitals that are specifically designated as ACHD tertiary care centers? The centers theoretically have duplicated all of the necessary essentials for success as present in children's hospitals, including personnel and equipment. They should have optimal results versus any other centers, but these conditions are difficult to develop because of the paucity of trained ACHD specialists and the added expense of gearing up for ACHD care. Children's hospitals will have to continue to care for many of these patients with ACHD until more ACHD centers are developed.

T. P. Graham, Jr, MD

Birth Before 39 Weeks' Gestation Is Associated With Worse Outcomes in Neonates With Heart Disease
Costello JM, Polito A, Brown DW, et al (Children's Hosp Boston, MA; et al)
Pediatrics 126:e277-e284, 2010

Background.—Recent studies have revealed increased morbidity and mortality rates in term neonates without birth defects who were delivered before 39 weeks of completed gestation. We sought to determine if a similar association exists between gestational age at delivery and adverse outcomes in neonates with critical congenital heart disease, with particular interest in those born at 37 to 38 weeks' gestation.

Patients and Methods.—We studied 971 consecutive neonates who had critical congenital heart disease and a known gestational age and were admitted to our cardiac ICU from 2002 through 2008. Gestational age was stratified into 5 groups: >41, 39 to 40, 37 to 38, 34 to 36, and <34 completed weeks. Multivariate logistic regression analyses were used to evaluate mortality and a composite morbidity variable. Multivariate Poisson regression was used to evaluate duration of ventilation, intensive care, and hospitalization.

Results.—Compared with the referent group of neonates who were delivered at 39 to 40 completed weeks' gestation, neonates born at 37 to 38 weeks had increased mortality (6.9% vs 2.6%; adjusted $P = .049$) and morbidity (49.7% vs 39.7%; adjusted $P = .02$) rates and tended to require a longer duration of mechanical ventilation (adjusted $P = .05$). Patients born after 40 or before 37 weeks also had greater adjusted mortality rates, and those born before 37 weeks had increased morbidity rates and required more days of mechanical ventilation and intensive care.

Conclusions.—For neonates with critical congenital heart disease, delivery before 39 weeks' gestation is associated with greater mortality and morbidity rates and more resource use. With respect to neonatal mortality, the ideal gestational age for delivery of these patients may be 39 to 40 completed weeks.

▶ This article has the intriguing finding that infants with critical congenital heart disease delivered at 39 to 40 weeks had clearly improved outcomes over those delivered earlier or later than this rather short window of optimal timing. I would have predicted that those infants who were delivered between 37 to 38 weeks would not differ in adjusted risk. This kind of thinking without data can be dangerous, as we have to relearn the lesson that practicing without data can be dangerous to your patients' health. Kudos to this group for helping the field to again question any practice that is not data driven.

T. P. Graham, Jr, MD

Biventricular Repair of Atrioventricular Septal Defect With Common Atrioventricular Valve and Double-Outlet Right Ventricle
Devaney EJ, Lee T, Gelehrter S, et al (Univ of Michigan School of Medicine, Ann Arbor; Univ College, London, UK)
Ann Thorac Surg 89:537-543, 2010

Background.—The combination of an atrioventricular septal defect with a common atrioventricular junction guarded by a common valve, and double-outlet right ventricle, is a rare lesion that presents a challenge for surgical repair. This report describes our surgical approach and results in 16 patients undergoing biventricular repair for such a combination of lesions.

Methods.—A retrospective analysis was performed for all patients undergoing biventricular repair of atrioventricular septal defect with common atrioventricular valve and double-outlet right ventricle between 1991 and 2008. Patients with tetralogy of Fallot and common atrioventricular valve were excluded from analysis. Early and actuarial outcomes were evaluated using the χ^2 test for categorical variables and Wilcoxon rank sum for ordinal variables.

Results.—The median age at operation was 16 months. Heterotaxy syndrome was present in 12 of the 16 patients (9 right isomerism and 3 left isomerism), and 6 had concurrent totally anomalous pulmonary venous connections. Primary repair was achieved in 6 patients, and 10 underwent one or more prior operations (most frequently a shunt, banding of the pulmonary trunk, or repair of the anomalous pulmonary venous connections). Enlargement of the ventricular septal defect by resection of the muscular outlet septum was required in 11 patients, in whom the ventricular septal defect emptied entirely or primarily to the inlet of the right ventricle. A conduit was placed from the right ventricle to the pulmonary arteries in 13. There was 1 death before discharge from hospital, 1 late death, and 2 episodes of heart block. Among survivors, follow-up was complete with a median follow-up of 66 months. No patient had late obstruction of the left ventricular outflow tract. The presence of heterotaxy with totally anomalous pulmonary venous connections was associated with combined mortality and significant morbidity ($p = 0.008$).

Conclusions.—Although technically challenging, the surgical repair can be accomplished with acceptable early results. Heterotaxy syndrome, with concurrent anomalous connections of the pulmonary veins, represented the strongest identified risk factor for death or significant complication.

▶ These are excellent results in a very difficult group of patients. The surgery is very difficult and long with pump times of 232 minutes and cross clamp times of 156 minutes. In addition, conduits, complex intracardiac baffles, and ventricular septal defect enlargement were necessary in the majority of patients. I marvel at these results and congratulate the group on their success as well as their ability to do this surgery with incredibly good myocardial protection.

T. P. Graham, Jr, MD

Clinically silent preoperative brain injuries do not worsen with surgery in neonates with congenital heart disease
Block AJ, McQuillen PS, Chau V, et al (Univ of British Columbia, Vancouver, Canada; The Univ of California San Francisco)
J Thorac Cardiovasc Surg 140:550-557, 2010

Objective.—Preoperative brain injury, particularly stroke and white matter injury, is common in neonates with congenital heart disease. The objective of this study was to determine the risk of hemorrhage or extension of preoperative brain injury with cardiac surgery.

Methods.—This dual-center prospective cohort study recruited 92 term neonates, 62 with transposition of the great arteries and 30 with single ventricle physiology, from 2 tertiary referral centers. Neonates underwent brain magnetic resonance imaging scans before and after cardiac surgery.

Results.—Brain injury was identified in 40 (43%) neonates on the preoperative magnetic resonance imaging scan (median 5 days after birth): stroke in 23, white matter injury in 21, and intraventricular hemorrhage in 7. None of the brain lesions presented clinically with overt signs or seizures. Preoperative brain injury was associated with balloon atrial septostomy ($P = .003$) and lowest arterial oxygen saturation ($P = .007$); in a multivariable model, only the effect of balloon atrial septostomy remained significant when adjusting for lowest arterial oxygen saturation. On postoperative magnetic resonance imaging in 78 neonates (median 21 days after birth), none of the preoperative lesions showed evidence of extension or hemorrhagic transformation (0/40 [95% confidence interval: 0%−7%]). The presence of preoperative brain injury was not a significant risk factor for acquiring new injury on postoperative magnetic resonance imaging ($P = .8$).

Conclusions.—Clinically silent brain injuries identified preoperatively in neonates with congenital heart disease, including stroke, have a low risk of progression with surgery and cardiopulmonary bypass and should therefore not delay clinically indicated cardiac surgery. In this multicenter cohort, balloon atrial septostomy remains an important risk factor for preoperative brain injury, particularly stroke.

▶ This is both a reassuring as well as a somewhat frightening report. Thank goodness the brains of these neonates are apparently very resilient and MRI central nervous system (CNS) lesions do not correlate with clinical symptoms in most instances. The lack of progression of MRI lesions with complex cardiac surgery is good news. The long-term follow-up of patients with clinically silent CNS lesions will be extremely important.

T. P. Graham, Jr, MD

Influence of Tracheobronchomalacia on Outcome of Surgery in Children With Congenital Heart Disease and Its Management
Chen Q, Langton-Hewer S, Marriage S, et al (Bristol Royal Hosp for Children, UK)
Ann Thorac Surg 88:1970-1974, 2009

Background.—Patients with complex congenital heart disease associated with tracheobronchomalacia (TBM) remain difficult to manage after cardiac surgery. We studied the influence of TBM on the outcomes of pediatric patients after cardiac surgery for congenital heart disease to determine how to manage these patients better.

Methods.—Twenty-two consecutive pediatric patients who had TBM diagnosed by bronchoscopy or dynamic contrast bronchography before or after cardiac surgery for congenital heart disease during a 5.5-year period were compared with an age- and procedure-matched control group operated on during the same period. Patients diagnosed postoperatively were investigated after a second failed extubation. Patients were managed by oxygen administration, endotracheal suctioning, and positive end-expiratory or continuous positive airway pressure through a nasotracheal tube or tracheostomy.

Results.—There were 4 deaths within 1 year of surgery, all in the study group, with 2 early (neither of which appeared related to TBM) and 2 late. The estimated survival at 5 years was 82% (95% confidence interval, 59% to 93%) for the study group compared with 100% for control patients ($p = 0.012$). All deaths occurred in patients undergoing palliative procedures ($p = 0.0004$), and both children who underwent redo operations died ($p = 0.02$). Postoperatively, 50% of children with TBM required prolonged ventilation and tracheostomy. Compared with control patients the average postoperative ventilation time, pediatric intensive care unit stay, and hospital stay were 6.5, 11.5, and 20 days versus 1, 2, and 6.5 days, respectively ($p < 0.001$).

Conclusions.—Although associated with longer postoperative ventilation time, pediatric intensive care unit stay, hospital stay, and mortality, outcomes after cardiac procedures in children with TBM are acceptable. Palliative and redo procedures in this group of patients are associated with significantly higher risk of death.

▶ Tracheobronchomalacia in conjunction with congenital heart disease can significantly compromise postoperative care and be a common cause of prolonged ventilatory support and need for tracheostomy. These investigators outline a plan of care by incorporating early consideration for this diagnosis in patients who fail early extubation postoperatively and who have not had this diagnosis made before surgery. The good news is that infants will usually grow out of this condition after infancy. Thus, perseverance is the name of the game.

T. P. Graham, Jr, MD

Lesion-specific outcomes in neonates undergoing congenital heart surgery are related predominantly to patient and management factors rather than institution or surgeon experience: A Congenital Heart Surgeons Society Study

Karamlou T, McCrindle BW, Blackstone EH, et al (Hosp for Sick Children, Toronto, Ontario, Canada; Cleveland Clinic Foundation, OH; et al)
J Thorac Cardiovasc Surg 139:569-577, 2010

Objective.—To identify the role of institution and surgeon factors, including case volume and experience, on survival of neonates with complex congenital heart disease.

Methods.—A total of 2421 neonates from 4 groups—transposition of the great arteries (n = 829), pulmonary atresia with intact ventricular septum (n = 408), Norwood (n = 710), and interrupted aortic arch (n = 474)—were prospectively enrolled from Congenital Heart Surgeons Society institutions. Multivariable analysis of risk-adjusted survival was performed for each group, entering each institution or surgeon into the multivariable analysis separately. Institutional performance was defined as [predicted survival − actual survival]. Neutralization of risk factors within each institution was evaluated using complex interaction terms. Institution and surgeon experience, defined by 5 domains (total case volume, total time each operation was performed, cases per year, rank-order of cases, case velocity), were also investigated.

Results.—Institutional performance varied among all groups. Improved outcomes in Norwood and pulmonary atresia with intact ventricular septum were unrelated to any "experience" domains, whereas improved outcomes in transposition of the great arteries were significantly related to increased experience in most domains. No institution enrolling in all 4 studies ranked number 1 in performance for all groups. Neutralization of low birth weight as a risk factor contributed to decreased mortality after Norwood in one institution.

Conclusion.—Survival of neonates with complex congenital heart disease is influenced more by patient and management factors than by institution or surgeon experience. Institutional excellence in managing some diagnostic groups does not indicate similar performance for all diagnostic groups. Weighted risk-adjusted comparisons could provide a mechanism to improve results in institutions with less than optimal outcomes.

▶ This is a complex article with interesting conclusions. First, surgical superiority in 1 complex procedure, such as a Norwood operation, does not carry over to other complex procedures. There appears to be a definite learning curve with the arterial switch—less of an effect with other lesions—a fact that seems counterintuitive. Second, it appears that small patient size and earlier gestational age is a definite risk factor for death in the hypoplastic left heart group; and 1 surgical group stood out by neutralizing this effect—hopefully, other groups can learn from their experience.

T. P. Graham, Jr, MD

Management and long-term outcome of neonatal Ebstein anomaly
Shinkawa T, Polimenakos AC, Gomez-Fifer CA, et al (Univ of Michigan Med School, Ann Arbor)
J Thorac Cardiovasc Surg 139:354-358, 2010

Objective.—The objective of this study was to review the long-term results of symptomatic patients with Ebstein anomaly in the neonatal period.

Methods.—The medical records of 40 neonates with a diagnosis of Ebstein anomaly who were admitted to our institution between January 1988 and June 2008 were retrospectively reviewed. Primary outcomes studied included patient survival and need for reintervention.

Results.—No early intervention was required in 16 of the 40 patients with a hospital survival of 94% (15/16) and no late mortality. The remaining 24 patients underwent surgical intervention in the neonatal period. A shunt alone was performed in 9 patients with an actuarial survival of 88.9% at 1 year and 76.2% at 5 and 10 years. For the patients undergoing intervention on the tricuspid valve, survival estimates for the 11 patients with a right ventricular exclusion procedure were 63.6% at 1, 5, and 10 years and 47.7% at 15 years compared with 25.0% at 1, 5, and 10 years for the 4 patients with tricuspid valve repair. All long-term survivors were in New York Heart Association class I or II, and only 1 patient required antiarrhythmic medication.

Conclusion.—Symptomatic neonates with Ebstein anomaly requiring no intervention or shunting alone have good long-term survival. For patients needing intervention on the tricuspid valve, overall survival is lower. For these patients, right ventricular exclusion may be superior to tricuspid valve repair.

▶ This is an excellent report on the results of management of 40 consecutive neonates with symptomatic Ebstein anomaly. NO surgery was required in

16 (40 %) of the infants; of whom 9 required prostaglandin (PGE1) infusion and then were successfully weaned to an O_2 saturation greater than 75%. Only 3 of these patients have required tricuspid valve (TV) repair to date at 4, 8, and 13 years of age. TV repair in infancy was performed in 4 patients, with only 1 survivor. These authors favor right ventricle exclusion for patients who could not be weaned from PGE1 and hospital care for cyanosis plus congestive heart failure—73 % early survival in this series.

T. P. Graham, Jr, MD

Selective Right Ventricular Unloading and Novel Technical Concepts in Ebstein's Anomaly
Malhotra SP, Petrossian E, Reddy VM, et al (Stanford Univ School of Medicine, CA)
Ann Thorac Surg 88:1975-1981, 2009

Background.—Favorable outcomes in Ebstein's anomaly are predicated on tricuspid valve competence and right ventricular function. Successful valve repair should be aggressively pursued to avoid the morbidity of prosthetic tricuspid valve replacement. We report our experience with valve-sparing intracardiac repair, emphasizing novel concepts and techniques of valve repair supplemented by selective bidirectional Glenn (BDG).

Methods.—Between June 1993 and December 2008, 57 nonneonatal patients underwent Ebstein's anomaly repairs. The median age at operation was 8.1 years. All were symptomatic in New York Heart Association (NYHA) functional class II (n = 38), III (n = 17), or IV (n = 1). Preoperatively, 26 had mild or moderate cyanosis at rest. We used a number of valve reconstructive techniques that differed substantially from those currently described. BDG was performed in 31 patients (55%) who met specific criteria.

Results.—No early or late deaths occurred. At the initial repair, 3 patients received a prosthetic valve. Four patients required reoperation for severe tricuspid regurgitation. Repeat repairs were successful in 2 patients. At follow-up (range, 3 months to 6 years), all patients were acyanotic and in NYHA class I. Tricuspid regurgitation was mild or less in 49 (86%) and moderate in 6 (11%). Freedom from a prosthesis was 91% (52 of 57).

Conclusions.—Following a protocol using BDG for ventricular unloading in selected patients with Ebstein's anomaly can achieve a durable valve-sparing repair using the techniques described. Excellent functional midterm outcomes can be obtained with a selective one and a half ventricle approach to Ebstein's anomaly.

▶ This article details the use of several different methods to improve surgical repair of nonneonatal Ebstein anomaly. These include limited valvuloplasty by different techniques to decrease tricuspid regurgitation, incorporating a strategy to decrease valve diameter to 25 mm for an adult, and achieving appropriately sized diameters normalized for body surface area in younger patients. Part of this strategy included a limited plication of the atrialized right ventricle (RV) in 55 of 57 patients—attempting to stay well away from the true TV annulus and thus prevent the potential distortion of the right coronary artery that has been considered as the probable cause of life-threatening ventricular arrhythmias. This complication has occurred in only one of the patients in this study—treated successfully with an implantable cardioverter defibrillator. Finally, the authors used the bidirectional Glenn in 55% of patients to unload the RV in patients with cyanosis at rest preoperatively, with right atrial pressure > 1.5 times left atrial pressure immediately after bypass, or in an adult in whom they had to make the tricuspid valve (TV) diameter considerably less than 2.5 cm and who exhibits evidence of TV obstruction by transesophageal echocardiography Doppler early after bypass. The early results are very encouraging and hopefully will stand the test of time.

T. P. Graham, Jr, MD

Follow-up and Outcome Studies

Cardiac outcomes after pregnancy in women with congenital heart disease

Balint OH, Siu SC, Mason J, et al (Univ of Toronto Pregnancy and Heart Disease Res Program, Ontario, Canada)
Heart 96:1656-1661, 2010

Objective.—Women with congenital heart disease (CHD) are at risk for adverse cardiac events during pregnancy; however, the risk of events late after pregnancy (late cardiac events; LCE) has not been well studied. A study was undertaken to examine the frequency and determinants of LCE in a large cohort of women with CHD.

Design.—Baseline characteristics and pregnancy were prospectively recorded. LCE (>6 months after delivery) were determined by chart review. Survival analysis was used to determine the risk factors for LCE.

Setting.—A tertiary care referral hospital.

Patients.—The outcomes of 405 pregnancies were studied (318 women; median follow-up 2.6 years).

Main Outcome Measures.—LCE included cardiac death/ arrest, pulmonary oedema, arrhythmia or stroke.

Results.—LCE occurred after 12% (50/405) of pregnancies. The 5-year rate of LCE was higher in women with adverse cardiac events during pregnancy than in those without ($27 \pm 9\%$ vs $15 \pm 3\%$, HR 2.2, p=0.02). Women at highest risk for LCE were those with functional limitations/cyanosis (HR 3.9, 95% CI 1.2 to 13.0), subaortic ventricular dysfunction (HR 3.0, 95% CI 1.4 to 6.6), subpulmonary ventricular dysfunction and/or significant pulmonary regurgitation (HR 3.2, 95% CI 1.6 to 6.6), left heart obstruction (HR 2.6, 95% CI 1.2 to 5.2) and cardiac events before or during pregnancy (HR 2.6, 95% CI 1.3 to 4.9). In women with 0, 1 or >1 risk predictors the 5-year rate of LCE was $7 \pm 2\%$, $23 \pm 5\%$ and $44 \pm 10\%$, respectively (p<0.001).

Conclusions.—In women with CHD, pre-pregnancy maternal characteristics can help to identify women at increased risk for LCE. Adverse cardiac events during pregnancy are important and are associated with an increased risk of LCE.

▶ This report highlights baseline characteristics of women with congenital heart disease (CHD) who developed late adverse cardiac events following pregnancy. As might be expected, functional limitations, cyanosis, ventricular dysfunction, left heart obstruction, and cardiac events before or during pregnancy predicted a higher incidence of laparoscopic cholecystectomies. Women with CHD deserve to know the potential risk for trouble if they do decide to attempt to become pregnant. Most acute CHD centers now have experts in this area who can help them with making informed decisions and obtaining state-of-the-art care during and after pregnancy.

T. P. Graham, Jr, MD

Atrial Septal Defect/Ventricular Septal Defect

Atrial septal defect: waiting for symptoms remains an unsolved medical anachronism
Berger F, Ewert P (German Heart Inst Berlin, Germany)
Eur Heart J 32:531-534, 2011

Background.—Atrial septal defect (ASD) is the most underdiagnosed congenital heart disease among adults. Closure by intervention for selected patients is the standard treatment, chosen because it is less invasive and carries a lower complication rate. A study of a relatively large cohort of adult patients, age 20 to 80 years, showed that defects can be closed successfully by intervention regardless of age with excellent results and no significant complications. Nearly all patients had improved New York Heart Association functional class and rapid right ventricular (RV) remodeling that produced significant improvement in RV measurements and a decline in pulmonary artery (PA) pressure levels for patients whose pressures and resistances had been elevated. The best outcome is seen in patients with no symptoms when the treatment is performed. The consequences that accompany disease untreated until symptoms develop were noted.

Progress of Disease.—Most patients are free of symptoms until their mid 40s or early 50s. The onset of symptoms is a function of time that expresses the duration of the volume load. By age 50 years, patients become clinically symptomatic and suffer a higher incidence of atrial tachyarrhythmia and increased PA pressure values. Closure of the ASD in these patients does not significantly prolong life expectancy or restore sinus rhythm, but it improves symptoms and right heart load conditions. The result is a significant improvement in quality of life that justifies closure at any age. For patients over age 60 years, the restrictive properties of the left ventricular (LV) myocardium with increasing diastolic stiffness can be underestimated or completely obscured by the ASD. The diastolic stiffness can eventually increase pulmonary vascular resistance even after ASD closure. However, most patients who undergo ASD closure even at this age have lower PA pressure levels and pulmonary vascular resistance, perhaps because of the removal of the shunt but also as a result of the remodeling and adaptation of the left ventricle, possibly supported by the delayed and occasionally prolonged course required to normalize PA pressures.

To Be Determined.—Limited data document the results of surgical or catheter closure of ASDs in older patients, especially those who have chronic atrial fibrillation. These elderly patients can safely undergo the intervention and achieve an impressive improvement in hemodynamic measurements, with both the right and left ventricles adapting to the change. The functional class of nearly all patients is dramatically improved because the volume load disappears. Nearly all patients over age 60 years who have chronic atrial fibrillation remain in atrial fibrillation even after ASD closure. However, it is unknown whether the surgical approach combined with a MAZE procedure offers a better approach for these patients. The outcomes for patients with paroxysmal atrial tachycardia is also unknown. Limited data show that patients benefit from closure in terms of preventing arrhythmia, but the possible contribution of an ablational treatment before ASD closure remains unclear. It is also unknown whether the incidence of atrial tachyarrhymia will approximate the statistical frequency seen in the general population if ASD is treated in early childhood. If the incidence of atrial tachyarrhythmia remains elevated, ablational procedures may be of benefit and influence the choice to implant large devices and complicate access to the left atrium long term.

Conclusions.—Currently the interventional approach to ASD is the method of choice. Future directions should include developing totally resorbable devices that can occlude defects up to 40 mm in diameter, which would overcome the theoretical disadvantages of diminishing access to the left atrium with age. Children should be treated before reaching school age if they have a hemodynamically significant ASD. Complete closure of the defect is the goal regardless of which approach is chosen for selected patients. Optimally an intelligent screening program will be developed to detect all patients suffering from asymptomatic but hemodynamically significant ASD before they become adults and develop clinical symptoms. It is important to recognize that ASD is not a benign disease, and waiting for symptoms to develop is not the best approach to treatment.

▶ This is an excellent review of the current state of knowledge regarding the increasing morbidity of a clinically significant atrial septal defect with increasing age. This is one condition that can be not only repaired but also corrected by childhood therapy. Hopefully, with diligent use of a complete cardiovascular exam by each caregiver who provides primary care for children, there will be only rare instances of this missed diagnosis before reaching adolescence. The findings can be subtle, but the use of an electrocardiogram is a relatively inexpensive way to decide whether or not to refer a patient for a cardiac workup. There should be at least a suggestion of right ventricular hypertrophy in any patient with a moderate or large left to right atrial level shunt.

T. P. Graham, Jr, MD

Do Patients With Complete Transposition of the Great Arteries and Severe Pulmonary Hypertension Benefit From an Arterial Switch Operation?

Fan H, Hu S, Zheng Z, et al (Cardiovascular Inst and Fu Wai Hosp, Beijing, China)

Ann Thorac Surg 91:181-186, 2011

Background.—Whether an arterial switch operation benefits patients with transposition of the great arteries and severe pulmonary hypertension (PH) remains controversial. Therefore, we evaluated the relationship between preoperative PH and early and midterm clinical outcomes after an arterial switch procedure.

Methods.—In this retrospective study, 101 consecutive patients with transposition of the great arteries underwent an arterial switch operation between February 2004 and October 2007. Seventy had a ventricular septal defect as well; patients with intact ventricular septum and complicated concomitant abnormities were excluded. Preoperative medical records were reviewed and mean follow-up was 22.4 ± 15.2 months. After sternotomy, we directly measured pulmonary artery pressure before and after instituting extracorporeal circulation. Patients were divided into three groups according to mean pulmonary artery pressure (mPAP): control group (mPAP < 25 mm Hg, n = 23), moderate PH group (mPAP 25 to 50 mm Hg, n = 37), and severe PH group (mPAP ≥ 50 mm Hg, n = 10). Early and midterm results were compared among groups.

Results.—Postoperatively, pulmonary artery pressure of both the moderate and severe PH groups decreased significantly. There were no significant differences in occurrence of postoperative complications or in-hospital mortality in the three groups (control group, 8.7%; moderate PH group, 8.1%; severe PH group, 10%; $p = 0.98$). However, midterm mortality differed significantly (control group, 4.3%; moderate PH group, 2.7%; severe PH group, 40%; $p < 0.01$).

Conclusions.—Patients with transposition of the great arteries and mPAP less than 50 mm Hg can achieve satisfying results after an arterial switch operation. However, even though the operation can decrease pulmonary artery pressure, patients with preoperative mPAP greater than 50 mm Hg still suffer from high midterm mortality.

▶ Although pulmonary artery pressure fell postoperatively in the patients in the moderate and high pressure groups, it did not prevent late complications and increased mortality in the high pressure group. All patients had large ventricular septal defects (VSDs); 70% of the severe pulmonary arterial hypertension group had a patent ductus arteriosus, and all were operated upon after 6 months of age.

When such patients come to operation this late, as the authors suggest, alternate management strategies such as the use of pulmonary vasodilators preoperatively and postoperatively and the use of a VSD patch should be considered.

T. P. Graham, Jr, MD

Aortic Valve Disorders

Assessment of Left Ventricular Endocardial Fibroelastosis in Fetuses With Aortic Stenosis and Evolving Hypoplastic Left Heart Syndrome
McElhinney DB, Vogel M, Benson CB, et al (Children's Hosp Boston, MA; Brigham and Women's Hosp and Harvard Med School, Boston, MA)
Am J Cardiol 106:1792-1797, 2010

Systematic evaluation of left ventricular (LV) endocardial fibroelastosis (EFE) in the fetus has not been reported. The role of EFE in the pre- and postnatal evolution of hypoplastic left heart disease, and the implications of EFE for outcomes after prenatal intervention for fetal aortic stenosis with evolving hypoplastic left heart syndrome have also not been determined. A 4-point grading system (0-3) was devised for the assessment of fetal LV echogenicity, which was presumed to be due to EFE. Two reviewers independently graded EFE on the preintervention echocardiograms of fetuses treated with in utero aortic valvuloplasty for evolving hypoplastic left heart syndrome from 2000 to 2008. Intra- and interobserver reproducibility was determined for the EFE grade and characterization of related echocardiographic features. The relations among EFE severity, other left heart anatomic and physiologic variables, and postintervention outcomes were analyzed. The assessment and grading of EFE was possible for both observers in all 74 fetuses studied. By consensus, the EFE severity was grade 1 in 31 patients, grade 2 in 32, and grade 3 in 11. Fetuses with mild (grade 1) EFE had significantly greater maximum instantaneous aortic stenosis gradients (e.g., higher LV pressures) and less globular LV geometry than patients with grade 2 or 3 EFE on preintervention echocardiogram. The severity of EFE was not associated with the size of the aortic valve or LV. From preintervention to late gestation, the time-indexed change in LV end-diastolic volume was significantly greater in fetuses with grade 1 EFE than those with more severe EFE. Incorporation of EFE severity into our previously published threshold score improved the sensitivity and positive predictive value for the postnatal biventricular outcomes. In conclusion, echocardiographic grading of EFE is possible, with reasonable intra- and interobserver reliability in midgestation fetuses with evolving hypoplastic left heart syndrome. EFE severity corresponded to some indexes of left heart size, geometry, and function and with the probability of a biventricular outcome postnatally. Additional experience and external validation of the EFE grading scoring system are necessary.

▶ This is another step in prenatal evaluation of aortic stenosis and endocardial fibroelastosis (EFE) for outcome. The severity of EFE was associated with less growth of the left ventricle and when added to the ability to predict a univentricular versus biventricular outcome. These studies hopefully can aid in determining the etiology of EFE, and if successful, in utero valvuloplasty can prevent or ameliorate the effects of this complication on outcome.

T. P. Graham, Jr, MD

Current Expectations for Surgical Repair of Isolated Ventricular Septal Defects

Scully BB, Morales DLS, Zafar F, et al (Texas Children's Hosp, Houston)
Ann Thorac Surg 89:544-551, 2010

Background.—Ventricular septal defect (VSD) is the most commonly recognized congenital heart defect. With the development of device closure for intracardiac defects, we sought to evaluate current expectations for surgical closure of isolated VSD.

Methods.—Between January 1, 2000, and December 31, 2006, 215 patients underwent isolated VSD repair at a median age of 10 months (range, 20 days to 18 years) and a median weight of 7 kg (range, 2 to 66 kg). The following VSD types were found: 172 perimembranous (80%), 28 supracristal (13%), 6 inlet (3%), and 9 muscular (4%). One hundred eight patients (50%) had evidence of congestive heart failure or failure to thrive preoperatively. Thirty-one patients (14%) had aortic valve cusp prolapse, and 63 (29%) had genetic abnormalities.

Results.—Incidence of significant postoperative complications was extremely low. No patient underwent reoperation for a residual VSD. None had complete heart block. One operative mortality (0.5%) and 2 late deaths (0.9%) occurred. Median postoperative hospital length of stay was 5 days (range, 2 to 187 days). In the immediate postoperative period, 6 patients (2.8%) required reoperation. No patients were discharged on antiarrhythmic agents, had complete heart block, or required permanent pacing. At mean follow-up of 2.1 ± 2.0 years, 99.5% (211 of 212) of patients were asymptomatic from a cardiac standpoint. None exhibited greater than mild new-onset tricuspid valve regurgitation. No aortic valve injuries occurred.

Conclusions.—Surgical closure of isolated VSD is a safe, effective therapy. Risk of death, complete heart block, and reoperation is minimal. As new technologies for VSD closure evolve, results such as these should be considered when evaluating patients, choosing therapeutic options, and counseling families.

▶ This study provides excellent results for surgical ventricular septal defect (VSD) closure and excellent benchmarks for surgical or interventional closure. Hopefully, long-term follow-up data can be obtained from this group for a more complete picture of any further implications of the questions of tricuspid regurgitation, small residual VSDs, aortic regurgitation, and neurological/developmental findings.

T. P. Graham, Jr, MD

Coarctation, Interrupted Arch

Balloon expandable stent implantation for native and recurrent coarctation of the aorta—prospective computed tomography assessment of stent integrity, aneurysm formation and stenosis relief
Chakrabarti S, Kenny D, Morgan G, et al (Bristol Royal Hosp for Children and Bristol Royal Infirmary, UK)
Heart 96:1212-1216, 2010

Background.—Stenting for aortic coarctation is known to be effective in the medium term. Aneurysm formation following stent implantation is a recognised complication. However, data regarding aortic wall injury and stent integrity following stent placement are sparse.

Objectives.—We report comprehensive clinical, echocardiographic and prospective CT follow-up data following stenting for aortic coarctation from a single centre.

Methods.—Full data analysis of all patients undergoing balloon expandable stent implantation and follow-up procedures in a single tertiary congenital cardiac unit.

Results.—Between October 2002 and April 2008, we performed 102 coarctation stent procedures on 88 patients. Median age was 20.6 years (range 8.5—65) and median weight 65 kg (range 34—101). 94 stents (26 covered) were implanted. 12 procedures were re-dilatations. Stenting resulted in a reduction of the gradient across the site of coarctation, from a median of 20 mm Hg to 4 mm Hg. There were no procedure-related deaths. Four patients had immediate complications (one requiring emergency surgery). During median follow-up of 34.5 months (range 4.2—72.8), two patients had late complications requiring additional stent procedures. Follow-up CT data are available in 84 patients with MRI in one patient (96.5%). Only one patient developed a procedure-related aortic aneurysm. All stent fractures (n = 7) occurred with a single stent design.

Conclusions.—Stenting for aortic coarctation and recoarctation is effective with low immediate complication rates. CT is useful in the longer term for assessment of stent integrity and post-procedural aneurysm formation. Overall incidence of post-procedural aneurysm is rare and stent fractures were not seen with newer generation stents.

▶ This is a detailed study regarding the use and follow-up of 88 patients who had stenting of native coarctation (n = 45) or recoarctations with covered stents used in 28% of cases. This procedure is not for the fainthearted; immediate complications occurred in 4 cases, including embolization of the stent, ventricular fibrillation, aortic dissection, and rupture. Only 1 patient required emergency surgery. There were no procedure-related deaths. There was only 1 aneurysm. Follow-up CT studies were available in 84/88. Stent fractures (n = 7) were all present with the Genesis stent, which is no longer used. Covered stents were used to treat stent fractures and 1 aneurysm. Follow-up by CT is now the procedure of choice because MRI studies have significant dropout of images due to stent artifact, which can mask stenosis or aneurysm. This is unfortunate because most patients are relatively young and repeated CT studies could increase the risk of malignancy. Hopefully, someone is working on a stent that does not cause artifact or an MRI modification that does not have such a distortion from these stents.

T. P. Graham, Jr, MD

Do High-Risk Infants Have a Poorer Outcome From Primary Repair of Coarctation? Analysis of 192 Infants Over 20 Years
McGuinness JG, Elhassan Y, Lee SY, et al (Our Lady's Childrens Hosp, Crumlin, Dublin, Ireland)
Ann Thorac Surg 90:2023-2027, 2010

Background.—Balloon angioplasty for infant coarctation is associated with a high recurrence rate, making operative repair the gold standard for low-risk infants. Debate exists as to whether high-risk infants might be better served with primary angioplasty. We compared the outcome in high-risk versus low-risk infants over 20 years, in a center that always used surgical repair as the primary intervention.

Methods.—Of 192 infants from 1986 to 2005, 56 were considered "high-risk," defined as requiring prostaglandin infusion together with either epinephrine infusion for 24 hours preoperatively, or ventilation and milrinone infusion for 24 hours preoperatively. All high-risk patients had a period of ventricular dysfunction prior to surgery, ranging from mild to severe. Outcomes were compared using Bonferroni comparison of means or the Fischer exact test as appropriate.

Results.—Although the high-risk patients were smaller (3.3 ± 0.1 vs 4.2 ± 0.2 kg, $p < 0.01$), younger (18 ± 4 vs 57 ± 7 days, $p < 0.01$), and more often required a concomitant pulmonary artery band (25% vs 15%, $p = 0.05$), their cross-clamp times were the same as the low-risk patients (18.9 ± 0.9 vs 18.0 ± 0.4 minutes, $p = 0.27$) and there was no difference in postoperative morbidity (7% vs 3%, $p = 0.11$). However, there was a trend toward higher perioperative mortality (7% vs 2%, $p = 0.07$). When compared with the published studies of primary angioplasty in comparable high-risk infants, the mortality rate in our surgically treated high-risk group is much lower. Additionally, only 11% of our high-risk group required reintervention, with two-thirds treated successfully with a single angioplasty at 3.8 ± 2.2 years later, far lower than recurrence rates with primary angioplasty.

Conclusions.—We propose that primary surgical repair of coarctation in infants who are high risk should be the primary treatment, with angioplasty reserved for recurrent coarctation.

▶ This study indicates that surgery provides better results for primary repair for high-risk infants with coarctation of the aorta. Comparisons were made for the majority present in Ireland from 1986 to 2005 with all operations performed in 1 institution by 1 of 3 surgeons. Comparisons of low- and high-risk infants were made with similar results in cross-clamp times and perioperative morbidity and minimal differences (Ns) in mortality. Only 11% of high-risk infants required reintervention with the majority of those having a single angioplasty. These results are quite good; all were done from a left lateral thoracotomy. Comparisons with studies published in the last 10 years with primary angioplasty for infants showed a much higher recurrence rate for coarctation and higher morbidity, particularly with decreased or absent femoral pulses. The current plan in many institutions includes primary repair of associated lesions, such as a ventricular septal defect, at the initial operation. Hopefully, 1 of these groups can provide comparisons of results for such a protocol for similar high-risk patients. The Irish infants appear to be getting excellent care currently with this protocol.

T. P. Graham, Jr, MD

Cardiomyopathy

Percutaneous closure of hypertensive ductus arteriosus

Zabal C, García-Montes JA, Buendía-Hernández A, et al (Natl Inst of Cardiology "Ignacio Chavez", Mexico City)
Heart 96:625-629, 2010

Background.—The Amplatzer duct occluder (ADO) has been used with success to close large patent ductus arteriosus (PDA), but some problems exist especially with hypertensive PDAs, such as incomplete closure, haemolysis, left pulmonary artery stenosis, obstruction of the descending aorta and progressive pulmonary vascular disease.

Methods and Results.—We analysed a group of 168 patients with isolated PDA and pulmonary artery systolic pressure (PSAP) $\geq$50 mm Hg. Mean age was 10.3 $\pm$ 14.3 years (median 3.9), PDA diameter was 6.4 $\pm$ 2.9 mm (median 5.9), PASP was 63.5 $\pm$ 16.2 mm Hg (median 60), Qp/Qs was 2.7 $\pm$ 1.2 (median 2.5), total pulmonary resistance index (PRI) was 3.69 $\pm$ 2.15 (median 3.35) and vascular PRI was 2.73 $\pm$ 1.72 (median 2.37). We used ADOs in 145 (86.3%) cases, Amplatzer muscular ventricular septal defect occluders (AMVSDO) in 18 (10.7%), Amplatzer septal occluders (ASO) in three (1.8%) and the Gianturco-Grifka device in two (1.2%) cases. Device diameter was 106.3% $\pm$ 51% higher than PDA diameter. PASP decreased after occlusion to 42.5 $\pm$ 13.3 mm Hg (p<0.00001). Immediately after closure, no or trivial shunt was present in 123 (74.5%) cases. Immediate complications were device embolisation in five (3%) cases and descending aortic obstruction in one case. The overall success rate was 98.2%. Follow-up in 145 (86.3%) cases for 37.1 $\pm$ 24 months (median 34.1) showed further decrease of the PASP to 30.1 $\pm$ 7.7 mm Hg (p<0.0001).

Conclusions.—Percutaneous treatment of hypertensive PDA is safe and effective. ADO works well for most cases, but sometimes other devices

(MVSDO or ASO) have to be used. When cases are selected adequately, pulmonary pressures decrease immediately and continue to fall with time.

▶ This is a relatively large study of catheter-based closure of hypertensive patent ductus arteriosus (PDAs) with quite good overall results. The authors chose not to close 3 PDAs because of high pulmonary vascular resistance, no response to test occlusion, and unfavorable anatomy on pulmonary wedge anatomy; these patients are being treated with Bosentan and plans are to recatheterize them in the future to assess for possible improvement in the results of test occlusion. A number of different devices were used for closure. This is a real tour de force; anyone attempting this therapy would do well to carefully read this report. It certainly would seem to be the treatment of choice over surgery if an experienced group of congenital heart defect interventionalists are available.

T. P. Graham, Jr, MD

Imaging

Dilated cardiomyopathy in children with ventricular preexcitation: the location of the accessory pathway is predictive of this association

Udink ten Cate FEA, Kruessell MA, Wagner K, et al (Univ Hosp of Cologne, Germany; Centre Hospitalier de Luxembourg)
J Electrocardiol 43:146-154, 2010

Background.—Ventricular preexcitation may be associated with dilated cardiomyopathy, even in the absence of recurrent and incessant tachycardia.

Methods.—This report describes the clinical and electrophysiologic characteristics of 10 consecutive children (6 males), with median age of 8 years (range, 1-17 years), who presented with dilated cardiomyopathy and overt ventricular preexcitation on the 12-lead electrocardiogram. Incessant tachycardia as the cause of dilated cardiomyopathy could be excluded. Coronary angiography, right ventricular endomyocardial biopsy (4/10 patients), and metabolic and microbiologic screening were nondiagnostic.

Results.—The electrocardiograms suggested right-sided pathways in all patients. A right-sided accessory pathway was demonstrated in 8 patients during invasive electrophysiologic study (superoparaseptal, n = 5; septal, n = 2; fasciculoventricular, n = 1). All pathways were successfully ablated (radiofrequency ablation in 7, cryoablation in 1). Two patients had spontaneous loss of ventricular preexcitation during follow-up. Left ventricular (LV) function completely recovered after a loss of preexcitation in all patients.

Conclusions.—Right-sided accessory pathways with overt ventricular preexcitation and LV dyssynchrony may cause dilated cardiomyopathy. An association between such pathways and dilated cardiomyopathy is suggested by the rapid normalization of ventricular function and reverse LV remodeling after a loss of ventricular preexcitation.

▶ This represents another potential cause of cardiomyopathy that appears treatable with excellent results. We had several patients who questionably fit this profile a number of years ago, but we never were certain of the association and the causative nature of the preexcitation.

T. P. Graham, Jr, MD

Recommendations for cardiovascular magnetic resonance in adults with congenital heart disease from the respective working groups of the European Society of Cardiology
Kilner PJ, Geva T, Kaemmerer H, et al (Royal Brompton Hosp, London, UK; Childen's Hosp Boston, MA; Dept of Pediatric Cardiology and Congenital Heart Disease, Deutsches Herzzentrum, Munich, Germany; et al)
Eur Heart J 31:794-805, 2010

This paper aims to provide information and explanations regarding the clinically relevant options, strengths, and limitations of cardiovascular magnetic resonance (CMR) in relation to adults with congenital heart disease (CHD). Cardiovascular magnetic resonance can provide assessments of anatomical connections, biventricular function, myocardial viability, measurements of flow, angiography, and more, without ionizing radiation. It should be regarded as a necessary facility in a centre specializing in the care of adults with CHD. Also, those using CMR to investigate acquired heart disease should be able to recognize and evaluate previously unsuspected CHD such as septal defects, anomalously connected pulmonary veins, or double-chambered right ventricle. To realize its full potential and to avoid pitfalls, however, CMR of CHD requires training and experience. Appropriate pathophysiological understanding is needed to evaluate cardiovascular function after surgery for tetralogy of Fallot, transposition of the great arteries, and after Fontan operations. For these and other complex CHD, CMR should be undertaken by specialists committed to long-term collaboration with the clinicians and surgeons managing the patients. We provide a table of CMR acquisition protocols in relation to CHD categories as a guide towards appropriate use of this uniquely versatile imaging modality.

▶ This is an excellent summary with a lot of details about the use of cardiovascular magnetic resonance in adult congenital heart disease patients. This modality is quite an attractive option for diagnosis and management of these patients in situations where less expensive options do not provide the data required. It does not provide the very important information on clinical indications for these studies but refers to a previous publication for this essential information.[1]

T. P. Graham, Jr, MD

Reference

1. Pennell DJ, Sechtem UP, Higgins CB, et al. Clinical indications for cardiovascular magnetic resonance (CMR): Consensus Panel report. *Eur Heart J.* 2004;25: 1940-1965.

Interventional Catheterization

Cardiac Operations After Patent Ductus Arteriosus Stenting in Duct-Dependent Pulmonary Circulation

Vida VL, Speggiorin S, Maschietto N, et al (Univ of Padua, Italy)
Ann Thorac Surg 90:605-609, 2010

Background.—Stenting of the patent ductus arteriosus (PDA) has been recently introduced to palliate patients with duct-dependent pulmonary circulations. We evaluated the surgical outcome of patients who had a previous PDA stent, focusing on their pulmonary arteries status.

Methods.—This study included 15 patients (11 boys, 4 girls) who underwent cardiac operations after PDA stenting between August 2004 and April 2009. Outcomes included hospital mortality, morbidity, and need for reintervention or operation on the PDA and on the pulmonary artery branches.

Results.—Thirteen patients underwent elective cardiac operations at a median of 11 months (range, 0.3 months to 3.7 years) from PDA stenting. Two patients underwent emergency operations due to stent migration during percutaneous positioning. Six patients (46%) required a preoperative interventional cardiology procedure, including PDA stent dilatation in 5 and multiple left pulmonary artery dilatations in 1. During elective surgical repair, PDA stents were completely retrieved in 3 patients (23%) and partially removed in 10 (77%) due to the fusion of the stent to the vascular wall. Seven patients (53.8%) required surgical pulmonary artery plasty. One in-hospital death (6%) occurred after an emergency operation. Median follow-up was 16.7 months (range, 1 month to 2.5 years). Two late deaths (14%) occurred at 4 and 9 months. Four patients required additional interventional procedures on the left pulmonary artery after surgical repair.

Conclusions.—Operations after PDA stenting are safe and low-risk. The presence of PDA stents requires additional surgical maneuvers on pulmonary arteries in near half of the patients, and postoperative interventions can be required.

▶ Patent ductus arteriosus stenting in complex congenital heart disease appears to be experiencing a renewal in interest probably because of the increased expertise of interventionalists and the hybrid procedure proponents in a number of centers. It is not for the faint of heart as stent migration, tissue proliferation at the duct site and/or left pulmonary artery, and significant difficulty at stent removal at the time of later surgery are some of the issues to deal with. Despite these problems, it may become a procedure of choice for many complex conditions in the future.

T. P. Graham, Jr, MD

Clinical, echocardiographic and histopathologic findings in nine patients with surgically explanted ASD/PFO devices: Do we know enough about the healing process in humans?
Vogt MO, Kühn A, Hörer J, et al (Technical Univ, Munich, Germany; et al)
Int J Cardiol 147:398-404, 2011

Background.—Atrial septal defects (ASD) and persistent foramen ovale (PFO) are managed in increasing numbers by catheter interventions as an attractive alternative to surgery. Early complications have been described in clinical series whereas late complications are rare. No series are reported with clinical, echocardiographic and histological data.

Methods and Results.—We collected clinical, echocardiographic, and histolological data of nine patients with surgically explanted devices. Occlusion devices were explanted after a mean interval of 3.4 ± 2.4 years (range 0.9–8.3). Indications were recurrent thromboembolic events in five, residual shunt/dislocation in three, and growing mass on echocardiography despite oral anticoagulation in one patient. Two patients suffered potentially life threatening events due to coronary embolism. One of them had to be resuscitated due to ventricular fibrillation. Histologically, residues of superficial thrombus formation could be demonstrated in two of the devices. In another patient, hyperplastic tissue formation was related to a local inflammatory process but not to a thrombus as suspected by echocardiography.

Conclusion.—Late complications after device implantation may occur up to 8 years after device implantation and may be potentially life threatening. Echocardiographic controls should be prolonged beyond the first year after implantation and every explanted device should be histologically worked up in an experienced center. Up to now, the mechanisms of late thrombogenesis are not fully understood.

▶ This comprehensive report of late complications of percutaneous delivered atrial septal defects (ASD) devices from 4 different manufacturers merit attention to the need for long-term follow-up despite early success without any sign to predict late problems. Recurrent coronary and/or cerebral embolism with catastrophic results can occur. The authors should be commended for their extensive workups of the explanted material. Again, there is no free lunch; despite outstanding success with percutaneous ASD closure, some patients will show up with late complications. Perhaps there are genetic differences that predispose this small number of patients to these complications. In the meantime, diligence in continued follow-up of patients with an implanted device with a high index of suspicion for abnormalities around the implanted device with any new arrhythmia, possible embolic episode, and/or change in ventricular function is in order.

T. P. Graham, Jr, MD

Kawasaki Disease

Increased Detection Rate of Kawasaki Disease Using New Diagnostic Algorithm, Including Early Use of Echocardiography
Heuclin T, the Hospital Network for Evaluating the Management of Common Childhood Diseases (Lille Univ Hosp, France; et al)
J Pediatr 155:695-699, 2009

Objective.—To determine the incidence of Kawasaki disease (KD) in Northern France by using new American Heart Association (AHA) criteria.

Study Design.—A 1-year prospective multicenter cohort study was performed in all pediatric departments. Patients <18 years old, who were admitted for prolonged but initially unexplained fever or suspected KD were included. All patients received the standard treatment considered appropriate by their physicians. A descriptive analysis and comparison of patients with complete and incomplete forms of KD were performed. The incidence of confirmed cases of KD (complete and incomplete forms) was calculated.

Results.—Seventy-seven children were included (39 in whom KD was diagnosed). Of the patients with KD, 26 (67%) met the classic AHA case definition, and 7 (18%) had incomplete KD. Cardiac ultrasound scanning was helpful in the diagnosis of 6 of 7 patients with incomplete KD (86%). The final incidence of confirmed KD was 9 of 100 000 children <5 years of age. In 6 children (15%) the diagnosis of KD was uncertain, but they were successfully treated for it. Coronary disease was identified in 48% of patients with confirmed KD.

Conclusion.—The incidence of KD is higher than previously reported, in part because earlier reports did not include incomplete forms. New AHA criteria (laboratory tests and early echocardiography) were helpful for the diagnosis of incomplete forms of KD.

▶ This study appears to affirm the decision of the newer American Heart Association criteria for diagnosis of Kawasaki disease (KD) in the absence of the complete classic picture. This change in diagnostic criteria hopefully will lead to earlier treatment of KD and reduced incidence of severe and long-standing coronary complications.

T. P. Graham, Jr, MD

Medical Therapy

Cardiovascular Abnormalities, Interventions, and Long-term Outcomes in Infantile Williams Syndrome

Collins RT II, Kaplan P, Somes GW, et al (Univ of Pennsylvania School of Medicine, Philadelphia; The Univ of Tennessee Health Sciences Ctr Dept of Preventive Medicine, Memphis, TN)

J Pediatr 156:253-258, 2010

Objective.—To determine the prevalence of cardiovascular abnormalities (CVA) and outcomes in patients with Williams syndrome presenting before 1 year of age.

Study Design.—A retrospective review was undertaken of consecutive patients with WS at our institution from January 1, 1980, through December 31, 2007. WS was diagnosed by an experienced medical geneticist and/or by fluorescence in situ hybridization. CVA were diagnosed with the use of echocardiography, cardiac catheterization, or computerized tomographic angiography. Freedom from intervention was determined using Kaplan-Meier analysis.

Results.—The study group was 129 patients with CVA. Age at presentation was 127 ± 116 days, with follow-up of 8.0 ± 7.5 years (0 to 42 years). The most common lesions were peripheral pulmonary artery stenosis (62%) and supravalvar aortic stenosis (57%). Other CVA were common. CV interventions were performed in 29%, with 58% of those before 1 year. Freedom from intervention was 85%, 73%, and 66% at 1, 5, and 25 years, respectively. Four patients died.

Conclusions.—CVA are the most common manifestations of infantile Williams syndrome and occur with greater frequency than previously reported. In those with CVA, interventions are common and usually occur by 5 years of age. Most of these patients do not require intervention on long-term follow-up, and overall mortality is low.

▶ This relatively large review of cardiovascular abnormalities in infants with Williams Syndrome provides some new insight and reinforces some other concepts. As others have found, mild and some moderate peripheral pulmonary arterial stenoses frequently improve or resolve. In addition, some patients with localized mild supravalvar aortic stenosis improved or resolved. Coronary anomalies were relatively common at 11% and can be lethal. Males and females were affected equally in terms of severity in contrast to previous reports of worse prognosis in males.

T. P. Graham, Jr, MD

Miscellaneous

Franklin H. Epstein Lecture. Cardiac Development and Implications for Heart Disease
Epstein JA (Univ of Pennsylvania School of Medicine, Philadelphia)
N Engl J Med 363:1638-1647, 2010

Recent studies have revealed a surprising number of previously unappreciated aspects of cardiac morphogenesis that are relevant to both congenital and adult cardiovascular disease. It is now clear that cell populations extrinsic to the primary heart field and the linear heart tube of the embryo contribute to the development of the mature heart and modulate cardiac morphogenesis. These cell populations include neural-crest cells, the cells arising from a second heart field, and epicardial cells. The full developmental potential and unique defining characteristics of various cardiac progenitor cells are only partially known, and specific stages of the progressive lineage restriction of these cardiac progenitors require further characterization. The ability to expand cardiac progenitor populations, either in situ or ex vivo, and to direct cell fate will have important implications for regenerative cardiovascular therapies. The cell biology of myocyte maturation and the effects of the transition from the fetal heart to the adult heart remain areas of investigation that are likely to inform our understanding of heart failure. Studies of the regulation of gene-expression programs in the heart are likely to suggest new therapeutic targets for cardiovascular disease.

▶ This is an outstanding review of cardiac development including new concepts, new avenues for research, and potential avenues for bold new approaches for treatment of both acquired and congenital cardiac disease. It should be required reading for all cardiology trainees as well as their mentors.

T. P. Graham, Jr, MD

Cardiovascular Anomalies in Turner Syndrome: Spectrum, Prevalence, and Cardiac MRI Findings in a Pediatric and Young Adult Population
Kim HK, Gottliebson W, Hor K, et al (Cincinnati Children's Hosp Med Ctr, OH)
AJR Am J Roentgenol 196:454-460, 2011

Objective.—Turner syndrome affects one in 2,500 girls and women and is associated with cardiovascular anomalies. Visualizing the descending thoracic aorta in adults with Turner syndrome with echocardiography is difficult. Therefore, cardiac MRI is the preferred imaging modality for surveillance. Our goals were to use cardiac MRI describe the spectrum and frequency of cardiovascular abnormalities and to evaluate aortic dilatation and associated abnormalities in pediatric patients with Turner syndrome.

Materials and Methods.—The cases of 51 patients with Turner syndrome (median age, 18.4 years; range, 6—36 years) were evaluated with cardiac MRI. The characteristics assessed included aortic structure, elongation of the transverse aortic arch, aortic diameter at multiple locations, and coarctation of the aorta (CoA). Additional evaluations were made for presence of bicuspid aortic valve (BAV), and partial anomalous pulmonary venous return (PAPVR). Associations between the cardiac MRI data and the following factors were assessed: age, karyotype, body surface area, blood pressure, and ventricular sizes and function.

Results.—Sixteen patients (31.4%) had elongation of the transverse aortic arch, eight (15.7%) had CoA, 20 (39.2%) had BAV, and eight (15.7%) had PAPVR. Aortic dilatation was most common at the aortic sinus (30%). Elongation of the transverse aortic arch was associated with CoA ($p < 0.01$) and BAV ($p < 0.05$). Patients with elongation of the transverse aortic arch had dilated aortic sinus ($p < 0.05$). Patients with PAPVR had increased right heart mass ($p < 0.05$), increased ratio of main pulmonary artery to aortic valve blood flow ($p = 0.0014$), and increased right ventricular volume ($p < 0.05$).

Conclusion.—Cardiovascular anomalies in pediatric patients with Turner syndrome include aortic abnormalities and PAPVR. The significant association between elongation of the transverse aortic arch and CoA, BAV, and aortic sinus dilatation may contribute to increased risk of aortic dissection. The presence of PAPVR can be hemodynamically significant. These findings indicate that periodic cardiac MRI screening of persons with Turner syndrome is beneficial.

▶ This moderate-sized cohort of patients with Turner syndrome provides a very useful spectrum of the prevalence of cardiovascular abnormalities and clear evidence that MRI studies in asymptomatic patients is a valuable procedure. The differential of partial anomalous pulmonary venous return and quantification of degree of left to right shunting as well as data on degree of aortic dilatation are important findings to plan future follow-up and cardiovascular care.

T. P. Graham, Jr, MD

Cerebrovascular accidents in adult patients with congenital heart disease
Hoffmann A, Chockalingam P, Balint OH, et al (Univ Hosp, Basel, Switzerland; Academic Med Ctr, Amsterdam, Netherlands; Univ Health Network/Toronto General Hosp, Canada; et al)
Heart 96:1223-1226, 2010

Objective.—To investigate the prevalence and characteristics of cerebrovascular accidents (CVA) in a large population of adults with congenital heart disease (CHD).

Methods and Results.—In a retrospective analysis of aggregated European and Canadian databases a total population of 23 153 patients with CHD was followed up to the age of 16—91 years (mean 36.4 years). Among them, 458 patients (2.0%) had one or more CVA, with an estimated event rate of 0.05% per patient-year. Permanent neurological sequelae were noted in 116 patients (25.3%). The prevalence of CVA in selected diagnostic categories was as follows: open atrial septal defect 93/2351 (4.0%); closed atrial or ventricular septal defect 57/4035 (1.4%); corrected tetralogy of Fallot 52/2196 (2.4%); Eisenmenger physiology 24/467 (5.1%); other cyanotic 50/215 (23.3%); mechanical prostheses (29/882 (3.3%). Associated conditions in patients with CVA were absence of sinus rhythm (25%), transvenous pacemakers (7%), endocarditis (2%), cardiac surgery (11%) and catheter intervention (2%), but with the exception of absent sinus rhythm these were not significantly more prevalent in patients with CVA.

Conclusion.—CVA are a major contributor to morbidity in this young population despite absence of classical cardiovascular risk factors. Although the prevalence of CVA in patients with CHD appears low, it is 10—100 times higher than expected in control populations of comparable age. Residua occur in a strong minority of patients. The subjects at highest risk are those patients with CHD with cyanotic lesions, in whom the prevalence is over 10-fold above the average.

▶ This retrospective analysis of cerebrovascular accident (CVA) prevalence in adults with congenital heart disease (CHD) shows that these patients have a risk of 1 in 50 of having a CVA in early or midlife. This risk is doubled in several instances such as open atrial septal defect and up to 10 times higher in certain cyanotic groups. These data are very important to be cognizant of by all adult CHD providers in order to try to minimize risk where possible and make patients aware of the possibility of these potentially devastating events in order to try to ensure their cooperation in preventive strategies.

T. P. Graham, Jr, MD

Comparison of Clinical Presentations and Outcomes Between Patients With *TGFBR2* and *FBN1* Mutations in Marfan Syndrome and Related Disorders

Attias D, Stheneur C, Roy C, et al (Hôpital Bichat, Paris, France; et al)
Circulation 120:2541-2549, 2009

Background.—TGFBR2 mutations were recognized recently among patients with a Marfan-like phenotype. The associated clinical and prognostic spectra remain unclear.

Methods and Results.—Clinical features and outcomes of 71 patients with a TGFBR2 mutation (TGFBR2 group) were compared with 50 age-and sex-matched unaffected family members (control subjects) and 243 patients harboring FBN1 mutations (FBN1 group). Aortic dilatation was present in a similar proportion of patients in both the TGFBR2 and FBN1 groups (78% versus 79%, respectively) but was highly variable.

The incidence and average age for thoracic aortic surgery (31% versus 27% and 35 ± 16 versus 39 ± 13 years, respectively) and aortic dissection (14% versus 10% and 38 ± 12 versus 39 ± 9 years) were also similar in the 2 groups. Mitral valve involvement (myxomatous, prolapse, mitral regurgitation) was less frequent in the TGFBR2 than in the FBN1 group (all $P < 0.05$). Aortic dilatation, dissection, or sudden death was the index event leading to genetic diagnosis in 65% of families with *TGFBR2* mutations, versus 32% with *FBN1* mutations ($P = 0.002$). The rate of death was greater in TGFBR2 families before diagnosis but similar once the disease had been recognized. Most pregnancies were uneventful (without death or aortic dissection) in both TGFBR2 and FBN1 families (38 of 39 versus 213 of 217; $P = 1$). Seven patients (10%) with a *TGFBR2* mutation fulfilled international criteria for Marfan syndrome, 3 of whom presented with features specific for Loeys-Dietz syndrome.

Conclusions.—Clinical outcomes appear similar between treated patients with *TGFBR2* mutations and individuals with *FBN1* mutations. Prognosis depends on clinical disease expression and treatment rather than simply the presence of a *TGFBR2* gene mutation.

▶ These authors provide data indicating the importance of genetic testing and early detection of aortic abnormalities in patients in whom the recently recognized *TGFBR2* mutations are suspected. It does appear that treatment can be effective in either of the groups with these known mutations.

T. P. Graham, Jr, MD

Equivalent Outcomes for Pediatric Heart Transplantation Recipients: ABO-Blood Group Incompatible versus ABO-Compatible
Dipchand AI, Pollock BarZiv SM, Manlhiot C, et al (Univ of Toronto, Canada; et al)
Am J Transplant 10:389-397, 2010

ABO-blood group incompatible infant heart transplantation has had excellent short-term outcomes. Uncertainties about long-term outcomes have been a barrier to the adoption of this strategy worldwide. We report a nonrandomized comparison of clinical outcomes over 10 years of the largest cohort of ABO-incompatible recipients. ABO-incompatible (n = 35) and ABO-compatible (n = 45) infant heart transplantation recipients (≤14 months old, 1996—2006) showed no important differences in pretransplantation characteristics. There was no difference in incidence of and time to moderate acute cellular rejection. Despite either the presence (seven patients) or development (eight patients) of donor-specific antibodies against blood group antigens, in only two ABO-incompatible patients were these antibodies implicated in antibody-mediated rejection (which occurred early posttransplantation, was easily managed and did not recur in follow-up). Occurrence of graft vasculopathy (11%), malignancy (11%) and freedom from severe renal dysfunction were identical in both groups. Survival was identical (74% at 7 years posttransplantation). ABO-blood group incompatible heart transplantation has excellent outcomes that are indistinguishable from those of the ABO-compatible population and there is no clinical justification for withholding this lifesaving strategy from all infants listed for heart transplantation. Further studies into observed differing responses in the development of donor-specific isohemagglutinins and the implications for graft accommodation are warranted.

▶ This study provides further data that infants have nondiscernible differences in short or midterm outcomes for incompatible ABO versus compatible graft recipients. This could widen the availability of grafts in this age group if algorithms can be agreed upon on the use of these hearts.

T. P. Graham, Jr, MD

Human Cord Blood Stem Cells Enhance Neonatal Right Ventricular Function in an Ovine Model of Right Ventricular Training

Davies B, Elwood NJ, Li S, et al (Univ of Melbourne, Australia; Univ of Nottingham Med School, UK)
Ann Thorac Surg 89:585-593, 2010

Background.—Nonischemic right ventricular dysfunction and cardiac failure is a source of considerable morbidity in children with congenital heart disease. Cell transplantation has not previously been studied in the pediatric setting in which enhancing ventricular function in response to supraphysiologic workloads might be beneficial.

Methods.—Engraftment and differentiation of human cord blood stem cells were studied in an immunosuppressed neonatal ovine model of right ventricular training. Week-old sheep underwent pulmonary artery banding and epicardial injection of cord blood stem cells (n = 8) or pulmonary artery banding and placebo injection (n = 8). Control groups received cord blood stem cells (n = 6) or placebo (n = 6) injection without pulmonary artery banding. Right ventricular function was measured at baseline and 1 month later using conductance catheter.

Results.—Cord blood stem cells were detected in the myocardium, spleen, kidney, and bone marrow up to 6 weeks after transplantation and expressed the hematopoietic markers CD45 and CD23. We identified neither differentiation nor fusion of transplanted human cells. In the groups undergoing pulmonary artery banding, cord blood stem cell transplantation was accompanied by functional benefits compared with placebo injection: end-systolic elastance increased by a mean of 1.4 ± 0.2 mm Hg/mL compared with 0.9 ± 0.1 mm Hg/mL, and the slope of preload recruitable stroke work increased by 21.1 ± 2.9 mm Hg compared with 15.8 ± 2.5 mm Hg. Cord blood stem cell transplantation had no significant effect on right ventricular function in the absence of pulmonary artery banding.

Conclusions.—Our data demonstrate that in the presence of increased workload, cord blood stem cells engraft and augment right ventricular function. Transplanted cells adopt hematopoietic fates in the myocardium, bone marrow, and spleen.

▶ This is exciting news. There is a great deal of research using stem cells to try to enhance cardiac function in a variety of settings. The data here suggest a paracrine function of the stem cells since there was no differentiation of the stem cells into myocardial cells. This group has found a potential use in pressure-loaded right ventricles—obviously a subject of great interest to physicians dealing with patients with congenital heart disease.

T. P. Graham, Jr, MD

Protective effect of periconceptional folic acid supplements on the risk of congenital heart defects: a registry-based case—control study in the northern Netherlands

van Beynum IM, Kapusta L, Bakker MK, et al (Radboud Univ Nijmegen Med Centre, The Netherlands; Univ of Groningen, The Netherlands)
Eur Heart J 31:464-471, 2010

Aims.—To investigate the potentially protective of periconceptional folic acid use on the risk of congenital heart defects (CHDs) relative to other non-folate related malformations.

Methods and Results.—We analysed data from a large regional register of birth defects (EUROCAT—Northern Netherlands), over a 10 year period (1996—2005) for a case—control study. The cases were mothers who had delivered infants with isolated or complex heart defects, without any related syndrome or genetic abnormality ($n = 611$). We used two control groups; one from the EUROCAT database and another from the general population. The registry controls consisted of mothers of children with a known chromosomal or genetic defect, and with infants with other non-folate related congenital malformations ($n = 2401$). Additional folic acid was taken as a single supplement or as a multivitamin containing folic acid in a dose of ≥ 400 μg daily. Mothers who had used folate antagonists or who had diabetes, and mothers of children with oral clefts, hypospadias, limb reduction- or neural tube defects, were excluded from both groups. Potentially confounding factors of periconceptional folic acid use in relation to CHD were explored, including baby's birth year, maternal body mass index, education, maternal age at delivery of index baby, smoking behaviour, and alcohol use during pregnancy. Periconceptional folic acid use revealed an odds ratio (OR) of 0.82 (95% CI 0.68—0.98) for all types of CHD relative to other malformations. The estimated relative risk for CHDs of additional folic acid use compared with the general population was comparable [OR 0.74 (95%CI 0.62—0.88)]. Subgroup analysis showed an OR of 0.62 (95% CI 0.47—0.82) for isolated septal defects. The proportions of the potential confounders between mothers of case and control infants did not differ significantly.

Conclusion.—Our results support the hypothesis that additional periconceptional folic acid use reduces CHD risk in infants. Use of periconceptional folic acid supplements was related to ~20% reduction in the prevalence of any CHD. Given the relatively high prevalence of CHD worldwide, our findings are important for public health.

▶ This observational study indicates that periconceptional folic acid supplements can reduce the prevalence of congenital heart defects by 20 %, which adds to the growing evidence of the positive effects of this supplement to potentially prevent congenital defects of major significance. Hopefully, this type of low-cost preventive care can be widely used worldwide in the near future.

T. P. Graham, Jr, MD

3 Cardiac Surgery

Aortic Disease

Have hybrid procedures replaced open aortic arch reconstruction in high-risk patients? A comparative study of elective open arch debranching with endovascular stent graft placement and conventional elective open total and distal aortic arch reconstruction

Milewski RK, Szeto WY, Pochettino A, et al (Hosp of the Univ of Pennsylvania, Philadelphia)

J Thorac Cardiovasc Surg 140:590-597, 2010

Objective.—Open total arch procedures have been associated with significant morbidity and mortality in patients with multiple comorbidities. Aortic arch debranching with endovascular graft placement, the hybrid arch procedure, has emerged as a surgical option in this patient population. This study evaluates the outcomes of a contemporary comparative series from one institution of open total arch and hybrid arch procedures for extensive aortic arch pathology.

Methods.—From July 2000 to March 2009, 1196 open arch procedures were performed, including 45 elective and 7 emergency open total arch procedures. From 2005 to 2009, 64 hybrid arch procedures were performed: 37 emergency type A dissections and 27 elective open arch debranchings. Hemiarch procedures were excluded.

Results.—The hybrid arch cohort was significantly older (*P* =.008) and had greater predominance of atherosclerotic pathophysiology (*P* < .001). The incidence of permanent cerebral neurologic deficit was similar at 4% (1/27) for the hybrid arch cohort and 9% (4/45) for the open aortic arch cohort. In-hospital mortality was similar at 11% (3/27) for the hybrid arch cohort and 16% (7/45) for the open aortic arch cohort. However, in the open arch group, there was a significant difference in mortality between patients aged less than 75 years at 9% (3/34) and patients aged more than 75 years at 36% (4/11) (*P* =.05).

Conclusions.—Hybrid arch procedures provide a safe alternative to open repair. This study suggests the hybrid arch approach has a lower mortality for high-risk patients aged more than 75 years. This extends the indication for the hybrid arch approach in patients with complex aortic arch pathology previously considered prohibitively high risk for conventional open total arch repair.

▶ Advancements in medical technology have allowed for diversification of operative procedures on the thoracic aorta. Innovative stent technologies have led to the development of branched stents, debranching procedures, and the so-called frozen elephant trunk. This article focused on outcomes of total aortic arch replacement in high-risk patients via either the traditional open approach or a hybrid approach using aortic debranching and thoracic stent grafting. Hybrid arch procedures combine open brachiocephalic debranching with concomitant antegrade endovascular stent graft placement in the aortic arch in a single-stage procedure. Despite the hybrid patients being considerably older, outcomes were similar. In-hospital and long-term mortality did not differ between the open and hybrid groups. Mortality was increased, however, for patients older than 75 years who underwent open repair, prompting the authors to conclude that this procedure may be preferred in elderly and other high-risk patients with aortic arch pathology.

V. H. Thourani, MD

Spectrum and Outcome of Reoperations After the Ross Procedure
Stulak JM, Burkhart HM, Sundt TM III, et al (Mayo Clinic and Foundation, Rochester, MN)
Circulation 122:1153-1158, 2010

Background.—Proposed advantages to the Ross procedure included presumed increased freedom from reoperation and simpler reoperation for pulmonary conduit replacement if needed. It is increasingly apparent, however, that reoperations are frequent after the Ross procedure and that when required, they may be more complex than previously thought.

Methods and Results.—Between September 1991 and August 2008, 56 patients underwent reoperation at our institution after a Ross procedure performed by ourselves (n = 13) or elsewhere (n = 43). Median age at first reoperation at our institution was 26 years (range 1 to 69 years). The 4 most common indications for reoperation were isolated autograft (neoaortic) regurgitation in 11 cases (20%), isolated pulmonary conduit regurgitation/stenosis in 9 (16%), combined autograft regurgitation/ dilatation in 8 (14%), and combined autograft regurgitation and pulmonary conduit regurgitation/ stenosis in 6 (11%). A total of 144 procedures were performed in these 56 patients during first reoperation at our institution. The autograft valve required replacement in 21 cases (38%) and aortic root replacement in 21 (38%), with ascending aortic/arch reconstruction in 13 (23%) and mitral valve surgery in 5 (9%). The pulmonary valve was replaced in 33 cases (59%) and the tricuspid valve was repaired/ replaced in 10 (18%). Early mortality was 1.8% (1 of 56 patients), and morbidity included 6 patients with respiratory failure and 3 who required postcardiotomy extracorporeal membrane oxygenation. There were 4 late deaths during the median follow-up of 8 months (range 1 to 179 months).

Conclusions.—A broad spectrum of complex reoperations may be required after the Ross procedure. Patients and family members considering the procedure should be informed of the potential for associated morbidity should reoperation be necessary.

▶ This article provides valuable information to cardiologists and surgeons alike because they are involved in the preoperative consultation and the long-term follow-up of patients being considered for the Ross procedure. The Ross procedure is performed for aortic valve disease and offered to patients in all age groups: infants, children, and adults. The operation is palliative, and the need for reintervention (percutaneous or surgical) over a lifetime is inevitable for most patients. This study represents the largest reported series of patients undergoing reoperation after the Ross procedure to date. Although literature is available that quantifies the incidence of reoperation after the Ross procedure, there are no published reports that address the qualitative nature and risks associated with reoperation when it is required. This article provides that missing information so the clinician can properly counsel patients about not only the potential need for reoperation but also the nature of the reoperation when it is necessary. The authors detail their experience with reoperations following the Ross procedure and explain modes of failure. Often, complex multiprocedure repair is necessary during reoperation, and reoperation was not without significant morbidity.

V. H. Thourani, MD

Superior nationwide outcomes of endovascular versus open repair for isolated descending thoracic aortic aneurysm in 11,669 patients
Gopaldas RR, Huh J, Dao TK, et al (Baylor College of Medicine, Houston, TX; Univ of Houston, TX)
J Thorac Cardiovasc Surg 140:1001-1010, 2010

Objectives.—Thoracic endovascular aneurysm repair (TEVAR) was introduced in 2005 to treat descending thoracic aortic aneurysms. Little is known about TEVAR's nationwide effect on patient outcomes. We evaluated nationwide data regarding the short-term outcomes of TEVAR and open aortic repair (OAR) procedures performed in the United States during a 2-year period.

Methods.—From the Nationwide Inpatient Sample data, we identified patients who had undergone surgery for an isolated descending thoracic aortic aneurysm from 2006 to 2007. Patients with aneurysm rupture, aortic dissection, vasculitis, connective tissue disorders, or concomitant aneurysms in other aortic segments were excluded. Of the remaining 11,669 patients, 9106 had undergone conventional OAR and 2563 had undergone TEVAR. Hierarchic regression analysis was used to assess the effect of TEVAR versus OAR after adjusting for confounding factors. The primary outcomes were mortality and the hospital length of stay (LOS). The secondary outcomes were the discharge status, morbidity, and hospital charges.

Results.—The patients who had undergone TEVAR were older (69.5 ± 12.7 vs 60.2 ± 14.2 years; $P < .001$) and had higher Deyo comorbidity scores (4.6 ± 1.8 vs 3.3 ± 1.8; $P < .001$). The unadjusted LOS was shorter for the TEVAR patients (7.7 ± 11 vs 8.8 ± 7.9 days), but the unadjusted mortality was similar (TEVAR 2.3% vs OAR 2.3%; $P = 1.0$). The proportion of nonelective interventions was similar between the 2 groups (TEVAR 15.9% vs OAR 15.8%; $P = .9$). The TEVAR and OAR techniques produced similar risk-adjusted mortality rates; however, the TEVAR patients had 60% fewer complications overall (odds ratio, 0.39; $P < .001$) and a shorter LOS (by 1.3 days). The TEVAR patients' hospital charges were greater by $6713 (95% confidence interval $1869 to $11,556; $P < .001$). However, the TEVAR patients were 4 times more likely to have a routine discharge to home.

Conclusions.—The nationwide data on TEVAR for descending thoracic aortic aneurysms have associated this procedure with better in-hospital outcomes than OAR, even though TEVAR was selectively performed in patients who were almost 1 decade older than the OAR patients. Compared with OAR, TEVAR was associated with a shorter hospital LOS and fewer complications but significantly greater hospital charges.

▶ Open repair of the descending thoracic aorta carries significant morbidity and mortality. Recent technology has allowed for intraluminal stenting of the thoracic aorta to exclude blood flow to the aneurysm, thus depressurizing the excluded segment and significantly decreasing if not eliminating the risk of rupture. While stenting of the thoracic aorta has up-front advantages in avoiding important morbidities associated with open repair, secondary interventions are greater and hospital costs remain higher. This large study used a national inpatient database to compare open repair of the thoracic aorta with stent grafting. Patients who underwent stenting were almost 10 years older than those who underwent open repair. While length of stay was shorter in the group who underwent stent grafting, in-hospital mortality was similar to open repair. The authors concluded that despite an older patient population, stenting of the descending thoracic aorta was superior to open repair and was associated with lower rates of morbidity and a shorter length of stay in spite of greater hospital charges. Although this report is not randomized, it does provide a review of a large database of thoracic aortic aneurysm surgery.

V. H. Thourani, MD

Importance of Refractory Pain and Hypertension in Acute Type B Aortic Dissection: Insights From the International Registry of Acute Aortic Dissection (IRAD)

Trimarchi S, on behalf of the International Registry of Acute Aortic Dissection (IRAD) Investigators (Univ of Milano, San Donato Milanese, Italy; et al)
Circulation 122:1283-1289, 2010

Background.—In patients with acute type B aortic dissection, presence of recurrent or refractory pain and/or refractory hypertension on medical therapy is sometimes used as an indication for invasive treatment. The International Registry of Acute Aortic Dissection (IRAD) was used to investigate the impact of refractory pain and/or refractory hypertension on the outcomes of acute type B aortic dissection.

Methods and Results.—Three hundred sixty-five patients affected by uncomplicated acute type B aortic dissection, enrolled in IRAD from 1996 to 2004, were categorized according to risk profile into 2 groups. Patients with recurrent and/or refractory pain or refractory hypertension (group I; n=69) and patients without clinical complications at presentation (group II; n=296) were compared. "High-risk" patients with classic complications were excluded from this analysis. The overall in-hospital mortality was 6.5% and was increased in group I compared with group II (17.4% versus 4.0%; $P=0.0003$). The in-hospital mortality after medical management was significantly increased in group I compared with group II (35.6% versus 1.5%; $P=0.0003$). Mortality rates after surgical (20% versus 28%; $P=0.74$) or endovascular management (3.7% versus 9.1%; $P=0.50$) did not differ significantly between group I and group II, respectively. A multivariable logistic regression model confirmed that recurrent and/or refractory pain or refractory hypertension was a predictor of in-hospital mortality (odds ratio, 3.31; 95% confidence interval, 1.04 to 10.45; $P=0.041$).

Conclusions.—Recurrent pain and refractory hypertension appeared as clinical signs associated with increased in-hospital mortality, particularly when managed medically. These observations suggest that aortic intervention, such as via an endovascular approach, may be indicated in this intermediate-risk group.

▶ For patients presenting with an uncomplicated acute type B aortic dissection (ABAD), medical management (specifically blood pressure control) has been the mainstay of treatment. Surgical management (open or endovascular) has been reserved in those patients with complications, including malperfusion syndromes, extending dissection, or aortic rupture. The optimal approach for patients with uncomplicated ABAD who develop recurrent/refractory pain or refractory hypertension remains unclear. Using the International Registry of Acute Aortic Dissection, this study suggests that patients with ABAD presenting with uncomplicated ABAD should continue to undergo medical management. However, refractory hypertension and/or pain symptoms in these patients, in the absence of other complications, are at intermediate risk for an adverse in-hospital outcome. The authors have concluded that aortic intervention may be appropriate in this intermediate-risk group of patients with ABAD with the use of endovascular techniques in lieu of medical management.

V. H. Thourani, MD

Surgical Management of Descending Thoracic Aortic Disease: Open and Endovascular Approaches: A Scientific Statement From the American Heart Association

Coady MA, on behalf of the American Heart Association Council on Cardiovascular Surgery and Anesthesia and Council on Peripheral Vascular Disease

Circulation 121:2780-2804, 2010

Recent years have witnessed the emergence of novel technologies that enable less invasive endovascular treatment of descending thoracic aortic disease (TAD). This has occurred against a backdrop of improved identification of various disease processes and better results with open surgical repair. The natural history of the specific acute aortic syndromes that affect the descending thoracic aorta has also been described with more clarity and has become more commonly recognized. This is in part secondary to the widespread availability and application of advanced imaging technologies that permit precise diagnoses. As data are accumulating, these pathological processes involving the descending thoracic aorta are no longer thought of as simply variants of one another but as distinct entities with well-defined clinical behavior. As the technology for endovascular repair continues to mature and its utilization increases, there is a need for a careful assessment of the current state of medical management, traditional open therapy, and evolving endovascular treatment of distinct thoracic aortic pathologies.

The purpose of this scientific statement is to present a contemporary review of the various pathological processes that affect the descending thoracic aorta: Aneurysms, dissections, intramural hematomas (IMHs), penetrating atherosclerotic ulcers (PAUs), and aortic transections. These disorders will be considered in detail, with an exploration of the natural history, available treatment options, and controversies regarding management. Current intervention criteria will be reviewed with respect to both open surgical repair and endovascular treatment.

Our goal is to provide the healthcare professional with a better understanding of the pathophysiology of the various disease processes that involve the descending thoracic aorta and to review current outcomes and technical pitfalls associated with these therapies to facilitate strong, evidence-based decision making in the care of these patients.

▶ The surgical management of the thoracic aorta has evolved into a variety of treatment options: open, endovascular, or a hybrid approach. The scientific statement from Coady et al for the surgical management of descending thoracic aortic disease (TAD) is an excellent review of all of these options. Important aspects of this article include: (1) open surgical intervention for descending TAD is associated with a paraplegia rate of approximately 3% and mortality of 4% to 9%; (2) thoracic endovascular aortic repair (TEVAR) when feasible may provide an excellent option for these patients because of lower published risks of mortality and paraplegia; (3) in those undergoing TEVAR: long-term data (> 5 years) are not available, there is a lack of prospective randomized trials to directly compare open with endovascular therapy, reintervention rates for endoleaks are not insignificant, the risk of stroke approaches 4%, and patients with connective tissue diseases were excluded; (4) open surgery for complicated acute type B dissection continues to carry significant morbidity and mortality, and endovascular therapy is emerging as an alternative; prophylactic stent grafting to prevent complications of chronic type B dissection is compared with medical management in the Investigation of Stent grafts in patients with type B Aortic Dissections and Acute uncomplicated aortic Dissection type B: evaluating Stent-graft placement Or Best medical treatment alone trials, but long-term data are not yet available; and (5) treatment of traumatic aortic transaction with stent grafts is an alternative to surgery in high-risk cases, but open surgery should be entertained in younger patients.

V. H. Thourani, MD

Coronary Artery Disease

Aspirin Plus Clopidogrel Versus Aspirin Alone After Coronary Artery Bypass Grafting: The Clopidogrel After Surgery for Coronary Artery Disease (CASCADE) Trial

Kulik A, Le May MR, Voisine P, et al (Boca Raton Regional Hosp, FL; Univ of Ottawa Heart Inst, Ontario, Canada; Hôpital Laval, Quebec City, Quebec, Canada; et al)
Circulation 122:2680-2687, 2010

Background.—Clopidogrel inhibits intimal hyperplasia in animal studies and therefore may reduce saphenous vein graft (SVG) intimal hyperplasia after coronary artery bypass grafting. The Clopidogrel After Surgery for Coronary Artery DiseasE (CASCADE) study was undertaken to evaluate whether the addition of clopidogrel to aspirin inhibits SVG disease after coronary artery bypass grafting, as assessed at 1 year by intravascular ultrasound.

Methods and Results.—In this double-blind phase II trial, 113 patients undergoing coronary artery bypass grafting with SVGs were randomized to receive aspirin 162 mg plus clopidogrel 75 mg daily or aspirin 162 mg plus placebo daily for 1 year. The primary outcome was SVG intimal hyperplasia (mean intimal area) as determined by intravascular ultrasound at 1 year. Secondary outcomes were graft patency, major adverse cardiovascular events, and major bleeding. One-year intravascular ultrasound and coronary angiography were performed in 92 patients (81.4%). At 1 year, SVG intimal area did not differ significantly between the 2 groups

(4.1 ± 2.0 versus 4.5 ± 2.1 mm², aspirin-clopidogrel versus aspirin-placebo, $P=0.44$). Overall 1-year graft patency was 95.2% in the aspirin-clopidogrel group compared with 95.5% in the aspirin-placebo group ($P=0.90$), and SVG patency was 94.3% in the aspirin-clopidogrel group versus 93.2% in the aspirin-placebo group ($P=0.69$). Freedom from major adverse cardiovascular events at 1 year was 92.9 ± 3.4% in the aspirin-clopidogrel group and 91.1 ± 3.8% in the aspirin-placebo group ($P=0.76$). The incidence of major bleeding at 1 year was similar for the 2 groups (1.8% versus 0%, aspirin-clopidogrel versus aspirin-placebo, $P=0.50$).

Conclusions.—Compared with aspirin monotherapy, the combination of aspirin plus clopidogrel did not significantly reduce the process of SVG intimal hyperplasia 1 year after coronary artery bypass grafting.

▶ Coronary artery bypass grafting (CABG) is an effective treatment for ischemic heart disease, but its long-term results are compromised by the development of saphenous vein graft (SVG) disease. After surgery, a platelet-mediated thickening of the SVG wall occurs, with smooth muscle cell proliferation and extracellular matrix protein synthesis. This process, termed intimal hyperplasia, forms a template for the development of SVG atherosclerosis and eventual occlusion. Clopidogrel has been shown to inhibit intimal hyperplasia in animal studies and therefore may reduce SVG intimal hyperplasia after CABG. The Clopidogrel After Surgery for Coronary Artery Disease study, a double-blind placebo-controlled trial, evaluates whether the addition of clopidogrel to aspirin inhibits the development of SVG disease. A total of 113 patients undergoing CABG with SVGs were randomized to receive either aspirin 162 mg plus clopidogrel 75 mg daily (n = 56) or aspirin 162 mg plus placebo (n = 57) daily for 1 year, followed by SVG intravascular ultrasound and coronary angiography. The primary outcome, SVG intimal area at 1 year, did not differ significantly between the 2 groups. Moreover, graft patency and freedom from major adverse cardiovascular events also did not significantly differ between the 2 groups. Although this trial is well designed, its power remains too small for closing the door on the aspect of dual versus mono antiplatelet therapy following CABG. Newer antiplatelet agents with purported advantages over clopidogrel may constitute important areas for future research to target the inhibition of SVG disease after CABG.

V. H. Thourani, MD

Clinical Characteristics of Patients Undergoing Surgical Ventricular Reconstruction by Choice and by Randomization
Zembala M, Michler RE, Rynkiewicz A, et al (Silesian Ctr for Heart Diseases/ Med Univ of Silesia, Zabrze-Katowice, Poland; Montefiore Med Ctr/Albert Einstein College of Medicine, Bronx, NY; Med Univ of Gdansk, Poland; et al)
J Am Coll Cardiol 56:499-507, 2010

Objectives.—The aim of this study was to confirm the generalizability of the conclusions of the STICH (Surgical Treatment for Ischemic Heart Failure) trial.

Background.—Surgical ventricular reconstruction (SVR) added to coronary artery bypass grafting (CABG) did not decrease death or cardiac hospitalization in STICH patients randomized to CABG with (n = 501) or without (n = 499) SVR.

Methods.—Baseline clinical characteristics of 1,000 STICH SVR hypothesis patients and 1,036 STICH-eligible Society of Thoracic Surgeons (STS) National Cardiac Database patients undergoing CABG plus SVR were entered into a multivariate model equation to predict a mortality that placed these 2,036 patients in 1 of 32 risk at randomization (RAR) groups. The number of patients in each RAR group profiled the risk of STICH treatment arms and of STICH and STS STICH-eligible patients.

Results.—That 85% of the 1,000 STICH patients known to have no significant differences in baseline characteristics between the 2 treatment arms shared the same RAR group suggests that the RAR methodology has sufficient accuracy to compare RAR profiles of STICH and STS patients. RAR group was shared by 1,522 of 2,036 STICH and STS STICH-eligible patients (75%) who underwent CABG plus SVR. Differences in baseline characteristics responsible for more low-risk STICH patients and more high-risk STS patients were modest. Cox proportional hazard ratios of 1,000 STICH patients in 3 RAR groups suggested by STICH and STS RAR differences showed no differential treatment effect on survival across the low-, intermediate-, and high-risk groups.

Conclusions.—The STICH conclusion of no benefit from adding SVR to CABG applies to a broad spectrum of CABG-eligible patients with ischemic cardiomyopathy. (Comparison of Surgical and Medical Treatment for Congestive Heart Failure and Coronary Artery Disease; NCT00023595).

▶ Over the past 2 decades, improved treatments for acute myocardial infarction have improved survival. Survivors often have reduced left ventricular (LV) function, with immediate ramifications for functional capacity as well as future progressive remodeling changes occurring in LV chamber size and/or LV geometry. Because preliminary data from a case-control study indicated promising improvements in LV function after surgical ventricular reconstruction (SVR), the Surgical Treatment for Ischemic Heart Failure (STICH) trial was designed to evaluate whether coronary artery bypass grafting (CABG) either alone or in combination with SVR might improve outcomes in patients with heart failure. Zembala and colleagues extracted STICH-eligible patient records (the closest match of patients with ischemic heart failure meeting STICH inclusion and exclusion criteria) from the Society of Thoracic Surgeons (STS) National Cardiac Database, identifying 104 135 STICH-eligible STS patients, of whom 1092 (1%) underwent CABG with SVR. This report has provided a partial assurance that for most patients enrolled, there appears to be general concordance of their providers' assessments of SVR treatment eligibility, both within the STICH trial and comparing STICH patients with STS CABG plus SVR patients.

V. H. Thourani, MD

Comparable patencies of the radial artery and right internal thoracic artery or saphenous vein beyond 5 years: Results from the Radial Artery Patency and Clinical Outcomes trial

Hayward PAR, Gordon IR, Hare DL, et al (Austin Hosp and Univ of Melbourne, Victoria, Australia; Univ of Melbourne, Parkville, Victoria, Australia)
J Thorac Cardiovasc Surg 139:60-67, 2010

Objective.—To investigate the optimum conduit for coronary targets other than the left anterior descending artery, we evaluated long-term patencies and clinical outcomes of the radial artery, right internal thoracic artery, and saphenous vein through the Radial Artery Patency and Clinical Outcomes trial.

Methods.—As part of a 10-year prospective, randomized, single-center trial, patients undergoing primary coronary surgery were allocated to the radial artery (n = 198) or free right internal thoracic artery (n = 196) if aged less than 70 years (group 1), or radial artery (n = 113) or saphenous vein (n = 112) if aged at least 70 years (group 2). All patients received a left internal thoracic artery to the left anterior descending, and the randomized conduit was used to graft the second largest target. Protocol-directed angiography has been performed at randomly assigned intervals, weighted toward the end of the study period. Grafts are defined as failed if there was occlusion, string sign, or greater than 80% stenosis, independently reported by 3 assessors. Analysis is by intention to treat.

Results.—At mean follow up of 5.5 years, protocol angiography has been performed in groups 1 and 2 in 237 and 113 patients, respectively. There are no significant differences within each group in preoperative comorbidity, age, or urgency. Patencies were similar for either of the 2 conduits in each group (log rank analysis, $P = .06$ and $P = .54$, respectively). The differences in estimated 5-year patencies were 6.6% (radial minus right internal thoracic artery) in group 1 and 2.9% (radial minus saphenous vein graft) in group 2.

Conclusion.—At mean 5-year angiography in largely asymptomatic patients, the selection of arterial or venous conduit for the second graft has not significantly affected patency. This finding offers surgeons, for now, enhanced flexibility in planning revascularization.

▶ The Radial Artery Patency and Clinical Outcomes trial has been designed to identify the place of the radial artery (RA) in the hierarchy of conduit options available to the modern surgeon to supplement the gold standard left internal thoracic artery to left anterior descending (LAD) graft. Comparable angiographic and clinical outcomes at mean 5- to 6-year follow-up can be achieved with any free arterial graft in patients younger than 70 years and with an RA or a saphenous vein (SV) in older patients when grafted to the largest non-LAD target. This finding allows the surgeon considerable flexibility in the selection of conduits according to other patient comorbidities or factors. Whether the free arterial grafts are equivalent or superior to SV grafts in younger patients is not known, and caution should be expressed in extrapolation of patency results from second-order coronary targets to lesser targets, although the likely clinical impact of graft failure in the territories of lesser targets diminishes accordingly. This trial offered surgeons flexibility in their choices of arterial versus venous routes for revascularization; at a mean follow-up of 5 years, venous versus arterial did not affect patency significantly. This trial is important because there has been some controversy regarding the utility of radial artery grafts for coronary artery bypass surgery (CABG) because of concerns about spasm and occlusion. This trial refutes these concerns and establishes the use of the radial artery as a truly reasonable and desirable conduit for CABG.

V. H. Thourani, MD

Diabetic and Nondiabetic Patients With Left Main and/or 3-Vessel Coronary Artery Disease: Comparison of Outcomes With Cardiac Surgery and Paclitaxel-Eluting Stents

Banning AP, Westaby S, Morice M-C, et al (John Radcliffe Hosp, Oxford, UK; Institut Hospitalier Jacques Cartier, Massy, France; et al)

J Am Coll Cardiol 55:1067-1075, 2010

Objectives.—This study was designed to compare contemporary surgical revascularization (coronary artery bypass graft surgery [CABG]) versus TAXUS Express (Boston Scientific, Natick, Massachusetts) paclitaxel-eluting stents (PES) in diabetic and nondiabetic patients with left main and/or 3-vessel disease.

Background.—Although the prevalence of diabetes mellitus is increasing, the optimal coronary revascularization strategy in diabetic patients with complex multivessel disease remains controversial.

Methods.—The SYNTAX (SYNergy between percutaneous coronary intervention with TAXus and cardiac surgery) study randomly assigned 1,800 patients (452 with medically treated diabetes) to receive PES or CABG.

Results.—The overall 1-year major adverse cardiac and cerebrovascular event rate was higher among diabetic patients treated with PES compared with CABG, but the revascularization method did not impact the death/stroke/myocardial infarction rate for nondiabetic patients (6.8% CABG vs. 6.8% PES, $p = 0.97$) or for diabetic patients (10.3% CABG vs. 10.1% PES, $p = 0.96$). The presence of diabetes was associated with significantly increased mortality after either revascularization treatment. The incidence of stroke was higher among nondiabetic patients after CABG (2.2% vs. PES 0.5%, $p = 0.006$). Compared with CABG, mortality was higher after PES use for diabetic patients with highly complex lesions (4.1% vs. 13.5%, $p = 0.04$). Revascularization with PES resulted in higher repeat revascularization for nondiabetic patients (5.7% vs. 11.1%, $p < 0.001$) and diabetic patients (6.4% vs. 20.3%, $p < 0.001$).

Conclusions.—Subgroup analyses suggest that the 1-year major adverse cardiac and cerebrovascular event rate is higher among diabetic patients with left main and/or 3-vessel disease treated with PES compared with

CABG, driven by an increase in repeat revascularization. However, the composite safety end point (death/stroke/myocardial infarction) is comparable between the 2 treatment options for diabetic and nondiabetic patients. Although further study is needed, these exploratory results may extend the evidence for PES use in selected patients with less complex left main and/or 3-vessel lesions. (SYNergy Between PCI With TAXus and Cardiac Surgery [SYNTAX]; NCT00114972).

▶ It is well known that diabetes increases the risk of developing cardiovascular disease and is a consistent predictor of mortality, myocardial infarction, and restenosis after percutaneous coronary intervention (PCI) and coronary artery bypass grafting (CABG). The SYNTAX (SYNergy between percutaneous coronary intervention with TAXus and cardiac surgery) study is the first to compare CABG with the TAXUS Express paclitaxel-eluting stent (PES) in nondiabetic and diabetic patients with complex left main and/or 3-vessel coronary disease. The 1-year SYNTAX results suggest that in patients with left main and/or 3-vessel disease, major adverse cardiac and cerebrovascular event is increased for PES-treated diabetic patients compared with CABG-treated patients, driven by an increase in repeat revascularization. Composite safety and mortality end points are comparable between the CABG and PES arms.

The SYNTAX study presents PCI as a viable general option with the following caveats: (1) multivessel PCI for diabetic patients performed without drug-eluting stents (DES) is likely associated with increased death and should not be done unless there is no reasonable surgical option and (2) diabetic patients undergoing PCI with DES remain at higher risk for repeat revascularization with PCI versus CABG. This is an excellent study performed by high-volume centers.

V. H. Thourani, MD

Outcomes in Patients With De Novo Left Main Disease Treated With Either Percutaneous Coronary Intervention Using Paclitaxel-Eluting Stents or Coronary Artery Bypass Graft Treatment in the Synergy Between Percutaneous Coronary Intervention With TAXUS and Cardiac Surgery (SYNTAX) Trial

Morice M-C, Serruys PW, Kappetein AP, et al (Institut Hospitalier Jacques Cartier, Massy, France; Erasmus Univ Med Ctr Rotterdam, the Netherlands; et al)
Circulation 121:2645-2653, 2010

Background.—The prospective, multinational, randomized Synergy Between Percutaneous Coronary Intervention With TAXUS and Cardiac Surgery (SYNTAX) trial was designed to assess the optimal revascularization strategy between percutaneous coronary intervention (PCI) and coronary artery bypass grafting (CABG), for patients with left main (LM) and/or 3-vessel coronary disease.

Methods and Results.—This observational hypothesis-generating analysis reports the results of a prespecified powered subgroup of 705 randomized patients who had LM disease among the 1800 patients with de novo 3-vessel disease and/or LM disease randomized to PCI with paclitaxel-eluting stents or CABG in the SYNTAX trial. Major adverse cardiac and cerebrovascular event rates at 1 year in LM patients were similar for CABG and PCI (13.7% versus 15.8%; Δ2.1% [95% confidence interval −3.2% to 7.4%]; P=0.44). At 1 year, stroke was significantly higher in the CABG arm (2.7% versus 0.3%; Δ−2.4% [95% confidence interval −4.2% to −0.1%]; P=0.009]), whereas repeat revascularization was significantly higher in the PCI arm (6.5% versus 11.8%; Δ5.3% [95% confidence interval 1.0% to 9.6%]; P=0.02); there was no observed difference between groups for other end points. When patients were scored for anatomic complexity, those with higher baseline SYNTAX scores had significantly worse outcomes with PCI than did patients with low or intermediate SYNTAX scores; outcomes for patients with CABG did not correlate with baseline SYNTAX score, but baseline EuroSCORE significantly predicted outcomes for both treatments.

Conclusions.—Patients with LM disease who had revascularization with PCI had safety and efficacy outcomes comparable to CABG at 1 year; longer follow-up is required to determine whether these 2 revascularization strategies offer comparable medium-term outcomes in this group of complex patients.

▶ In the United States, the consensus treatment guidelines continue to recommend coronary artery bypass grafting (CABG) as the gold standard for revascularization of an unprotected left main (LM) coronary stenosis. Percutaneous coronary intervention (PCI) is feasible and appropriately recommended for high-risk patients who are not candidates for CABG. In the absence of a large randomized controlled trial, interventional cardiologists have had difficulty developing objective evidence-based criteria for determining the optimal revascularization strategy for a given patient. The Synergy Between Percutaneous Coronary Intervention With TAXUS and Cardiac Surgery (SYNTAX) trial is the first large trial to randomize patients suitable for revascularization by either CABG or PCI using drug-eluting stents for the treatment of LM and/or 3-vessel disease. This article presents outcomes in the prespecified subgroup of patients (N = 705) with LM disease. Patients with LM disease had comparable overall 12-month major adverse cardiovascular and cerebrovascular events in both the PCI and the CABG group (14% CABG vs 16% PCI). When patients were scored for anatomic complexity, those with higher baseline SYNTAX scores had significantly worse outcomes with PCI than those with low or intermediate SYNTAX scores; outcomes for patients with CABG did not correlate with baseline SYNTAX score. It is important to note that stroke was higher in the CABG group while repeat revascularization was significantly higher in the PCI arm. These results are consistent with findings of the only other randomized LM trial to compare PCI with CABG, the Study of Unprotected Left Main Stenting Versus Bypass Surgery.[1] Longer term follow-up and additional prospective studies are required to determine whether these 2 revascularization strategies offer comparable outcomes, especially over the next 3 to 5 years, when you expect the differences in outcomes between patients treated with CABG and those treated with PCI may begin to emerge.

V. H. Thourani, MD

Reference

1. Buszman PE, Kiesz SR, Bochenek A, et al. Acute and late outcomes of unprotected left main stenting in comparison with surgical revascularization. *J Am Coll Cardiol.* 2008;51:538-545.

Randomized trial to compare bilateral vs. single internal mammary coronary artery bypass grafting: 1-year results of the Arterial Revascularisation Trial (ART)

Taggart DP, on behalf of the ART Investigators (Univ of Oxford, UK; et al)
Eur Heart J 31:2470-2481, 2010

Aims.—Observational data suggest that the use of bilateral internal mammary arteries (BIMA) during coronary artery bypass graft surgery provides superior revascularization to a single internal mammary artery (SIMA), but concerns about safety have prevented the widespread use of BIMA. The Arterial Revascularisation Trial (ART) is a randomized trial of BIMA vs. SIMA, with a primary outcome of survival at 10 years. This paper reports mortality, morbidity, and resource use data at 1 year.

Methods and Results.—Coronary artery bypass graft patients were enrolled in 28 hospitals in seven countries. Three thousand one hundred and two patients were randomly assigned to SIMA ($n = 1554$) or BIMA ($n = 1548$). The mean number of grafts was 3 for both groups. Forty per cent of the SIMA procedures and 42% of the BIMA were performed off-pump. Mortality at 30 days was 18 of 1548 (1.2%) for SIMA and 19 of 1537 (1.2%) for BIMA, and at 1 year was 36 of 1540 (2.3%) and 38 of 1529 (2.5%), respectively. The rates of stroke, myocardial infarction, and repeat revascularization were all ≤2% at 1 year and similar between the two groups. Sternal wound reconstruction was required in 0.6 and 1.9% of the SIMA and BIMA groups, respectively.

Conclusion.—Data from ART demonstrate similar clinical outcomes for SIMA and BIMA at 1 year but BIMA grafts are associated with a small absolute increase (1.3%) in the need for sternal wound reconstruction. The results suggest that the use of BIMA grafts is feasible on a routine basis. The 10-year results of the ART will confirm whether BIMA grafting results in lower mortality and the need for repeat intervention.

Trial Registration.—Controlled-trials.com (ISRCTN46552265).

▶ Numerous compelling retrospective studies have documented a clear benefit for bilateral internal mammary arteries (BIMA) grafting over single internal mammary artery (SIMA) grafting in reducing the long-term risk of death, cardiac death, and late cardiac events. Nevertheless, there is a wide discrepancy between these findings in the literature and clinical practice. BIMA usage is only around 4% in the United States and 12% in Europe. The primary objective of the Arterial Revascularisation Trial (ART) is to assess whether the use of BIMA grafts during coronary artery bypass graft (CABG) improves 10-year survival and reduces the need for further interventions compared with a SIMA graft. The secondary outcome measures include clinical events and quality of life and health economic assessments. The ART is unique in not only being the largest randomized trial of 2 surgical operations ever undertaken in cardiac surgery but also having a primary outcome at 10 years of follow-up. It is designed to specifically answer the question of whether BIMA grafts offer additional survival benefit and freedom from reintervention at 10 years to that already provided by a SIMA graft. There are 2 key findings of the 1-year interim analyses of ART: (1) the overall very low mortality and major morbidity of contemporary CABG, irrespective of whether the procedure was BIMA or SIMA, with a 30-day mortality of around 1% and a 1-year mortality of around 2.5% and (2) a 1.3% increase in the incidence of sternal wound reconstruction associated with the BIMA. Although BIMA grafting appears to offer superior revascularization to SIMA, it is technically more challenging, and concerns that it leads to a longer operation and increases the risk of early mortality and major morbidity, in particular impaired wound healing, have prevented widespread use. This is an important and timely study performed with an excellent and reliable surgical group. The progression of management of these patients long term will provide incredible insight of this arterial conduit dilemma.

V. H. Thourani, MD

Valve Disease

Late Outcomes Following Freestyle Versus Homograft Aortic Root Replacement: Results From a Prospective Randomized Trial

El-Hamamsy I, Clark L, Stevens LM, et al (Imperial College London, UK; Harvard Univ, Boston, MA; et al)
J Am Coll Cardiol 55:368-376, 2010

Objectives.—The aims of this study were to compare long-term results after homograft versus Freestyle (Medtronic Inc., Minneapolis, Minnesota) aortic root replacement.

Background.—The ideal substitute for aortic root replacement remains undetermined.

Methods.—Between 1997 and 2005, 166 patients (age 65 ± 8 years) undergoing total aortic root replacement were randomized to receive a homograft (n = 76) or a Freestyle bioprosthesis (n = 90). Six patients randomly assigned to homograft crossed over to Freestyle because of unavailability of suitably sized homografts. Median follow-up was 7.6 years (maximum 11 years; 1,035 patient-years). "Evolving" aortic valve dysfunction was defined as aortic regurgitation ≥2/4 and/or peak gradient >20 mm Hg.

Results.—Patient characteristics were comparable between groups. Concomitant procedures were performed in 44% and 47% of Freestyle and homograft patients, respectively (p = 0.5). Overall hospital mortality was 4.8% (1% for isolated root replacement). Eight-year survival was 80 ± 5% in the Freestyle group versus 77 ± 6% in the homograft group (p = 0.9). Freedom from need for reoperation at 8 years was significantly higher after Freestyle root replacement (100 ± 0% vs. 90 ± 5% after homograft replacement; p = 0.02). All reoperations were secondary to structural valve deterioration (n = 6). At last echocardiographic follow-up, actuarial freedom from evolving aortic valve dysfunction was 86 ± 5% for Freestyle bioprostheses versus 37 ± 7% for homografts (p < 0.001). Clinically, freedom from New York Heart Association functional class III to IV and freedom from valve-related complications were similar between groups (p = 0.7 and p = 0.9, respectively).

Conclusions.—In this patient group, late survival is similar after homograft versus Freestyle root replacement. However, Freestyle aortic root replacement is associated with significantly less progressive aortic valve dysfunction and a lower need for reoperations.

▶ The exact choice of prosthesis for an aortic root replacement remains undetermined. The authors of the article sought to partly clarify this issue by conducting a randomized trial comparing homograft roots versus stentless porcine aortic roots. Importantly, median follow-up was 7.6 years, thus allowing comment on durability of the given prostheses. The main findings of the study include the following: (1) there was no difference in hospital mortality between the stentless porcine and homograft groups; (2) there was no difference in late valve-related complications; (3) there was no difference in late functional class; (4) there was no difference in late survival (which, in both groups, approached that of an age- and sex-matched general population); and (5) there was a marked difference in valve performance, with the homografts showing a much higher incidence of aortic valve dysfunction and need for reoperation. This is a well-designed randomized trial by an excellent surgical group.

W. B. Keeling, MD

Outcomes of the RESTOR-MV Trial (Randomized Evaluation of a Surgical Treatment for Off-Pump Repair of the Mitral Valve)
Grossi EA, for the RESTOR-MV Study Group (New York Univ School of Medicine and New York Harbor Veterans Healthcare System; et al)
J Am Coll Cardiol 56:1984-1993, 2010

Objectives.—We sought to determine whether patients with functional mitral regurgitation (FMR) would benefit from ventricular reshaping by the Coapsys device (Myocor, Inc., Maple Grove, Minnesota).

Background.—FMR occurs when ventricular remodeling impairs valve function. Coapsys is a ventricular shape change device placed without cardiopulmonary bypass to reduce FMR. It compresses the mitral annulus and reshapes the ventricle. We hypothesized that Coapsys for FMR would improve clinical outcomes compared with standard therapies.

Methods.—RESTOR-MV (Randomized Evaluation of a Surgical Treatment for Off-Pump Repair of the Mitral Valve) was a randomized, prospective, multicenter study of patients with FMR and coronary disease with core laboratory analysis. After enrollment, patients were stratified to the standard indicated surgery: either coronary artery bypass graft alone or coronary artery bypass graft with mitral valve repair. In each stratum, randomization was to either control (indicated surgery) or treatment (coronary artery bypass graft with Coapsys ventricular reshaping).

Results.—The study was terminated when the sponsor failed to secure ongoing funding; 165 patients were randomized. Control and Coapsys both produced decreases in left ventricular (LV) end-diastolic dimension and MR at 2 years ($p < 0.001$); Coapsys provided a greater decrease in LV end-diastolic dimension ($p = 0.021$). Control had lower MR grades during follow-up ($p = 0.01$). Coapsys showed a survival advantage compared with control at 2 years (87% vs. 77%) (hazard ratio: 0.421; 95% confidence interval: 0.200 to 0.886; stratified log-rank test; $p = 0.038$). Complication-free survival (including death, stroke, myocardial infarction, and valve reoperation) was significantly greater with Coapsys at 2 years (85% vs. 71%) (hazard ratio: 0.372; 95% confidence interval: 0.185 to 0.749; adjusted log-rank test; $p = 0.019$).

Conclusions.—Analysis of RESTOR-MV indicates that patients with FMR requiring revascularization treated with ventricular reshaping rather than standard surgery had improved survival and a significant decrease in major adverse outcomes. This trial validates the concept of the ventricular reshaping strategy in this subset of patients with heart failure. (Randomized Evaluation of a Surgical Treatment for Off-Pump Repair of the Mitral Valve [RESTOR-MV]; NCT00120276).

▶ Current treatments for left ventricular dysfunction with functional mitral regurgitation (FMR) include medical therapy and/or surgery. Medical therapy includes unloading the ventricle and downregulating the metabolic pathways that cause progression of ventricular failure. For patients with viable ischemic myocardium, revascularization is a first step, with the objectives of preventing further damage, relieving the ischemia that may contribute to FMR, and perhaps arresting or reversing the remodeling process. The effect of correcting ischemia on mitral valve (MV) function has been unpredictable and often transient, leaving most patients with residual, recurrent, or progressive mitral regurgitation. Alternatively, FMR is treated by MV surgery, consisting of either MV repair or prosthetic replacement. The Randomized Evaluation of a Surgical Treatment for Off-Pump Repair of the Mitral Valve (RESTOR-MV) was a randomized, prospective, multicenter study of patients with FMR and coronary disease. After enrollment, patients were stratified to the standard indicated surgery: either coronary artery bypass graft alone or coronary artery bypass graft with MV repair. In each stratum, randomization was to either control (indicated surgery) or treatment (coronary artery bypass graft with Coapsys ventricular reshaping). A total of 165 patients were randomized prior to study termination when the sponsor failed to secure ongoing funding. The analysis of RESTOR-MV indicates that patients with FMR requiring revascularization treated with ventricular reshaping rather than standard surgery had improved survival and a significant decrease in major adverse outcomes. This very well performed trial validates the concept of the ventricular reshaping strategy in this subset of patients with heart failure.

W. B. Keeling, MD

Should Patients With Severe Degenerative Mitral Regurgitation Delay Surgery Until Symptoms Develop?
Gillinov AM, Mihaljevic T, Blackstone EH, et al (Heart and Vascular Inst, Cleveland, OH; Cleveland Clinic, OH)
Ann Thorac Surg 90:481-488, 2010

Background.—The American College of Cardiology/American Heart Association practice guidelines recommending surgery for asymptomatic patients with severe mitral regurgitation caused by degenerative disease remain controversial. This study examined whether delaying surgery until symptoms occur causes adverse cardiac changes and jeopardizes outcome.

Methods.—From January 1985 to January 2008, 4,586 patients had primary isolated mitral valve surgery for degenerative mitral regurgitation; 4,253 (93%) underwent repair. Preoperatively, 30% were in New York Heart Association (NYHA) class I (asymptomatic), 56% in class II, 13% in class III, and 2% in class IV. Multivariable analysis and propensity matching were used to assess association of symptoms (NYHA class) with cardiac structure and function and postoperative outcomes.

Results.—Increasing NYHA class was associated with progressive reduction in left ventricular function, left atrial enlargement, and development of atrial fibrillation and tricuspid regurgitation. These findings were evident even in class II patients (mild symptoms). Repair was accomplished in 96% of asymptomatic patients, and in progressively fewer as NYHA class increased (93%, 86%, and 85% in classes II to IV, respectively; $p < 0.0001$). Hospital mortality was 0.37%, but was particularly high in class IV (0.29%, 0.20%, 0.67%, and 5.1% for classes I to IV, respectively; $p = 0.004$). Although long-term survival progressively diminished with increasing NHYA class, these differences were largely related to differences in left ventricular function and increased comorbidity.

Conclusions.—In patients with severe degenerative mitral regurgitation, the development of even mild symptoms by the time of surgical referral is associated with deleterious changes in cardiac structure and function. Therefore, particularly because successful repair is highly likely, early surgery is justified in asymptomatic patients with degenerative disease and severe mitral regurgitation.

▶ The American College of Cardiology/American Heart Association (ACC/AHA) practice guidelines recommending surgery for asymptomatic patients with severe mitral regurgitation caused by degenerative disease remain controversial. With this controversy in mind, researchers from the Cleveland Clinic shared their broad experience in mitral valve repair and documented results based on New York Heart Association (NYHA) classification. With increasing NYHA class, the likelihood of repair decreased significantly and the subsequent in-hospital mortality increased. Long-term survival was also decreased in patients with increased NYHA class, but this was likely related to decreases in left ventricular ejection fraction. This article stands as a seminal work to fortify the ACC/AHA guidelines for early surgical intervention in patients with severe asymptomatic mitral regurgitation.

W. B. Keeling, MD

Transapical transcatheter aortic valve implantation: Follow-up to 3 years
Ye J, Cheung A, Lichtenstein SV, et al (Univ of British Columbia, Vancouver, Canada)
J Thorac Cardiovasc Surg 139:1107-1113, 2010

Background.—We performed the first human case of successful transapical transcatheter aortic valve implantation on a beating heart in October 2005, and therefore we have the longest follow-up on transapical aortic valve implantation in humans. We now report clinical and echocardiographic outcomes of transapical aortic valve implantation in 71 patients.

Methods.—Between October 2005 and February 2009, 71 patients (44 female) underwent transcatheter transapical aortic valve implantation with either 23- or 26-mm Edwards Lifesciences transcatheter bioprostheses. All patients with symptomatic aortic stenosis were declined for conventional aortic valve replacement owing to unacceptable operative risks and were not candidates for transfemoral aortic valve implantation because of poor arterial access. Clinical and echocardiographic follow-ups were performed before discharge, at 1 and 6 months, and then yearly. The mean follow-up was 12.9 ± 11.5 months with a total of 917.3 months of follow-up.

Results.—Mean age was 80.0 ± 8.1 years and predicted operative mortality was $34.5\% \pm 20.4\%$ by logistic EuroSCORE and $12.1\% \pm 7.7\%$ by The Society of Thoracic Surgeons Risk Calculator. Valves were successfully implanted in all patients. Twelve patients died within 30 days (30-day mortality: 16.9% in all patients, 33% in the first 15 patients, and 12.5% in the remainder), and 10 patients died subsequently. Overall survival at 24 and 36 months was $66.3\% \pm 6.4\%$ and $58.0\% \pm 9.5\%$, respectively. Among 59 patients who survived at least 30 days, 24- and

36-month survivals were 79.8% ± 6.4%and 69.8% ± 10.9%, respectively. Late valve-related complications were rare. New York Heart Association functional class improved significantly from preoperative 3.3 ± 0.8 to 1.8 ± 0.8 at 24 months. The aortic valve area and mean gradient remained stable at 24 months (1.6 ± 0.3 cm² and 10.3 ± 5.9 mm Hg, respectively).

Conclusion.—Our outcome suggests that transapical transcatheter aortic valve implantation provides sustained clinical and hemodynamic benefits for up to 36 months in selected high-risk patients with symptomatic severe aortic stenosis.

▶ Transcatheter aortic valve implantation (TAVI) has been well described in patients with severe aortic stenosis and considered high risk. This retrospective review from one of the largest sites of TAVI in the world suggests that the transapical approach, in the right hands and after a significant initial learning curve, appears to be a viable option for what may be the highest risk patients, in those in which vascular access is inadequate for retrograde transfemoral TAVI. In the lessons learned in this patient population at very high risk, the authors have noted that (1) patients with end-stage organ diseases should not be recommended for transapical TAVI since correcting aortic stenosis would not necessarily reverse their poor outcome; (2) hybrid operating room with a high-quality imaging system is preferable to the portable C-arm fluoroscope that provides suboptimal images during the procedure; (3) surgical technique is particularly important in avoiding fatal complications, such as massive apical bleeding; (4) operators should understand potential major complications and appropriate ways to deal with these complications on an emergency basis; and (5) postoperative care in this patient population is extremely important, especially in preventing and managing pneumonia, line infection, sepsis, or acute renal failure.

W. B. Keeling, MD

Transcatheter Aortic-Valve Implantation for Aortic Stenosis in Patients Who Cannot Undergo Surgery
Leon MB, for the PARTNER Trial Investigators (Columbia Univ Med Ctr/ New York—Presbyterian Hosp; et al)
N Engl J Med 363:1597-1607, 2010

Background.—Many patients with severe aortic stenosis and coexisting conditions are not candidates for surgical replacement of the aortic valve. Recently, transcatheter aortic-valve implantation (TAVI) has been suggested as a less invasive treatment for high-risk patients with aortic stenosis.

Methods.—We randomly assigned patients with severe aortic stenosis, whom surgeons considered not to be suitable candidates for surgery, to standard therapy (including balloon aortic valvuloplasty) or transfemoral transcatheter implantation of a balloon-expandable bovine pericardial valve. The primary end point was the rate of death from any cause.

Results.—A total of 358 patients with aortic stenosis who were not considered to be suitable candidates for surgery underwent randomization at 21 centers (17 in the United States). At 1 year, the rate of death from any cause (Kaplan—Meier analysis) was 30.7% with TAVI, as compared with 50.7% with standard therapy (hazard ratio with TAVI, 0.55; 95% confidence interval [CI], 0.40 to 0.74; P<0.001). The rate of the composite end point of death from any cause or repeat hospitalization was 42.5% with TAVI as compared with 71.6% with standard therapy (hazard ratio, 0.46; 95% CI, 0.35 to 0.59; P<0.001). Among survivors at 1 year, the rate of cardiac symptoms (New York Heart Association class III or IV) was lower among patients who had undergone TAVI than among those who had received standard therapy (25.2% vs. 58.0%, P<0.001). At 30 days, TAVI, as compared with standard therapy, was associated with a higher incidence of major strokes (5.0% vs. 1.1%, P = 0.06) and major vascular complications (16.2% vs. 1.1%, P<0.001). In the year after TAVI, there was no deterioration in the functioning of the bioprosthetic valve, as assessed by evidence of stenosis or regurgitation on an echocardiogram.

Conclusions.—In patients with severe aortic stenosis who were not suitable candidates for surgery, TAVI, as compared with standard therapy, significantly reduced the rates of death from any cause, the composite end point of death from any cause or repeat hospitalization, and cardiac symptoms, despite the higher incidence of major strokes and major vascular events. (Funded by Edwards Lifesciences; ClinicalTrials.gov number, NCT00530894.)

▶ Transcatheter aortic-valve implantation (TAVI) has emerged as an alternative treatment for aortic stenosis in patients who are considered to have a high or prohibitive surgical risk. TAVI can be performed by either a retrograde approach, in which a catheter is inserted through the common femoral artery, or an antegrade transapical approach, in which a catheter is inserted through the apex of the left ventricle with the use of an anterolateral thoracotomy. Single-center nonrandomized trials have shown the feasibility of TAVI in patients who are not suitable candidates for surgical replacement of the aortic valve; however, there has been a paucity of data from randomized trials comparing TAVI with medical management in this population. Leon and his colleagues report the results of the Placement of Aortic Transcatheter Valves trial, a prospective, randomized, multicenter trial to determine the optimal method of treating patients with critical aortic stenosis who are considered not to be suitable candidates for surgery. This is a well-designed study that confirms that untreated severe aortic stenosis has a poor outcome, and TAVI is associated with a dramatic improvement in survival and symptoms. While TAVI was associated with a high risk of stroke and vascular complications in this trial, these rates are likely to improve with better technology and greater operator experience. The absolute reduction in mortality seen in this trial is unparalleled in the modern era and establishes TAVI as the standard of care in patients with aortic stenosis, who are not surgical candidates.

W. B. Keeling, MD

Transplantation/Ventricular Assist Devices

A United Network for Organ Sharing analysis of heart transplantation in adults with congenital heart disease: Outcomes and factors associated with mortality and retransplantation
Karamlou T, Hirsch J, Welke K, et al (Univ of Michigan, Ann Arbor; Oregon Health & Science Univ, Portland)
J Thorac Cardiovasc Surg 140:161-168, 2010

Objectives.—Heart transplantation in patients with adult congenital heart disease is increasing, yet no large studies have defined how this subgroup differs from other adult recipients. We investigated outcomes and risk factors for mortality and retransplantation among patients with adult congenital heart disease compared with adult recipients.

Methods.—A review was performed of 18- to 45-year-old patients undergoing heart transplantation from 1990–2008 reported to the United Network for Organ Sharing database. Trends were compared between 2 eras: era 1 (1990–1998) and era 2 (1999–2008). Multivariable semiparametric hazard models identified factors associated with time-related death and retransplantation.

Results.—Of 8496 patients identified, 575 had adult congenital heart disease. The prevalence of heart transplantation among adult recipients decreased by 28% over time ($P < .001$) and increased among patients with adult congenital heart disease by 41% ($P < .001$). Induction therapy use was less in patients with adult congenital heart disease (66%) compared with that seen in adult recipients (71%, $P = .02$). Steroid maintenance was less in patients with adult congenital heart disease (92%) compared with that seen in adult recipients (97%, $P < .001$). Post–heart transplantation survival among adult recipients improved over time ($P = .02$) but not among patients with adult congenital heart disease ($P = .81$). Overall post–heart transplantation mortality ($P = .006$) and retransplantation ($P = .03$) were significantly higher for patients with adult congenital heart disease than for adult recipients, mainly because of an early hazard phase. Adult congenital heart disease was a risk factor for both death ($P < .001$) and retransplantation ($P = .04$). Any induction therapy and steroid maintenance was associated with improved survival for all recipients ($P = .001$).

Conclusions.—Adult congenital heart disease represents an increasing proportion of heart transplant recipients. Compared with adult recipients, patients with adult congenital heart disease experience higher post–heart transplantation mortality and retransplantation. Immunosuppression differs among patients with adult congenital heart disease and adult recipients. Further studies should investigate whether post–heart transplantation outcomes would be improved by more aggressive induction therapy or judicious steroid tapers.

▶ Advances in surgical and medical management have greatly improved the long-term survival of patients with congenital heart disease. Coupled with the added complexity of heart transplantation (HTx) in patients with adult congenital heart disease (ACHD) compared with other adult recipients (ARs), patients with ACHD are likely to comprise an increasing number of HTx recipients in the near future. Many of these are anticipated to be single-ventricle patients, a subgroup whose outcomes might be less favorable than those patients with biventricular physiology. Despite these changes in the ACHD recipient pool, preoperative selection and postoperative management of patients with ACHD and ARs have been similar without evidence supporting this approach. Thus only small single-institution reports for posttransplantation outcomes in patients with ACHD have been reported. The study by Karamlou and colleagues based on cumulative United Network for Organ Sharing experience, which is a large retrospective study with prospectively collected data, is very timely. They have concluded that patients with ACHD represent an increasing proportion of HTx recipients. Higher post—heart transplant mortality and retransplant rates among patients with ACHD compared with ARs are persistent over time. Furthermore, management of immunosuppression differs among patients with ACHD and ARs. This study opens the door for more invasive analysis of this patient cohort.

V. H. Thourani, MD

Early and late outcomes of 517 consecutive adult patients treated with extracorporeal membrane oxygenation for refractory postcardiotomy cardiogenic shock
Rastan AJ, Dege A, Mohr M, et al (Univ of Leipzig, Germany)
J Thorac Cardiovasc Surg 139:302-311, 2010

Objective.—Adult postcardiotomy cardiogenic shock potentially requiring mechanical circulatory support occurs in 0.5% to 1.5% of cases. Risk factors influencing early or long-term outcome after extracorporeal membrane oxygenation implantation are not well described.

Methods.—Between May 1996 and May 2008, 517 adult patients received extracorporeal membrane oxygenation support for postcardiotomy cardiogenic shock. Procedures were isolated coronary artery bypass grafting (37.4%), isolated valve surgery (14.3%), coronary artery bypass grafting plus valve surgery (16.8%), thoracic organ transplantion (6.5%), and other combinations (25.0%). Fifty-four preoperative and 42 procedural risk factors concerning in-hospital mortality were evaluated by logistic regression analyses.

Results.—Mean age was 63.5 years, 71.5% were male, ejection fraction was 45.9% ± 17.6%, logistic EuroSCORE was 21.6% ± 20.7%. Extracorporeal membrane oxygenation was established through thoracic (60.8%) or extrathoracic (39.2%) cannulation. Extracorporeal membrane oxygenation support was 3.28 ± 2.85 days. Intra-aortic balloon pumps were implanted in 74.1%. Weaning from extracorporeal membrane oxygenation was successful for 63.3%, and 24.8%were discharged.

Cerebrovascular events occurred in 17.4%, gastrointestinal complications in 18.8%, and renal replacement therapy in 65.0%. Risk factors for hospital mortality were age older than 70 years (odds ratio, 1.6), diabetes (odds ratio, 2.5), preoperative renal insufficiency (odds ratio, 2.1), obesity (odds ratio, 1.8), logistic EuroSCORE greater than 20% (odds ratio, 1.8), operative lactate greater than 4 mmol/L (odds ratio, 2.2). Isolated coronary artery bypass grafting (odds ratio, 0.44) was protective. Cumulative survivals were 17.6% after 6 months, 16.5% after 1 year, and 13.7% after 5 years.

Conclusions.—Extracorporeal membrane oxygenation support is an acceptable option for patients with postcardiotomy cardiogenic shock who otherwise would die and is justified by good long-term outcome of hospital survivors. Because of high morbidity and mortality, extracorporeal membrane oxygenation must be decided by individual risk profile.

▶ Patients with persistent refractory postcardiotomy cardiogenic shock (PCS) despite optimal medical treatment and intra-aortic balloon pump face almost certain death, and all treatment alternatives have to be assessed in the light of an otherwise dismal prognosis. Although the incidence of PCS in adult cardiac surgical patients only ranges from 0.5% to 1.5%, it is a dreaded complication following cardiac surgery. Rastan and colleagues have reported on a large cohort of patients with PCS supported by extracorporeal membrane oxygenation (ECMO). Not surprisingly, for this difficult group of patients, this experience featured substantial mortality and morbidity, particularly bleeding and thromboembolic complications. The hospital survival of approximately 25% is similar to numerous previous reports as well as to registry data, which are approximately in the 30% to 35% range. They have shown that in these high-risk patients, the implantation of an ECMO device is an easily applicable and widely accepted option for temporary mechanical circulatory support allowing cardiac and pulmonary recovery or bridging until further therapeutic alternatives can be carefully considered. During the last 20 years however, ECMO results in these patients have not been satisfactory. Successful ECMO weaning rate ranges from 31% to 60% and corresponds with an in-hospital mortality of 59% to 84%. By indication, acute myocardial failure is the major cause of mortality, although a significant number of other primary causes of death have also been reported. A major disadvantage of ECMO is the need for anticoagulation and the requirement of high amounts of transfused blood products, increasing the systemic inflammatory response that is induced by the initial surgery, the ECMO components, and PCS itself. Thus, indication for temporary ECMO support for PCS always depends on patient-specific characteristics and center experience, balancing risks and benefits.

V. H. Thourani, MD

Post–cardiac transplant survival after support with a continuous-flow left ventricular assist device: Impact of duration of left ventricular assist device support and other variables

John R, Pagani FD, Naka Y, et al (Univ of Minnesota, Minneapolis; Univ of Michigan, Ann Arbor; Columbia Univ, NY; et al)
J Thorac Cardiovasc Surg 140:174-181, 2010

Objective.—Although left ventricular assist devices (LVADs) are associated with excellent outcomes in patients with end-stage heart failure, there are conflicting reports on posttransplant survival in these patients. Furthermore, prior studies with pulsatile LVADs have shown that transplantation, either early (<6 weeks) or late (>6 months) after LVAD implantation, adversely affected post–cardiac transplant survival. We sought to determine factors related to posttransplant survival in patients supported with continuous-flow LVADs.

Methods.—The HeartMate II LVAD (Thoratec Corporation, Pleasanton, Calif) was implanted in 468 patients as a bridge to transplant at 36 centers in a multicenter trial. Patients who underwent transplantation after support were stratified by demographics: gender, age, etiology, body mass index, duration of device support, and by adverse events during support. The median age was 54 years (range 18–73 years); 43% had ischemic etiology, and 18% were women. Survival was determined at the specific intervals of 30 days and 1 year after transplantation.

Results.—Of 468 patients, 250 (53%) underwent cardiac transplant after a median duration of LVAD support of 151 days (longest: 3.2 years), 106 (23%) died, 12 (2.6%) recovered ventricular function and the device was removed, and 100 (21%) were still receiving LVAD support. The overall 30-day and 1-year posttransplant survivals were 97% and 87%. There were no significant differences in survival based on demographic factors or LVAD duration of less than 30 days, 30 to 90 days, 90 to 180 days, and more than 180 days. Patients requiring more than 2 units of packed red blood cells in 24 hours during LVAD support had a statistically significant decreased 1-year survival (82% vs 94%) when compared with patients who did not require more than 2 units of packed red blood cells in 24 hours during LVAD support ($P = .03$). There was a trend for slightly lower survival at 1 year in patients with percutaneous lead infections during LVAD support versus no infection (75% vs 89%; $P = .07$).

Conclusions.—Post–cardiac transplant survival in patients supported with continuous-flow devices such as the HeartMate II LVAD is equivalent to that with conventional transplantation. Furthermore, posttransplant survival is not influenced by the duration of LVAD support. The improved durability and reduced short- and long-term morbidity associated with the HeartMate II LVAD has reduced the need for urgent cardiac transplantation, which may have adversely influenced survival in the pulsatile LVAD era. This information may have significant implications for changing the current

United Network for Organ Sharing criteria regarding listing of heart transplant candidates.

▶ Heart transplantation remains the gold standard treatment modality for patients with advanced heart failure. However, the limited availability of donor hearts has led to an increasing number of patients who are being successfully bridged to a heart transplant with a left ventricular assist device (LVAD). Most patients who have undergone LVAD placement as a bridge to transplant (BTT) in the United States have been supported by pulsatile volume-displacement devices such as the HeartMate XVE device. The new HeartMate II LVAD, which incorporates continuous-flow rotary pump technology, represents the next generation of devices. Continuous-flow rotary pumps are thought to have enhanced durability and provide improved quality of life for extended periods of support. The HeartMate II LVAD has recently concluded a Food and Drug Administration (FDA)—approved pivotal trial in 133 patients designed to evaluate outcomes at 6 months. In this report by John and colleagues, 335 additional patients have undergone implantation of the HeartMate II LVAD through a continued-access protocol approved by the FDA and 250 have received transplants. They have reported on the results of posttransplant survival in patients who have undergone heart transplantation from this large observational clinical study using the HeartMate II LVAD as a BTT. The findings from this study support and validate the use of the HeartMate II as BTT.

V. H. Thourani, MD

Right ventricular failure in patients with the HeartMate II continuous-flow left ventricular assist device: Incidence, risk factors, and effect on outcomes
Kormos RL, for the HeartMate II Clinical Investigators (Univ of Pittsburgh Med Ctr, PA; et al)
J Thorac Cardiovasc Surg 139:1316-1324, 2010

Objective.—The aim of this study was to evaluate the incidence, risk factors, and effect on outcomes of right ventricular failure in a large population of patients implanted with continuous-flow left ventricular assist devices.

Methods.—Patients (n = 484) enrolled in the HeartMate II left ventricular assist device (Thoratec, Pleasanton, Calif) bridge-to-transplantation clinical trial were examined for the occurrence of right ventricular failure. Right ventricular failure was defined as requiring a right ventricular assist device, 14 or more days of inotropic support after implantation, and/or inotropic support starting more than 14 days after implantation. Demographics, along with clinical, laboratory, and hemodynamic data, were compared between patients with and without right ventricular failure, and risk factors were identified.

Results.—Overall, 30 (6%) patients receiving left ventricular assist devices required a right ventricular assist device, 35 (7%) required extended inotropes, and 33 (7%) required late inotropes. A significantly greater percentage of patients without right ventricular failure survived to transplantation, recovery, or ongoing device support at 180 days compared with patients with right ventricular failure (89% vs 71%, P < .001). Multivariate analysis revealed that a central venous pressure/pulmonary capillary wedge pressure ratio of greater than 0.63 (odds ratio, 2.3; 95% confidence interval, 1.2–4.3; P = .009), need for preoperative ventilator support (odds ratio, 5.5; 95% confidence interval, 2.3–13.2; P < .001), and blood urea nitrogen level of greater than 39 mg/dL (odds ratio, 2.1; 95% confidence interval, 1.1–4.1; P = .02) were independent predictors of right ventricular failure after left ventricular assist device implantation.

Conclusions.—The incidence of right ventricular failure in patients with a HeartMate II ventricular assist device is comparable or less than that of patients with pulsatile-flow devices. Its occurrence is associated with worse outcomes than seen in patients without right ventricular failure. Patients at risk for right ventricular failure might benefit from preoperative optimization of right heart function or planned biventricular support.

▶ Mechanical circulatory support and, more specifically, left ventricular assist devices (LVADs) can be used as destination therapy for patients who are not suitable for transplantation and as temporary support for patients whose cardiac function is expected to recover. Outcomes of patients are critically dependent on right ventricular function (RVF), which must provide sufficient flow through the pulmonary vasculature to fill the LVAD and ensure optimal performance. Most of the current studies describing RVF in patients with LVADs are limited by either a small sample size or a single-center experience or were done on earlier generation pulsatile devices. However, a detailed analysis of multicenter data for the risks of RVF with the continuous-flow devices has not been established for a large group of patients. This study is the first to examine RVF in a large cohort undergoing implant of a commonly used, contemporary, continuous-flow device. Although preoperative univariable predictors may have been correlated, variable dichotomization was potentially biased and power was limited to perform detailed multivariable analyses required to identify truly independent RVF risk predictors. This study again highlights the importance of closely examining preoperative laboratory and cardiopulmonary hemodynamics to gauge RVF risk. It also reveals that rates of RVF and right ventricular assist device requirements in patients with the HeartMate II are low relative to previous results with pulsatile LVADs and support the use of this device in those with end-stage heart failure.

V. H. Thourani, MD

Miscellaneous

Where does atrial fibrillation surgery fail? Implications for increasing effectiveness of ablation

McCarthy PM, Kruse J, Shalli S, et al (Northwestern Univ Feinberg School of Medicine and Northwestern Memorial Hosp, Chicago, IL)
J Thorac Cardiovasc Surg 139:860-867, 2010

Objective.—Surgical ablation of atrial fibrillation is generally safe and effective, but atrial fibrillation redevelops in approximately 20% of patients. We sought to determine anatomic factors, technology factors, or both that contribute to these failures.

Methods.—Four hundred eight patients underwent 5 types of atrial fibrillation ablation depending on their atrial fibrillation history and need for concomitant surgical intervention: the classic maze procedure, high-intensity focused ultrasound, the left atrial maze procedure, the biatrial maze procedure, and pulmonary vein isolation. Ninety-five percent of patients with preoperative atrial fibrillation underwent surgical ablation.

Results.—Patients undergoing high-intensity focused ultrasound had a high rate of late postoperative percutaneous ablation (37.5%) after surgical intervention ($P < .001$ vs the other groups). At last follow-up, freedom from atrial fibrillation and need for ablation was as follows: classic maze procedure, 90%; high-intensity focused ultrasound, 43%; left atrial maze procedure, 79%; biatrial maze procedure, 79%; and pulmonary vein isolation, 69% ($P < .001$ between groups). For those with atrial fibrillation, mapping and ablation were performed in 23.6% (n = 27), and all patients with high-intensity focused ultrasound had failure of the box lesion around the pulmonary veins. Of those with just the left atrial maze procedure or pulmonary vein isolation, the right atrium was the source for failure in 75% (6/8).

Conclusions.—Patients undergoing high-intensity focused ultrasound had a high need for postoperative ablation and low freedom from atrial fibrillation. The classic maze procedure had the best results. Left atrial ablation might allow failure from right atrial foci. Matching the technology and lesion set to the patient yields good results and can be applied in 95% of patients. We suggest others obtain late catheter ablation to correct remaining atrial fibrillation, and add to the paucity of late data regarding failure mode.

▶ From the Society of Thoracic Surgeons Database, concomitant atrial fibrillation (AF) ablation surgery increased from 28.1% in 2004 to 39% in 2007 and was performed during mitral valve (MV) surgery (in those with preoperative AF) in 54.7% of cases. Six prospective randomized trials have also demonstrated a statistically significantly better return to sinus rhythm (44%-94%) for those patients who were treated with AF ablation versus control subjects. However, it appears that failures occur in approximately 20% of patients who undergo AF ablation with MV surgery. The sources of energy and techniques of AF ablation vary widely among surgeons. In the study by McCarthy and colleagues, they analyzed the patterns of ablation failure and determined whether there are identifiable causes, such as incomplete lesion sets or unreliable technologies. The principal findings of this study confirm the general success of surgical treatments for AF with a low perioperative risk and 84% of antiarrhythmia drugs at the last follow-up, that there was a high failure rate using high-intensity focused ultrasound technology related to incomplete transmural encircling lesions, that left atrial lesions alone allow for AF failure from right atrial foci, and that the mitral isthmus lesion is another potential source of failure. This retrospective study was a real-world study using various techniques and technologies adapted for a variety of concomitant or stand-alone operations. However, there is obvious inherent patient selection bias with significantly differing subsets, each of which have different mechanisms for AF. The study design is complicated, attempting to delineate 5 techniques (3 different surgical approaches), each with a modality of having inherent modes of failure, different ability to deliver transmurality, inadequate design of the instrument, and varying ability to produce lesion sets. Despite the limitations, this important article considers many of the factors that are important in the decision-making process for the surgical treatment of AF. A clear treatment algorithm is offered that can help surgeons increase their success, with an obvious potential benefit for patients.

V. H. Thourani, MD

.

4 Coronary Heart Disease

Acute ST-Segment Elevation Myocardial Infarction

Association Between Timeliness of Reperfusion Therapy and Clinical Outcomes in ST-Elevation Myocardial Infarction
Lambert L, Brown K, Segal E, et al (McGill Univ, Montreal, Québec, Canada; et al)
JAMA 303:2148-2155, 2010

Context.—Guidelines emphasize the importance of rapid reperfusion of patients with ST-elevation myocardial infarction (STEMI) and specify a maximum delay of 30 minutes for fibrinolysis and 90 minutes for primary percutaneous coronary intervention (PPCI). However, randomized trials and selective registries are limited in their ability to assess the effect of timeliness of reperfusion on outcomes in real-world STEMI patients.

Objectives.—To obtain a complete interregional portrait of contemporary STEMI care and to investigate timeliness of reperfusion and outcomes.

Design, Setting, and Patients.—Systematic evaluation of STEMI care for 6 months during 2006-2007 in 80 hospitals that treated more than 95% of patients with acute myocardial infarction in the province of Quebec, Canada (population, 7.8 million).

Main Outcome Measures.—Death at 30 days and at 1 year and the combined end point of death or hospital readmission for acute myocardial infarction or congestive heart failure at 1 year by linkage to Quebec's medicoadministrative databases.

Results.—Of 1832 patients treated with reperfusion, 392 (21.4%) received fibrinolysis and 1440 (78.6%) received PPCI. Fibrinolysis was untimely (>30 minutes) in 54% and PPCI was untimely (>90 minutes) in 68%. Death or readmission for acute myocardial infarction or heart failure at 1 year occurred in 13.5% of fibrinolysis patients and 13.6% of PPCI patients. When the 2 treatment groups were combined, patients treated outside of recommended delays had an adjusted higher risk of death at 30 days (6.6% vs 3.3%; odds ratio [OR], 2.14; 95% confidence interval [CI], 1.21-3.93) and a statistically nonsignificant increase in risk of death at 1 year (9.3% vs 5.2%; OR, 1.61; 95% CI, 1.00-2.66) compared with patients who received timely treatment. Patients treated outside of recommended delays also had an adjusted higher risk for the combined outcome of death or hospital readmission for congestive heart failure or acute myocardial infarction at 1 year (15.0% vs 9.2%; OR, 1.57; 95% CI, 1.08-2.30). At the regional level, after adjustment, each 10% increase in patients treated within the recommended time was associated with a decrease in the region-level odds of overall 30-day mortality (OR, 0.80; 95% CI, 0.65-0.98).

Conclusion.—Among patients in Quebec with STEMI, reperfusion delivered outside guideline-recommend delays was associated with significantly increased 30-day mortality, a statistically nonsignificant increase in 1-year mortality, and significantly increased risk of the composite of mortality or readmission for acute myocardial infarction or heart failure at 1 year (Table 3).

▶ This is an important article based upon a systematic evaluation of ST-segment elevation myocardial infarction (STEMI) care for a 6-month period for all patients in the province of Quebec, Canada. A strength of this study is

TABLE 3.—Adverse Outcomes by Type and Timeliness of Treatment

Outcomes	No. (%) of Patients		OR (95% CI)[a]
	Fibrinolysis		
	≤30 min (n = 182)	>30 min (n = 210)	
Mortality at 30 d	6 (3.3)	18 (8.6)	2.75 (1.07-7.08)
Mortality at 1 y	8 (4.4)	21 (10.0)	2.41 (1.04-5.60)
Readmission for AMI at 1 y	7 (3.3)	7 (3.8)	0.86 (0.29-2.51)
Readmission for CHF at 1 y	2 (1.1)	9 (4.3)	4.02 (0.86-18.90)
Mortality, CHF, or AMI at 1 y	16 (8.8)	37 (17.6)	2.22 (1.19-4.14)
	PPCI[b]		
	≤90 min (n = 417)	<90 min (n = 870)	
Mortality at 30 d	14 (3.4)	53 (6.1)	1.87 (1.02-3.41)
Mortality at 1 y	23 (5.5)	79 (9.1)	1.71 (1.06-2.76)
Readmission for AMI at 1 y	8 (1.9)	21 (2.4)	1.26 (0.56-2.88)
Readmission for CHF at 1 y	8 (1.9)	33 (3.8)	2.02 (0.92-4.40)
Mortality, CHF, or AMI at 1 y	39 (9.4)	125 (14.4)	1.63 (1.11-2.38)
	Combined Fibrinolysis and PPCI[b]		
	≤ Recommended Delay (n = 599)	< Recommended Delay (n = 1080)	
Mortality at 30 d	20 (3.3)	71 (6.6)	2.04 (1.22-3.38) 2.14 (1.21-3.93)[c]
Mortality at 1 y	31 (5.2)	100 (9.3)	1.87 (1.23-2.83) 1.61 (1.00-2.66)[c]
Mortality, CHF, or AMI at 1 y	55 (9.2)	162 (15.0)	1.75 (1.26-2.41) 1.57 (1.08-2.30)[c]

Abbreviations: AMI, acute myocardial infarction; CHF, congestive heart failure; CI, confidence interval; OR, odds ratio; PPCI, primary percutaneous coronary intervention.
[a]Odds ratios are unadjusted unless otherwise indicated.
[b]Patients sent to the catheterization laboratory but who did not receive PPCI were excluded from these analyses.
[c]Adjusted OR.

the inclusion of all patients with STEMI since prior registry studies have demonstrated bias in that eligible patients who were not enrolled received poorer quality care and sustained a 3-fold greater mortality.[1,2] Another limitation of some registries is that the predominance of centers may be academic and highly motivated and as such not representative of the wider world of clinical practice.

Of 2356 patients with STEMI, 61.1% were treated with primary percutaneous coronary intervention (PPCI), 16.6% with fibrinolysis, and 22.2% received no reperfusion therapy. This article focuses on reperfusion therapy so we do not have much information on those who received either PPCI or fibrinolytics, but other studies would suggest that such patients constitute a sicker group.

The major point of the article is that patients treated outside the guideline-recommended delays of less than 30 minutes with fibrinolysis (door-to-needle time) and less than 90 minutes for PPCI (door-to-balloon time) had a higher 30-day mortality, a nonsignificant increased 1-year mortality, and a statistically significant increase in the composite of mortality or readmission for heart failure at 1 year. It should be emphasized, however, that most patients actually did receive untimely treatment because of excessive delays, 54% with lytics and 68% with PPCI.

In an analysis by region, it is interesting that the timeliness of treatment was associated with lower mortality rates irrespective of whether patients had PPCI or fibrinolytics. Moreover, this was not because of selection bias incurred by treating healthier patients more quickly. This is reassuring news for those living in areas where PPCI is not an option.

What is, however, lacking in this and many other data sets is information on treatment delays stratified by total ischemia time from the onset of symptoms. Based upon the slope of the curve correlating duration of ischemia prior to reperfusion and mortality,[3] one would expect that the major impact of treatment delay would be in patients with the shortest duration of symptoms when time is muscle.

B. J. Gersh, MB, ChB, DPhil, FRCP

References

1. Ferreira-González I, Marsal JR, Mitvavila F, et al. Patient registries of acute coronary syndrome: assessing or biasing the clinical real world data? *Circ Cardiovasc Qual Outcomes.* 2009;2:540-547.
2. Krumholz HM. Registries and selection bias: the need for accountability. *Circ Cardiovasc Qual Outcomes.* 2009;2:517-518.
3. Gersh BJ, Stone GW, White HD, Holmes DR Jr. Pharmacological facilitation of primary percutaneous coronary intervention for acute myocardial infarction: is the slope of the curve the shape of the future? *JAMA.* 2005;293:979-986.

Culprit Vessel Percutaneous Coronary Intervention Versus Multivessel and Staged Percutaneous Coronary Intervention for ST-Segment Elevation Myocardial Infarction Patients With Multivessel Disease

Hannan EL, Samadashvili Z, Walford G, et al (Univ at Albany, NY; St Joseph's Hosp, Syracuse, NY; et al)
J AM Coll Cardiol Intr 3:22-31, 2010

Objectives.—The purpose of this study was to examine the differences in in-hospital and longer-term mortality for ST-segment elevation myocardial infarction (STEMI) patients with multivessel disease as a function of whether they underwent single-vessel (culprit vessel) percutaneous coronary interventions (PCIs) or multivessel PCI.

Background.—The optimal treatment of patients with STEMI and multivessel disease is of continuing interest in the era of drug-eluting stents.

Methods.—STEMI patients with multivessel disease undergoing PCIs in New York between January 1, 2003, and June 30, 2006, were subdivided into those who underwent culprit vessel PCI and those who underwent multivessel PCI during the index procedure, during the index admission, or staged within 60 days of the index admission. Patients were propensity-matched and mortality rates were calculated at 12, 24, and 42 months.

Results.—A total of 3,521 patients (87.5%) underwent culprit vessel PCI during the index procedure. A total of 259 of them underwent staged PCI during the index admission and 538 patients underwent staged PCI within 60 days of the index procedure. For patients without hemodynamic compromise, culprit vessel PCI during the index procedure was associated with lower in-hospital mortality than multivessel PCI during the index procedure (0.9% vs. 2.4%, p = 0.04). Patients undergoing staged multivessel PCI within 60 days after the index procedure had a significantly lower 12-month mortality rate than patients undergoing culprit vessel PCI only (1.3% vs. 3.3%, p = 0.04).

Conclusions.—Our findings support the American College of Cardiology/American Heart Association (ACC/AHA) recommendation that culprit vessel PCI be used for STEMI patients with multivessel disease at the time of the index PCI when patients are not hemodynamically compromised. However, staged PCI within 60 days after the index procedure, including during the index admission, is associated with risk-adjusted mortality rates that are comparable with the rate for culprit vessel PCI alone.

▶ Current American College of Cardiology/American Heart Association guidelines for primary percutaneous coronary intervention (PPCI) in patients with ST-segment elevation myocardial infarction recommend PPCI as the treatment of choice. In patients with multivessel disease, PPCI of the culprit vessel (CV) only is recommended, unless patients are hemodynamically compromised.[1] This remains an area of controversy, which is addressed by this interesting article from the large New York State registry database.

The vast majority of the patients were treated with CV PCI, and in comparison with those undergoing multivessel PCI at the time of the index procedure, CV patients were younger with a lower proportion of ejection fractions at 50% or more but also with a lower proportion with poor ejection fractions of 19% or less. In addition, CV PCI patients had a lower likelihood of a chronic total occlusion, had a better thrombolysis in myocardial infarction (TIMI) flow grades in the CV, and were more likely to receive drug-eluting stents. Propensity matching was carried out to minimize the impact of these baseline differences. Overall, mortality rates were lower in patients undergoing CV PCI alone in comparison with those undergoing multivessel PCI during the same procedure. This would tend to support the guidelines, but one cannot discount the role of confounders. Were patients undergoing multivessel PCI at the time of the index procedure a sicker group? This would not clearly appear to be the case using measured parameters, but this remains, nonetheless, the Achilles heel of all observational studies and despite the statistical adjustment, residual bias might still exist. This is particularly the case, as pointed out by the authors, when there are many potential confounders that were unmeasured, including persistent pain, ST-segment elevation after dilatation of the CV, or the presence of another lesion compromising TIMI flow.

What was interesting in this study is the apparently lower mortality in 1 year in patients who underwent a staged multivessel PCI within 60 days or less but not during the index admission. What is also interesting is that there is no mortality difference between patients undergoing CV PCI and staged multivessel PCI during the same admission but not during the index procedure. It would appear, therefore, that in the absence of a trial, it is reasonable to perform CV PCI in most patients with multivessel disease undergoing PPCI, and if it is felt that multivessel PCI is necessary, this can be done as a staged procedure during the initial hospitalization or at a later stage. In some patients with severe hemodynamic compromise, including cardiogenic shock, multivessel PCI at the time of the initial procedure may still be a reasonable option.

B. J. Gersh, MB, ChB, DPhil, FRCP

Reference

1. Smith SC Jr, Feldman TE, Hirshfield JW Jr, et al. ACC/AHA/SCAI 2005 guideline update for percutaneous coronary intervention: a report of the American College of Cardiology/American Heart Association Task force on Practice Guidelines (ACC/AHA/SCAI Writing Committee to Update the 2001 Guidelines for Percutaneous Coronary Intervention). *J Am Coll Cardiol.* 2006;47:e1-121.

Early routine percutaneous coronary intervention after fibrinolysis vs. standard therapy in ST-segment elevation myocardial infarction: a meta-analysis
Borgia F, Goodman SG, Halvorsen S, et al (Royal Brompton Hosp and Imperial College, London, UK; Univ of Toronto, Canada; Oslo Univ Hosp, Ulleval, Norway; et al)
Eur Heart J 31:2156-2169, 2010

Aims.—Multiple trials in patients with ST-segment elevation myocardial infarction (STEMI) compared early routine percutaneous coronary intervention (PCI) after successful fibrinolysis vs. standard therapy limiting PCI only to patients without evidence of reperfusion (rescue PCI). These trials suggest that all patients receiving fibrinolysis should receive mechanical revascularization within 24 h from initial hospitalization. However, individual trials could not demonstrate a significant reduction in 'hard' endpoints such as death and reinfarction. We performed a meta-analysis of randomized controlled trials to define the benefits of early PCI after fibrinolysis over standard therapy on clinical and safety endpoints in STEMI.

Methods and Results.—We identified seven eligible trials, enrolling a total of 2961 patients. No difference was found in the incidence of death at 30 days between the two strategies. Early PCI after successful fibrinolysis reduced the rate of reinfarction (OR: 0.55, 95% CI: 0.36−0.82; $P = 0.003$), the combined endpoint death/reinfarction (OR: 0.65, 95% CI: 0.49−0.88; $P = 0.004$) and recurrent ischaemia (OR: 0.25, 95% CI: 0.13−0.49; $P < 0.001$) at 30-day follow-up. These advantages were achieved without a significant increase in major bleeding (OR: 0.93, 96% CI: 0.67−1.34; $P = 0.70$) or stroke (OR: 0.63, 95% CI: 0.31−1.26; $P = 0.21$). The benefits of a routine invasive strategy over standard therapy were maintained at 6−12 months, with persistent significant reduction in the endpoints reinfarction (OR: 0.64, 95% CI: 0.40−0.98; $P = 0.01$) and combined death/reinfarction (OR: 0.71, 95% CI: 0.52−0.97; $P = 0.03$).

Conclusion.—Early routine PCI after fibrinolysis in STEMI patients significantly reduced reinfarction and recurrent ischaemia at 1 month, with no significant increase in adverse bleeding events compared to standard therapy. Benefits of early PCI persist at 6−12 month follow-up (Fig 5).

▶ Many of the questions posed by the evolution of reperfusion therapy for ST-segment elevation myocardial infarction have been answered, but there remain areas of controversy. While it is widely accepted that primary percutaneous coronary intervention (PCI) is the best form of reperfusion therapy, an unanswered questions is what degree of delay is acceptable in patients transferred directly to a PCI center.[1] Nonetheless, the geography of the United States and logistical constraints imposed by weather and long distances in rural areas will ensure a role for the initial administration of fibrinolytic drugs in many situations. The initial approach or reperfusion strategy will therefore vary markedly between regions and countries.

The optimal approach to the patient who has received fibrinolytic therapy in a community hospital has been a subject of some debate. The trials of facilitated PCI in which PCI is routinely performed as an emergency on arrival at the referral hospital fail to show a benefit, and there were some signals suggesting potential harm due to bleeding and perhaps balloon inflation in a thrombolytic milieu.

Subsequently, several trials strongly suggest that a routine invasive approach with angiography performed 3 to 24 hours following fibrinolytic drug

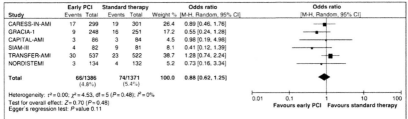

FIGURE 5.—Clinical endpoints at 6–12 months. Odds ratios and 95% confidence interval for death, reinfarction, and combined death/reinfarction between early PCI and standard therapy. Size of data markers indicates the weight of each trial. Benefits observed after early PCI on reduction of reinfarction and combined endpoint death/reinfarction are maintained in longer follow-up. (Reprinted from Borgia F, Goodman SG, Halvorsen S, et al. Early routine percutaneous coronary intervention after fibrinolysis vs. standard therapy in ST-segment elevation myocardial infarction: a meta-analysis. *Eur Heart J.* 2010;31:2156-2169, by permission of The European Society of Cardiology.)

administration is the preferred strategy in patients who are clinically stable with evidence of successful reperfusion therapy. This meta-analysis of 7 trials involving approximately 2900 patients strongly suggests that a routine invasive strategy performed early (3-24 hours), as opposed to immediate PCI, reduces reinfarction and recurrent ischemia with no significant increase in bleeding events. The umbrella term for this strategy is the pharmacoinvasive approach. A key component, however, of the pharmacoinvasive strategy is the ability to perform rescue PCI. The best approach, therefore, following lytic drugs administered in a non-PCI-capable hospital is immediate transfer if at all possible.

B. J. Gersh, MB, ChB, DPhil, FRCP

Reference

1. Gersh BJ, Stone GW, White HD, Holmes DR Jr. Pharmacological facilitation of primary percutaneous coronary intervention for acute myocardial infarction: is the slope of the curve the shape of the future? *JAMA.* 2005;293:979-986.

Comparative Effectiveness of ST-Segment−Elevation Myocardial Infarction Regionalization Strategies

Concannon TW, Kent DM, Normand S-L, et al (Tufts Med Ctr and Tufts Univ School of Medicine, Boston, MA; Harvard Med School, Boston, MA; et al)
Circ Cardiovasc Qual Outcomes 3:506-513, 2010

Background.—Primary percutaneous coronary intervention (PCI) is more effective on average than fibrinolytic therapy in the treatment of ST-segment−elevation myocardial infarction. Yet, most US hospitals are not equipped for PCI, and fibrinolytic therapy is still widely used. This study evaluated the comparative effectiveness of ST-segment−elevation myocardial infarction regionalization strategies to increase the use of PCI against standard emergency transport and care.

Methods and Results.—We estimated incremental treatment costs and quality-adjusted life expectancies of 2000 patients with ST-segment−elevation myocardial infarction who received PCI or fibrinolytic therapy in simulations of emergency care in a regional hospital system. To increase access to PCI across the system, we compared a base case strategy with 12 hospital-based strategies of building new PCI laboratories or extending the hours of existing laboratories and 1 emergency medical services−based strategy of transporting all patients with ST-segment−elevation myocardial infarction to existing PCI-capable hospitals. The base case resulted in 609 (95% CI, 569−647) patients getting PCI. Hospital-based strategies increased the number of patients receiving PCI, the costs of care, and quality-adjusted life years saved and were cost-effective under a variety of conditions. An emergency medical services−based strategy of transporting every patient to an existing PCI facility was less costly and more effective than all hospital expansion options.

Conclusion.—Our results suggest that new construction and staffing of PCI laboratories may not be warranted if an emergency medical services strategy is both available and feasible.

▶ This is an interesting cost-effectiveness analysis that has potentially major implications for the development of regional strategies for the delivery of reperfusion therapy.

It is increasingly accepted that if administered in a timely manner, primary percutaneous coronary intervention (PPCI) is the preferred form of reperfusion therapy. Nonetheless, since PPCI is not available in many hospitals, the key question is what degree of delay is acceptable during transfer to a PPCI facility as opposed to giving fibrinolytics at the primary presenting institution.[1] There is understandable interest, therefore, in increasing access to PPCI, and a number of regionalization strategies have been proposed.

This analysis using a recently developed triage and allocation model[2] compares the incremental benefits and costs of 2 approaches for increasing access to PPCI:

1. hospital-based in which new PPCI-capable facilities would be added;
2. emergency medical service (EMS)-based in which the key element is rapid transport to PCI-capable systems.

The bottom line is that providing additional catheterization laboratories does increase the number of patients receiving PPCI and could be cost effective in a variety of conditions. Nonetheless, the EMS-based strategy was less costly and more effective in all the scenarios that were tested.

What should be emphasized is that one size does not fit all, and the optimal strategy for a particular region will vary according to available resources, ambulance services, geographical constraints, including weather and distance. For many parts of the United States and other countries around the world, there will remain an important role for fibrinolytic therapy.[3]

B. J. Gersh, MB, ChB, DPhil, FRCP

References

1. Gersh BJ, Antman EM. Selection of the optimal reperfusion strategy for STEMI: does time matter? *Eur Heart J*. 2006;27:761-763.
2. Nallamothu BK, Bates ER, Wang Y, Bradley EH, Krumholz HM. Driving times and distances to hospitals with percutaneous coronary intervention in the United States: implications for prehospital triage of patients with ST-elevation myocardial infarction. *Circulation*. 2006;113:1189-1195.
3. Ting HH, Rihal CS, Gersh BJ, et al. Regional systems of care to optimize timeliness of reperfusion therapy for ST-elevation myocardial infarction: the Mayo Clinic STEMI Protocol. *Circulation*. 2007;116:729-736.

Health Care Insurance, Financial Concerns in Accessing Care, and Delays to Hospital Presentation in Acute Myocardial Infarction

Smolderen KG, Spertus JA, Nallamothu BK, et al (Tilburg Univ, the Netherlands; Saint Luke's Mid America Heart Inst, Kansas City, MO; Univ of Michigan Med School, Ann Arbor; et al)
JAMA 303:1392-1400, 2010

Context.—Little is known about how health insurance status affects decisions to seek care during emergency medical conditions such as acute myocardial infarction (AMI).

Objective.—To examine the association between lack of health insurance and financial concerns about accessing care among those with health insurance, and the time from symptom onset to hospital presentation (prehospital delays) during AMI.

Design, Setting, and Patients.—Multicenter, prospective study using a registry of 3721 AMI patients enrolled between April 11, 2005, and December 31, 2008, at 24 US hospitals. Health insurance status was categorized as insured without financial concerns, insured but have financial concerns about accessing care, and uninsured. Insurance information was determined from medical records while financial concerns among those with health insurance were determined from structured interviews.

Main Outcome Measure.—Prehospital delay times (≤2 hours, >2-6 hours, or >6 hours), adjusted for demographic, clinical, and social and psychological factors using hierarchical ordinal regression models.

Results.—Of 3721 patients, 2294 were insured without financial concerns (61.7%), 689 were insured but had financial concerns about accessing care (18.5%), and 738 were uninsured (19.8%). Uninsured and insured patients with financial concerns were more likely to delay seeking care during AMI and had prehospital delays of greater than 6 hours among 48.6% of uninsured patients and 44.6% of insured patients with financial concerns compared with only 39.3% of insured patients without financial concerns. Prehospital delays of less than 2 hours during AMI occurred among 36.6% of those insured without financial concerns compared with 33.5% of insured patients with financial concerns and 27.5% of uninsured patients (P < .001). After adjusting for potential confounders, prehospital delays were associated with insured patients with financial concerns (adjusted odds ratio, 1.21 [95% confidence interval, 1.05-1.41]; P = .01) and with uninsured patients (adjusted odds ratio, 1.38 [95% confidence interval, 1.17-1.63]; P < .001).

Conclusion.—Lack of health insurance and financial concerns about accessing care among those with health insurance were each associated with delays in seeking emergency care for AMI (Table 3).

▶ In regard to the management of myocardial infarction and, in particular, ST-segment elevation myocardial infarction, almost 3 decades of randomized controlled trials have taught us what to do, and most of the questions have been answered. Recently, there has been a shift in emphasis in that it is not just the nature of the therapy but also the efficacy of its delivery that is important. This has resulted in the formation of networks to enhance the speed of delivery of reperfusion therapy and its delivery to all eligible patients. The structure of these networks is markedly influenced by local and regional factors, including weather, facilities, logistical constraints, and ambulance services.

Although many aspects of care, including door-to-needle and door-balloon times, have improved, what has been frustrating is the relative lack of change in the time from symptom onset to presentation for medical care. In a recent large study utilizing a national registry, the median delay was 114 minutes, and this is shortened by only 10 minutes from 1996-2004.[1] The results of a trial of a community intervention program aimed at reducing patient delay were also disappointing.[2] Given the results of the current analysis, perhaps the inability to address patient concerns about the cost of emergency care contributed to the lack of any shortening in the time to presentation in the trial.

TABLE 3.—Association Between Insurance Status and Prehospital Delays[a]

	Adjusted OR (95% CI)	P Value
Adjusted for study site		
Insured without financial concerns	1 [Reference]	
Insured with financial concerns	1.22 (1.06-1.40)	.005
No insurance	1.30 (1.12-1.51)	<.001
Adjusted for study site, age, sex, race, and residential area		
Insured without financial concerns	1 [Reference]	
Insured with financial concerns	1.27 (1.10-1.47)	<.001
No insurance	1.44 (1.23-1.68)	<.001
Adjusted for variables above plus comorbidities and clinical characteristics		
Insured without financial concerns	1 [Reference]	
Insured with financial concerns	1.25 (1.08-1.45)	.003
No insurance	1.41 (1.20-1.66)	<.001
Adjusted for variables above plus baseline CAD health status and social and psychological factors		
Insured without financial concerns	1 [Reference]	
Insured with financial concerns	1.21 (1.05-1.41)	.01
No insurance	1.38 (1.17-1.63)	<.001

Abbreviations: CAD, coronary artery disease; CI, confidence interval; OR, odds ratio.
[a]The OR reflects the cumulative probabilities of a hospital presentation time of greater than 6 hours vs 6 hours or less and greater than 2 hours vs 2 hours or less.

It is well established that socioeconomic status is associated with patient delay. In the registry study,[1] factors associated with increased delay were older age, women, Hispanic or black race, or diabetes. This analysis provides additional information that a lack of health insurance and financial concerns about accessing care among those with insurance were each contributors to the delay in seeking emergency medical care. The strength of this article is that these 2 variables remain strong predictors of delay even after adjustment for age, sex, race, residential area, comorbidities, and social and psychological factors. Other studies have shown that avoidance of care because of costs is associated with more symptoms, poorer health status, and higher rates of rehospitalization,[3] and it is likely that patients who delay seeking care for myocardial infarction also delayed care for other conditions.

Efforts to reduce patient delays for myocardial infarction and other conditions in the current climate of US health care insurance are likely to have limited benefit unless coverage is expanded and improved.

B. J. Gersh, MB, ChB, DPhil, FRCP

References

1. Ting HH, Bradley EH, Wang Y, et al. Factors associated with longer time from symptom onset to hospital presentation for patients with ST-elevation myocardial infarction. *Arch Intern Med.* 2008;168:959-968.
2. Luepker RV, Raczynski JM, Osganian S, et al. Effect of a community intervention on patient delay and emergency medical service use in acute coronary heart disease: The Rapid Early Action for Coronary Treatment (REACT) trial. *JAMA.* 2000;284:60-67.
3. Tamblyn R, Laprise R, Hanley JA, et al. Adverse events associated with prescription drug cost-sharing among poor and elderly persons. *JAMA.* 2001;285:421-429.

Immediate Percutaneous Coronary Intervention Is Associated With Better Survival After Out-of-Hospital Cardiac Arrest: Insights From the PROCAT (Parisian Region Out of Hospital Cardiac Arrest) Registry

Dumas F, Cariou A, Manzo-Silberman S, et al (European Georges Pompidou Hosp, Paris, France; Paris Descartes Univ Med School, France)

Circ Cardiovasc Interv 3:200-207, 2010

Background.—Acute coronary occlusion is the leading cause of cardiac arrest. Because of limited data, the indications and timing of coronary angiography and angioplasty in patients with out-of-hospital cardiac arrest are controversial. Using data from the Parisian Region Out of hospital Cardiac ArresT prospective registry, we performed an analysis to assess the effect of an invasive strategy on hospital survival.

Methods and Results.—Between January 2003 and December 2008, 714 patients with out-of-hospital cardiac arrest were referred to a tertiary center in Paris, France. In 435 patients with no obvious extracardiac cause of arrest, an immediate coronary angiogram was performed at admission followed, if indicated, by coronary angioplasty. At least 1 significant coronary artery lesion was found in 304 (70%) patients, in 128 (96%) of 134 patients with ST-segment elevation on the ECG performed after the return of spontaneous circulation, and in 176 (58%) of 301 patients without ST-segment elevation. The hospital survival rate was 40%. Multivariable analysis showed successful coronary angioplasty to be an independent predictive factor of survival, regardless of the postresuscitation ECG pattern (odds ratio, 2.06; 95% CI, 1.16 to 3.66).

Conclusions.—Successful immediate coronary angioplasty is associated with improved hospital survival in patients with or without ST-segment elevation. Therefore, our findings support the use of immediate coronary angiography in patients with out-of-hospital cardiac arrest with no obvious noncardiac cause of arrest regardless of the ECG pattern.

▶ It is well documented from a variety of sources that acute ischemia is the cause of primary ventricular fibrillation in a substantial portion of patients with sudden cardiac death. The approach to the survivor of out-of-hospital cardiac arrest is an issue of increasing importance given the results of recent studies demonstrating the success of bystander cardiopulmonary resuscitation (CPR) and particularly in conjunction with highly organized regional care systems, as documented in Olmsted County Minnesota and in this study.[1]

Among patients with ST-segment elevation, the yield from emergency angiography and immediate percutaneous intervention (PCI) is high (at least 1 significant coronary lesion in 96% and successful PCI in 74%). PCI success was an independent predictor of survival, irrespective of electrocardiogram (ECG) presentation. These data support the 2008 consensus statement on postcardiac arrest syndrome, which recommends immediate angiography and subsequent PCI or thrombolytic therapy if PCI is unavailable in patients resuscitated from cardiac arrest who have ECG criteria for ST-segment elevation myocardial infarction.

An accompanying editorial, however, raises questions about the role of immediate angiography in patients without ST-segment elevation.[2] The yield in terms of the identification of critical lesions is much lower, as are PCI success rates in patients without ST-segment elevation. Although survival in this subset is similar to those with ST-segment elevation, the question is to what extent this is because of the performance of PCI, as opposed to this being a benefit of excellent regional care systems with a fast response time, etc. Given the relatively low yield of angiography and the fact that the neurologic status of many of these patients is uncertain at least in the early hours after resuscitation, perhaps immediate angiography should be confined to those with a high index of suspicion of acute coronary occlusion, that is, circumflex coronary artery occlusion or left main coronary artery disease. For those patients who do not undergo emergency angiography but subsequently regain neurologic function, I would recommend routine angiography before discharge. Irrespectively, the benefits of developing regional systems of care to streamline the process and promote rapid bystander CPR are not in doubt.

B. J. Gersh, MB, ChB, DPhil, FRCP

References

1. Bunch TJ, White RD, Gersh BJ, et al. Long-term outcomes of out-of-hospital cardiac arrest after successful early defibrillation. *N Engl J Med.* 2003;348: 2626-2633.
2. Bangalore S, Hochman JS. A routine invasive strategy for out-of-hospital cardiac arrest survivors: are we there yet? *Circ Cardiovasc Interv.* 2010;3:197-199.

Initial Clinical Results Using Intracardiac Electrogram Monitoring to Detect and Alert Patients During Coronary Plaque Rupture and Ischemia

Fischell TA, Fischell DR, Avezum A, et al (Borgess Heart Inst, Kalamazoo, MI; Angel Med Systems, Inc., Shrewsbury, NJ; Dante Pazzanese Inst of Cardiology, São Paulo, Brazil; et al)
J Am Coll Cardiol 56:1089-1098, 2010

Objectives.—We report the first clinical studies of intracardiac ST-segment monitoring in ambulatory humans to alert them to significant ST-segment shifts associated with thrombotic occlusion.

Background.—Despite improvements in door-to-balloon times, delays in symptom-to-door times of 2 to 3 h remain. Early alerting of the presence of acute myocardial infarction could prompt patients to seek immediate medical evaluation.

Methods.—Intracardiac monitoring was performed in 37 patients at high risk for acute coronary syndromes. The implanted monitor continuously evaluated the patients' ST segments sensed from a conventional pacemaker right ventricle apical lead, and alerted patients to detected ischemic events.

Results.—During follow-up (median 1.52 years, range 126 to 974 days), 4 patients had ST-segment changes of ≥3 SDs of their normal daily range, in the absence of an elevated heart rate. This in combination with immediate hospital monitoring led to angiogram and/or intravascular ultrasonography, which confirmed thrombotic coronary occlusion/ruptured plaque. The median alarm-to-door time was 19.5 min (6, 18, 21, and 60 min, respectively). Alerting for demand-related ischemia at elevated heart rates, reflective of flow-limiting coronary obstructions, occurred in 4 patients. There were 2 false-positive ischemia alarms related to arrhythmias, and 1 alarm due to a programming error that did not prompt cardiac catheterization.

Conclusions.—Shifts exceeding 3 SD from a patient's daily intracardiac ST-segment range may be a sensitive/specific marker for thrombotic coronary occlusion. Patient alerting was associated with a median alert-to-door time of 19.5 min for patients at high risk of recurrent coronary syndromes who typically present with 2- to 3-h delays (Fig 6).

▶ This is a rather intriguing idea. The "Achilles heel" of reperfusion therapy is the lengthy time from symptom onset to first medical contact, which in the United States ranges from 2.5 to 3 hours. That this has not changed over the last decade is frustrating, and community-based efforts to reduce this have

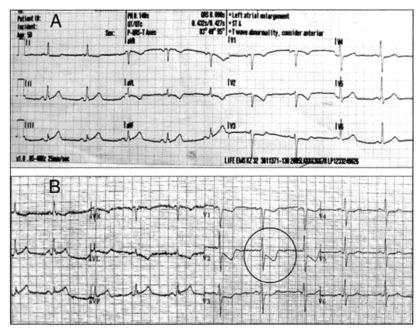

FIGURE 6.—Case 4: Surface 12-Lead ECG. (**A**) The 12-lead electrocardiogram (ECG) at ambulance arrival (7:00 AM) is shown. (**B**) The evolution to "true posterior" ST-segment elevation myocardial infarction (**circled beat** in lead V$_2$) is shown at 7:20 AM, during hospital arrival. (Reprinted from the Journal of the American College of Cardiology, Fischell TA, Fischell DR, Avezum A, et al. Initial clinical results using intracardiac electrogram monitoring to detect and alert patients during coronary plaque rupture and ischemia. *J Am Coll Cardiol.* 2010;56:1089-1098. Copyright 2010, with permission from the American College of Cardiology Foundation.)

been of avail.[1,2] Since the results of reperfusion therapy within the first hour of symptoms are outstanding, one way to reduce the community mortality of STEMI would be to get patients to seek treatment earlier.

The rationale for this study is that rapidly progressive ST-segment shifts are a highly specific and early marker of thrombotic or vasospastic coronary occlusion, and this may precede or even occur in the absence of symptoms. In this respect, continuous monitoring of the patient's electrocardiographic ST-segments by an implanted device using telemetry to an external device might provide advanced warning of an impending occlusion and promote a reduction in symptom-to-door time.

This study is the first-in-humans clinical experience with intracardiac ischemic monitoring. Safety and feasibility are documented, and the ability of the device to detect significant ST-segment changes and to sound an alarm is quite impressive. The mean alarm-to-door time was 26.5 minutes (medium 19.5 minutes) is short and would facilitate reperfusion therapy within the golden window of opportunity. This pilot study, however, is too small to assess the clinical impact of the device and the need for angiography following an alarm, and this is now being addressed by a prospective (phase II) study of 1000 patients. This is certainly an interesting approach and to be watched with interest.[1,2]

B. J. Gersh, MB, ChB, DPhil, FRCP

References

1. Luepker RV, Raczynski JM, Osganian S, et al. Effect of a community intervention on patient delay in emergency medical service use in acute coronary heart disease; The Rapid Early Action for Coronary Treatment (REACT) trial. *JAMA.* 2000;284: 60-67.
2. Brown AL, Mann NC, Daya M, et al. Demographic, belief, and situational factors influencing the decision to utilize emergency medical services among chest pain patients Rapid Early Action for Coronary Treatment (REACT) study. *Circulation.* 2000;102:173-178.

Lack of Effect of Oral Beta-Blocker Therapy at Discharge on Long-Term Clinical Outcomes of ST-Segment Elevation Acute Myocardial Infarction After Primary Percutaneous Coronary Intervention

Ozasa N, on behalf of the j-Cypher Registry Investigators (Kyoto Univ, Japan; et al)

Am J Cardiol 106:1225-1233, 2010

Beta-blocker therapy is recommended after ST-segment elevation acute myocardial infarction (STEMI) in current guidelines, although its efficacy in those patients who have undergone primary percutaneous coronary intervention (PCI) has not been adequately evaluated. Of 12,824 consecutive patients who underwent sirolimus-eluting stent implantation in the J-Cypher registry, we identified 910 patients who underwent PCI within 24 hours from onset of STEMI. Three-year outcomes were evaluated according to use of β blockers at hospital discharge (349 patients in β-blocker group and 561 patients in no–β-blocker group). Patients in the β-blocker group more frequently had hypertension, low left ventricular ejection fraction (LVEF), a left anterior descending artery infarct, and statin use than those in the no-β-blocker group. No difference was observed between the β-blocker and no–β-blocker groups in mortality (6.6% vs 6.6%, p = 0.85; propensity score adjusted hazard ratio 1.10, 95% confidence interval 0.64 to 1.90, p = 0.70) or in incidence of major adverse cardiac events (all-cause death, recurrent myocardial infarction, and heart failure hospitalization, 13.5% vs 12.1%, p = 0.91; hazard ratio 1.13, 95% confidence interval 0.76 to 1.66, p = 0.53). Better outcomes were observed in the β-blocker group than in the no–β-blocker group in a subgroup of patients with LVEF ≤40% (n = 125, death 6.4% vs 17.4%, p = 0.04; major adverse cardiac events 14.5% vs 31.8%, p = 0.009). In conclusion, β-blocker therapy was not associated with better 3-year clinical outcomes in patients with STEMI who underwent primary PCI and had preserved LVEF (Figs 3 and 4).

▶ Based upon randomized controlled trials and meta-analyses, the guidelines strongly recommend the use of β-blockers to improve long-term survival after ST-segment elevation acute myocardial infarction. Nonetheless, we need to appreciate that the bulk of the data emanate from the prereperfusion era or in patients who had received fibrinolytic drugs and not primary percutaneous coronary intervention (PPCI).[1] The issue is not whether or not to administer

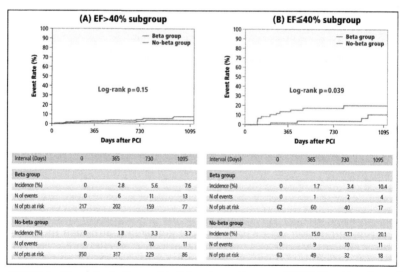

FIGURE 3.—Cumulative incidences of death in patients with preserved LVEF *(A)* and in patients with low LVEF *(B)* were compared according to use of β blockers. (Reprinted from Ozasa N, on behalf of the j-Cypher Registry Investigators. Lack of effect of oral beta-blocker therapy at discharge on long-term clinical outcomes of ST-segment elevation acute myocardial infarction after primary percutaneous coronary intervention. *Am J Cardiol.* 2010;106:1225-1233, with permission from Elsevier Inc.)

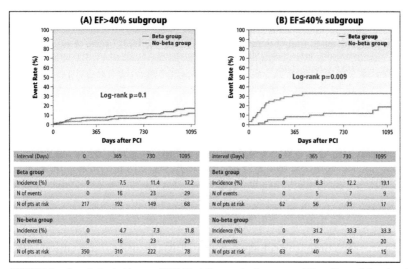

FIGURE 4.—Cumulative incidences of MACEs (all-cause death, recurrent MI, and heart failure hospitalization) in patients with preserved LVEF *(A)* and in patients with low LVEF *(B)* were compared according to use of β blockers. (Reprinted from Ozasa N, on behalf of the j-Cypher Registry Investigators. Lack of effect of oral beta-blocker therapy at discharge on long-term clinical outcomes of ST-segment elevation acute myocardial infarction after primary percutaneous coronary intervention. *Am J Cardiol.* 2010;106:1225-1233, with permission from Elsevier Inc.)

β-blockers to patients undergoing PPCI because the use is extremely logical in terms of reducing myocardial oxygen demands, perhaps bleeding and perhaps cardiac rupture.[2] What is more germane to current practice, particularly among an increasingly elderly population, is the multiplicity of drugs prescribed at the time of discharge and the potential for hypotension, bradycardia, dizziness, and fatigue with β-blockers. These are all symptoms that could also compromise the rehabilitation period. In certain individuals, 1 has to choose 1 drug as opposed to a combination, and this often applies to patients who are prescribed both β-blockers and agents that block the renin-angiotensin-aldosterone system. In this respect, this retrospective study from a large drug-eluting stent registry provides some useful information.

The study focused on 3-year outcomes after drug-eluting stenting using PPCI and demonstrated a benefit from β-blockers on late mortality and major adverse cardiac events only in sicker patients as defined by an ejection fraction of less than 40%. This is consistent with previous studies demonstrating a benefit in patients with systolic dysfunction and in heart failure. Nonetheless, there are limitations to the study, including selection bias, as is the case with all observational studies, lack of data on the type of β-blockers and dose, and the duration of β-blocker use after discharge. Nonetheless, in these complex patients with multiple comorbidities and the potential for adverse side effects, these data may help individual decision making.

B. J. Gersh, MB, ChB, DPhil, FRCP

References

1. Randomised trial of intravenous atenolol among 16,027 cases of suspected acute myocardial infarction: ISIS-1. First International Study of Infarct Survival Collaborative Group. *Lancet.* 1986;2:57-66.
2. Faxon DP. Beta-blocker therapy and primary angioplasty: what is the controversy? *J Am Coll Cardiol.* 2004;43:1788-1790.

Primary angioplasty vs. fibrinolysis in very old patients with acute myocardial infarction: TRIANA (TRatamiento del Infarto Agudo de miocardio eN Ancianos) randomized trial and pooled analysis with previous studies
Bueno H, on behalf of the TRIANA Investigators (Hospital General Universitario Gregorio Marañón, Madrid, Spain; et al)
Eur Heart J 32:51-60, 2011

Aims.—To compare primary percutaneous coronary intervention (pPCI) and fibrinolysis in very old patients with ST-segment elevation myocardial infarction (STEMI), in whom head-to-head comparisons between both strategies are scarce.

Methods and Results.—Patients $\geq$75 years old with STEMI <6 h were randomized to pPCI or fibrinolysis. The primary endpoint was a composite of all-cause mortality, re-infarction, or disabling stroke at 30 days. The trial was prematurely stopped due to slow recruitment after enroling 266 patients (134 allocated to pPCI and 132 to fibrinolysis). Both groups were well balanced in baseline characteristics. Mean age was 81 years. The primary endpoint was reached in 25 patients in the pPCI group (18.9%) and 34 (25.4%) in the fibrinolysis arm [odds ratio (OR), 0.69; 95% confidence interval (CI) 0.38−1.23; $P = 0.21$]. Similarly, non-significant reductions were found in death (13.6 vs. 17.2%, $P = 0.43$), re-infarction (5.3 vs. 8.2%, $P = 0.35$), or disabling stroke (0.8 vs. 3.0%, $P = 0.18$). Recurrent ischaemia was less common in pPCI-treated patients (0.8 vs. 9.7%, $P < 0.001$). No differences were found in major bleeds. A pooled analysis with the two previous reperfusion trials performed in older patients showed an advantage of pPCI over fibrinolysis in reducing death, re-infarction, or stroke at 30 days (OR, 0.64; 95% CI 0.45−0.91).

Conclusion.—Primary PCI seems to be the best reperfusion therapy for STEMI even for the oldest patients. Early contemporary fibrinolytic therapy may be a safe alternative to pPCI in the elderly when this is not available.

▶ No one would dispute that primary percutaneous coronary intervention (pPCI) is the treatment of choice for patients presenting with ST-segment elevation myocardial infarction, providing the facilities and the expertise are available. Nonetheless, prior trials comparing pPCI with fibrinolysis either excluded or really enrolled patients in the elderly (age, $\geq$75 years) subgroup, and in fact, only 2 such trials have been performed and are with conflicting results.[1]

This trial from Spain was confined to patients age 75 years or older (mean age, 81 years) treated within 6 hours of symptoms. The trial was prematurely terminated because of slow recruitment, but in total, 266 patients were recruited. Patient's characteristics differ somewhat from those in the senior Primary Angioplasty in Myocardial Infarction trial in which the age cutoff was 70 years and above. The period of enrollment took 5 years, and the time limit was less than 12 hours in contrast to the enrollment period of 2 to 3 years in this trial.[2]

Although underpowered to provide definitive answers, the trends in regard to mortality, reinfarction, and stroke at 30 days (the primary end point) were in favor of pPCI as was recurrent ischemia. There was no difference in bleeding rates. A pooled analysis for the 2 other trials demonstrated statistical significance for the primary composite end point. Although a large community-based trial would be desirable, from a practical standpoint, this is unlikely to happen. Irrespective of the therapy, advanced stages are a powerful predictor of mortality and morbidity, but the risks of reperfusion therapy is more than outweighed from the potential for gain, as the elderly are a sicker group. Although the prompt early use of fibrinolytic therapy is a reasonable alternative to pPCI in the elderly in areas where the facilities for percutaneous coronary intervention are not available, it would appear that in the elderly and younger patients, pPCI remains the optimal therapeutic strategy.

B. J. Gersh, MB, ChB, DPhil, FRCP

References

1. Alexander KP, Newby LK, Armstrong PW, et al. American Heart Association Council on Clinical Cardiology, Society of Geriatric Cardiology. Acute coronary care in the elderly, part II: ST-segment-elevation myocardial infarction: a scientific statement for healthcare professionals from the American Heart Association Council on Clinical Cardiology: in collaboration with the Society of Geriatric Cardiology. *Circulation.* 2007;115:2570-2589.
2. Senior PAMI. Primary PCI not better than lytic therapy in elderly patients. http://www.theheart.org/article/581549.do. Accessed May 14, 2010.

Remote ischaemic conditioning before hospital admission, as a complement to angioplasty, and effect on myocardial salvage in patients with acute myocardial infarction: a randomised trial

Bøtker HE, Kharbanda R, Schmidt MR, et al (Aarhus Univ Hosp Skejby, Aarhus N, Denmark; John Radcliffe Hosp, Headington, Oxford, UK; et al)
Lancet 375:727-734, 2010

Background.—Remote ischaemic preconditioning attenuates cardiac injury at elective surgery and angioplasty. We tested the hypothesis that remote ischaemic conditioning during evolving ST-elevation myocardial infarction, and done before primary percutaneous coronary intervention, increases myocardial salvage.

Methods.—333 consecutive adult patients with a suspected first acute myocardial infarction were randomly assigned in a 1:1 ratio by computerised block randomisation to receive primary percutaneous coronary intervention with (n=166 patients) versus without (n=167) remote conditioning (intermittent arm ischaemia through four cycles of 5-min inflation and 5-min deflation of a blood-pressure cuff). Allocation was concealed with opaque sealed envelopes. Patients received remote conditioning during transport to hospital, and primary percutaneous coronary intervention in hospital. The primary endpoint was myocardial salvage index at 30 days after primary percutaneous coronary intervention, measured by myocardial perfusion imaging as the proportion of the area at risk salvaged by treatment; analysis was per protocol. This study is registered with ClinicalTrials.gov, number NCT00435266.

Findings.—82 patients were excluded on arrival at hospital because they did not meet inclusion criteria, 32 were lost to follow-up, and 77 did not complete the follow-up with data for salvage index. Median salvage index was 0·75 (IQR 0·50—0·93, n=73) in the remote conditioning group versus 0·55 (0·35—0·88, n=69) in the control group, with median difference of 0·10 (95% CI 0·01—0·22; p=0·0333); mean salvage index was 0·69 (SD 0·27) versus 0·57 (0·26), with mean difference of 0·12 (95% CI 0·01—0·21; p=0·0333). Major adverse coronary events were death (n=3 per group), reinfarction (n=1 per group), and heart failure (n=3 per group).

Interpretation.—Remote ischaemic conditioning before hospital admission increases myocardial salvage, and has a favourable safety profile. Our findings merit a larger trial to establish the effect of remote conditioning on clinical outcomes (Fig 2).

▶ Primary percutaneous coronary intervention (pPCI) has been extraordinarily successful in restoring flow in the epicardial infarct-related artery, and the last 20 to 30 years have witnessed a great success story. Nonetheless, many patients with patent artery still experience suboptimal myocardial perfusion and significant myocardial necrosis. Whether this is because of reperfusion injury or microvascular dysfunction—and the mechanisms underlying these phenomena are uncertain—but the search for better myocardial protection continues.

The list of agents and procedures that have been successful in the experimental model is lengthy, but despite a large clinical agenda, the results of trials have been generally disappointing.[1] Explanations for the dichotomy between the animal model and the clinical situation are multifactorial and not that well understood.

An alternative approach uses innate cardiovascular cytoprotective mechanisms such as ischemic pre-and postconditioning. In several animal models and small clinical studies, this has been associated with a reduction in infarct size.[2] Here again the mechanisms are uncertain but might involve signaling cascades that protect myocardial function.[3] What is fascinating is that the same benefits appear to be obtained by remote conditioning as opposed to using the inflation and deflation of a balloon catheter in a coronary artery to provide a local preconditioning.[4]

This very innovative study takes the field a step further by demonstrating the value of remote conditioning provided by intermittent arm ischemia, during

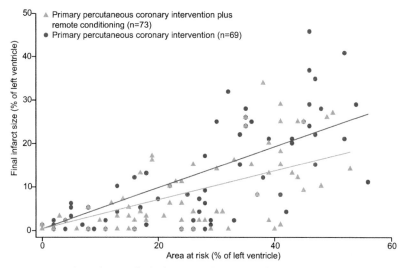

FIGURE 2.—Relation between final infarct size and area at risk for patients receiving primary percutaneous coronary intervention with or without remote conditioning (per-protocol analysis). (Reprinted from Bøtker HE, Kharbanda R, Schmidt MR, et al. Remote ischaemic conditioning before hospital admission, as a complement to angioplasty, and effect on myocardial salvage in patients with acute myocardial infarction: a randomised trial. *Lancet.* 2010;375:727-734, with permission from Elsevier.)

transport for pPCI. This is a small study in a substantial number of patients who were lost to follow-up, but the results are impressive and merit a much larger trial. The implications are potentially far reaching for both myocardial infarction and stroke, and the mechanisms of benefit remain intriguing.

B. J. Gersh, MB, ChB, DPhil, FRCP

References

1. Prasad A, Stone GW, Holmes DR, Gersh B. Reperfusion injury, microvascular dysfunction, and cardioprotection: the "dark side" of reperfusion. *Circulation.* 2009;120:2105-2112.
2. Staat P, Rioufol G, Piot C, et al. Postconditioning the human heart. *Circulation.* 2005;112:2143-2148.
3. Hausenloy DJ, Yellon DM. Time to take myocardial reperfusion injury seriously. *N Engl J Med.* 2008;359:518-520.
4. Schmidt MR, Smerup M, Konstantinov IE, et al. Intermittent peripheral tissue ischemic during coronary ischemia reduces myocardial infarction through a KATP-dependent mechanism: first demonstration of remote ischemic preconditioning. *Am J Physiol Heart Circ Physiol.* 2007;292:H1883-H1890.

Right Ventricular Ischemic Injury in Patients With Acute ST-Segment Elevation Myocardial Infarction: Characterization With Cardiovascular Magnetic Resonance

Masci PG, Francone M, Desmet W, et al (Fondazione G. Monasterio CNR Regione Toscana, Pisa, Italy; Sapienza Univ, Rome, Italy; Univ Hosp Leuven, Belgium; et al)

Circulation 122:1405-1412, 2010

Background.—Experimental data show that the right ventricle (RV) is more resistant to ischemia than the left ventricle. To date, limited data are available in humans because of the difficulty of discriminating reversible from irreversible ischemic damage. We sought to characterize RV ischemic injury in patients with reperfused myocardial infarction using cardiovascular magnetic resonance.

Methods and Results.—In 3 tertiary centers, 242 consecutive patients with reperfused acute ST-segment elevation myocardial infarction were studied with cardiovascular magnetic resonance at 1 week and 4 months after myocardial infarction. T2-weighted and postcontrast cardiovascular magnetic resonance scans were used to depict myocardial edema and late gadolinium enhancement, respectively. Early after infarction, RV edema was common (51% of patients), often associated with late gadolinium enhancement (31% of patients). Remarkably, RV edema and late gadolinium enhancement were found in 33% and 12% of anterior left ventricular infarcts, respectively. Baseline regional and global RV functions were inversely related to the presence and extent of RV edema and RV late gadolinium enhancement. At follow-up, a significant decrease in frequency (25/242 patients; 10%) and extent of RV late gadolinium enhancement was observed (P<0.001). With the use of multivariable analysis, the presence of RV edema was an independent predictor of RV global function improvement during follow-up (β-coefficient=0.221, P=0.003).

Conclusions.—Early postinfarction RV ischemic injury is common and is characterized by the presence of myocardial edema, late gadolinium enhancement, and functional abnormalities. RV injury is not limited to inferior infarcts but is commonly found in anterior infarcts as well. Cardiovascular magnetic resonance findings suggest reversibility of acute RV dysfunction with limited permanent myocardial damage at 4-month follow-up.

▶ This study using cardiovascular magnetic resonance (CMR) imaging provides new information about the natural history and pathophysiology of right ventricular (RV) dysfunction in patients with ST-segment elevation myocardial infarction. Previous studies have suggested that after ischemic injury, the RV recovers more rapidly and completely than the left ventricle, despite similar degrees of initial dysfunction, and this is reinforced by the findings of this study.[1]

Early after myocardial infarction, RV edema and late gadolinium enhancement (LGE) was common, occurring in 51% and 31% of patients, respectively.

It is interesting to note that this was frequently present in patients with anterior infarction in addition to the previously documented very common association with inferior infarct. Perhaps this should not be so surprising because it is reported that in pigs, 28% of RV mass is supplied by the left anterior descending coronary artery, and in about one-fourth of the patients, 30% or more of the RV free wall is supplied by the left anterior descending coronary artery branches.[2,3]

What is also of interest in a novel observation is the decrease over time in both RV edema (not surprising) and in the frequency of LGE, suggesting a limited extent of permanent damage. Moreover, the presence of RV edema initially was a predictor of RV improvement. In summary, this study using CMR strongly emphasizes the reversibility of RV dysfunction after ST-segment elevation myocardial infarction in reperfused patients.

Why does RV edema predict functional recovery? One explanation is that this is because of RV ischemic injury with limited extent of necrosis and that the RV dysfunction is not secondary to left ventricular dysfunction. These data agree closely with animal studies suggesting the reversibility of RV dysfunction, which could be because the RV faces a lower stroke work, extracts less oxygen at rest, and thereby has a greater oxygen reserve during stress and is a result of a more efficient circulation because of a high systolic/diastolic flow ratio and protective anatomic collaterals from the left coronary system.

From a management standpoint, one needs to remember that patients with RV infarction may be extraordinarily sensitive to volume depletion, particularly during the early days following infarction.[4]

B. J. Gersh, MB, ChB, DPhil, FRCP

References

1. Bowers TR, O'Neill WW, Grines C, Pica MC, Safian RD, Goldstein JA. Effect of reperfusion on biventricular function and survival after right ventricular infarction. *N Engl J Med.* 1998;338:933-940.
2. Weaver ME, Pantely GA, Bristow JD, Ladley HD. A quantitative study of the anatomy and distribution of coronary arteries in swine in comparison with other animals and man. *Cardiovasc Res.* 1986;20:907-917.
3. James TN. The arteries of the free ventricular walls in man. *Anat Rec.* 1960;136:371-384.
4. Lloyd EA, Gersh BJ, Kennelly BM. Hemodynamic spectrum of "dominant" right ventricular infarction in 19 patients. *Am J Cardiol.* 1981;48:1016-1022.

System Delay and Mortality Among Patients With STEMI Treated With Primary Percutaneous Coronary Intervention

Terkelsen CJ, Sørensen JT, Maeng M, et al (Aarhus Univ Hosp, Denmark; et al)
JAMA 304:763-771, 2010

Context.—Timely reperfusion therapy is recommended for patients with ST-segment elevation myocardial infarction (STEMI), and door-to-balloon delay has been proposed as a performance measure in triaging patients for primary percutaneous coronary intervention (PCI). However, focusing on the time from first contact with the health care system to the initiation of reperfusion therapy (system delay) may be more relevant, because it constitutes the total time to reperfusion modifiable by the health care system. No previous studies have focused on the association between system delay and outcome in patients with STEMI treated with primary PCI.

Objective.—To evaluate the associations between system, treatment, patient, and door-to-balloon delays and mortality in patients with STEMI.

Design, Setting, and Patients.—Historical follow-up study based on population-based Danish medical registries of patients with STEMI transported by the emergency medical service and treated with primary PCI from January 1, 2002, to December 31, 2008, at 3 high-volume PCI centers in Western Denmark. Patients (N = 6209) underwent primary PCI within 12 hours of symptom onset. The median follow-up time was 3.4 (interquartile range, 1.8-5.2) years.

Main Outcome Measures.—Crude and adjusted hazard ratios of mortality obtained by Cox proportional regression analysis.

Results.—A system delay of 0 through 60 minutes (n = 347) corresponded to a long-term mortality rate of 15.4% (n = 43); a delay of 61 through 120 minutes (n = 2643) to a rate of 23.3% (n = 380); a delay of 121 through 180 minutes (n = 2092) to a rate of 28.1% (n = 378); and a delay of 181 through 360 minutes (n = 1127) to a rate of 30.8% (n = 275) ($P < .001$). In multivariable analysis adjusted for other predictors of mortality, system delay was independently associated with mortality (adjusted hazard ratio, 1.10 [95% confidence interval, 1.04-1.16] per 1-hour delay), as was its components, prehospital system delay and door-to-balloon delay.

Conclusion.—System delay was associated with mortality in patients with STEMI treated with primary PCI.

▶ This study from Denmark makes a contribution to our understanding of the impact of factors attributing to the efficacy of the delivery of primary percutaneous coronary intervention (PPCI) and prognosis. Traditionally, measures that have been used include door-to-balloon time (D-B) and total ischemic time prior to reperfusion. The problem with D-B times is that the impact of shorter D-B time is markedly dependent on the duration of ischemia and the level of baseline risk. In patients who present after 90 to 120 minutes of ischemia, particularly in those at low risk, there is no significant relationship between D-B time and mortality.[1]

In regard to total ischemia time, this is confounded by the lack of precision in determining the onset of myocardial infarction. Moreover, patients who present late are typically at lower risk having already survived the prehospital period and are hemodynamically stable, and as such, the benefits of reperfusion therapy are less than with high-risk patients presenting earlier.

This study is confined to patients who are undergoing PPCI among whom, some are triaged in the field directly to a PCI center and others are transferred from the local hospital. The strength of the study is the evaluation of system delay, which incorporates all aspects of the time to reperfusion, beginning with the time to first contact with the health care system. The authors clearly demonstrate that system delay is associated with mortality, including the individual components, namely prehospital system delay and D-B times. These data demonstrate that system delay correlates with mortality, but is this a cause-and-effect relationship or simply a surrogate of good clinical care? I can understand that shorter times to treatment (within 60 minutes) will reduce mortality in patients reporting within 60 to 90 minutes of the onset of systems. Nonetheless, in the United States, the average time from symptom onset to presentation is almost 2 hours—at which point in time, the patient is on the flat portion of the curve and time-to-treatment is less critical.[2]

What this article also does not address is the issue of delay incurred during transport for PPCI as opposed to immediate administration of fibrinolytic therapy. Irrespectively, I agree that system delay is a valid and significant measure of health care performance.

B. J. Gersh, MB, ChB, DPhil, FRCP

References

1. Brodie BR, Gersh BJ, Stuckey TD, et al. When is door-to-balloon time critical? Analysis from the HORIZONS-AMI (Harmonizing Outcomes with Revascularization and Stents in Acute Myocardial Infarction) and CADILLAC (Controlled Abciximab and Device Investigation to Lower Late Angioplasty Complications) trials. *J Am Coll Cardiol.* 2010;56:407-413.
2. Gersh BJ, Stone GW, White HD, Holmes DR Jr. Pharmacological facilitation of primary percutaneous coronary intervention for acute myocardial infarction: is the slope of the curve the shape of the future? *JAMA.* 2005;293:979-986.

Trends in Door-to-Balloon Time and Mortality in Patients With ST-Elevation Myocardial Infarction Undergoing Primary Percutaneous Coronary Intervention

Flynn A, Moscucci M, Share D, et al (Univ of Michigan, Ann Arbor; Univ of Miami, FL; et al)
Arch Intern Med 170:1842-1849, 2010

Background.—In patients with acute ST-elevation myocardial infarction (STEMI) who are undergoing percutaneous coronary intervention, current guidelines for reperfusion therapy recommend a door-to-balloon (DTB) time of less than 90 minutes. Considerable effort has focused on reducing DTB time with the assumption that a reduction in DTB time translates into a significant reduction in mortality; however, the clinical impact of this effort has not been evaluated. Therefore, our objective was to determine whether a decline in DTB time in patients with STEMI was associated with an improvement in clinical outcomes.

Methods.—We assessed the yearly trend in DTB time for 8771 patients with STEMI who were undergoing primary percutaneous coronary intervention from 2003 to 2008 as part of the Blue Cross Blue Shield of Michigan Cardiovascular Consortium and correlated it with trends in in-hospital mortality. Patients were stratified according to risk of death using a mortality model to evaluate whether patient risk factors affect the relationship between DTB time and mortality.

Results.—Median DTB time decreased each year from 113 minutes in 2003 to 76 minutes in 2008 ($P < .001$), and the percentage of patients who were revascularized with a DTB time of less than 90 minutes increased from 28.5% in 2003 to 67.2% in 2008 ($P < .001$). In-hospital mortality remained unchanged at 4.10% in 2003, 4.02% in 2004, 4.40% in 2005, 4.42% in 2006, 4.73% in 2007, and 3.62% in 2008 ($P = .69$). After the differences in baseline characteristics were adjusted for, there was no difference in the standardized mortality ratios (SMRs) across the study period (SMR, 1.00; 95% confidence interval [CI], 0.74-1.26 in 2003 compared with SMR, 0.95; 95% CI, 0.77-1.13 in 2008).

Conclusions.—There has been a dramatic reduction in median DTB time and increased compliance with the related national guideline. Despite these improvements, in-hospital mortality was unchanged over the study period. Our results suggest that a successful implementation of efforts to reduce DTB time has not resulted in the expected survival benefit.

▶ This article is a mix of good and disappointing news. The study is based upon a regional consortium of hospitals in Michigan participating in a multihospital quality improvement collaborative. During the years 2003-2008, which encompassed the period of this analysis, there was a strong focus upon efforts to reduce the door-to-balloon (DTB) time.

Over the period of the study, mean age increased and patients were sicker due to increased comorbidities, but in contrast, there was an increase in the use of evidence-based medications and cardiogenic shock declined. Mean DTB steadily decreased from 113 minutes in 2003 to 76 minutes in 2008, and the proportion of patients with a DTB time of less than 90 minutes increased from 28.5% to 67.2%, respectively. Mortality, however, was unchanged being 4.1% in 2003, 4.3% in 2007, and 3.62% in 2008 ($P =$ not significant). These trends did not change when patients were stratified according to cortiles of risk, but I still would have liked to have seen a multivariant analysis incorporating the changes in baseline characteristics, but this was not done. The lack of correlation between DTB time shortening and a corresponding change in mortality is multifactorial. Healthier patients may be treated with shorter balloon times. Moreover, in these registry studies, there are multiple sources of bias. A major factor, however, is the lack of any change in the symptom onset to door time that is sufficiently long as to place the patient on the flat part of the curve (relating to the duration of ischemia prior to salvage) at the time of balloon inflation.[1] It has been noted previously that patients with higher risk characteristics or sicker patients have a longer symptom-to-door time, and it could be that the negative impact of the increased symptom-to-door time among high-risk patients is sufficient to mask any potential protective effect on the decreased DTB time. When one thinks of performance measures, what we need to do is consider total ischemic time, and in this respect, the persistently prolonged times from symptom onset to seeking medical help remain a source of frustration that seems to be resistant to change.[2] This remains the Achilles heel of reperfusion therapy.

B. J. Gersh, MB, ChB, DPhil, FRCP

References

1. Gersh BJ, Stone GW, White HD, Holmes DR Jr. Pharmacological facilitation of primary percutaneous coronary intervention for acute myocardial infarction: is the slope of the curve the shape of the future? *JAMA*. 2005;293:979-986.
2. Luepker RV, Raczynski JM, Osganian S, et al. Effect of a community intervention on patient delay in emergency medical service use in acute coronary heart disease. The Rapid Early Action for Coronary Treatment (REACT) trial. *JAMA*. 2000;284: 60-67.

Treatments, Trends, and Outcomes of Acute Myocardial Infarction and Percutaneous Coronary Intervention

Roe MT, Messenger JC, Weintraub WS, et al (Duke Univ Med Ctr, Durham, NC; Univ of Colorado—Denver, Aurora; Christiana Care Health System, Newark, DE; et al)
J Am Coll Cardiol 56:254-263, 2010

Coronary artery disease remains a major public health problem in the U.S. as many Americans experience an acute myocardial infarction (MI) and/or undergo percutaneous coronary intervention (PCI) each year. Given the attendant risks of mortality and morbidity, acute MI remains a principal focus of cardiovascular therapeutics. Moreover, 30-day mortality and rehospitalization rates for acute MI are publicly reported in an effort to promote optimal acute MI care, and aspects of MI care delivery are the focus of local, regional, and national quality initiatives. PCI remains a central therapy for patients with symptomatic coronary artery disease, particularly among patients with acute MI, and has garnered tremendous attention in the last decade with issues such as the risks and benefits of drug-eluting stents (DES) and adjunctive antithrombotic therapies.

However, there are few representative data describing contemporary patterns of care and outcomes trends for patients with acute MI and/or those undergoing PCI. This is of particular importance because the process of updating clinical practice guidelines and quality metrics for acute MI and PCI has accelerated. Updates or revisions to the American College of Cardiology (ACC)/American Heart Association (AHA) practice guidelines for PCI, STsegment elevation myocardial infarction (STEMI), and unstable angina (UA)/non—ST-segment elevation myocardial infarction (NSTEMI) have been published within the last 3 years, building upon prior versions published earlier in the decade. The ACC and AHA have also published performance measures to direct quality assessment and improvement activities. However, data are lacking on current guideline adherence as well as on trends in the patients in the U.S. with symptomatic coronary artery disease.

Large-scale, national clinical registries provide an important opportunity to evaluate current clinical practice. The American College of Cardiology's National Cardiovascular Data Registry (NCDR) comprises a suite of programs involving >2,400 hospitals in the U.S. (www.ncdr.com). We analyzed the NCDR Acute Coronary Treatment and Intervention Outcomes Network (ACTION) Registry—Get With The Guidelines (AR-G) and Catheterization PCI (CathPCI) databases to characterize recent trends in treatment and outcomes among patients with acute MI and those undergoing PCI. More specifically, we sought to evaluate patient and hospital characteristics, rates of guideline adherence, procedural details, and in-hospital outcomes related to acute MI and PCI care over the last several years.

▶ This study from a large national database provides an interesting and relevant perspective of the in-hospital treatment of ST segment elevation myocardial infarction (STEMI) and non-STEMI in the United States between 2005 and 2009, including a large registry of patients undergoing cardiac catheterization and percutaneous coronary intervention.[1]

There is much in this report that is gratifying. There were considerable improvements in the provision and timeliness of reperfusion therapy for patients with STEMI. This reflects widespread efforts to enhance the efficacy of the delivery of reperfusion therapies and as many patients who are eligible. There is also an improvement in the use of guideline-based therapies and performance measures for both STEMI and non-STEMI and a reduction in procedural-related vascular complications. Overall, the results are encouraging but also point to areas that need quality improvement. These data demonstrate what can be done in participating hospitals that receive the benefits of quarterly feedback reports that profile and benchmark performance. Participation is, however, voluntary and as such these results may not be generalized to all US hospitals because of the potential for bias toward a greater participation of high performing hospitals. We need to be cautious therefore in generalization of these data given the marked differences and baseline variables and socioeconomic status among patients in hospitals across the United States.

The bottom line is that these results serve as a benchmark for the ongoing process of evaluating evidence-based strategies and their impact upon outcomes. In regard to STEMI, perhaps the greatest barrier to further improvement is the persistent Achilles' heel of delay from symptom onset to seeking medical care.[2]

B. J. Gersh, MB, ChB, DPhil, FRCP

References

1. Brindis RG, Fitzgerald S, Anderson HV, Shaw RE, Weintraub WS, Williams JF. The American College of Cardiology-National Cardiovascular Data Registry (ACC-NCDR): building a national clinical data repository. *J Am Coll Cardiol.* 2001;37:2240-2245.
2. Luepker RV, Raczynski JM, Osganian S, et al. Effect of a community intervention on patient delay and emergency medical service use in acute coronary heart disease; The Rapid Early Action for Coronary Treatment (REACT) Trial. *JAMA.* 2000;284:60-67.

When Is Door-to-Balloon Time Critical? Analysis From the HORIZONS-AMI (Harmonizing Outcomes with Revascularization and Stents in Acute Myocardial Infarction) and CADILLAC (Controlled Abciximab and Device Investigation to Lower Late Angioplasty Complications) Trials

Brodie BR, Gersh BJ, Stuckey T, et al (LeBauer Cardiovascular Res Foundation, Greensboro, NC; Mayo Clinic, Rochester, MN; et al)

J Am Coll Cardiol 56:407-413, 2010

Objectives.—Our objective was to evaluate the impact of door-to-balloon time (DBT) on mortality depending on clinical risk and time to presentation.

Background.—DBT affects the mortality rate in ST-segment elevation myocardial infarction treated with primary percutaneous coronary intervention, but the impact may vary across subgroups.

Methods.—The CADILLAC (Controlled Abciximab and Device Investigation to Lower Late Angioplasty Complications) and HORIZONS-AMI (Harmonizing Outcomes with Revascularization and Stents in Acute Myocardial Infarction) trials evaluated stent and antithrombotic therapy in patients undergoing primary percutaneous coronary intervention. We studied the impact of DBT on mortality in 4,548 patients based on time to presentation and clinical risk.

Results.—The 1-year mortality rate was lower in patients with short versus long DBT ($\leq$90 min vs. >90 min, 3.1% vs. 4.3%, p = 0.045). Short DBTs were associated with a lower mortality rate in patients with early presentation ($\leq$90 min: 1.9% vs. 3.8%, p = 0.029) but not those with later presentation (>90 min: 4.0% vs. 4.6%, p = 0.47). Short DBTs showed similar trends for a lower mortality rate in high-risk (5.7% vs. 7.4%, p = 0.12) and low-risk (1.1% vs. 1.6%, p = 0.25) patients. Short DBTs had similar relative risk reductions in patients with early presentation in high-risk (3.7% vs. 7.0%, p = 0.08) and low-risk (0.8% vs. 1.5%, p = 0.32) patients, although the absolute benefit was greatest in high-risk patients.

Conclusions.—Short DBTs ($\leq$90 min) are associated with a lower mortality rate in patients with early presentation but have less impact on the mortality rate in patients presenting later. The absolute mortality rate reduction with short DBT is greatest in high-risk patients presenting early. These data may be helpful in designing triage strategies for reperfusion therapy in patients presenting to non—percutaneous coronary intervention hospitals.

▶ Several decades of clinical trials have taught us much about the benefits of reperfusion therapy and in regard to which groups will benefit from which reperfusion modality. The remaining controversy resolves around the acceptable duration of delay involved in transporting a patient for primary percutaneous coronary intervention (PCI) versus immediate administration of a thrombolytic agent.

In general, we have the answers for much of what we do, and the emphasis more recently has shifted somewhat from the nature of the therapy to the efficacy of its delivery and to as many eligible patients as possible. The association between door-to-balloon (D-B) times on mortality has led to a national initiative to shorten D-B times and as such to deliver primary PCI more promptly. This is certainly a worthwhile objective, but the impact of short D-B times may vary substantially with a total duration of ischemia and is consistent with the concept that the greatest benefit of reperfusion therapy occurs within the first 3 hours, and during this narrow window of opportunity, time to treatment is critical.[1] After that period during the flat part of the curve, incremental delays have less impact on outcome.

One potential drawback of the rush to get the patient to the catheter laboratory is the performance of angiography in patients without ST-segment elevation myocardial infarction—so called false positives.[2] The data in this analysis reinforce the criticality of delays in patients presenting early and particularly in those at high risk. In patients with a longer duration of symptoms and who are at lower risk, perhaps an extra 10 to 15 minutes for taking a history might be a good idea before transfer to the catheterization laboratory. One problem that is difficult to get around, however, is the lack of precision in determining the precise onset of myocardial infarction. Whether these data will have any impact on the role of facilitated PCI remains to be proven.

B. J. Gersh, MB, ChB, DPhil, FRCP

References

1. Gersh BJ, Stone GW, White HD, Holmes DR Jr. Pharmacological facilitation of primary percutaneous coronary intervention for acute myocardial infarction. is the shape of the curve the shape of the future? *JAMA.* 2005;293:979-986.
2. Larson DM, Menssen KM, Sharkey SW. "False-positive" cardiac catheterization laboratory activation among patients with suspected ST-segment elevation myocardial infarction. *JAMA.* 2007;298:2754-2760.

Chronic Coronary Artery Disease

Early Reperfusion During Acute Myocardial Infarction Affects Ventricular Tachycardia Characteristics and the Chronic Electroanatomic and Histological Substrate

Wijnmaalen AP, Schalij MJ, von der Thüsen JH, et al (Leiden Univ Med Ctr, the Netherlands; Academic Med Ctr, Amsterdam, the Netherlands)
Circulation 121:1887-1895, 2010

Background.—Reperfusion therapy during acute myocardial infarction results in myocardial salvage and improved ventricular function but may also influence the arrhythmogenic substrate for ventricular tachycardia (VT). This study used electroanatomic mapping and infarct histology to assess the impact of reperfusion on the substrate and on VT characteristics late after acute myocardial infarction.

Methods and Results.—The study population consisted of 36 patients (32 men; age, 63 ± 15 years) referred for treatment of VT 13 ± 9 years after acute myocardial infarction. Fourteen patients with early reperfusion during acute myocardial infarction were compared with 22 nonreperfused patients. Spontaneous and induced VTs and the characteristics of electro-anatomic voltage maps were analyzed. Twenty-seven patients were treated by radiofrequency catheter ablation. Ten patients (6 nonreperfused) were treated by ventricular restoration with intraoperative cryoablation in 9. During surgery, biopsies were obtained from the resected core of the infarct. VT cycle length of spontaneous and induced VTs was shorter in reperfused patients (reperfused, $299 \pm 52/270 \pm 58$ ms; nonreperfused, $378 \pm 77/362 \pm 74$ ms; $P = 0.01$). An electroanatomic patchy scar pattern was present in 71% of reperfused and 14% of nonreperfused patients ($P = 0.004$). The proportion of electroanatomic dense scar was smaller in reperfused patients ($24 \pm 18\%$ versus $45 \pm 21\%$; $P = 0.02$). Histological assessment in 10 patients revealed thick layers of surviving myocardium in 75% of reperfused but in none of the nonreperfused patients.

Conclusions.—Scar size and pattern defined by electroanatomic mapping are different between VT patients with and without reperfusion during acute myocardial infarction. Less confluent electroanatomic scars match with thick layers of surviving myocardium on histology. Early reperfusion and less confluent electroanatomic scar are associated with faster VTs.

▶ This interesting and difficult study adds to our knowledge of the effects of early reperfusion therapy on the characteristics and the electroanatomic and histologic findings in patients presenting late following a myocardial infarction with sustained monomorphic ventricular tachycardia (VT). Prior studies that have characterized the VT substrate using electroanatomic mapping have been essential steps in the development of techniques of radiofrequency ablation. Most of these studies, however, were performed in an animal model of a chronically occluded infarct-related artery, which resulted in homogenous dense scar surrounded by a small scar border zone.[1]

There is a general perception that current approaches to reperfusion therapy plus adjunctive pharmacotherapy have reduced the incidence of VT after myocardial infarction. Nonetheless, there is a lack of data on the influence of reperfusion therapy on the mechanisms and structural basis of VT and the methods by which treatment can modify the pathophysiology. This carefully performed study does demonstrate that early reperfusion is associated with smaller, less dense, and less confluent electroanatomic scars consisting of thicker layers of viable myocardium that appeared to give rise to faster spontaneous and inducible VTs. The implications for radiofrequency ablation are particularly important in that these data suggest that in reperfused patients, techniques that use voltage and pace mapping to locate an extensive scar border zone may not be applicable for these smaller, less dense, and patchy areas of scar tissue.

An accompanying editorial by Callans[2] emphasizes that there is much more that needs to be understood in regard to the relationship of the VT circuit to the underlying VT substrate. Answers to these ongoing questions are essential to our understanding and treatment of VT in patients who have undergone reperfusion therapy. The benefits of reperfusion therapy are undisputed, but it should be emphasized that for most patients, the myocardial infarction substrate is modified but not eliminated and as such, the risk of VT persists.

B. J. Gersh, MB, ChB, DPhil, FRCP

References

1. Reddy VY, Wrobleski D, Houghtaling C, Josephson ME, Ruskin JN. Combined epicardial and endocardial electroanatomic mapping in a porcine model of healed myocardial infarction. *Circulation.* 2003;107:3236-3242.
2. Callans DJ. On the nature of ventricular tachycardia in coronary heart disease. *Circulation.* 2010;121:1881-1883.

Adherence of Catheterization Laboratory Cardiologists to American College of Cardiology/American Heart Association Guidelines for Percutaneous Coronary Interventions and Coronary Artery Bypass Graft Surgery: What Happens in Actual Practice?

Hannan EL, Racz MJ, Gold J, et al (Univ at Albany, NY; Med Univ of Ohio, Toledo; et al)

Circulation 121:267-275, 2010

Background.—The American College of Cardiology and the American Heart Association have issued guidelines for the use of coronary artery bypass graft surgery (CABG) and percutaneous coronary interventions (PCI) for many years, but little is known about the impact of these evidence-based guidelines on referral decisions.

Methods and Results.—A cardiac catheterization laboratory database used by 19 hospitals in New York State was used to identify treatment (CABG surgery, PCI, medical treatment, or nothing) recommended by the catheterization laboratory cardiologist for patients undergoing catheterization with asymptomatic/mild angina, stable angina, and unstable angina/non–ST-elevation myocardial infarction between January 1, 2005, and August 31, 2007. The recommended treatment was compared with indications for these patients based on American College of Cardiology/American Heart Association guidelines. Of the 16 142 patients undergoing catheterization who were found to have coronary artery disease, the catheterization laboratory cardiologist was the final source of recommendation for 10 333 patients (64%). Of these 10 333 patients, 13% had indications for CABG surgery, 59% for PCI, and 17% for both CABG surgery and PCI. Of the patients who had indications for CABG surgery, 53% were recommended for CABG and 34% for PCI. Of the patients with indications for PCI, 94% were recommended for PCI. For the patients who had indications for both CABG surgery and PCI, 93% were recommended for PCI and 5% for CABG surgery. Catheterization laboratory cardiologists in hospitals with PCI capability were more likely to recommend patients for PCI than hospitals in which only catheterization was performed.

Conclusions.—Patients with coronary artery disease receive more recommendations for PCI and fewer recommendations for CABG surgery than indicated in the American College of Cardiology/American Heart Association guidelines (Tables 1 and 2).

▶ Current American College of Cardiology/American Heart Association guidelines for primary percutaneous coronary intervention (PPCI) in patients with ST-segment elevation myocardial infarction recommend PPCI as the treatment of choice. In patients with multivessel disease, PPCI of the culprit vessel (CV) alone is recommended, unless patients are hemodynamically compromised.[1] This remains an area of controversy that is addressed by this interesting article from the large New York State registry database.

The vast majority of the patients were treated with CV PCI, and in comparison with those undergoing multivessel PCI at the time of the index procedure, CV patients were younger with a lower proportion of ejection fractions at 50% or more but also a lower proportion with poor ejection fractions of 19% or less. In addition, CV PCI patients had a lower likelihood of a chronic total occlusion, better thrombolysis in myocardial infarction (TIMI) flow grades in the CV and were more likely to receive drug-eluting stents. Propensity matching was carried out to minimize the impact of these baseline differences. Overall, mortality rates were lower in patients undergoing CV PCI alone in comparison with those undergoing multivessel PCI during the same procedure. This would tend to support the guidelines, but one cannot discount the role of confounders. Were patients undergoing multivessel PCI at the time of the index procedure, a sicker group? This would not clearly appear to be the case using measured parameters, but this remains, nonetheless, the Achilles heel of all observational studies and despite the statistical adjustment, residual bias might still exist. This is particularly the case, as pointed out by the authors, when there are many potential confounders that were unmeasured, including persistent pain, ST-segment elevation after dilatation of the CV, or the presence of another lesion compromising TIMI flow.

What was interesting in this study is the apparently lower mortality in 1 year in patients who underwent a staged multivessel PCI within 60 days or less but not during the index admission. What is also interesting is that there is no

TABLE 1.—ACC/AHA Indications vs Catheterization Laboratory Recommendations, New York, January 1, 2005—December 31, 2007: Indications for ACC/AHA Class I and Class IIa Regarded as Equal

ACC/AHA Indication/Cath Lab Recommendation	CABG, n (%)	PCI, n (%)	Medical Treatment, n (%)	None, n (%)	Total, n (%)
CABG	712 (53)	455 (34)	156 (12)	14 (1)	1337 (100)
PCI	124 (2)	5660 (94)	255 (4)	12 (<1)	6051 (100)
CABG and PCI	84 (5)	1608 (93)	26 (2)	4 (<1)	1722 (100)
Neither CABG or PCI	70 (6)	261 (21)	873 (71)	19 (2)	1223 (100)
Total	990 (10)	7984 (77)	1310 (13)	49 (<1)	10 333 (100)

Cath Lab indicates catheterization laboratory.

TABLE 2.—ACC/AHA Indications vs Catheterization Laboratory Recommendations, New York, January 1, 2005—December 31, 2007: Indications for Class I for 1 Procedure Regarded as Superior to Indications for Class IIa for Another Procedure

ACC/AHA Indication/Cath Lab Recommendation	CABG, n (%)	PCI, n (%)	Medical Treatment, n (%)	None, n (%)	Total, n (%)
CABG	748 (43)	800 (46)	160 (9)	15 (1)	1723 (100)
PCI	132 (2)	6086 (94)	259 (4)	14 (<1)	6491 (100)
CABG and PCI	40 (4)	837 (93)	18 (2)	1 (<1)	896 (100)
Neither CABG or PCI	70 (6)	261 (21)	873 (71)	19 (2)	1223 (100)
Total	990 (10)	7984 (77)	1310 (13)	49 (<1)	10 333 (100)

Cath Lab indicates catheterization laboratory.

mortality difference between patients undergoing CV PCI and staged PCI during the same admission but not during the index procedure. It would appear, therefore, that in the absence of a trial, it is reasonable to perform CV PCI in most patients with multivessel disease undergoing PPCI, and if it is felt that multivessel PCI is necessary, this can be done as a staged procedure during the initial hospitalization or at a later stage. In some patients with severe hemodynamic compromise, including cardiogenic shock, multivessel PCI at the time of the initial procedure may still be a reasonable option.

B. J. Gersh, MB, ChB, DPhil, FRCP

Reference

1. Smith SC Jr, Feldman TE, Hirshfield JW Jr, et al. ACC/AHA/SCAI 2005 guideline update for percutaneous coronary intervention: a report of the American College of Cardiology/American Heart Association Task force on Practice Guidelines (ACC/AHA/SCAI Writing Committee to Update the 2001 Guidelines for Percutaneous Coronary Intervention). *J Am Coll Cardiol.* 2006;47:e1-121.

Angiographic Versus Functional Severity of Coronary Artery Stenoses in the FAME Study: Fractional Flow Reserve Versus Angiography in Multivessel Evaluation

Tonino PAL, Fearon WF, De Bruyne B, et al (Catharina Hosp, Eindhoven, the Netherlands; Stanford Univ Med Ctr and Palo Alto Veterans Affairs Health Care Systems, CA; Cardiovascular Ctr Aalst, Belgium; et al)

J Am Coll Cardiol 55:2816-2821, 2010

Objectives.—The purpose of this study was to investigate the relationship between angiographic and functional severity of coronary artery stenoses in the FAME (Fractional Flow Reserve Versus Angiography in Multivessel Evaluation) study.

Background.—It can be difficult to determine on the coronary angiogram which lesions cause ischemia. Revascularization of coronary stenoses that induce ischemia improves a patient's functional status and outcome.

For stenoses that do not induce ischemia, however, the benefit of revascularization is less clear.

Methods.—In the FAME study, routine measurement of the fractional flow reserve (FFR) was compared with angiography for guiding percutaneous coronary intervention in patients with multivessel coronary artery disease. The use of the FFR in addition to angiography significantly reduced the rate of all major adverse cardiac events at 1 year. Of the 1,414 lesions (509 patients) in the FFR-guided arm of the FAME study, 1,329 were successfully assessed by the FFR and are included in this analysis.

Results.—Before FFR measurement, these lesions were categorized into 50% to 70% (47% of all lesions), 71% to 90% (39% of all lesions), and 91% to 99% (15% of all lesions) diameter stenosis by visual assessment. In the category 50% to 70% stenosis, 35% were functionally significant (FFR ≤0.80) and 65% were not (FFR >0.80). In the category 71% to 90% stenosis, 80% were functionally significant and 20% were not. In the category of subtotal stenoses, 96% were functionally significant. Of all 509 patients with angiographically defined multivessel disease, only 235 (46%) had functional multivessel disease (≥2 coronary arteries with an FFR ≤0.80).

Conclusions.—Angiography is inaccurate in assessing the functional significance of a coronary stenosis when compared with the FFR, not only in the 50% to 70% category but also in the 70% to 90% angiographic severity category.

▶ This is an interesting analysis from the Fractional Flow Reserve Versus Angiography in Multivessel Evaluation (FAME) trial, which demonstrated that in patients with stable angina and multivessel disease (MVD), fractional flow reserve (FFR)-guided percutaneous coronary intervention (PCI) was associated with a lower event rate at 1 year in comparison to patients treated with angiographically guided PCI.[1] Moreover, in the FFR-guided group, fewer stents were used, but freedom from angina at 1 year was greater. FFR is an accurate and selected index of the physiologic significance of a coronary stenosis. The visual assessment of the significance of the stenosis at angiography is subject to both under- and overestimation and may be inaccurate in determining which events cause ischemia.[2]

This substudy demonstrates that angiography may be inaccurate in assessing the functional significance of a coronary stenosis, not only in the 50% to 70% category but also in the 70% to 90% category. Moreover, of 509 patients with MVD as determined by angiography (stenosis greater than or equal to 50%), only 46% had functional MVD as defined by a FFR of ≤0.80.

An accompanying editorial appropriately emphasizes the need to demonstrate reproducibility of the FAME results in other studies, but before routinely transitioning from an angiographically based to a physiologically based approach to stenting.[3] Moreover, these observations may not apply to patients with acute coronary syndromes in which the underlying pathology is plaque rupture as opposed to flow-limiting stenoses in patients with chronic stable angina.

Nonetheless, it is well recognized that interobserver variability in the evaluation of stenosis severity, particularly in the 50% to 70% range, is wide, and there is a need for better methods of assessing the functional and hemodynamic significance of stenoses.[4] The attraction of the FFR-based approach is the use of fewer stents and a reduced likelihood of both early and late stent complications. Moreover, such an approach may lead to more appropriate use of angiography, which is in itself important.

B. J. Gersh, MB, ChB, DPhil, FRCP

References

1. Tonino PA, De Bruyne B, Pijls NH, et al. Fractional flow reserve versus angiography for guiding percutaneous coronary intervention. *N Engl J Med.* 2009;360: 213-224.
2. Topol EJ, Nissen SE. Our preoccupation with coronary luminology. The dissociation between clinical and angiographic findings in ischemic heart disease. *Circulation.* 1995;92:2333-2342.
3. Applegate RJ. Fractional flow reserve-guided stent therapy for multivessel disease: taking a closer look. *J Am Coll Cardiol.* 2010;55:2822-2824.
4. Lima RS, Watson DD, Goode AR, et al. Incremental value of combined perfusion and function over perfusion alone by gated SPECT myocardial perfusion imaging for detection of severe three-vessel coronary artery disease. *J Am Coll Cardiol.* 2003;42:64-70.

Diabetic and Nondiabetic Patients With Left Main and/or 3-Vessel Coronary Artery Disease: Comparison of Outcomes With Cardiac Surgery and Paclitaxel-Eluting Stents

Banning AP, Westaby S, Morice MC, et al (John Radcliffe Hosp, Oxford, UK; Institut Hospitalier Jacques Cartier, Massy, France; et al)
J Am Coll Cardiol 55:1067-1075, 2010

Objectives.—This study was designed to compare contemporary surgical revascularization (coronary artery bypass graft surgery [CABG]) versus TAXUS Express (Boston Scientific, Natick, Massachusetts) paclitaxel-eluting stents (PES) in diabetic and nondiabetic patients with left main and/or 3-vessel disease.

Background.—Although the prevalence of diabetes mellitus is increasing, the optimal coronary revascularization strategy in diabetic patients with complex multivessel disease remains controversial.

Methods.—The SYNTAX (SYNergy between percutaneous coronary intervention with TAXus and cardiac surgery) study randomly assigned 1,800 patients (452 with medically treated diabetes) to receive PES or CABG.

Results.—The overall 1-year major adverse cardiac and cerebrovascular event rate was higher among diabetic patients treated with PES compared with CABG, but the revascularization method did not impact the death/stroke/myocardial infarction rate for nondiabetic patients (6.8% CABG vs. 6.8% PES, p = 0.97) or for diabetic patients (10.3% CABG vs. 10.1%

PES, p = 0.96). The presence of diabetes was associated with significantly increased mortality after either revascularization treatment. The incidence of stroke was higher among nondiabetic patients after CABG (2.2% vs. PES 0.5%, p = 0.006). Compared with CABG, mortality was higher after PES use for diabetic patients with highly complex lesions (4.1% vs. 13.5%, p = 0.04). Revascularization with PES resulted in higher repeat revascularization for nondiabetic patients (5.7% vs. 11.1%, p < 0.001) and diabetic patients (6.4% vs. 20.3%, p < 0.001).

Conclusions.—Subgroup analyses suggest that the 1-year major adverse cardiac and cerebrovascular event rate is higher among diabetic patients with left main and/or 3-vessel disease treated with PES compared with CABG, driven by an increase in repeat revascularization. However, the composite safety end point (death/stroke/myocardial infarction) is comparable between the 2 treatment options for diabetic and nondiabetic patients. Although further study is needed, these exploratory results may extend the evidence for PES use in selected patients with less complex left main and/or 3-vessel lesions. (SYNergy Between PCI With TAXus and Cardiac Surgery [SYNTAX]; NCT00114972).

▶ The results of coronary revascularization are of major interest, particularly given the projected increase in the world's population with diabetes over the coming 2 decades. In regard to the indications for revascularization, the recent Bypass Angioplasty Revascularization Investigation (BARI)-2D trial among patients with type 2 diabetes demonstrated no benefit from routine revascularization versus optimal medical therapy in patients who have mild to moderate chronic stable coronary disease.[1] This is similar to the results of the Clinical Outcomes Utilizing Revascularization and Aggressive Drug Evaluation trial, where a minority had diabetes.

Obviously, there are many subsets of patients at much higher risk on the basis of coronary anatomy, left ventricular (LV) function, and the severity of symptoms in ischemia, and in this subgroup the benefits of revascularization are generally accepted.

In the original BARI trial, which compared percutaneous transluminal coronary angioplasty to coronary bypass surgery in patients with multivessel disease, this demonstrated a significant mortality benefit with coronary artery bypass grafting (CABG), although among patients with no diabetes, no differences were noted.[2] The explanation was that the diabetic subgroup was sicker with more diffuse disease, triple vessel disease, proximal left anterior descending coronary artery disease, or LV dysfunction. It was speculated that the benefit from CABG may have related to the fact that surgery bypasses the entire epicardial vessel, which includes both culprit lesions and future culprits as opposed to percutaneous coronary intervention (PCI), which targets primarily the culprit lesions or lesion.[3]

The SYNergy between percutaneous coronary intervention with TAXus and cardiac surgery (SYNTAX) trial, which is confined to patients with triple vessel and left main coronary artery disease, adds further to our knowledge of PCI and CABG in the era of drug-eluting stents. As in other studies, event rates are higher in diabetics, and this is consistent with a concept that coronary disease is more aggressive and diffuse in patients with diabetes. In regard to the results of PCI versus CABG, there are no differences overall in rates of death, myocardial infarction, and stroke in patients with diabetes versus patients without diabetes, but repeat revascularization rates were almost doubled among patients with diabetes. The use of the SYNTAX score, however, identifies a lowered risk subgroup in which drug-eluting stents might provide equivalent benefit to bypass surgery. In contrast among those with a higher SYNTAX score, bypass surgery appears to be markedly superior both in regard to repeat revascularization, but there is also a statistically significant mortality difference. It will be interesting to see these results over the next 5 years because this is certainly a high-risk subgroup of patients who underwent extensive stenting both in terms of the number and the length of the stent, and the extent to which this will influence long-term outcomes remains to be determined.

For the present, I believe the choice of revascularization strategy for patients with diabetes needs to be individualized on the basis of the coronary anatomy, suitability for PCI, LV function, comorbidities, and the patient's lifestyle and expectations.

B. J. Gersh, MB, ChB, DPhil, FRCP

References

1. BARI-IID Study Group, Frye RL, August P, Brooks MM, et al. A randomized trial of therapies for type 2 diabetes and coronary artery disease. *N Engl J Med.* 2009; 360:2503-2515.
2. Influence of diabetes on 5-year mortality and morbidity in a randomized trial comparing CABG and PTCA in patients with multivessel disease: the Bypass Angioplasty Revascularization Investigations (BARI). *Circulation.* 1997;96: 1761-1769.
3. Gersh BJ, Frye RL. Methods of coronary revascularization—things may not be as they seem. *N Eng J Med.* 2005;353:2235-2237.

Single-Photon Emission Computed Tomography Myocardial Perfusion Imaging and the Risk of Sudden Cardiac Death in Patients With Coronary Disease and Left Ventricular Ejection Fraction >35%
Piccini JP, Starr AZ, Horton JR, et al (Duke Univ Med Ctr, Durham, NC; Duke Clinical Res Inst, Durham, NC; et al)
J Am Coll Cardiol 56:206-214, 2010

Objectives.—The aim of this study was to determine whether single-photon emission computed tomography (SPECT) myocardial perfusion imaging (MPI) is an effective method of risk stratification for sudden cardiac death (SCD) in patients with coronary artery disease (CAD) and left ventricular ejection fraction (LVEF) >35%.

Background.—Most victims of SCD have an LVEF >35%.

Methods.—The study population included 4,865 patients with CAD and LVEF >35% who underwent gated SPECT MPI. We used Cox proportional hazard modeling to examine the relationship between patient characteristics and SCD.

Results.—The median age of the population was 63 years (25th, 75th percentile: 54, 71 years), and the median LVEF was 56% (25th, 75th percentile: 50%, 64%). The median follow-up for all patients was 6.5 years (25th, 75th percentile: 3.6, 9.3 years). During follow-up, there were 161 SCDs (3.3%). After multivariable adjustment, LVEF, the Charlson index, hypertension, smoking, antiarrhythmic drug therapy, and the summed stress score (SSS) were associated with SCD (all $p < 0.05$). For each 3-U increase in the SSS, the hazard ratio for SCD was 1.13 (95% confidence interval: 1.04 to 1.23). The addition of perfusion data to the clinical history and LVEF was associated with increased discrimination for SCD events (*c*-index 0.728). Risk stratification with a derived SPECT nomogram did not result in statistically significant net reclassification improvement ($p = 0.26$) or integrated discrimination improvement ($p = 0.38$).

Conclusions.—Among patients with CAD and LVEF >35%, the extent of stress MPI perfusion defects is associated with an increased risk of SCD. Future large prospective studies should address the role of perfusion imaging in the identification of high-risk patients with LVEF >35% who might benefit from ICD implantation.

▶ This database study is interesting from the perspective of the pathophysiology of sudden cardiac death in patients with coronary artery disease. Guidelines and risk stratification for implantable cardioverter defibrillator (ICD) implantation for primary prevention use ejection fraction and particularly an ejection fraction of ≤0.35 as the gold standard. We need to realize, however, that there is a lack of precision in the measurement of ejection fraction. Moreover, although patients with an ejection fraction of greater than 0.35 may be at lower risk for sudden cardiac death, most sudden cardiac death events do occur in patients with relatively preserved left ventricular (LV) systolic function.[1]

What I found particularly interesting in this article is the powerful prognostic effect in regard to sudden cardiac death of the Summed Stress Score (reflecting both reversible and fixed perfusion defects). This was present even after adjusting for revascularization and emphasizes the role of both scar and ischemia as the substrate for malignant ventricular arrhythmia. In this respect, it is interesting that the Summed Difference Score (as an index of reversible defects alone) was not an independent predictor of sudden cardiac death. Although acute ischemia alone is undoubtedly a cause of sudden cardiac death[2] in this patient population with presumably stable disease who underwent stress-rest perfusion imaging, the presence of scar in addition to ischemia was important in the prediction of sudden cardiac death.

These data point to the need for prospective studies to identify patients with preserved or mildly impaired LV function and coronary artery disease who may benefit from ICD implantation. Nonetheless, from a public health perspective, the 30% to 50% of sudden cardiac deaths that occur as first cardiac events, most of whom have silent coronary artery disease, will escape detection and prevention.[3] We can at least, however, focus our efforts in identifying which patients with known coronary artery disease who are considered at lower risk may in fact be at higher risk warranting a prophylactic ICD.

B. J. Gersh, MB, ChB, DPhil, FRCP

References

1. Stecker EC, Vickers C, Waltz J, et al. Population-based analysis of sudden cardiac death with and without left ventricular systolic dysfunction: two-year findings from the Oregon Sudden Unexpected Death Study. *J Am Coll Cardiol.* 2006;47: 1161-1166.
2. Bunch TJ, Hohnloser SH, Gersh BJ. Mechanisms of sudden cardiac death in myocardial infarction survivors: insights from the randomized trials of implantable cardioverter-defibrillators. *Circulation.* 2007;115:2451-2457.
3. Myerburg RJ, Hendel RC. Expanding risk-profiling strategies for prediction and prevention for sudden cardiac death. *J Am Coll Cardiol.* 2010;56:215-217.

No Major Differences in 30-Day Outcomes in High-Risk Patients Randomized to Off-Pump Versus On-Pump Coronary Bypass Surgery: The Best Bypass Surgery Trial

Møller CH, Perko MJ, Lund JT, et al (Copenhagen Univ Hosp, Denmark)
Circulation 121:498-504, 2010

Background.—Off-pump coronary artery bypass grafting compared with coronary revascularization with cardiopulmonary bypass seems safe and results in about the same outcome in low-risk patients. Observational studies indicate that off-pump surgery may provide more benefit in high-risk patients. Our objective was to compare 30-day outcomes in high-risk patients randomized to coronary artery bypass grafting without or with cardiopulmonary bypass.

Methods and Results.—We randomly assigned 341 patients with a EuroSCORE ≥5 and 3-vessel coronary disease to undergo coronary artery bypass grafting without or with cardiopulmonary bypass. Patients were followed through the Danish National Patient Registry. The primary outcome was a composite of adverse cardiac and cerebrovascular events (ie, all-cause mortality, acute myocardial infarction, cardiac arrest with successful resuscitation, low cardiac output syndrome/cardiogenic shock, stroke, and coronary reintervention). An independent adjudication committee blinded to treatment allocation assessed the outcomes. Baseline characteristics were well balanced between groups. The mean number of grafts per patient did not differ significantly between groups (3.22 in off-pump group and 3.34 in on-pump group; $P=0.11$). Fewer grafts were performed to the lateral part of the left ventricle territory during off-pump surgery (0.97 versus 1.14 after on-pump surgery; $P=0.01$). No significant differences in the composite primary outcome (15% versus 17%; $P=0.48$) or the individual components were found at 30-day follow-up.

Conclusions.—Both off- and on-pump coronary artery bypass grafting can be performed in high-risk patients with low short-term complications. *Clinical Trial Registration.*—clinicaltrials.gov. Identifier: NCT00120991 (Table 4).

▶ Off-pump coronary artery bypass grafting CABG (OP-CAB) is an intuitively attractive concept, given the wealth of data on the adverse effects of cardiopulmonary bypass (CPB), including the possibility that this could predispose to cognitive dysfunction.

Subsequent randomized trials have been somewhat disappointing for the proponents of OP-CAB. In 3 trials, the technique was shown to be safe and effective when performed by surgeons with expertise and experience, but avoiding CPB and cardioplegic arrest did not result in any reduction in mortality, myocardial infarction, and stroke.[1,2] In regard to the softer end points of quality of life, duration of hospitalization, and development of atrial fibrillation, the results were variable.[3,4] A criticism of past trials, however, is that these included mainly low-risk patients as defined by younger age, preserved left ventricular function, and without extensive systemic comorbidities. Prior observational studies, however, suggested that the major benefit of OP-CAB would be among those considered at high risk.

This well-conducted single-center trial of 341 patients from Denmark with triple vessel disease and higher risk based on a EuroSCORE of ≥5 did not show any difference in a 30-day composite of individual outcomes, including all-cause mortality, myocardial infarction, cardiac arrest with successful resuscitation, low cardiac output syndrome/cardiogenic shock, stroke, and coronary reintervention. Duration of hospital stay was also no different as was renal insufficiency or the need for dialysis. There was a higher rate of incomplete revascularization in the OP-CAB group in regard to the lateral territory of the left ventricle, but whether this will have any effect on long-term outcomes is uncertain since the major benefit, at least for survival as opposed to symptoms, is via grafting the territory to the region of the anterior left ventricle.

TABLE 4.—Primary Outcome After 30 Days

Variable	Off-Pump (n=176)	On-Pump (n=163)	RR	95% CI	P
Composite primary outcome*	27 (15)	30 (18)	0.83	0.52–1.34	0.47
All-cause mortality	6 (3.4)	11 (6.7)	0.51	0.19–1.34	0.21
Myocardial infarction	9 (5.1)	15 (9.2)	0.56	0.25–1.24	0.20
Cardiac arrest with successful resuscitation	2 (1.1)	3 (1.8)	0.62	0.10–3.65	0.67
Low cardiac output syndrome	7 (4.0)	10 (6.1)	0.65	0.25–1.66	0.46
Stroke	7 (4.0)	6 (3.7)	1.08	0.37–3.15	1.00
Coronary reintervention†	1 (0.6)	3 (1.8)	0.31	0.03–2.94	0.36

Values are numbers (percentages). RR indicates relative risk; CI, confidence interval.
*All-cause mortality, acute myocardial infarction, cardiac arrest with successful resuscitation, low cardiac output syndrome/cardiogenic shock, stroke, and coronary reintervention.
†Coronary artery bypass grafting or percutaneous coronary intervention.

OP-CAB will continue to have its proponents and may be effective for the right patient and in the right hands, but its use in the United States has plateaued and is currently in the region of 21% overall and approximately 33% in large academic centers.

B. J. Gersh, MB, ChB, DPhil, FRCP

References

1. Puskas JD, Williams WH, Mahoney EM, et al. Off-pump vs conventional coronary artery bypass grafting: early and 1-year graft patency, cost, and quality-of-life outcomes: a randomized trial. *JAMA.* 2004;291:1841-1849.
2. Møller CH, Penninga L, Wetterslev J, Steinbrüchel DA, Gluud C. Clinical outcomes in randomized trials of off- vs. on-pump coronary artery bypass surgery: systematic review with meta-analyses and trial sequential analyses. *Eur Heart J.* 2008;29:2601-2616.
3. Angelini GD, Taylor FC, Reeves BC, Ascione R. Early and midterm outcome after off-pump and on-pump surgery in Beating Heart Against Cardioplegic Arrest Studies (BHACAS 1 and 2): a pooled analysis of two randomized controlled trials. *Lancet.* 2002;359:1194-1199.
4. Al-Ruzzeh S, George S, Bustami M, et al. Effect of off-pump coronary artery bypass surgery on clinical, angiographic, neurocognitive, and quality of life outcomes: randomized controlled trial. *BMJ.* 2006;332:1365.

Percutaneous Revascularization for Stable Coronary Artery Disease: Temporal Trends and Impact of Drug-Eluting Stents
Hilliard AA, From AM, Lennon RJ, et al (Mayo Clinic and Mayo Foundation, Rochester, MN)
J AM Coll Cardiol Intr 3:172-179, 2010

Objectives.—We sought to determine the characteristics, outcomes, and temporal trends among patients undergoing percutaneous coronary intervention (PCI) for stable coronary artery disease (CAD) from a single-center registry.

Background.—There is controversy regarding the generalizability of the findings from randomized trials of PCI for stable CAD to daily practice. An important perspective on the significance of the trial results can be achieved by clearly documenting past and present practice of PCI.

Methods.—This was a retrospective analysis of 8,912 consecutive patients undergoing elective PCI from 1979 through 2006 at a tertiary referral center. Clinical, angiographic, and procedural characteristics as well as in-hospital and long-term outcomes were measured in patients grouped into 4 eras depending on the dominant interventional strategy of that time: percutaneous transluminal coronary angioplasty, early stent, bare-metal stent, and drug-eluting stent.

Results.—Procedural success rates have improved (81%, 92%, 96%, and 97%, respectively, p < 0.001), and in-hospital mortality has decreased significantly (1.0%, 0.8%, 0.1%, and 0.1%, respectively, p < 0.001) over time. Kaplan-Meier estimates of mortality at 4 years were 11%, 13%,

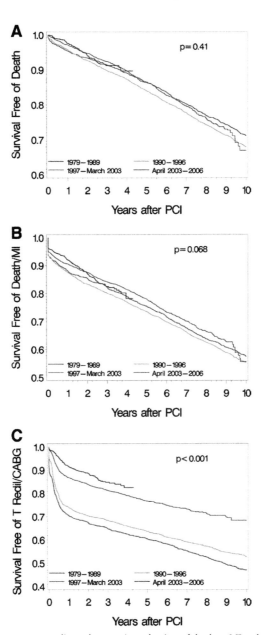

FIGURE 2.—Long-term mortality and composite end points of death or MI and repeat target lesion redilation or CABG. Kaplan-Meier curves showing survival free of (**A**) death, (**B**) death/myocardial infarction (MI), and (**C**) target lesion redilation (T Redil)/coronary artery bypass grafting (CABG). PCI = percutaneous coronary intervention. (Reprinted from Hilliard AA, From AM, Lennon RJ, et al. Percutaneous revascularization for stable coronary artery disease: temporal trends and impact of drug-eluting stents. *JACC Cardiovasc Interv.* 2010;3:172-179, with permission The American College Of Cardiology Foundation.)

10%, and 10%, respectively (p = 0.4). The 1-year target lesion revascularization rates in the 4 groups were 29%, 26%, 13%, and 8%, respectively (p < 0.001).

Conclusions.—Procedural success rates in contemporary practice of PCI for stable CAD are excellent with very low in-hospital mortality. Introduction of drug-eluting stents has reduced target lesion revascularization but not mortality among all comers. Outcomes similar to that observed in recent clinical trials are being achieved in routine clinical practice (Fig 2).

▶ This study from the Mayo Clinic provides a sweeping perspective of the results of percutaneous coronary intervention in patients with stable coronary artery disease over almost 3 decades. Patients were divided into 4 groups that reflect the dominant interventional strategy at the time, beginning in 1976 through 2006. As shown in other studies, patients have been getting progressively older and sicker with an increased number of comorbid conditions, heavier, and the frequency of reduced ejection fraction and symptomatic heart failure has increased. Despite this, procedural success rates have steadily improved, in-hospital mortality has fallen from 1% to 0.1%, and the rate of repeat revascularization has declined following the introduction of stents, particularly drug-eluting stents. Nonetheless, Kaplan Meier estimates of mortality at 4 years were basically unchanged being 11%, 13%, 10%, and 10% in the 4 cohorts.

Of note, the composite end point of death and myocardial infarction at 4 years was almost identical to that reported in the Clinical Outcomes Utilizing Revascularization and Aggressive Drug Evaluation (COURAGE) trial.[1] This is interesting from a number of different perspectives. Firstly, these data suggest that the population enrolled in the COURAGE trial was probably very representative of patients seen in clinical practice. Secondly, the lack of any change in late death or myocardial infarction despite higher procedural success rates and the development of drug-eluting stents would suggest that late events are the consequence of disease progression and unrelated to the original target lesion.[2] Another factor underlying the lack of improvement in late mortality could be that the more recent cohort is a sicker subgroup and that late survival might have been increased in the event that the baseline characteristics were similar.

Irrespectively, these data provide a roadmap for the future. New developments in stent technology will probably improve success rates even further, particularly if innovative approaches to chronic total occlusions bear fruit. On the other hand, these developments need to go hand in hand with one other new technology in interventional cardiology, and that is secondary prevention and optimal medical therapy.

B. J. Gersh, MB, ChB, DPhil, FRCP

References

1. Boden WE, O'Rourke RA, Teo KK, et al. Optimal medical therapy with or without PCI for stable coronary artery disease. *N Engl J Med.* 2007;356: 1503-1516.
2. Cutlip DE, Chhabra AG, Baim DS, et al. Beyond restenosis: five-year clinical outcomes from second-generation coronary stent trials. *Circulation.* 2004;110: 1226-1230.

Coronary Bypass Surgery and Percutaneous Coronary Intervention

Outcomes in Patients With De Novo Left Main Disease Treated With Either Percutaneous Coronary Intervention Using Paclitaxel-Eluting Stents or Coronary Artery Bypass Graft Treatment in the Synergy Between Percutaneous Coronary Intervention With TAXUS and Cardiac Surgery (SYNTAX) Trial

Morice M-C, Serruys PW, Kappetein AP, et al (Institut Hospitalier Jacques Cartier, Massy, France; Erasmus Univ Med Ctr Rotterdam, the Netherlands; et al)
Circulation 121:2645-2653, 2010

Background.—The prospective, multinational, randomized Synergy Between Percutaneous Coronary Intervention With TAXUS and Cardiac Surgery (SYNTAX) trial was designed to assess the optimal revascularization strategy between percutaneous coronary intervention (PCI) and coronary artery bypass grafting (CABG), for patients with left main (LM) and/or 3-vessel coronary disease.

Methods and Results.—This observational hypothesis-generating analysis reports the results of a prespecified powered subgroup of 705 randomized patients who had LM disease among the 1800 patients with de novo 3-vessel disease and/or LM disease randomized to PCI with paclitaxel-eluting stents or CABG in the SYNTAX trial. Major adverse cardiac and cerebrovascular event rates at 1 year in LM patients were similar for CABG and PCI (13.7% versus 15.8%; Δ2.1% [95% confidence interval −3.2% to 7.4%]; $P=0.44$). At 1 year, stroke was significantly higher in the CABG arm (2.7% versus 0.3%; Δ−2.4% [95% confidence interval −4.2% to −0.1%]; $P=0.009$]), whereas repeat revascularization was significantly higher in the PCI arm (6.5% versus 11.8%; Δ5.3% [95% confidence interval 1.0% to 9.6%]; $P=0.02$); there was no observed difference between groups for other end points. When patients were scored for anatomic complexity, those with higher baseline SYNTAX scores had significantly worse outcomes with PCI than did patients with low or intermediate SYNTAX scores; outcomes for patients with CABG did not correlate with baseline SYNTAX score, but baseline EuroSCORE significantly predicted outcomes for both treatments.

Conclusions.—Patients with LM disease who had revascularization with PCI had safety and efficacy outcomes comparable to CABG at 1 year; longer follow-up is required to determine whether these 2 revascularization strategies offer comparable medium-term outcomes in this group of complex patients.

▶ This is an important substudy from the Synergy Between Percutaneous Coronary Intervention With TAXUS and Cardiac Surgery (SYNTAX) trial that reflects the expanding indications for stent use for more complex lesions, including left main coronary artery disease. Left main disease has traditionally been the bastion of the surgeon, but several studies have demonstrated good results with stents, and in particular drug-eluting stents.[1] Moreover, such studies have demonstrated a low risk of sudden cardiac death or stent thrombosis in moderate and long-term follow-up.

Nonetheless, these are primarily (with one exception) registry studies and single-center studies in the majority and as such are subject to selection bias. The guidelines consider that bypass surgery is the gold standard for unprotected left main coronary disease, but percutaneous coronary intervention (PCI) is considered a feasible and promising strategy.[2]

This analysis is confined to a subgroup of 705 patients with left main disease, the majority having associated 2- or 3-vessel disease. The data demonstrate similar outcomes at 1 year for death and myocardial infarction but with a higher rate of stroke after bypass surgery and repeat revascularization after PCI, as was the case in the main trial.[3] It is interesting but not surprising that the SYNTAX score, as a measure of anatomic complexity, influenced the outcomes of PCI but not surgery.

These data are encouraging for PCI, but we need to remember that these are 1-year follow-up data. Patients in this trial have multiple stents (4.6 mean) and average stent length was approximately 86.1 mm; this may certainly affect the results over a longer period of time, during which differences between coronary surgery and PCI may emerge. In this respect, a recent study with 4 years of follow-up of drug-eluting stents demonstrated a significant and concerning increase in late events between 1 and 4 years.[4] We also need larger trials that can address detailed subsets of patients with left main disease, for example, ostial versus distal lesions. Such trials are in the planning phase.

Careful follow-up is therefore mandatory, but until further data are available, clinicians should follow the American College of Cardiology/American Heart Association guidelines, which state that the presence of a stenosis in the left main coronary artery is a class IIb indication for PCI unless the patient has clinical conditions that predict an increase risk of adverse surgical outcomes.

B. J. Gersh, MB, ChB, DPhil, FRCP

References

1. Park SJ, Kim YH, Lee BK, et al. Sirolimus-eluting stent implantation for unprotected left main coronary artery stenosis: comparison with bare metal stent implantation. *J Am Coll Cardiol.* 2005;45:351-356.
2. Smith SC Jr, Feldman TE, Hirshfeld JW Jr, et al. ACC/AHA/SCAI 2005 guideline update for percutaneous coronary intervention: a report of the American College of Cardiology/American Heart Association Task Force on Practice Guidelines (ACC/AHA/SCAI Writing Committee to Update the 2001 Guidelines for Percutaneous Coronary Intervention). *J Am Coll Cardiol.* 2006;47:e1-e121.
3. Serruys PW, Morice MC, Kappetein AP, et al. Percutaneous coronary intervention versus coronary-artery bypass grafting for severe coronary artery disease. *N Eng J Med.* 2009;360:961-972.
4. Onuma Y, Girasis C, Piazza N, et al. Long-term clinical results following stenting of the left main stem: insights from RESEARCH (Rapamycin-Eluting Stent Evaluated at Rotterdam Cardiology Hospital) and T-SEARCH (Taxus-Stent Evaluated at Rotterdam Cardiology Hospital) Registries. *JACC Cardiovasc Interv.* 2010;3:584-594.

Ten-Year Follow-Up Survival of the Medicine, Angioplasty, or Surgery Study (MASS II): A Randomized Controlled Clinical Trial of 3 Therapeutic Strategies for Multivessel Coronary Artery Disease
Hueb W, Lopes N, Gersh BJ, et al (Heart Inst of the Univ of São Paulo, Brazil; Mayo Clinic, Rochester, MN)
Circulation 122:949-957, 2010

Background.—This study compared the 10-year follow-up of percutaneous coronary intervention (PCI), coronary artery surgery (CABG), and medical treatment (MT) in patients with multivessel coronary artery disease, stable angina, and preserved ventricular function.

Methods and Results.—The primary end points were overall mortality, Q-wave myocardial infarction, or refractory angina that required revascularization. All data were analyzed according to the intention-to-treat principle. At a single institution, 611 patients were randomly assigned to CABG (n=203), PCI (n=205), or MT (n=203). The 10-year survival rates were 74.9% with CABG, 75.1% with PCI, and 69% with MT ($P=0.089$). The 10-year rates of myocardial infarction were 10.3% with CABG, 13.3% with PCI, and 20.7% with MT ($P<0.010$). The 10-year rates of additional revascularizations were 7.4% with CABG, 41.9% with PCI, and 39.4% with MT ($P<0.001$). Relative to the composite end point, Cox regression analysis showed a higher incidence of primary events in MT than in CABG (hazard ratio 2.35, 95% confidence interval 1.78 to 3.11) and in PCI than in CABG (hazard ratio 1.85, 95% confidence interval 1.39 to 2.47). Furthermore, 10-year rates of freedom from angina were 64% with CABG, 59% with PCI, and 43% with MT ($P<0.001$).

Conclusions.—Compared with CABG, MT was associated with a significantly higher incidence of subsequent myocardial infarction, a higher rate of additional revascularization, a higher incidence of cardiac death, and consequently a 2.29-fold increased risk of combined events. PCI was associated with an increased need for further revascularization, a higher incidence of myocardial infarction, and a 1.46-fold increased risk of combined events compared with CABG. Additionally, CABG was better than MT at eliminating anginal symptoms.

Clinical Trial Registration Information.—URL: http://www.controlled-trials.com. Registration number: ISRCTN66068876.

▶ Trials of coronary revascularization in patients with chronic stable angina are difficult to perform and by their very nature are highly selective in that patients have to be considered amenable to all therapies, for example, coronary artery bypass grafting (CABG), percutaneous coronary intervention (PCI), or medical treatment. This state of clinical equipoise, which is ethically necessary, imposes a form of entry bias tilted toward the selection of lower risk patient subsets.[1]

Most trials of PCI and CABG have been neutral, and this also has been the case in trials of PCI versus medical therapy, for example, Clinical Outcomes Utilizing Revascularization and Aggressive Drug Evaluation (COURAGE) trial and Bypass Angioplasty Revascularization Investigation IID trial. Previous trials of bypass surgery versus medical therapy identified a benefit for revascularization only in those patients at higher risk as defined by left main coronary artery disease, left ventricular dysfunction, and in patients with severe angina. In any event, these trials are approximately 30 years old and do not reflect contemporary care. Some subsets that were not addressed by the trials have been included in registries, and it is important to consider registry and randomized trial data as complementary as both have their advantages and disadvantages.[2]

The Multicentre Aneurysm Screening Study (MASS) II trial is the only randomized trial that has compared all 3 treatment arms, and the 10-year data are of interest as there is 100% follow-up. Limitations are the small size and the fact that it is a single-center study. Moreover, medical therapy may not be considered optimal by today's standards, and PCI has also changed substantially over the last 10 years, particularly with the introduction of drug-eluting stents.[3]

Nonetheless, MASS II has potentially important implications because prior to the publication of these data, the large trials have been neutral in regard to the benefits of revascularization over medical therapy. The MASS II population is perhaps at higher risk than those in the COURAGE trial because all had multivessel disease. The event rate after bypass surgery was significantly less than with medical therapy, although there were no significant differences in mortality. In comparison with PCI, a nonsignificant trend in favor of coronary bypass surgery was noted for most end points. Nonetheless, cardiovascular therapies evolve over time, and we await with interest for other results of ongoing trials, such as Fracture Reduction Evaluation of Denosumab in Osteoporosis Every 6 Months trial and the 5-year follow-up of the SYNTAX trial.

B. J. Gersh, MB, ChB, DPhil, FRCP

References

1. Brown ML, Gersh BJ, Holmes DR, Bailey KR, Sundt TM 3rd. From randomized trials to registry studies: translating data into clinical information. *Nat Clin Pract Cardiovasc Med.* 2008;5:613-620.
2. Gersh BJ, Frye RL. Methods of coronary revascularization – things may not be as they seem. *N Engl J Med.* 2005;352:2235-2237.
3. Williams DO, Vasaiwala SC, Boden WE. Is optimal medical therapy "optimal therapy" for multivessel coronary artery disease? Optimal management of multivessel coronary artery disease. *Circulation.* 2010;122:943-945.

Duration of Dual Antiplatelet Therapy after Implantation of Drug-Eluting Stents
Park S-J, Park D-W, Kim Y-H, et al (Univ of Ulsan College of Medicine, Seoul, South Korea; et al)
N Engl J Med 362:1374-1382, 2010

Background.—The potential benefits and risks of the use of dual antiplatelet therapy beyond a 12-month period in patients receiving drug-eluting stents have not been clearly established.

Methods.—In two trials, we randomly assigned a total of 2701 patients who had received drugeluting stents and had been free of major adverse cardiac or cerebrovascular events and major bleeding for a period of at least 12 months to receive clopidogrel plus aspirin or aspirin alone. The primary end point was a composite of myocardial infarction or death from cardiac causes. Data from the two trials were merged for analysis.

Results.—The median duration of follow-up was 19.2 months. The cumulative risk of the primary outcome at 2 years was 1.8% with dual antiplatelet therapy, as compared with 1.2% with aspirin monotherapy (hazard ratio, 1.65; 95% confidence interval [CI], 0.80 to 3.36; P = 0.17). The individual risks of myocardial infarction, stroke, stent thrombosis, need for repeat revascularization, major bleeding, and death from any cause did not differ significantly between the two groups. However, in the dual-therapy group as compared with the aspirin-alone group, there was a nonsignificant increase in the composite risk of myocardial infarction, stroke, or death from any cause (hazard ratio, 1.73; 95% CI, 0.99 to 3.00; P = 0.051) and in the composite risk of myocardial infarction, stroke, or death from cardiac causes (hazard ratio, 1.84; 95% CI, 0.99 to 3.45; P = 0.06).

Conclusions.—The use of dual antiplatelet therapy for a period longer than 12 months in patients who had received drug-eluting stents was not significantly more effective than aspirin monotherapy in reducing the rate of myocardial infarction or death from cardiac causes. These findings should be confirmed or refuted through larger, randomized clinical trials with longer-term follow-up. (ClinicalTrials.gov numbers, NCT00484926 and NCT00590174.) (Fig 1).

▶ Multiple clinical trials have indisputably shown a benefit from drug-eluting stents (DESs) over bare-metal stents in regard to the prevention of restenosis.[1] In contrast, DESs have been shown to have a higher rate of late stent thrombosis and myocardial infarction,[2] although data suggesting an increase in late mortality were flawed by the inclusion of confounder variables in large registry studies. Nonetheless, there is strong pathological evidence that the occurrence of late clinical events following DES may be caused by delayed arterial healing.[3] This has led to recommendations that dual antiplatelet therapy be continued for at least 12 months in patients not considered at high risk for bleeding. However, the optimal duration of dual antiplatelet therapy is unknown, and this is the first of several randomized controlled trials designed to address this issue. This analysis is actually based upon the merging of 2 concurrent randomized trials that were experiencing slower-than-expected enrollment.

Patients who had been treated for at least 12 months and were free of major adverse cardiac events, including bleeds, were randomized to continued aspirin/clopidogrel versus aspirin alone. Over a median duration of approximately 19 months, there was a nonsignificant trend favoring aspirin in regard to the composite end point of myocardial infarction, stroke, or death from any cause or cardiac causes. This is somewhat surprising since I would have expected a lower rate of these events in patients treated with aspirin and Plavix based upon prior studies in patients without DESs. The limitations are that the event rate was low, and the trial was statistically underpowered. Moreover, the patients comprised a low-risk group since they had already received the drug

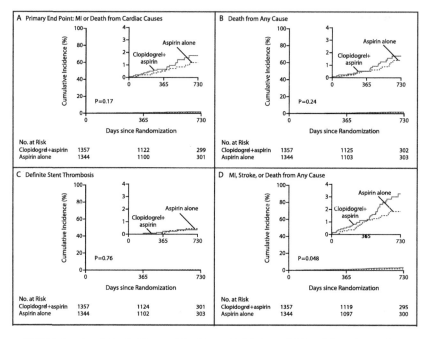

FIGURE 1.—Cumulative Incidence of the Primary End Point and Selected Secondary End Points, According to Treatment Group. Cumulative-incidence curves are shown for the primary end point of myocardial infarction (MI) or death from cardiac causes (Panel A), death from any cause (Panel B), definite stent thrombosis (Panel C), and the secondary composite end point of death from any cause, MI, or stroke (Panel D). P values were calculated with the use of the log-rank test. (Reprinted from Park S-J, Park D-W, Kim Y-H, et al. Duration of dual antiplatelet therapy after implantation of drug-eluting stents. *N Engl J Med.* 2010;362:1374-1382, Copyright © 2010 Massachusetts Medical Society. All rights reserved.)

for 24 months without experiencing an event. In addition, during the trial, 17% of patients discontinued clopidogrel, and this was initiated in 6% of the aspirin-alone group. In addition, the interval between the index procedure and enrollment varied among patients so the precise optimal time for drug discontinuation remains unclear. For all of these reasons, the results of this trial should be interpreted with caution.

Nonetheless, large clinical trials are necessary and ongoing and hopefully will show conclusively that clopidogrel can be discontinued after 12 months. For the present, the decision whether to discontinue after 12 months needs to be individualized as is the initial decision whether to use a DES or a bare-metal stent.

B. J. Gersh, MB, ChB, DPhil, FRCP

References

1. Williams DO, Abbott JD, Kip KE. Outcomes of 6906 patients undergoing percutaneous coronary intervention in the era of drug-eluting stents: report of the DEScover Registry. *Circulation.* 2006;114:2154-2162.
2. Lagerqvist B, James SK, Stenestrand U, Lindbäck J, Nilsson T, Wallentin L. Long-term outcomes with drug-eluting stents versus bare-metal stents in Sweden. *N Engl J Med.* 2007;356:1009-1019.

3. Nakazawa G, Finn AV, Joner M, et al. Delayed arterial healing and increased late stent thrombosis at culprit sites after drug-eluting stent placement for acute myocardial infarction patients: an autopsy study. *Circulation.* 2008;118:1138-1145.

Clinical Pharmacology

Effect of high-dose allopurinol on exercise in patients with chronic stable angina: a randomised, placebo controlled crossover trial

Noman A, Ang DSC, Ogston S, et al (Univ of Dundee, UK)
Lancet 375:2161-2167, 2010

Background.—Experimental evidence suggests that xanthine oxidase inhibitors can reduce myocardial oxygen consumption for a particular stroke volume. If such an effect also occurs in man, this class of inhibitors could become a new treatment for ischaemia in patients with angina pectoris. We ascertained whether high-dose allopurinol prolongs exercise capability in patients with chronic stable angina.

Methods.—65 patients (aged 18−85 years) with angiographically documented coronary artery disease, a positive exercise tolerance test, and stable chronic angina pectoris (for at least 2 months) were recruited into a double-blind, randomised, placebo-controlled, crossover study in a hospital and two infirmaries in the UK. We used computer-generated randomisation to assign patients to allopurinol (600 mg per day) or placebo for 6 weeks before crossover. Our primary endpoint was the time to ST depression, and the secondary endpoints were total exercise time and time to chest pain. We did a completed case analysis. This study is registered as an International Standard Randomised Controlled Trial, number ISRCTN 82040078.

Findings.—In the first treatment period, 31 patients were allocated to allopurinol and 28 were analysed, and 34 were allocated to placebo and 32 were analysed. In the second period, all 60 patients were analysed. Allopurinol increased the median time to ST depression to 298 s (IQR 211−408) from a baseline of 232 s (182−380), and placebo increased it to 249 s (200−375; p=0·0002). The point estimate (absolute difference between allopurinol and placebo) was 43 s (95% CI 31−58). Allopurinol increased median total exercise time to 393 s (IQR 280−519) from a baseline of 301 s (251−447), and placebo increased it to 307 s (232−430; p=0·0003); the point estimate was 58 s (95% CI 45−77). Allopurinol increased the time to chest pain from a baseline of 234 s (IQR 189−382) to 304 s (222−421), and placebo increased it to 272 s (200−380; p=0·001); the point estimate was 38 s (95% CI 17−55). No adverse effects of treatment were reported.

Interpretation.—Allopurinol seems to be a useful, inexpensive, well tolerated, and safe anti-ischaemic drug for patients with angina (Figs 2 and 3).

▶ This is an interesting and unique small trial, and if these findings are confirmed, this could lead to the addition of a useful, inexpensive, and safe drug to our current therapeutic armamentarium for patients with angina.

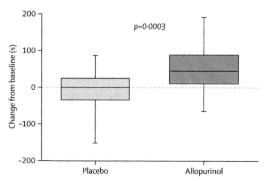

FIGURE 2.—Change in total exercise time from baseline. Data are median (IQR). (Reprinted from Noman A, Ang DSC, Ogston S, et al. Effect of high-dose allopurinol on exercise in patients with chronic stable angina: a randomised, placebo controlled crossover trial. *Lancet.* 2010;375:2161-2167, copyright 2010, with permission from Elsevier.)

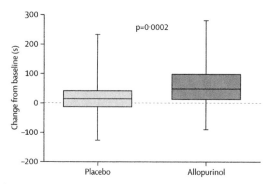

FIGURE 3.—Change in time to ST depression from baseline. Data are median (IQR). (Reprinted from Noman A, Ang DSC, Ogston S, et al. Effect of high-dose allopurinol on exercise in patients with chronic stable angina: a randomised, placebo controlled crossover trial. *Lancet.* 2010;375:2161-2167, copyright 2010, with permission from Elsevier.)

Allopurinol has previously been shown to improve myocardial energetics in heart failure and, in particular, experimental heart failure.[1] The mechanisms whereby allopurinol reduces myocardial oxygen demands are not well understood, but the potential for this to benefit patients with angina pectoris is certainly logical. This double-blinded randomized and placebo-controlled crossover study of 65 patients with stable angina and a positive stress test demonstrated that high-dose allopurinol (600 mg per day) increased the median time to ST-segment depression, total exercise time, and also time to the onset of chest pain. The magnitude of the effect was similar to that noted with standard antianginal drugs.[2]

The data suggest that in some way endogenous xanthine oxidase actively contributes to exercise-induced ischemia. The mechanism of benefit is not related to a reduction in cardiac work as defined by rate pressure product as is the case with beta-blockers. Presumably, reduced oxidative stress with allopurinol can result in a reduction in myocardial oxygen demands for a particular stroke volume, and in addition, perhaps there are direct anti-ischemic effects. Other actions on endothelial function, both coronary and peripheral, have been postulated.[3]

There is certainly a need for new antianginal drugs, and it remains to be seen whether allopurinol will stay the course. Nonetheless it is always interesting, however, when new actions and benefits are identified for old drugs, for example, spironolactone for heart failure.

B. J. Gersh, MB, ChB, DPhil, FRCP

References

1. Stull LB, Leppo MK, Szweda L, Gao WD, Marbán E. Chronic treatment with allopurinol boosts survival and cardiac contractility in murine postischemic cardiomyopathy. *Circ Res.* 2004;95:1005-1011.
2. Rousseau MF, Pouleur H, Cocco G, Wolff AA. Comparative efficacy of ranolazine versus atenolol for chronic angina pectoris. *Am J Cardiol.* 2005;95:311-316.
3. George J, Carr E, Davies J, Belch JJ, Struthers A. High-dose allopurinol improves endothelial function by profoundly reducing vascular oxidative stress and not by lowering uric acid. *Circulation.* 2006;114:2508-2516.

Safety of Anacetrapib in Patients with or at High Risk for Coronary Heart Disease

Cannon CP, for the DEFINE Investigators (Brigham and Women's Hosp, Boston, MA; et al)

N Engl J Med 363:2406-2415, 2010

Background.—Anacetrapib is a cholesteryl ester transfer protein inhibitor that raises high-density lipoprotein (HDL) cholesterol and reduces low-density lipoprotein (LDL) cholesterol.

Methods.—We conducted a randomized, double-blind, placebo-controlled trial to assess the efficacy and safety profile of anacetrapib in patients with coronary heart disease or at high risk for coronary heart disease. Eligible patients who were taking a statin and who had an LDL cholesterol level that was consistent with that recommended in guidelines were assigned to receive 100 mg of anacetrapib or placebo daily for 18 months. The primary end points were the percent change from baseline in LDL cholesterol at 24 weeks (HDL cholesterol level was a secondary end point) and the safety and side-effect profile of anacetrapib through 76 weeks. Cardiovascular events and deaths were prospectively adjudicated.

Results.—A total of 1623 patients underwent randomization. By 24 weeks, the LDL cholesterol level had been reduced from 81 mg per deciliter (2.1 mmol per liter) to 45 mg per deciliter (1.2 mmol per liter) in the anacetrapib group, as compared with a reduction from 82 mg per deciliter (2.1 mmol per liter) to 77 mg per deciliter (2.0 mmol per liter) in the placebo group (P<0.001) — a 39.8% reduction with anacetrapib beyond that seen with placebo. In addition, the HDL cholesterol level increased from 41 mg per deciliter (1.0 mmol per liter) to 101 mg per deciliter (2.6 mmol per liter) in the anacetrapib group, as compared with an increase from 40 mg per deciliter (1.0 mmol per liter) to 46 mg per deciliter (1.2 mmol per liter) in the placebo group (P<0.001) — a 138.1% increase with anacetrapib beyond that seen with placebo. Through 76 weeks, no changes were noted in blood pressure or electrolyte or aldosterone levels with anacetrapib as compared with placebo. Prespecified adjudicated cardiovascular events occurred in 16 patients treated with anacetrapib (2.0%) and 21 patients receiving placebo (2.6%) (P=0.40). The prespecified Bayesian analysis indicated that this event distribution provided a predictive probability (confidence) of 94% that anacetrapib would not be associated with a 25% increase in cardiovascular events, as seen with torcetrapib.

Conclusions.—Treatment with anacetrapib had robust effects on LDL and HDL cholesterol, had an acceptable side-effect profile, and, within the limits of the power of this study, did not result in the adverse cardiovascular effects observed with torcetrapib. (Funded by Merck Research Laboratories; ClinicalTrials.gov number, NCT00685776.)

▶ Will the Details of the Determining the Efficacy and Tolerability of CETP Inhibition with Anacetrapib (DEFINE) trial be looked upon in the future as a defining moment in cardiology? We will all know in time, but for the present, this trial points us in the new clinical directions.

There is an abundant epidemiologic evidence to show that elevated low-density lipoprotein (LDL) cholesterol and reduced high-density lipoprotein (HDL) cholesterol levels are major risk factors for the development of cardiovascular disease. Despite the remarkable success of statins in reducing LDL cholesterol and cardiovascular events, in patients with and without coronary artery disease, it should be appreciated that a high residual risk of cardiovascular events persists even while on statins and particularly in the presence of other lipid abnormalities, that is, a low HDL cholesterol.[1]

One approach to raising HDL cholesterol is to inhibit the cholesteryl ester transfer protein (CETP), as this protein promotes the transfer of cholesteryl esters from HDL and other lipoprotein fractions. A previous trial with a CETP inhibitor or cetrapib was terminated because of an excess of deaths and cardiovascular events thought subsequently to be caused by drug-induced increases in aldosterone levels and blood pressure .[2] These adverse effects are thought, however, not to be related to CETP inhibition and as such are not necessarily shared by other members of the class of CETP inhibitors.

The DEFINE trial demonstrated quite emphatically a striking effect of anacetrapib on reducing LDL cholesterol and increasing HDL cholesterol (in patients already on statins) but without changes in blood pressure, aldosterone, or electrolyte levels.

This is a moderate sized safety study and demonstrates efficacy in regard to lipid levels, but this does not necessarily translate into a reduction in clinical events. A legitimate question is whether the HDL particles generated by inhibition of CETP are as protective functionally as naturally occurring HDL, which does appear to be atheroprotective. Preliminary in vitro studies in this respect are, however, encouraging.[3] It is interesting that in this study anacetrapib did not have any effect on C-reactive protein levels; what this means in terms of future clinical effectiveness is uncertain.

Whether elevating HDL cholesterol with CETP inhibitors would lead to a reduction in cardiovascular events awaits the results of large phase III studies. If these are positive, this will certainly usher in a new era in preventive cardiology, and it goes without saying that the results of these trials will be eagerly awaited.

B. J. Gersh, MB, ChB, DPhil, FRCP

References

1. LaRosa JC, Grundy SM, Waters DD, et al. Intensive lipid lowering with atorvastatin in patients with stable coronary disease. *N Engl J Med.* 2005;352:1425-1435.
2. Barter PJ, Caulfield M, Eriksson M, et al. Effects of torcetrapib in patients at high risk for coronary events. *N Engl J Med.* 2007;357:2109-2122.
3. Yvan-Charvet L, Kling J, Pagler T, et al. Cholesterol efflux potential and anti-inflammatory properties of high-density lipoprotein after treatment with niacin or anacetrapib. *Arterioscler Thromb Vasc Biol.* 2010;30:1430-1438.

Epidemiology

Association of Marine Omega-3 Fatty Acid Levels With Telomeric Aging in Patients With Coronary Heart Disease

Farzaneh-Far R, Lin J, Epel ES, et al (San Francisco General Hosp, CA; Univ of California; et al)
JAMA 303:250-257, 2010

Context.—Increased dietary intake of marine omega-3 fatty acids is associated with prolonged survival in patients with coronary heart disease. However, the mechanisms underlying this protective effect are poorly understood.

Objective.—To investigate the association of omega-3 fatty acid blood levels with temporal changes in telomere length, an emerging marker of biological age.

Design, Setting, and Participants.—Prospective cohort study of 608 ambulatory outpatients in California with stable coronary artery disease recruited from the Heart and Soul Study between September 2000 and December 2002 and followed up to January 2009 (median, 6.0 years; range, 5.0-8.1 years).

Main Outcome Measures.—We measured leukocyte telomere length at baseline and again after 5 years of follow-up. Multivariable linear and logistic regression models were used to investigate the association of baseline levels of omega-3 fatty acids (docosahexaenoic acid [DHA] and eicosapentaenoic acid [EPA]) with subsequent change in telomere length.

Results.—Individuals in the lowest quartile of DHA + EPA experienced the fastest rate of telomere shortening (0.13 telomere-to-single-copy gene ratio

[T/S] units over 5 years; 95% confidence interval [CI], 0.09-0.17), whereas those in the highest quartile experienced the slowest rate of telomere shortening (0.05 T/S units over 5 years; 95% CI, 0.02-0.08; $P < .001$ for linear trend across quartiles). Levels of DHA + EPA were associated with less telomere shortening before (unadjusted β coefficient $\times 10^{-3} = 0.06$; 95% CI, 0.02-0.10) and after (adjusted β coefficient $\times 10^{-3} = 0.05$; 95% CI, 0.01-0.08) sequential adjustment for established risk factors and potential confounders. Each 1-SD increase in DHA + EPA levels was associated with a 32% reduction in the odds of telomere shortening (adjusted odds ratio, 0.68; 95% CI, 0.47-0.98).

Conclusion.—Among this cohort of patients with coronary artery disease, there was an inverse relationship between baseline blood levels of marine omega-3 fatty acids and the rate of telomere shortening over 5 years.

▶ This is a fascinating study that attempts to link the benefits of omega-3 fatty acid levels with reduced aging of telomeres. A number of epidemiological studies and randomized trials have suggested that omega-3 fatty acids are associated with improved survival in patients with established cardiovascular disease.[1] These studies form the basis for the American Heart Association recommendations for the increased intake of oily fish and the use of omega-3 fatty acid supplements in the primary and secondary prevention of coronary heart disease.[2] The mechanisms underlying these apparently protective effects are, however, poorly understood and potentially include antiarrhythmic, anti-inflammatory, and antiplatelet effects among others.

Telomeres that form a protective cap at the ends of eukaryotic chromosomes may play a major role in cellular senescence or apoptosis. This has led to the concept that telomeric length is a novel marker of biological aging, and with respect to telomeric length, longer is better. Moreover, there is a strong association between reduced telomeric length and cardiovascular morbidity and mortality in some populations.[3]

In this prospective cohort study of 600 ambulatory patients with stable coronary artery disease in California, the authors correlated baseline levels of omega-3 fatty acids with leukocyte telomeric length at baseline and again after 5 years of follow-up. There was a strong inverse relationship suggesting that higher levels of omega-3 fatty acids were associated with reduced telomere shortening, which in a biological context is a favorable effect. Potential mechanisms are that the delayed telomere attrition is caused by a reduction in oxidative stress as reactive oxygen species significantly target telomeric DNA. Another possibility is that fish oils increase the activity of the enzyme telomerase, which may be beneficial in noncancerous lesions.

The findings in this study are purely observational and do not prove causality because it may well be that other favorable lifestyle behaviors are associated with a higher intake of omega-3 fatty acids, and no amount of statistical judgment can eliminate the potential bias. Nonetheless, the association is of great potential interest. It has been said that one is as old as the state of our arteries, but perhaps we need to add to this that we are as old as the length of our telomeres.

B. J. Gersh, MB, ChB, DPhil, FRCP

References

1. Lee JH, O'Keefe JH, Lavie CJ, Marchioli R, Harris WS. Omega-3 fatty acids for cardioprotection. *Mayo Clin Proc.* 2008;83:324-332.
2. Kris-Etherton PM, Harris WS, Appel LJ, American Heart Association Nutrition Committee. Fish consumption, fish oil, omega-3 fatty acids, and cardiovascular disease. *Circulation.* 2002;106:2747-2757.
3. Cawthon RM, Smith KR, O'Brien E, Sivatchenko A, Kerber RA. Association between telomere length in blood and mortality in people aged 60 years or older. *Lancet.* 2003;361:393-395.

Alcohol Consumption and Cardiovascular Mortality Among U.S. Adults, 1987 to 2002

Mukamal KJ, Chen CM, Rao SR, et al (Beth Israel Deaconess Med Ctr, Boston, MA; CSR Incorporated, Arlington, VA; Massachusetts General Hosp, Boston; et al)
J Am Coll Cardiol 55:1328-1335, 2010

Objectives.—The aim of this study was to determine the association of alcohol consumption and cardiovascular mortality in the U.S. population.

Background.—Alcohol consumption has been associated with a lower risk of cardiovascular disease in cohort studies, but this association has not been prospectively examined in large, detailed, representative samples of the U.S. population.

Methods.—We analyzed 9 iterations of the National Health Interview Survey, an annual survey of a nationally representative sample of U.S. adults between 1987 and 2000. Exposures of interest included usual volume, frequency, and quantity of alcohol consumption and binge drinking. Mortality was ascertained through linkage to the National Death Index through 2002. Relative risks were derived from random-effects meta-analyses of weighted, multivariable-adjusted hazard ratios for cardiovascular mortality from individual survey administrations.

Results.—Light and moderate volumes of alcohol consumption were inversely associated with cardiovascular mortality. Compared with life-time abstainers, summary relative risks were 0.95 (95% confidence interval [CI]: 0.88 to 1.02) among lifetime infrequent drinkers, 1.02 (95% CI: 0.94 to 1.11) among former drinkers, 0.69 (95% CI: 0.59 to 0.82) among light drinkers, 0.62 (95% CI: 0.50 to 0.77) among moderate drinkers, and 0.95 (95% CI: 0.82 to 1.10) among heavy drinkers. The magnitude of lower risk was similar in subgroups of sex, age, or baseline health status. There was no simple relation of drinking pattern with risk, but risk was consistently higher among those who consumed ≥ 3 compared with 2 drinks/drinking day.

Conclusions.—In 9 nationally representative samples of U.S. adults, light and moderate alcohol consumption were inversely associated with CVD mortality, even when compared with lifetime abstainers, but consumption above recommended limits was not.

▶ This analysis of alcohol consumption and cardiovascular mortality from the National Health Survey of US adults from 1957 and 2000 reaffirms what we have learned from previous studies (the first of which was carried out approximately 50 years ago) as referenced in the accompanying editorial.[1] The totality of the evidence is consistent in that there appears to be a benefit in terms of cardiovascular mortality (which in turn is dominated by coronary artery disease mortality) from light and moderate alcohol consumption, even in comparison to lifetime abstainers, but drinking too much is bad for you on all counts.

As pointed out in the accompanying editorial, previous reports have undergone intense evaluation for methodologic flaws, and skepticism, particularly about the effects of confounding variables, remains and will continue to be an issue, particularly given that we are unlikely to see any randomized controlled trials. We need only to look at previous epidemiologic studies of hormone replacement therapy, vitamin E, and homocysteine levels to realize the gap between associations as documented in population studies and the rigorous scrutiny of a randomized controlled trial. The editorial points out, however, that confounding can cut both ways. Certain sources of bias might actually tend to reduce an apparent benefit, for example, smoking, which correlates with alcohol drinking. Another source of reverse bias is the imprecise categorization of alcohol intake because of underreporting by heavy drinkers.

This particular analysis has the strengths of a national sample and the ability to include past drinkers as one of the reference groups. In summary, the evidence that light to moderate alcohol consumption is beneficial from a cardiovascular and particularly coronary artery disease standpoint is quite compelling. Nonetheless, absolute proof is lacking, and it is difficult to see how the case could ever be settled one way or another because randomized trials are not possible. From a practical perspective therefore, moderation and sound judgment remain the watchword. It makes no sense to recommend alcohol to reduce coronary artery disease mortality, but for individuals who exercise judgment in regard to mild to moderate consumption of alcohol, there is no reason to dissuade them from continuing to do what they enjoy.

B. J. Gersh, MB, ChB, DPhil, FRCP

Reference

1. Klatsky AL. Alcohol and cardiovascular mortality: common sense and scientific truth. *J Am Coll Cardiol.* 2010;55:1336-1338.

Alcohol Intake and Risk of Coronary Heart Disease in Younger, Middle-Aged, and Older Adults

Hvidtfeldt UA, Tolstrup JS, Jakobsen MU, et al (Univ of Southern Denmark, Copenhagen, Denmark; Aarhus Univ Hosp, Aalborg, Denmark; et al)
Circulation 121:1589-1597, 2010

Background.—Light to moderate alcohol consumption is associated with a reduced risk of coronary heart disease. This protective effect of alcohol, however, may be confined to middle-aged or older individuals. Coronary heart disease incidence is low in men <40 years of age and in women <50 years of age; for this reason, study cohorts rarely have the power to investigate the effects of alcohol on coronary heart disease risk in younger adults. This study examined whether the beneficial effect of alcohol on coronary heart disease depends on age.

Methods and Results.—In this pooled analysis of 8 prospective studies from North America and Europe including 192 067 women and 74 919 men free of cardiovascular diseases, diabetes, and cancers at baseline, average daily alcohol intake was assessed at baseline with a food frequency or diet history questionnaire. An inverse association between alcohol and risk of coronary heart disease was observed in all age groups; hazard ratios among moderately drinking men (5.0 to 29.9 g/d) 39 to 50, 50 to 59, and ≥ 60 years of age were 0.58 (95% confidence interval [CI], 0.36 to 0.93), 0.72 (95% CI, 0.60 to 0.86), and 0.85 (95% CI, 0.75 to 0.97) compared with abstainers. However, the analyses indicated a smaller incidence rate difference between abstainers and moderate consumers in younger adults (incidence rate difference, 45 per 100 000; 90% CI, 8 to 84) than in middle-aged (incidence rate difference, 64 per 100 000; 90% CI, 24 to 102) and older (incidence rate difference, 89 per 100 000; 90% CI, 44 to 140) adults. Similar results were observed in women.

Conclusion.—Alcohol is also associated with a decreased risk of coronary heart disease in younger adults; however, the absolute risk was small compared with middle-aged and older adults.

▶ The association between moderate alcohol intake and coronary heart disease (CHD) has been the subject of multiple investigations and meta-analyses over several decades.[1] Although the influence of confounding variables has not been entirely excluded, there is a general consensus that moderate alcohol intake is linked to a lower risk of CHD.[2] Most results are obtained from cohorts consisting of middle-aged and older adults, and very few studies have addressed the impact of alcohol intake in younger adults. There is every reason to expect that the results may be different since the rates of CHD are low in younger individuals and genetic predisposition to premature cardiovascular disease may be present, thus modifying any potential benefit from alcohol intake.

This pooled analysis from 8 perspective studies, including over 200 000 subjects, demonstrates, as have many other studies, an inverse association between moderate alcohol intake versus abstainers and the risk of CHD in all age groups; however, the difference between moderate consumers and abstainers in younger adults was much smaller than among middle-aged and older adults (45/100 000; 64/100 000; 89/100 000; respectively).

Plausible mechanisms for the reduction in CHD risk include the potential for alcohol to increase high-density lipoprotein cholesterol and reduce plasma fibrinogen levels, thereby reducing platelet aggregatability and through an effect on plasminogen activator inhibitor-1 that could reduce the tendency to form thrombi.[3]

Limitations recognized by the authors include a lack of information on that pattern of consumption in different age groups, the type of alcohol consumed, and a lack of information in regard to confounding variables in both drinkers and abstainers (eg, quitting because of comorbid conditions or existing illness, such as hypertension—the sick-quitter hypothesis). Although the totality of the evidence favors moderate alcohol consumption in regard to the risk of CHD, the total picture needs to take into account total mortality, and this information was not available for the pooling project. Nonetheless, it is reasonable to assume that the protective effect of alcohol in middle and older age groups would have an impact on all-cause mortality since the mortality due to CHD is so high in these subsets. One also needs to remember, however, that excess alcohol consumption has an adverse effect on total mortality. Per the discussion of the issues, a recent editorial by Klatsky entitled "Alcohol and Cardiovascular Mortality Common Sense and Scientific Truth" is well worth reading.[4]

B. J. Gersh, MB, ChB, DPhil, FRCP

References

1. Costanzo S, Di Castelnuvo A, Donati MB, Iacoviello L, de Gaetano G. Alcohol consumption and mortality in patients with cardiovascular disease: a meta-analysis. *J Am Coll Cardiol.* 2010;55:1339-1347.
2. Mukamal JK, Conigrave KM, Mittleman MA, et al. Roles of drinking pattern and type of alcohol consumed in coronary heart disease in men. *N Engl J Med.* 2003; 348:109-118.
3. Rimm EB, Williams P, Fosher K, Criqui M, Stampfer MJ. Moderate alcohol intake and lower risk of coronary heart disease: meta-analysis of effects on lipids and haemostatic factors. *BMJ.* 1999;319:1523-1528.
4. Klatsky AL. Alcohol and cardiovascular mortality: common sense and scientific truth. *J Am Coll Cardiol.* 2010;55:1136-1138.

Attained Educational Level and Incident Atherothrombotic Events in Low- and Middle-Income Compared With High-Income Countries
Goyal A, for the Reduction of Atherothrombosis for Continued Health (REACH) Registry Investigators (Emory Rollins School of Public Health, Atlanta, GA; et al)
Circulation 122:1167-1175, 2010

Background.—Studies report a protective effect of higher attained educational level (AEL) on cardiovascular outcomes. However, most of these studies have been conducted in high-income countries (HICs) and lack representation from low and middle-income countries (LMICs), which bear >80% of the global burden of cardiovascular disease.

Methods and Results.—The Reduction of Atherothrombosis for Continued Health (REACH) Registry is a prospective study of 67 888 subjects with either established atherothrombotic (coronary, cerebrovascular, and/or peripheral arterial) disease or multiple atherothrombotic risk factors enrolled from 5587 physician practices in 44 countries. At baseline, AEL (0 to 8 years, 9 to 12 years, trade or technical school, and university) was self-reported for 61 332 subjects. Outcomes included the baseline prevalence of atherothrombotic risk factors and the rate of incident cardiovascular events (cardiovascular death, nonfatal myocardial infarction, or nonfatal stroke) through 23 months across AEL groups, stratified by sex and world region (LMICs or HICs). Educational attainment was inversely associated with age and diabetes mellitus and directly associated with hypercholesterolemia in all subjects. However, for other risk factors such as obesity, smoking, hypertension, and baseline burden of vascular disease, AEL was protective (inversely associated) in HICs but not protective in LMICs. The protective effect of greater AEL on incident cardiovascular events was strongest in men from HICs ($P<0.0001$), more modest in women from HICs ($P=0.0026$) and in men from LMICs ($P=0.082$), and essentially absent in women from LMICs ($P=0.32$).

Conclusion.—In contrast to HICs, higher AEL may not be protective against cardiovascular events in LMICs, particularly in women (Table 2).

▶ This analysis from a large international registry of patients with either established atherothrombotic coronary, cerebrovascular, or peripheral vascular disease or with multiple atherosclerotic risk factors provides a nice example of the epidemiologic transition.[1] The epidemiologic transition provides a framework for understanding the interactions between changing lifestyle and socioeconomic status and the development of cardiovascular disease.

In phase III of the epidemiologic transition (the United States between 1920 and the 1960s), cardiovascular disease was particularly evident in patients of higher socioeconomic status because these are the individuals who initially develop the risk factors associated with a western lifestyle and urbanization. In phase IV of the transition, as is the case in the United States and other high-income countries, premature coronary cardiovascular disease tends to occur in patients of lower socioeconomic status. This is because access to care and prevention delays the onset among those who are more socioeconomically advantaged and among whom cardiovascular disease tends to occur at an older age.[2]

In this analysis, attained educational levels (AELs) are in some ways a surrogate of socioeconomic status. In this respect, the protective effect of AEL on incident cardiovascular events and risk factors are strongest in men from the higher income countries (phase IV of the epidemiologic transition), more modest in women from high-income countries and in men from lower income countries (phase III), and essentially absent in women from lower income

TABLE 2.—Event Rates* at 23 Months by AEL Stratified by the Combination of Sex and Region

	AEL				P for Trend Adjusted for Age[†]
	0–8 y	9–12 y	Trade School	University	
Men in HICs					
n	9403	9853	5531	5522	...
Event rates					
CV death/MI/stroke (95% CI)	9.11 (8.25–9.95)	6.44 (5.78–7.09)	7.61 (6.56–8.65)	5.83 (5.04–6.62)	<0.0001
All-cause mortality (95% CI)	6.92 (6.16–7.67)	5.33 (4.65–6.01)	6.07 (5.08–7.06)	4.80 (3.93–5.65)	<0.0001
Men in LMICs					
n	2457	1932	1810	2700	...
Event rates					
CV death/MI/stroke (95% CI)	9.60 (8.24–10.94)	8.04 (6.64–9.43)	9.60 (8.02–11.15)	7.67 (6.49–8.83)	0.082
All-cause mortality (95% CI)	5.38 (4.34–6.41)	4.46 (3.37–5.52)	4.03 (2.97–5.08)	4.14 (3.26–5.02)	0.067
Women in HICs					
n	6895	6591	2002	1848	...
Event rates					
CV death/MI/stroke (95% CI)	7.93 (7.05–8.79)	6.94 (6.09–7.78)	6.46 (5.15–7.76)	6.32 (4.86–7.76)	0.003
All-cause mortality (95% CI)	5.69 (4.92–6.45)	5.62 (4.72–6.50)	3.82 (2.85–4.78)	5.22 (3.66–6.74)	0.007
Women in LMICs					
n	2079	1092	726	866	...
Event rates					
CV death/MI/stroke (95% CI)	7.47 (6.10–8.83)	7.21 (5.46–8.92)	8.35 (6.04–10.60)	8.29 (6.11–10.41)	0.32
All-cause mortality (95% CI)	4.43 (3.36–5.49)	3.76 (2.49–5.02)	4.14 (2.44–5.80)	4.41 (2.80–5.99)	0.94

CV indicates cardiovascular; CI, confidence interval.
*All event rates represent the percentage of the population with the event through 23 months after adjustment for age and were calculated with the corrected group prognosis method in the Cox proportional-hazard model as described in the text.
[†]P values for trend across education groups were calculated with the log-rank statistic.

countries. Whether data such as these can be used to shorten or telescope phase III of the epidemiologic transition is a critical yet unanswered question.

B. J. Gersh, MB, ChB, DPhil, FRCP

References

1. Yusuf S, Reddy S, Ounpuu S, Anand S. Global burden of cardiovascular diseases, part I: general considerations, the epidemiologic transition, risk factors, and the impact of urbanization. *Circulation.* 2001;104:2746-2753.
2. Gersh BJ, Sliwa K, Mayosi BM, Yusuf S. Novel therapeutic concept; the epidemic of cardiovascular disease in the developing world: global implications. *Eur Heart J.* 2010;31:642-648.

Efficacy and safety of more intensive lowering of LDL cholesterol: a meta-analysis of data from 170 000 participants in 26 randomised trials
Cholesterol Treatment Trialists' (CTT) Collaboration (Clinical Trial Service Unit and Epidemiological Studies Unit (CTSU), Oxford, UK)
Lancet 376:1670-1681, 2010

Background.—Lowering of LDL cholesterol with standard statin regimens reduces the risk of occlusive vascular events in a wide range of individuals. We aimed to assess the safety and efficacy of more intensive lowering of LDL cholesterol with statin therapy.

Methods.—We undertook meta-analyses of individual participant data from randomised trials involving at least 1000 participants and at least 2 years' treatment duration of more versus less intensive statin regimens (five trials; 39 612 individuals; median follow-up 5·1 years) and of statin versus control (21 trials; 129 526 individuals; median follow-up 4·8 years). For each type of trial, we calculated not only the average risk reduction, but also the average risk reduction per 1·0 mmol/L LDL cholesterol reduction at 1 year after randomisation.

Findings.—In the trials of more versus less intensive statin therapy, the weighted mean further reduction in LDL cholesterol at 1 year was 0·51 mmol/L. Compared with less intensive regimens, more intensive regimens produced a highly significant 15% (95% CI 11−18; p<0·0001) further reduction in major vascular events, consisting of separately significant reductions in coronary death or non-fatal myocardial infarction of 13% (95% CI 7−19; p<0·0001), in coronary revascularisation of 19% (95% CI 15−24; p<0·0001), and in ischaemic stroke of 16% (95% CI 5−26; p=0·005). Per 1·0 mmol/L reduction in LDL cholesterol, these further reductions in risk were similar to the proportional reductions in the trials of statin versus control. When both types of trial were combined, similar proportional reductions in major vascular events per 1·0 mmol/L LDL cholesterol reduction were found in all types of patient studied (rate ratio [RR] 0·78, 95% CI 0·76−0·80; p<0·0001), including those with LDL cholesterol lower than 2 mmol/L on the less intensive or control regimen. Across all 26 trials, all-cause mortality was reduced by 10% per

1·0 mmol/L LDL reduction (RR 0·90, 95% CI 0·87—0·93; p<0·0001), largely reflecting significant reductions in deaths due to coronary heart disease (RR 0·80, 99% CI 0·74—0·87; p<0·0001) and other cardiac causes (RR 0·89, 99% CI 0·81—0·98; p=0·002), with no significant effect on deaths due to stroke (RR 0·96, 95% CI 0·84—1·09; p=0·5) or other vascular causes (RR 0·98, 99% CI 0·81—1·18; p=0·8). No significant effects were observed on deaths due to cancer or other non-vascular causes (RR 0·97, 95% CI 0·92—1·03; p=0·3) or on cancer incidence (RR 1·00, 95% CI 0·96—1·04; p=0·9), even at low LDL cholesterol concentrations.

Interpretation.—Further reductions in LDL cholesterol safely produce definite further reductions in the incidence of heart attack, of revascularisation, and of ischaemic stroke, with each 1·0 mmol/L reduction reducing the annual rate of these major vascular events by just over a fifth. There was no evidence of any threshold within the cholesterol range studied, suggesting that reduction of LDL cholesterol by 2—3 mmol/L would reduce risk by about 40—50%.

▶ Statins have been in clinical use for almost 2 decades and their efficacy in reducing vascular events in addition to their safety is not in doubt. What this meta-analysis from the Cholesterol Treatment Trialists' Collaboration using individual patient rather than summary data tells us is that reducing low-density lipoprotein (LDL) cholesterol below current targets is beneficial. This adds to current knowledge by showing that we can indeed go lower and that patients who started out at a target level of 70 mg/dL had a further reduction in vascular events when going from 70 mg/dL to 50 mg/dL. What is important is the absolute and not the relative risk reductions, and we need to emphasize that the data really only apply to patients at a high risk of cardiovascular events. Nonetheless, in patients with low baseline LDL levels, statins may still be indicated, and this would depend in part on the presence of other markers of cardiovascular risk, at least when primary prevention is the goal. The argument for a statin, however, is much less persuasive for people at low cardiovascular risk, such as young people with no other cardiovascular risk factors.

Another study in the same issue of the journal suggested that 80 mg of simvastatin was associated with a much higher incidence of myopathy so that the more potent statins, such as atorvastatin or rosuvastatin, may be a better approach because they have better safety profiles and greater efficacy.[1]

It is encouraging that the increase in hemorrhagic stroke was small and far outweighed by the reduction in ischemic stroke. An accompanying editorial, however, makes the point that perhaps we cannot extrapolate these data to other populations that have much higher rates of hemorrhagic stroke, such as patients from Japan and China.[2] In a 10-year population-based observational study from Japan, a low LDL cholesterol level was also an independent predictor of hemorrhagic stroke.[3]

In summary, at the population level, statins are underused, so an urgent priority is to identify those people who will benefit most from statin therapy and to lower their LDL cholesterol aggressively with higher doses and more potent statins, if necessary.

B. J. Gersh, MB, ChB, DPhil, FRCP

References

1. Study of the Effectiveness of Additional Reductions in Cholesterol and Homocysteine (SEARCH) Collaborative Group. Intensive lowering of LDL cholesterol with 80-mg versus 20-mg simvastatin daily in 12,064 survivors of myocardial infarction: a double-blind randomized trial. *Lancet.* 2010;376:1658-1669.
2. Cheung BNY, Lamb KSL. Is intensive LDL-cholesterol lowering beneficial and safe? *Lancet.* 2010;376:1622-1624.
3. Kumana CR, Cheung BM, Leuder IJ. Gauging the impact of statins using number needed to treat. *JAMA.* 1999;282:1899-1901.

Orthostatic hypotension predicts all-cause mortality and coronary events in middle-aged individuals (The Malmö Preventive Project)
Fedorowski A, Stavenow L, Hedblad B, et al (Malmö Univ Hosp, Sweden)
Eur Heart J 31:85-91, 2010

Aims.—Orthostatic hypotension (OH) has been linked to increased mortality and incidence of cardiovascular disease in various risk groups, but determinants and consequences of OH in the general population are poorly studied.

Methods and Results.—Prospective data of the Swedish 'Malmö Preventive Project' ($n = 33\,346$, 67.3% men, mean age 45.7 ± 7.4 years, mean follow-up 22.7 ± 6.0 years) were analysed. Orthostatic hypotension was found in 6.2% of study participants and was associated with age, female gender, hypertension, antihypertensive treatment, increased heart rate, diabetes, low BMI, and current smoking. In Cox regression analysis, individuals with OH had significantly increased all-cause mortality (in particular those aged less than 42 years) and coronary event (CE) risk. Mortality and CE risk were distinctly higher in those with systolic blood pressure (BP) fall ≥30 mmHg [hazard ratio (HR): 1.6, 95% CI 1.3–1.9, $P < 0.0001$ and 1.6, 95% CI 1.2–2.1, $P = 0.001$] and diastolic BP fall ≥15 mmHg (HR: 1.4, 95% CI 1.1–1.9, $P = 0.024$ and 1.7, 95% CI 1.1–2.5, $P = 0.01$). In addition, impaired diastolic BP response had relatively greater impact (per mmHg) on CE incidence than systolic reaction.

Conclusion.—Orthostatic hypotension can be detected in ~6% of middle-aged individuals and is often associated with such comorbidities as hypertension or diabetes. Presence of OH increases mortality and CE risk, independently of traditional risk factors. Although both impaired systolic and diastolic responses predict adverse events, the diastolic impairment shows stronger association with coronary disease (Table 3).

▶ This analysis of a huge prospective database in Sweden identifies an unusual risk factor for mortality and cardiovascular events.

TABLE 3.—Relationships Between Orthostatic Blood Pressure Reaction and All-Cause Mortality, Coronary Event, Stroke, and Composite Endpoint in Crude and Adjusted Cox Regression Models (Hazard Ratio, 95% Confidence Interval, P-Value)

Endpoint	Systolic OBPR[a]	Diastolic OBPR[a]
All-cause mortality	1.21 (1.18−1.23), $P < 0.001$	1.18 (1.13−1.22), $P < 0.001$
	1.05 (1.02−1.07), $P = 0.001$[b]	1.05 (1.01−1.10), $P = 0.017$[b]
Coronary event	1.17 (1.13−1.21), $P < 0.001$	1.20 (1.14−1.26), $P < 0.001$
	1.02 (0.99−1.06), $P = 0.213$[b]	1.09 (1.03−1.15), $P = 0.003$[b]
Stroke	1.17 (1.12−1.22), $P < 0.001$	1.19 (1.11−1.27), $P < 0.001$
	0.98 (0.93−1.03), $P = 0.488$[b]	1.06 (0.99−1.14), $P = 0.111$[b]
Composite endpoint	1.18 (1.15−1.20), $P < 0.001$	1.17 (1.13−1.21), $P < 0.001$
(CE, stroke, or death)	1.04 (1.02−1.06), $P = 0.001$[b]	1.05 (1.01−1.09), $P = 0.011$[b]

[a]OBPR effects are presented for 10 mmHg difference.
[b]Cox proportional hazard model adjusted for age, gender, SBP, AHT, total cholesterol, diabetes, BMI, current smoking, previous CVD, and cancer (mortality only).

Orthostatic blood pressure control involves complex mechanisms, principally involving the autonomic nervous system. Orthostatic hypotension can result in debilitating symptoms and injuries caused by falls, and the clinical management is often difficult. In predominantly symptomatic patients considered at high risk, including the elderly, orthostatic hypotension has been associated with an increased mortality and an increased risk of cardiovascular disease.[1]

The importance of this study is that the data were obtained from the population at large and from participants who were middle aged (mean age 45.7 ± 7.4 years). Orthostatic hypotension defined by 20 mm Hg or greater fall in systolic blood pressure and by 10 mm Hg or greater fall in diastolic blood pressure was noted in 6.2% of study participants. This was strongly associated with a number of other variables, for example, age, hypertension, antihypertensive therapy, increased resting heart rate, diabetes, smoking, low body mass index, and female gender. Most, but not all, of these are known risk factors for cardiovascular disease. Nonetheless, after multivariate adjustment, individuals with orthostatic hypotension (particularly impaired diastolic blood pressure responses) had an increased all-cause mortality and an increased incidence of cardiovascular events.

Studies such as these are always subject to the limitations of confounders. A multivariant analysis tends to take these into account but cannot eliminate bias. Nonetheless, the results are of interest and suggest that improved autonomic control may be a marker of cardiovascular health. In this respect, the association with an elevated resting heart rate, which is reflective of increased sympathetic drive and reduced vagal influence, is of interest. Moreover, this provides a biologically plausible explanation for the increased cardiovascular risk and for the attenuation of the sympathetic responses required for blood pressure control.[2]

B. J. Gersh, MB, ChB, DPhil, FRCP

References

1. Hossain M, Ooi WL, Lipsitz LA. Intra-individual postural blood pressure variability and stroke in elderly nursing home residents. *J Clin Epidemiol.* 2001;54:488-494.
2. Mancia G, Grassi G. Orthostatic hypotension and cardiovascular risk: defining the epidemiological and prognostic relevance. *Eur Heart J.* 2010;31:12-14.

Outcomes After Acute Myocardial Infarction in South Asian, Chinese, and White Patients

Khan NA, Grubisic M, Hemmelgarn B, et al (Univ of British Columbia, Vancouver; Univ of Calgary, Alberta, Canada)
Circulation 122:1570-1577, 2010

Background.—Cardiac mortality rates vary substantially between countries and ethnic groups. It is unclear, however, whether South Asian, Chinese, and white populations have a variable prognosis after acute myocardial infarction (AMI). To clarify this association, we compared mortality, use of revascularization procedures, and risk of recurrent AMI and hospitalization for heart failure between these ethnic groups in a universal-access healthcare system.

Methods and Results.—We used a population cohort study design using hospital administrative data linked to cardiac procedure registries from British Columbia and the Calgary Health Region Area in Alberta (1994 to 2003) to identify AMI cases. Patient ethnicity was categorized using validated surname algorithms. There were 2190 South Asian, 946 Chinese, and 38479 white patients with AMI identified. There was no significant difference in use of revascularization procedures between ethnic groups at 30 d and 1 year. Short-term (30-day) mortality was higher among Chinese relative to white patients (odds ratio, 1.23; 95% confidence interval, 1.02 to 1.48). There was no significant difference in 30-day mortality between South Asian and white patients. South Asian patients had a 35% lower relative risk of long-term mortality compared with white patients (hazard ratio, 0.65; 95% confidence interval, 0.57 to 0.72). There was no significant difference in long-term mortality between Chinese and white patients. Among AMI survivors, Chinese patients had a lower risk of recurrent AMI, whereas there was no difference between South Asian and white patients.

Conclusion.—The ethnic groups studied have striking differences in outcomes after AMI, with South Asian patients having significantly lower long-term mortality after AMI.

▶ Approximately 40% of the world's population lives in China and the South Asian countries including India, Pakistan, and Bangladesh. Our own societies in North America are changing as a result of immigration from Europe but increasingly from China and South Asia. In Canada in 2006, people of Chinese and Indian descent accounted for 4.3% and 4.2% of the population, respectively.[1] Given the increasing diversity of our societies, racial differences in health care outcomes, delivery, and the quality of care are important and intriguing areas for analysis.

This study from an administrative database linked to large procedural registries in British Columbia and Alberta demonstrates interesting but puzzling differences in outcomes after acute myocardial infarction between South Asian, Chinese, and white patients.

An accompanying excellent editorial illustrates that there is a great deal we still need to know and also that unmeasured confounding variables may play a major role in accounting for these differences.[2] Understanding those cultural differences and obtaining access to care and in regard to the quality of care received could provide the key to our ability to deliver quality care to individuals with different cultural attitudes and languages. For instance, the higher early mortality in the Chinese could relate to delayed presentation leading to sicker patients, and there are multiple potential contributory reasons including language barriers, perceptions of racial discrimination, and lack of trust. Are the lower long-term mortality rates in South Asians because of their younger age or higher use of invasive procedures in the year following myocardial infarction? That in turn could lead to a higher use of secondary prevention measures and better outcomes.

In concert with the Institute of Medicine statement that health care organizations need to collect data related to ethnicity and other social factors, the state of Massachusetts has enacted a similar mandate.[3] This is in many ways a new and evolving area of research.

B. J. Gersh, MB, ChB, DPhil, FRCP

References

1. Statistics Canada stop population by selected ethnic origins, by providence and territory (2006 census), http://www.40.statcan.gc.ca/101/cst01/DENO26A-eng.htm. Accessed November 4, 2010.
2. Ayanian JZ. Diversity in cardiovascular outcomes among Chinese and South Asian patients. *Circulation.* 2010;122:1550-1552.
3. Ulmer C, McFadden B, Nerenz D, eds. Race, Ethnicity, and Language Data: Standardization for Healthcare Quality Improvements. Washington, DC: National Academy Press; 2009.

Population Trends in the Incidence and Outcomes of Acute Myocardial Infarction
Yeh RW, Sidney S, Chandra M, et al (Harvard Med School, Boston, MA; Kaiser Permanente Northern California, Oakland, CA)
N Engl J Med 362:2155-2165, 2010

Background.—Few studies have characterized recent population trends in the incidence and outcomes of myocardial infarction.

Methods.—We identified patients 30 years of age or older in a large, diverse, community-based population who were hospitalized for incident myocardial infarction between 1999 and 2008. Age- and sex-adjusted incidence rates were calculated for myocardial infarction overall and separately for ST-segment elevation and non—ST-segment elevation myocardial infarction. Patient characteristics, outpatient medications, and cardiac biomarker levels during hospitalization were identified from health plan databases, and 30-day mortality was ascertained from administrative databases, state death data, and Social Security Administration files.

Results.—We identified 46,086 hospitalizations for myocardial infarctions during 18,691,131 person-years of follow-up from 1999 to 2008. The age- and sex-adjusted incidence of myocardial infarction increased from 274 cases per 100,000 person-years in 1999 to 287 cases per 100,000 person-years in 2000, and it decreased each year thereafter, to 208 cases per 100,000 person-years in 2008, representing a 24% relative decrease over the study period. The age- and sex-adjusted incidence of ST-segment elevation myocardial infarction decreased throughout the study period (from 133 cases per 100,000 person-years in 1999 to 50 cases per 100,000 person-years in 2008, P<0.001 for linear trend). Thirty-day mortality was significantly lower in 2008 than in 1999 (adjusted odds ratio, 0.76; 95% confidence interval, 0.65 to 0.89).

Conclusions.—Within a large community-based population, the incidence of myocardial infarction decreased significantly after 2000, and the incidence of ST-segment elevation myocardial infarction decreased markedly after 1999. Reductions in short-term case fatality rates for myocardial infarction appear to be driven, in part, by a decrease in the incidence of ST-segment elevation myocardial infarction and a lower rate of death after non—ST-segment elevation myocardial infarction.

▶ This article delivers good news and illustrates the huge benefits to be gained by the implementation of evidence-based strategies for primary and secondary prevention.[1] This study is based upon the Kaiser Permanente Northern California Integrated Healthcare Delivery System database, but another recent article using Medicare fee-4-service beneficiaries also reported similar recent declines in hospitalizations for acute myocardial infarction.[2] Management of risk factors is in itself a benchmark of quality, but the reduction in the incidence of myocardial infarction and in case mortality rates is a better reflection of not just prevention strategies but also the impact of developments in the treatment of myocardial infarction. What is particularly interesting about this article is that the population under study is ethnically diverse and includes both ST-segment elevation myocardial infarction (STEMI) and non-STEMI in addition to encompassing the time period before and after the advent of the use of the troponins in diagnosis.

The data show a substantial decrease in the incidence of myocardial infarction after 2000 and a dramatic decrease in the incidence of STEMI. It is interesting that the decline in overall incidence has been noted despite the advent of the troponins, which would result in an increased frequency of detecting small but less severe myocardial infarction. In fact, there was an increase in the incidence of non-STEMI after troponin institution, but this stabilized after 2004 and declined thereafter.

An interesting related article in the same issue of this journal[3] points out that all is not well in the United States. Unfortunately, there remains a large geographical variation in rates of death because of heart disease in this country. The risk among residents in Oklahoma, the lower Mississippi corridor, and Appalachia is double that among other Americans, suggesting a powerful role of socioeconomic factors. The latter is a complex entity that includes disparities in risk factor reduction, access to care, and new treatments, such as coronary revascularization, compliance, and the frequency of seeking health care. Interestingly, and somewhat at variance with other studies, the increase in obesity and hypertension was less among individuals living below the poverty line.[4]

The decline in rates of myocardial infarction is extremely gratifying but over time may be balanced by the aging of our population. In addition, there remains a concern that the epidemic of obesity and diabetes in concert with an increase in prevalence of hypertension in some subgroups could result in an increase in the future or at least a flattening in the decline of coronary heart disease mortality.[5] If we had a hold on what we have gained over the last 50 years, society will have to translate the evidence base to promote relevant public policy and the encouragement of healthier lifestyles at a community and national level.

B. J. Gersh, MB, ChB, DPhil, FRCP

References

1. McWilliams JM, Meara E, Zaslavsky AM, Ayanian JZ. Differences in control of cardiovascular disease and diabetes by race, ethnicity, and education: U.S. trends from 1999 to 2006 and effects of Medicare coverage. *Ann Intern Med.* 2009; 150:505-515.
2. Chen J, Normand SL, Wang Y, Drye EE, Schreiner GC, Krumholz HM. Recent declines in hospitalizations for acute myocardial infarction for Medicare fee-for-service beneficiaries: progress and continuing challenges. *Circulation.* 2010; 121:1322-1328.
3. Brown JR, O'Connor GT. Coronary heart disease and prevention in the United States. *N Engl J Med.* 2010;362:2150-2153.
4. *Health, United States, 2009; Special Feature on Medical Technology.* Hyattsville, ND: National Center for Health Statistics; 2010.
5. Ford ES, Capewell S. Coronary heart disease mortality among young adults in the U.S. from 1980 through 2020: concealed leveling of mortality rates. *J Am Coll Cardiol.* 2007;50:2128-2132.

Prospective Study of Obstructive Sleep Apnea and Incident Coronary Heart Disease and Heart Failure: The Sleep Heart Health Study
Gottlieb DJ, Yenokyan G, Newman AB, et al (VA Boston Healthcare System, MA; Johns Hopkins Univ, Baltimore, MD; Univ of Pittsburgh, PA; et al)
Circulation 122:352-360, 2010

Background.—Clinic-based observational studies in men have reported that obstructive sleep apnea is associated with an increased incidence of coronary heart disease. The objective of this study was to assess the relation of obstructive sleep apnea to incident coronary heart disease and heart failure in a general community sample of adult men and women.

Methods and Results.—A total of 1927 men and 2495 women ≥40 years of age and free of coronary heart disease and heart failure at the time of baseline polysomnography were followed up for a median of 8.7 years in this prospective longitudinal epidemiological study. After adjustment for multiple risk factors, obstructive sleep apnea was a significant predictor of incident coronary heart disease (myocardial infarction, revascularization procedure, or coronary heart disease death) only in men ≤70 years of age (adjusted hazard ratio 1.10 [95% confidence interval 1.00 to 1.21] per 10-unit increase in apnea-hypopnea index [AHI]) but not in older men or in women of any age. Among men 40 to 70 years old, those with AHI ≥30 were 68% more likely to develop coronary heart disease than those with AHI <5. Obstructive sleep apnea predicted incident heart failure in men but not in women (adjusted hazard ratio 1.13 [95% confidence interval 1.02 to 1.26] per 10-unit increase in AHI). Men with AHI ≥30 were 58% more likely to develop heart failure than those with AHI <5.

Conclusions.—Obstructive sleep apnea is associated with an increased risk of incident heart failure in community-dwelling middle-aged and older men; its association with incident coronary heart disease in this sample is equivocal.

▶ Sleep-disordered breathing is a major problem in the United States and presumably in other countries. It is estimated that approximately 40 million Americans have sleep disorders of whom approximately 25 million or more have sleep apnea (60%-80% of whom have not been diagnosed). The prevalence of sleep apnea as defined by an Apnea/Hypopnea Index of 5% or greater is estimated to be 9% in women and 24% in men.[1] The impact on mortality is unknown, but morbidity, including accidents, is considerable, as is the cost to society.

There are multiple pathophysiological interactions with sleep apnea that have potentially deleterious cardiovascular consequences. These have been the subject of several comprehensive reviews and include the direct contributions associated with apnea and arousal and their effect on intermediary mechanisms as well as the presence of comorbidities.[2] This makes it very difficult to tease out the effects of sleep apnea on cardiovascular morbidity and mortality as opposed to the impact of comorbid conditions. Moreover, clinical trials in symptomatic patients will be extremely difficult to perform given that we do have an effective form of therapy in continuous positive airway pressure.

The Wisconsin Sleep Heart Study has been an extremely valuable resource in the area of sleep-related research because it is a large prospective community study of patients aged 40 years or older followed for a median of 8.7 years. All patients were free of overt coronary heart disease and heart failure at the time of entry polysomnography. This analysis demonstrates a strong correlation with incident congestive heart failure after adjustment for traditional risk factors, but the association with incident coronary heart disease is equivocal. Other studies, however, do demonstrate a strong association between obstructive sleep apnea and cardiovascular conditions, such as atrial fibrillation and a temporal relationship to the timing of myocardial infarction and sudden cardiac death.[3]

Irrespective of whether cause or consequence has been unequivocally established, sleep apnea is not good for you. It should be diagnosed and treated, and elimination of the other underlying risk factors, that is, obesity, is a logical target.

B. J. Gersh, MB, ChB, DPhil, FRCP

References

1. Young T, Palta M, Dempsey J, Skatrud J, Weber S, Badr S. The occurrence of sleep-disordered breathing among middle-aged adults. *N Engl J Med.* 1993;328: 1230-1235.
2. Shamsuzzaman AS, Gersh BJ, Somers VK. Obstructive sleep apnea: implications for cardiac and vascular disease. *JAMA.* 2003;290:1906-1914.
3. Gami AS, Howard DE, Olson EJ, Somers VK. Day-night pattern of sudden death in obstructive sleep apnea. *N Engl J Med.* 2005;352:1206-1214.

Sociodemographic patterning of non-communicable disease risk factors in rural India: a cross sectional study

Kinra S, Bowen LJ, Lyngdoh T, et al (London School of Hygiene and Tropical Medicine, UK; Centre for Chronic Disease Control, New Delhi, India; et al)
BMJ 341:c4974, 2010

Objectives.—To investigate the sociodemographic patterning of non-communicable disease risk factors in rural India.

Design.—Cross sectional study.

Setting.—About 1600 villages from 18 states in India. Most were from four large states due to a convenience sampling strategy.

Participants.—1983 (31% women) people aged 20–69 years (49% response rate).

Main Outcome Measures.—Prevalence of tobacco use, alcohol use, low fruit and vegetable intake, low physical activity, obesity, central adiposity, hypertension, dyslipidaemia, diabetes, and underweight.

Results.—Prevalence of most risk factors increased with age. Tobacco and alcohol use, low intake of fruit and vegetables, and underweight were more common in lower socioeconomic positions; whereas obesity, dyslipidaemia, and diabetes (men only) and hypertension (women only) were more prevalent in higher socioeconomic positions. For example, 37% (95% CI 30% to 44%) of men smoked tobacco in the lowest socioeconomic group compared with 15% (12% to 17%) in the highest, while 35% (30% to 40%) of women in the highest socioeconomic group were obese compared with 13% (7% to 19%) in the lowest. The age standardised prevalence of some risk factors was: tobacco use (40% (37% to 42%) men, 4% (3% to 6%) women); low fruit and vegetable intake (69% (66% to 71%) men, 75% (71% to 78%) women); obesity (19% (17% to 21%) men, 28% (24% to 31%) women); dyslipidaemia (33% (31% to 36%) men, 35% (31% to 38%) women); hypertension (20% (18% to 22%) men, 22% (19% to 25%) women); diabetes (6% (5% to 7%) men, 5% (4% to 7%) women); and underweight (21% (19% to 23%) men, 18% (15% to 21%) women). Risk factors were generally more prevalent in south Indians compared with north Indians. For example, the prevalence of dyslipidaemia was 21% (17% to 33%) in north Indian men compared with 33% (29% to 38%) in south Indian men, while the prevalence of obesity was 13% (9% to 17%) in north Indian women compared with 24% (19% to 30%) in south Indian women.

Conclusions.—The prevalence of most risk factors was generally high across a range of sociodemographic groups in this sample of rural villagers in India; in particular, the prevalence of tobacco use in men and obesity in women was striking. However, given the limitations of the study (convenience sampling design and low response rate), cautious interpretation of the results is warranted. These data highlight the need for careful monitoring and control of non-communicable disease risk factors in rural areas of India (Fig 1).

▶ Much has been written about the deleterious impact of urbanization in the genesis of the epidemic of cardiovascular disease in the developing world. The migration from rural to urban areas is associated with multiple potentially detrimental lifestyle changes, that is, changes in diet leading to increased caloric, fat, and salt intake, smoking, exposure to second-hand smoke, lack of exercise, industrial air pollution, and powerful socioeconomic stressors.[1] The environment in these settings of rural to urban migration is indeed hostile from a cardiovascular standpoint. Compounding the problem are the economic constraints and lack of infrastructure in most low- and middle-income countries.

This particular study is of both interest and of concern in that it demonstrates a high prevalence of cardiovascular risk factors in rural India. Noncommunicable diseases are already the commonest cause of deaths in some parts of rural India.[2] Moreover, the epidemic of cardiovascular disease in India is rampant, and two-thirds of India's one billion population live in the rural areas. What is also interesting are the socioeconomic differences in risk factors even among a rural population in that those in the highest socioeconomic group had a higher prevalence of dyslipidemia, diabetes, hypertension, and obesity, but the prevalence of

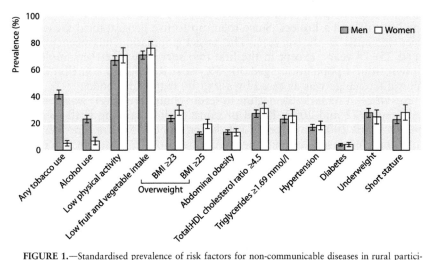

FIGURE 1.—Standardised prevalence of risk factors for non-communicable diseases in rural participants of the Indian Migration Study. (See table 3 for definitions of risk factors). (Reprinted from Kinra S, Bowen LJ, Lyngdoh T, et al. Sociodemographic patterning of non-communicable disease risk factors in rural India: a cross sectional study. *BMJ*. 2010;341:c4974, reproduced with permission from the BMJ Publishing Group Ltd.)

tobacco and alcohol use, low intake of fruits and vegetables, and being under-weight was less.

These data highlight a huge public health problem and the need to develop some systems of careful monitoring and, subsequently, control of noncommunicable disease risk factors in rural areas of India, but I am sure this applies to many other areas around the world.

B. J. Gersh, MB, ChB, DPhil, FRCP

References

1. Gersh BJ, Sliwa K, Mayosi BM, Yusuf S. Novel therapeutic concepts: the epidemic of cardiovascular disease in the developing world: global implications. *Eur Heart J.* 2010;31:642-648.
2. Joshi R, Cardona M, Iyengar S, et al. Chronic diseases now a leading cause of death in rural India—mortality data from the Andhra Pradesh Rural Health Initiative. *Int J Epidemiol.* 2006;35:1522-1529.

Thirty-five-year trends in cardiovascular risk factors in Finland
Vartiainen E, Laatikainen T, Peltonen M, et al (Natl Inst for Health and Welfare, Helsinki, Finland)
Int J Epidemiol 39:504-518, 2010

Background.—In the late 1960s, coronary heart disease (CHD) mortality among Finnish men was the highest in the world. From 1972 to 2007, risk factor surveys have been carried out to monitor risk factor trends and assess their contribution to declining mortality in Finland.

Methods.—The first risk factor survey was carried out in the North Karelia and Kuopio provinces in 1972 as the basis for the evaluation of the North Karelia Project. Since then, up to five geographical areas have been included in the surveys. The target population has been persons aged 25—74 years, except in the first two surveys where the sample was drawn from a population aged 30—59 years. Risk factor contribution on mortality change was assessed by a logistic regression model.

Results.—A remarkable decline in serum cholesterol levels was observed between 1972 and 2007. Blood pressure declined among both men and women until 2002 but levelled off during the last 5 years. Prevalence of smoking decreased among men. Among women, smoking increased throughout the survey years until 2002 but did not increase between 2002 and 2007. Body mass index (BMI) has continuously increased among men. Among women, BMI decreased until 1982, but since then an increasing trend has been observed. Risk factor changes explained a 60% reduction in coronary mortality in middle-aged men while the observed reduction was 80%.

Conclusions.—The 80% decline in coronary mortality in Finland mainly reflects a great reduction of the risk factor levels; these in turn have been associated with long-term comprehensive chronic disease prevention and health promotion interventions (Fig 1).

▶ One of the great success stories from the perspective of epidemiology and prevention has been the North Karelia Project in Finland, which was initiated in 1972.[1] At the end of the 1960s, Finnish men, particularly those in the North Karelia region had the highest cardiovascular mortality in the world. A key aspect of the program included a comprehensive survey of risk factors and health behaviors maintained at 5-year intervals in association with preventive medicine on a national scale. By 1995, North Karelia had experienced a staggering and gratifying 73% reduction in ischemic heart disease mortality, and between 53% and 76% of this was attributed to modification of risk factors.[2] From the mid-1980s onward, the new treatments for coronary artery disease including invasive procedures have become more common and can possibly explain most of the remaining decline in observed coronary heart disease (CHD) mortality. In other countries, although risk factor reduction is responsible for most of the decline in CHD mortality, the proportion attributed to therapies versus risk factor modification may vary.

This analysis of 35-year trends in risk factors showed that declines in population blood cholesterol levels continue, and this has been accompanied by substantial changes in the intake of saturated and polyunsaturated fats. In regard to blood pressures, the decline has leveled off, as is the case in the United States, and in this respect, obesity may play a major role. The prevalence of smoking decreased in men but not in women.

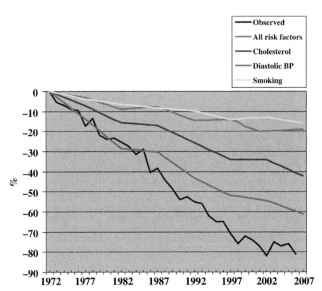

FIGURE 1.—Observed and predicted decline in CHD mortality in men. (Reprinted from Vartiainen E, Laatikainen T, Peltonen M, et al. Thirty-five-year trends in cardiovascular risk factors in Finland. *Int J Epidemiol.* 2010;39:504-518.)

In summary, the Finnish experience is a striking example of what can be achieved, and this has been witnessed in many other parts of the world. The concern is to what extent the epidemic of obesity and perhaps complacency could undermine these hard-won gains.

B. J. Gersh, MB, ChB, DPhil, FRCP

References

1. Puska P, Tuomilehto J, Salonen J, et al. *Community Control of Cardiovascular Diseases. The North Karelia Project. Evaluation of a Comprehensive Community Programme for Control of Cardiovascular Diseases in North Karelia, Finland 1972–1977*. Copenhagen, Denmark: WHO, Regional Office for Europe; 1981.
2. Ford E, Ajani U, Croft J, et al. Explaining the decrease in U.S. deaths from coronary disease, 1980–2000. *N Engl J Med.* 2007;356:2388-2398.

Trends in Incidence, Severity, and Outcome of Hospitalized Myocardial Infarction

Roger VL, Weston SA, Gerber Y, et al (Mayo Clinic, Rochester, MN; et al)
Circulation 121:863-869, 2010

Background.—In 2000, the definition of myocardial infarction (MI) changed to rely on troponin rather than creatine kinase (CK) and its MB fraction (CK-MB). The implications of this change on trends in MI incidence and outcome are not defined.

Methods and Results.—This was a community study of 2816 patients hospitalized with incident MI from 1987 to 2006 in Olmsted County, Minnesota, with prospective measurements of troponin and CK-MB from August 2000 forward. Outcomes were MI incidence, severity, and survival. After troponin was introduced, 278 (25%) of 1127 incident MIs met only troponin-based criteria. When cases meeting only troponin criteria were included, incidence did not change between 1987 and 2006. When restricted to cases defined by CK/CK-MB, the incidence of MI declined by 20%. The incidence of non–ST-segment elevation MI increased markedly by relying on troponin, whereas that of ST-segment elevation MI declined regardless of troponin. The age- and sex-adjusted hazard ratio of death within 30 days for an infarction occurring in 2006 (compared with 1987) was 0.44 (95% confidence interval, 0.30 to 0.64). Among 30-day survivors, survival did not improve, but causes of death shifted from cardiovascular to noncardiovascular ($P=0.001$). Trends in long-term survival among 30-day survivors were similar regardless of troponin.

Conclusions.—Over the last 2 decades, a substantial change in the epidemiology of MI occurred that was only partially mediated by the introduction of troponin. Non–ST-segment elevation MIs now constitute the majority of MIs. Although the 30-day case fatality improved markedly, long-term survival did not change, and the cause of death shifted from cardiovascular to noncardiovascular.

▶ A problem in evaluating temporal trends in the incidence and prognosis of myocardial infarction (MI) is that the definition of MI is evolving. The adoption of the more sensitive troponins in the revised definition of MI in 2000 raised the possibility that this would lead to the increase in the incidence of MI and a lower mortality because of the inclusion of patients with smaller infarcts.[1] A previous study from Olmsted County demonstrated a large increase in the number of infarctions related to the identification of cases by troponin-based criteria,[2] but this article adds to the literature by analyzing trends over time in both incidence and severity. The ability to look at patients included on the basis of the troponins and on traditional creatine kinase (CK) and its MB fraction (CK-MB) measurements allows for a comparison of like versus like.

The results of this study are encouraging in that the incidence of MI (based upon CK-MB criteria) has declined substantially (20%), although if one includes patients with smaller infarcts based upon troponins, the MI incidence has remained the same. A striking reduction in the incidence of ST-segment elevation MI is noted, as is the case in the much developed world in contrast to countries like India in which ST-segment elevation MI dominates.[3] There has also been a marked decline in 30-day mortality between 1987 and 2000, but late survival has not changed much because of a shift from cardiovascular disease to noncardiovascular deaths, which is perhaps not surprising in a much older population. Nonetheless, the reduction in 30-day mortality is encouraging and suggests that there could be an improvement in long-term survival in those patients with MI unaccompanied by other comorbidities.

Explanations for the decline in the severity of MI over time are speculative, but the increasing use of aspirin and beta blockers may play a role, in addition to the aging of the population, because older patients have a higher incidence of multivessel disease with collaterals and non-ST-segment elevation acute coronary syndromes . Another potential factor might be the increasing population of patients who have undergone coronary revascularization, and this perhaps predisposes to smaller infarcts at a later time. A limitation of this study is that patients with silent MIs who may comprise a third of all infarcts were not captured nor were sudden cardiac deaths. Nonetheless, a previous study from the same group has shown that there has been a decline in sudden cardiac death comparable with the decline of infarctions meeting CK-MB criteria, so the lack of sudden cardiac death capture would not affect the validity of the results in this study.[4]

B. J. Gersh, MB, ChB, DPhil, FRCP

References

1. Alpert JS, Thygesen K, Antman E, Bassand JP. Myocardial infarction redefined—a consensus document of The Joint European Society of Cardiology/American College of Cardiology Committee for the redefinition of myocardial infarction. *J Am Coll Cardiol.* 2000;36:959-969.
2. Roger VL, Killian JM, Weston SA, et al. Redefinition of myocardial infarction: prospective evaluation in the community. *Circulation.* 2006;114:790-797.

3. Xavier D, Bais P, Devereaux PJ, et al. Treatment and outcomes of acute coronary syndromes in India (CREATE): a prospective analysis of registry data. *Lancet.* 2008;371:1435-1442.
4. Goraya TY, Jacobsen SJ, Kottke TE, Frye RL, Weston SA, Roger VL. Coronary heart disease death and sudden cardiac death: a 20-year population-based study. *Am J Epidemiol.* 2003;157:763-770.

Miscellaneous

HDL cholesterol and residual risk of first cardiovascular events after treatment with potent statin therapy: an analysis from the JUPITER trial

Ridker PM, for the JUPITER Trial Study Group (Harvard Med School, Boston, MA; et al)
Lancet 376:333-339, 2010

Background.—HDL-cholesterol concentrations are inversely associated with occurrence of cardiovascular events. We addressed, using the JUPITER trial cohort, whether this association remains when LDL-cholesterol concentrations are reduced to the very low ranges with high-dose statin treatment.

Methods.—Participants in the randomised placebo-controlled JUPITER trial were adults without diabetes or previous cardiovascular disease, and had baseline concentrations of LDL cholesterol of less than 3·37 mmol/L and high-sensitivity C-reactive protein of 2 mg/L or more. Participants were randomly allocated by a computer-generated sequence to receive rosu-vastatin 20 mg per day or placebo, with participants and adjudicators masked to treatment assignment. In the present analysis, we divided the participants into quartiles of HDL-cholesterol or apolipoprotein A1 and sought evidence of association between these quartiles and the JUPITER primary endpoint of first non-fatal myocardial infarction or stroke, hospitalisation for unstable angina, arterial revascularisation, or cardiovascular death. This trial is registered with ClinicalTrials.gov, number NCT00239681.

Findings.—For 17 802 patients in the JUPITER trial, rosuvastatin 20 mg per day reduced the incidence of the primary endpoint by 44% (p<0·0001). In 8901 (50%) patients given placebo (who had a median on-treatment LDL-cholesterol concentration of 2·80 mmol/L [IQR 2·43–3·24]), HDL-cholesterol concentrations were inversely related to vascular risk both at baseline (top quartile *vs* bottom quartile hazard ratio [HR] 0·54, 95% CI 0·35–0·83, p=0·0039) and on-treatment (0·55, 0·35–0·87, p=0·0047). By contrast, among the 8900 (50%) patients given rosuvastatin 20 mg (who had a median on-treatment LDL-cholesterol concentration of 1·42 mmol/L [IQR 1·14–1·86]), no significant relationships were noted between quartiles of HDL-cholesterol concentration and vascular risk either at baseline (1·12, 0·62–2·03, p=0·82) or on-treatment (1·03, 0·57–1·87, p=0·97). Our analyses for apolipoprotein A1 showed an equivalent strong relation to frequency of primary outcomes in the placebo group but little association in the rosuvastatin group.

Interpretation.—Although measurement of HDL-cholesterol concentration is useful as part of initial cardiovascular risk assessment, HDL-cholesterol concentrations are not predictive of residual vascular risk among patients treated with potent statin therapy who attain very low concentrations of LDL cholesterol.

▶ Previous randomized trials of statin therapy have consistently reported large reductions in myocardial infarction, stroke, and vascular death in regard to both primary and secondary prevention. Nonetheless, significant vascular risk persists, and a legitimate question is whether this is related to low high-density lipoprotein (HDL) levels, which in themselves are a well-established baseline risk factor.

This intriguing substudy from the Justification for the Use of Statins in Primary Prevention: An Intervention Trial Evaluating Rosuvastatin (JUPITER) trial would suggest that the predictive value of HDL cholesterol is lost in patients given rosuvastatin who attain very low levels of low-density lipoprotein (LDL) cholesterol (in the range of 55 mg/dL). In contrast, another study demonstrated that the predictive value of HDL cholesterol was preserved even with LDL-cholesterol levels of less than 70 mg/dL.[1] Similarly, in the Framingham Offspring Study, the lower the pretreatment cholesterol, the greater the effect of increasing HDL cholesterol.[2] Moreover, in another study, HDL cholesterol remained a predictor of 1-year risk even when the LDL cholesterol was in the range of 62 mg/dL.[3]

An accompanying editorial speculates on why HDL-cholesterol concentrations did not predict cardiovascular risk in patients with low cardiovascular risk to begin with and who were then treated to very low concentrations of LDL cholesterol.[4] They do raise the question whether at very low LDL-cholesterol concentrations, other lipid measures, such as the apolipoprotein B to A1 ratio, would be of more benefit.

We also need to remember that this study does not mean that increasing HDL cholesterol levels in patients with low LDL levels will not be beneficial. This will require specifically designed randomized controlled trials. It should also be emphasized that the JUPITER trial was a trial of primary prevention in patients who did not have diabetes to begin with, and the study does not address the question of raising HDL cholesterol levels as part of a secondary prevention strategy. The findings should also not detract from the fact that raising HDL-cholesterol levels remains a major treatment strategy for the reduction of cardiovascular risks for most patients with elevated LDL-cholesterol concentrations, among whom many will not reach the concentrations obtained in this study. This remains a very interesting area, particularly given the ongoing development of HDL-elevating drugs that have the potential, but as yet unproven, to revolutionize the management of cardiovascular disease.[5]

B. J. Gersh, MB, ChB, DPhil, FRCP

References

1. Barter P, Gotto AM, LaRosa JC, et al. HDL cholesterol, very low levels of LDL cholesterol, and cardiovascular events. *N Engl J Med.* 2007;357:1301-1310.

2. Grover SA, Kaouache M, Joseph L, Barter P, Davignon J. Evaluating the incremental benefits of raising high-density lipoprotein cholesterol levels during lipid therapy after adjustment for the reductions in other blood lipid levels. *Arch Intern Med.* 2009;169:1775-1780.

3. deGoma EM, Leeper NJ, Heidenreich PA. Clinical significance of high-density lipoprotein cholesterol in patients with low low-density lipoprotein cholesterol. *J Am Coll Cardiol.* 2008;51:49-55.

4. Hausenloy DJ, Opie L, Yellon DM. Disassociating HDL cholesterol from cardiovascular risk. *Lancet.* 2010;376:305-306.

5. Natarajan P, Ray KK, Cannon CP. High-density lipoprotein in coronary heart disease: current and future therapies. *J Am Coll Cardiol.* 2010;55:1283-1299.

Projected Effect of Dietary Salt Reductions on Future Cardiovascular Disease

Bibbins-Domingo K, Chertow GM, Coxson PG, et al (Univ of California, San Francisco (UCSF); et al)
N Engl J Med 362:590-599, 2010

Background.—The U.S. diet is high in salt, with the majority coming from processed foods. Reducing dietary salt is a potentially important target for the improvement of public health.

Methods.—We used the Coronary Heart Disease (CHD) Policy Model to quantify the benefits of potentially achievable, population-wide reductions in dietary salt of up to 3 g per day (1200 mg of sodium per day). We estimated the rates and costs of cardiovascular disease in subgroups defined by age, sex, and race; compared the effects of salt reduction with those of other interventions intended to reduce the risk of cardiovascular disease; and determined the cost-effectiveness of salt reduction as compared with the treatment of hypertension with medications.

Results.—Reducing dietary salt by 3 g per day is projected to reduce the annual number of new cases of CHD by 60,000 to 120,000, stroke by 32,000 to 66,000, and myocardial infarction by 54,000 to 99,000 and to reduce the annual number of deaths from any cause by 44,000 to 92,000. All segments of the population would benefit, with blacks benefiting proportionately more, women benefiting particularly from stroke reduction, older adults from reductions in CHD events, and younger adults from lower mortality rates. The cardiovascular benefits of reduced salt intake are on par with the benefits of population-wide reductions in tobacco use, obesity, and cholesterol levels. A regulatory intervention designed to achieve a reduction in salt intake of 3 g per day would save 194,000 to 392,000 quality-adjusted life-years and $10 billion to $24 billion in health care costs annually. Such an intervention would be cost-saving even if only a modest reduction of 1 g per day were achieved gradually between 2010 and 2019 and would be more cost-effective than using medications to lower blood pressure in all persons with hypertension.

Conclusions.—Modest reductions in dietary salt could substantially reduce cardiovascular events and medical costs and should be a public health target.

▶ This complex study has huge potential ramifications for public health action by providing compelling evidence that reducing population-wide salt intake would markedly reduce the development of cardiovascular disease. The methodology is complicated and involves applying previously published data to a computer-simulation model. This model also involves a number of assumptions, namely that salt reduction lowers blood pressure and that this in turn reduces the incidence of stroke and cardiovascular disease. This is certainly a reasonable assumption, however, given much of the epidemiologic data and a few trials supporting this linkage.

The US diet is high in salt, and intake is much higher than the recommended target of 3.7 to 5.8 g of salt per day for individuals over the age of 40 years, those with hypertension, and in blacks.[1] The model suggests that a national effort to reduce salt intake by 3 g per day could translate into a massive impact upon the reduction of coronary heart disease, stroke, myocardial infarction, and all-cause mortality. These dramatic effects arising from an inexpensive intervention could be as beneficial as programs aimed at weight reduction, smoking cessation, and lipid lowering.

An accompanying editorial points out that even a reduction of 3 g per day would not achieve the desired targets for daily salt intake in many adults,[2] but the evidence to support a nationwide effort in the United States to reduce salt intake is nonetheless extremely strong. The same editorial, however, points out the magnitude of the problems involved in reducing salt intake. Given that the bulk of salt intake comes from processed foods, an individual approach would have relatively little impact. The level of salt in prepared and processed foods is excessively high, and this can only be changed by a national public health effort, which could be a relatively inexpensive but highly effective form of health care reform.

B. J. Gersh, MB, ChB, DPhil, FRCP

References

1. Centers for Disease Control and Prevention (CDC). Application of lower sodium intake recommendations to adults—United States, 1999–2006. *MMWR Morb Mortal Wkly Rep.* 2009;58:281-283.
2. Appel LJ, Anderson CAM. Compelling evidence for public health action to reduce salt intake. *N Engl J Med.* 2010;362:650-652.

Myocardial Infarction and Risk of Suicide: A Population-Based Case-Control Study
Larsen KK, Agerbo E, Christensen B, et al (Aarhus Univ, Denmark; et al)
Circulation 122:2388-2393, 2010

Background.—Myocardial infarction (MI) is associated with an increased risk of anxiety, depression, low quality of life, and all-cause mortality. Whether MI is associated with an increased risk of suicide is unknown. We examined the association between MI and suicide.

Methods and Results.—We conducted a population-based case-control study by retrieving data from 5 nationwide longitudinal registers in Denmark. As cases, we selected all persons aged 40 to 89 years who died by suicide from 1981 to 2006. As controls, we randomly selected up to 10 persons per case matched by sex, day of birth, and calendar time. We identified 19 857 persons who committed suicide and 190 058 controls. MI was associated with a marked increased risk of suicide. The risk of suicide was highest during the first month after discharge for MI for patients with no history of psychiatric illness (adjusted rate ratio, 3.25; 95% confidence interval, 1.61 to 6.56) and for patients with a history of psychiatric illness (adjusted rate ratio, 64.05; 95% confidence interval, 13.36 to 307.06) compared with those with no history of MI or psychiatric illness. However, the risk remained high for at least 5 years after MI.

Conclusions.—MI is followed by an increased risk of suicide for persons with and without psychiatric illness. Our results suggest the importance of screening patients with MI for depression and suicidal ideation.

▶ This is an interesting population-based, case-controlled study of myocardial infarction (MI) and the risk of suicide. Previous studies have found a broad range of chronic physical conditions, including MI/stroke, to be associated with increased suicidal attempts, regardless of whether persons have associated mental disorders or not.[1] A more recent large study demonstrated an association between the incidence of death from suicide and death from ischemic heart disease.[2]

This large study based upon data from 5 nationwide registries in Denmark is a case-controlled study of suicide patients compared with controls. MI was clearly associated with a marked increased risk of suicide, particularly during the first month after discharge and both in patients with and without a known history of psychiatric illness. Moreover, the risk remained high for at least 5 years after the onset of MI.

The clinical message is unequivocal. We need to be aware of the coexistence of depression and to be sure that at the time of discharge, patients and their families have the knowledge and the ability to seek further counseling if necessary.

On the other hand, there is not much evidence to show that treating depression can also reduce cardiovascular risk, although this is an attractive concept from a theoretical perspective.[3] Nonetheless, an accompanying editorial points out that there are exploratory analyses that suggest that pharmacological and behavioral interventions may have the potential to reduce cardiovascular morbidity and mortality.[4]

In summary, this recent report provides an additional impetus to develop randomized controlled trials testing the effects of interventions to reduce depression and other indicators of stress in post-MI patients.

B. J. Gersh, MB, ChB, DPhil, FRCP

References

1. Scott KM, Hwang I, Chiu WT, et al. Chronic physical conditions and their association with first onset of suicidal behavior in the world mental health surveys. *Psychosom Med.* 2010;72:712-719.
2. Placido A, Sposito AC. Association between suicide and cardiovascular disease: time series of 27 years. *Int J Cardiol.* 2009;135:261-262.
3. Berkman LF, Bluminthal J, Burg M, et al. Effects of treating depression and low perceived social support on clinical events after myocardial infarction: the Enhancing Recovery in Coronary Heart Disease Patients (ENRICHD) Randomized Trial. *JAMA.* 2003;289:3106-3116.
4. Williams RB. Myocardial infarction and risk of suicide: another reason to develop and test ways to reduce distress in postmyocardial-infarction patients? *Circulation.* 2010;122:2356-2358.

Relationship Between Cardiac Rehabilitation and Long-Term Risks of Death and Myocardial Infarction Among Elderly Medicare Beneficiaries

Hammill BG, Curtis LH, Schulman KA, et al (Duke Clinical Res Inst, Durham, NC)
Circulation 121:63-70, 2010

Background.—For patients with coronary heart disease, exercise-based cardiac rehabilitation improves survival rate and has beneficial effects on risk factors for coronary artery disease. The relationship between the number of sessions attended and long-term outcomes is unknown.

Methods and Results.—In a national 5% sample of Medicare beneficiaries, we identified 30 161 elderly patients who attended at least 1 cardiac rehabilitation session between January 1, 2000, and December 31, 2005. We used a Cox proportional hazards model to estimate the relationship between the number of sessions attended and death and myocardial infarction (MI) at 4 years. The cumulative number of sessions was a time-dependent covariate. After adjustment for demographic characteristics, comorbid conditions, and subsequent hospitalization, patients who attended 36 sessions had a 14% lower risk of death (hazard ratio [HR], 0.86; 95% confidence interval [CI], 0.77 to 0.97) and a 12% lower risk of MI (HR, 0.88; 95% CI, 0.83 to 0.93) than those who attended 24 sessions; a 22% lower risk of death (HR, 0.78; 95% CI, 0.71 to 0.87) and a 23% lower risk of MI (HR, 0.77; 95% CI, 0.69 to 0.87) than those who attended 12 sessions; and a 47% lower risk of death (HR, 0.53; 95% CI, 0.48 to 0.59) and a 31% lower risk of MI (HR, 0.69; 95% CI, 0.58 to 0.81) than those who attended 1 session.

Conclusions.—Among Medicare beneficiaries, a strong dose—response relationship existed between the number of cardiac rehabilitation sessions and long-term outcomes. Attending all 36 sessions reimbursed by Medicare was associated with lower risks of death and MI at 4 years compared with attending fewer sessions.

▶ It is well accepted that exercise-based cardiac rehabilitation has an important role to play in the management of patients with chronic stable angina, recent myocardial infarction, or prior bypass surgery among other conditions. Several trials and a meta-analysis have suggested that participation in a cardiac rehabilitation program improves survival and favorably modifies risk factors.[1] To what extent it is the exercise that is efficacious as opposed to the entire milieu of rehabilitation is uncertain, and there is also an obvious bias in favor of individuals who have both the time and the commitment to exercise and enter into a rehabilitation program.

One question addressed by this study is whether the optimal dose of cardiac rehabilitation and whether attending more cardiac rehabilitation sessions is better than attending fewer sessions and whether there is a specific threshold. This study on a national 5% sample of Medicare beneficiaries identified more than 30 000 elderly patients who had attended at least 1 cardiac rehabilitation session between 2000 and 2005. The qualifying indication for cardiac rehabilitation was coronary bypass surgery in the majority, recent myocardial infarction in 20.5%, stable angina in 14.9%, and unknown in 3.9%. Multivariant analysis using the number of sessions as a time-dependent covariant demonstrated that patients who attended all 36 sessions had a 14% lower incidence of death than those who attended 24 sessions, and there was also a lower risk of myocardial infarction. In summary, this study demonstrates at least on the surface a strong dose-response relationship and justifies the ongoing policy of Medicare reimbursement for cardiac rehabilitation.

An accompanying editorial appropriately emphasizes the potential for confounders in that sicker or severely disadvantaged patients were more likely to drop out of rehabilitation in addition to being at higher risk of events.[2] The conclusion is that the issue of causality remains uncertain and has not been proven by this study. This is certainly a subject for further investigation and perhaps a randomized trial. Nonetheless, for the present, cardiovascular rehabilitation should always be considered in the overall context of returning patients to a fully functional lifestyle, even though there is a need for more evidence-based medicine in this area.

B. J. Gersh, MB, ChB, DPhil, FRCP

References

1. Taylor RS, Brown A, Ebrahim S, et al. Exercise-based rehabilitation for patients with coronary heart disease: systematic review and meta-analysis of randomized controlled trials. *Am J Med.* 2004;116:682-692.
2. Weintraub WS. Do more cardiac rehabilitation visits reduce events compared with fewer visits? *Circulation.* 2010;121:8-9.

Enhanced External Counterpulsation Improves Peripheral Artery Flow-Mediated Dilation in Patients With Chronic Angina: A Randomized sham-Controlled Study
Braith RW, Conti CR, Nichols WW, et al (Univ of Florida, Gainesville; et al)
Circulation 122:1612-1620, 2010

Background.—Mechanisms responsible for anti-ischemic benefits of enhanced external counterpulsation (EECP) remain unknown. This was the first randomized sham-controlled study to investigate the extracardiac effects of EECP on peripheral artery flow-mediated dilation.

Methods and Results.—Forty-two symptomatic patients with coronary artery disease were randomized (2:1 ratio) to thirty-five 1-hour sessions of either EECP (n=28) or sham EECP (n=14). Flow-mediated dilation of the brachial and femoral arteries was performed with the use of ultrasound. Plasma levels of nitrate and nitrite, 6-keto-prostaglandin $F_{1\alpha}$, endothelin-1, asymmetrical dimethylarginine, tumor necrosis factor-α, monocyte chemo-attractant protein-1, soluble vascular cell adhesion molecule, high-sensitivity C-reactive protein, and 8-isoprostane were measured. EECP increased brachial (+51% versus +2%) and femoral (+30% versus +3%) artery flow-mediated dilation, the nitric oxide turnover/production markers nitrate and nitrite (+36% versus +2%), and 6-keto-prostaglandin $F_{1\alpha}$ (+71% versus +1%), whereas it decreased endothelin-1 (−25% versus +5%) and the nitric oxide synthase inhibitor asymmetrical dimethylarginine (−28% versus +0.2%) in treatment versus sham groups, respectively (all $P<0.05$). EECP decreased the proinflammatory cytokines tumor necrosis factor-α (−16% versus +12%), monocyte chemoattractant protein-1 (−13% versus +0.2%), soluble vascular cell adhesion molecule-1 (−6% versus +1%), high-sensitivity C-reactive protein (−32% versus +5%), and the lipid peroxidation marker 8-isoprostane (−21% versus +1.3%) in treat-ment versus sham groups, respectively (all $P<0.05$). EECP reduced angina classification (−62% versus 0%; $P<0.001$) in treatment versus sham groups, respectively.

Conclusions.—Our findings provide novel mechanistic evidence that EECP has a beneficial effect on peripheral artery flow-mediated dilation and endothelial-derived vasoactive agents in patients with symptomatic coronary artery disease.

▶ This is a very interesting proof-of-concept study because there is such a dearth of mechanistic data in regard to the relief of angina and functional improvement after enhanced external counterpulsation (EECP). Why it works has been a matter of some speculation. Skeptics have suggested that this was purely a placebo effect and to some extent a function of the close care that patients receive at the time of EECP sessions, although the magnitude of the benefit and frequency of responders would suggest that this is not the case. Another postulate is that EECP promotes coronary angiogenesis, but the data are just not there to support that hypothesis.[1]

In this randomized and blinded trial of 42 symptomatic patients with coro-nary artery disease, the authors provide novel mechanistic evidence using multiple biomarkers that EECP has a beneficial effect on peripheral artery flow-mediated dilation and endothelial-derived vasoactive agents. There was also a robust effect on endothelial function in the brachial artery that may be mediated by increased shear stress resulting in an increased production of nitric oxide and improvement in endothelial function.

These findings are particularly relevant from a clinical standpoint. The popu-lation of patients with symptomatic coronary artery disease who are not amenable to revascularization is large. Moreover, new antianginal therapies have been slow in coming and ranolazine is the only new antianginal drug that has been released in the United States in the last 2 decades. The attraction of EECP is that it is noninvasive and can be used in patients who are nonrevascularizable. This study provides a potential explanation for the mechanisms of benefit. Additional large studies are needed, but it would certainly be satisfying to know why this technique works and not just that it seems to work.

B. J. Gersh, MB, ChB, DPhil, FRCP

Reference

1. Michaels AD, Raisinghani A, Soran O, et al. The effects of enhanced external counterpulsation on myocardial perfusion in patients with stable angina: a multi-center radionuclide study. *Am Heart J.* 2005;150:1066-1073.

Low Diagnostic Yield of Elective Coronary Angiography
Patel MR, Peterson ED, Dai D, et al (Duke Univ, Durham, NC; et al)
N Engl J Med 362:886-895, 2010

Background.—Guidelines for triaging patients for cardiac catheterization recommend a risk assessment and noninvasive testing. We determined patterns of noninvasive testing and the diagnostic yield of catheterization among patients with suspected coronary artery disease in a contemporary national sample.

Methods.—From January 2004 through April 2008, at 663 hospitals in the American College of Cardiology National Cardiovascular Data Registry, we identified patients without known coronary artery disease who were undergoing elective catheterization. The patients' demographic characteristics, risk factors, and symptoms and the results of noninvasive testing were correlated with the presence of obstructive coronary artery disease, which was defined as stenosis of 50% or more of the diameter of the left main coronary artery or stenosis of 70% or more of the diameter of a major epicardial vessel.

Results.—A total of 398,978 patients were included in the study. The median age was 61 years; 52.7% of the patients were men, 26.0% had diabetes, and 69.6% had hypertension. Noninvasive testing was performed in 83.9% of the patients. At catheterization, 149,739 patients (37.6%) had obstructive coronary artery disease. No coronary artery disease (defined as <20% stenosis in all vessels) was reported in 39.2% of the patients. Independent predictors of obstructive coronary artery disease included male sex (odds ratio, 2.70; 95% confidence interval [CI], 2.64 to 2.76), older age (odds ratio per 5-year increment, 1.29; 95% CI, 1.28 to 1.30), presence of insulin-dependent diabetes (odds ratio, 2.14; 95% CI, 2.07 to 2.21), and presence of dyslipidemia (odds ratio, 1.62; 95% CI, 1.57 to 1.67). Patients with a positive result on a noninvasive test were moderately more likely to have obstructive coronary artery disease than those who did not undergo any testing (41.0% vs. 35.0%; P<0.001; adjusted odds ratio, 1.28; 95% CI, 1.19 to 1.37).

Conclusions.—In this study, slightly more than one third of patients without known disease who underwent elective cardiac catheterization had obstructive coronary artery disease. Better strategies for risk stratification are needed to inform decisions and to increase the diagnostic yield of cardiac catheterization in routine clinical practice.

▶ I was somewhat surprised by the results of this study in regard to the low rate of obstructive coronary artery disease as demonstrated by coronary angiography. If every coronary angiogram performed in an institution demonstrated obstructive coronary artery disease, this would indicate underutilization of angiography, and to my mind a negative or normal angiographic rate of approximately 20% would appear to be appropriate, but the 37.6% in this study seems to be quite high.

To understand this analysis, one really needs to go back to Bayesian principles, which require an appreciation of the baseline characteristics of the patients who were entered into the analysis. Firstly, patients with known coronary artery disease were excluded as were patients undergoing catheterization as an emergency or as part of the evaluation for another disease or procedure, for example, valve surgery, transplantation, etc. What should also be emphasized is that nonobstructive disease does not mean a normal coronary artery.

Patients with the traditional risk factors, including older age, diabetes, and dyslipidemia, were more likely to have obstructive coronary disease. Surprisingly, however, the presence of a previous positive result on noninvasive testing only moderately increased the likelihood of obstructive disease at angiography. It may be that many of these patients had atypical chest pain and possibly false positive stress tests, and this is what drove the performance of a coronary angiogram.

One limitation of this study is the inability to analyze the actual results of the noninvasive test in addition to an absence of any information and what specific test was used. If a high proportion of tests were equivocal or weakly positive, this might account for a low rate of obstructive disease, particularly, in patients with atypical symptoms or an absence of angina pectoris, and this again is simply consistent with Bayesian principles.[1]

Nonetheless, this study does suggest that a greater focus should be placed on the 30% of patients who had no symptoms among whom rates of obstructive coronary artery disease were really low. Because the overutilization of angiography could contribute to the overutilization of revascularization, one would need to know much more about what drove the decision to perform noninvasive testing in angiography in these asymptomatic patients without angina. These are essential steps to be taken in understanding and controlling health care costs.

B. J. Gersh, MB, ChB, DPhil, FRCP

Reference

1. Diamond GA, Forrester JS. Analysis of probability as an aid in the clinical diagnosis of coronary-artery disease. *N Engl J Med.* 1979;300:1350-1358.

Meta-analysis: Effects of Percutaneous Coronary Intervention Versus Medical Therapy on Angina Relief

Wijeysundera HC, Nallamothu BK, Krumholz HM, et al (Univ of Toronto, Ontario, Canada; Ann Arbor Veterans Affairs Med Ctr, MI; Yale Univ School of Medicine, New Haven, CT)
Ann Intern Med 152:370-379, 2010

Background.—Several meta-analyses have evaluated the efficacy of percutaneous coronary intervention (PCI) compared with medical therapy, but none has focused on angina relief.

Purpose.—To summarize the evidence on the degree of angina relief from PCI compared with medical therapy in patients with stable coronary artery disease.

Data Sources.—The Cochrane Library (1993 to June 2009), EMBASE (1980 to June 2009), and MEDLINE (1950 to June 2009), with no language restrictions.

Study Selection.—Two independent reviewers screened citations to identify randomized, controlled trials of PCI versus medical therapy in patients with stable coronary artery disease.

Data Extraction.—Two independent reviewers abstracted data on patient characteristics, study conduct, and outcomes. A random-effects model was used to combine data on freedom from angina and to perform stratified analyses based on duration of follow-up, inclusion of patients with recent myocardial infarction, coronary stent utilization, recruitment period, and utilization of evidence-based medications.

Data Synthesis.—A total of 14 trials, enrolling 7818 patients, met the inclusion criteria. Although PCI was associated with an overall benefit on angina relief (odds ratio, 1.69 [95% CI, 1.24 to 2.30]), important heterogeneity across trials was observed. The incremental benefit of PCI observed in older trials (odds ratio, 3.38 [CI, 1.89 to 6.04]) was substantially less and possibly absent in recent trials (odds ratio, 1.13 [CI, 0.76 to 1.68]). An inverse relationship between use of evidence-based therapies and the incremental benefit of PCI was observed.

Limitations.—Information about the long-term use of medication was incomplete in most trials. Few trials used drug-eluting stents. Meta-regression analyses used aggregated study-level data from few trials.

Conclusion.—Percutaneous coronary intervention was associated with greater freedom from angina compared with medical therapy, but this benefit was largely attenuated in contemporary studies. This observation may be related to greater use of evidence-based medications in contemporary trials.

▶ The benefits of percutaneous coronary intervention (PCI) versus medical therapy on death and myocardial infarction (MI) in patients with chronic stable angina have been the subject of over 15 years of randomized controlled trials involving approximately 10 000 patients. These have generated vigorous and sometimes fierce controversy, but the conclusions from the largest trials and meta-analyses are that PCI is not associated with any reduction in death/MI but that in general, it is accepted that PCI offers greater relief of angina, at least in the short term.[1] The implications are quite far reaching in that the indication for PCI in chronic stable angina is for the relief of angina after a trial of medical therapy, and this is reflected in the guidelines.

This meta-analysis is novel and summarizes the evidence for the degree of angina relief in the trials of patients with stable coronary disease, with and without the inclusion of patients with recent MI. Overall, 14 trials involving 7818 patients demonstrated that PCI was associated with a greater relief of angina in comparison to medical therapy alone (odds ratio 1.69, 95% confidence interval is 1.24-2.3), but there was considerable heterogeneity among the trials. Of interest, the benefit was not significant in trials with greater than 5 years follow-up, possibly because of crossover but also because of progression of disease in nontarget lesions and vessels.[2] Another interesting finding is that the benefits were greatest in the older trials and became substantially less and possibly absent in recent trials. This is likely the impact of evidence-based therapies and aggressive secondary prevention.

A limitation is the lack of drug-eluting stent use in these trials plus the inability to assess the degree of functional improvement as opposed to the end point of complete freedom from angina. Nonetheless, this is the most extensive review of the subject and supports guideline recommendations to optimize medical therapy before referral for PCI. Is this what is been widely carried out in clinical practice? There is certainly growing evidence that this is not the case.[3]

B. J. Gersh, MB, ChB, DPhil, FRCP

References

1. Boden WE, O'Rourke RA, Teo KK, et al. COURAGE Trial Research Group. Optimal medical therapy with or without PCI for stable coronary disease. *N Engl J Med.* 2007;356:1503-1516.
2. Cutlip DE, Chhabra AG, Baim DS, et al. Beyond restenosis: five-year clinical outcomes from second-generation coronary stent trials. *Circulation.* 2004;110: 1226-1230.
3. Holmes DR Jr, Gersh BJ, Whitlow P, King SB III, Dove JT. Percutaneous coronary intervention for chronic stable angina: a reassessment. *JACC Cardiovasc Interv.* 2008;1:34-43.

Effect of Sibutramine on Cardiovascular Outcomes in Overweight and Obese Subjects

James WPT, for the SCOUT Investigators (London School of Hygiene and Tropical Medicine, UK; et al)

N Engl J Med 363:905-917, 2010

Background.—The long-term effects of sibutramine treatment on the rates of cardiovascular events and cardiovascular death among subjects at high cardiovascular risk have not been established.

Methods.—We enrolled in our study 10,744 overweight or obese subjects, 55 years of age or older, with preexisting cardiovascular disease, type 2 diabetes mellitus, or both to assess the cardiovascular consequences of weight management with and without sibutramine in subjects at high risk for cardiovascular events. All the subjects received sibutramine in addition to participating in a weight-management program during a 6-week, single-blind, lead-in period, after which 9804 subjects underwent random assignment in a double-blind fashion to sibutramine (4906 subjects) or placebo (4898 subjects). The primary end point was the time from randomization to the first occurrence of a primary outcome event (nonfatal myocardial infarction, nonfatal stroke, resuscitation after cardiac arrest, or cardiovascular death).

Results.—The mean duration of treatment was 3.4 years. The mean weight loss during the lead-in period was 2.6 kg; after randomization, the subjects in the sibutramine group achieved and maintained further weight reduction (mean, 1.7 kg). The mean blood pressure decreased in both groups, with greater reductions in the placebo group than in the sibutramine group (mean difference, 1.2/1.4 mm Hg). The risk of a primary outcome event was 11.4% in the sibutramine group as compared with 10.0% in the placebo group (hazard ratio, 1.16; 95% confidence interval [CI], 1.03 to 1.31; P = 0.02). The rates of nonfatal myocardial infarction and nonfatal stroke were 4.1% and 2.6% in the sibutramine group and 3.2% and 1.9% in the placebo group, respectively (hazard ratio for nonfatal myocardial infarction, 1.28; 95% CI, 1.04 to 1.57; P = 0.02; hazard ratio for nonfatal stroke, 1.36; 95% CI, 1.04 to 1.77; P = 0.03). The rates of cardiovascular death and death from any cause were not increased.

Conclusions.—Subjects with preexisting cardiovascular conditions who were receiving long-term sibutramine treatment had an increased risk of nonfatal myocardial infarction and nonfatal stroke but not of cardiovascular death or death from any cause. (Funded by Abbott; ClinicalTrials. gov number, NCT00234832.)

▶ Given the magnitude of the epidemic of obesity and the link to diabetes and premature death, this remains an escalating public health concern.[1] Although it may be easy to identify the problem, the establishment of preventive measures and the treatment of obesity are difficult. More than 80% of well-motivated individuals are unable to achieve weight loss with dietary and lifestyle modifications alone.[2] The problem is, however, that new diet pills, although needed, have to date been seriously flawed.

Sibutramine is a norepinephrine and serotonin uptake inhibitor that has previously been approved for weight management for those who are unable to lose weight by diet and exercise alone. The drug apparently induces satiety, resulting in a reduction in caloric intake and an increase in energy expenditure.[3] Because the drug, however, has sympathomimetic effects, it increased heart rate and blood pressure, and for these reasons sibutramine has been excluded for use in patients with a history of cardiovascular disease. Moreover, the recommended duration of treatment is no more than 1 to 2 years, even in patients who lose weight.

The Sibutramine Cardiovascular Outcomes trial evaluated the long-term effects of sibutramine in patients with either a history of cardiovascular disease or those considered at high risk on the basis of diabetes plus the presence of one or more other risk factors. The results after a mean of 3.5 years follow-up are quite definitive and a statistically significant increase in nonfatal myocardial infarction and nonfatal stroke was noted, despite evidence of modest at best weight loss. The investigators have concluded that sibutramine should be avoided in patients with cardiovascular disease, but an accompanying editorial disagrees with the conclusion pointing out that we do not know whether patients without pre-existing cardiovascular disease would also have an increased risk of cardiovascular events. They argue that the efficacy of sub-tramine on weight loss is small. There is certainly no benefit in regard to clinical outcomes, and there is a plausible mechanism to explain the cardiovascular risk, and as such, perhaps the drug should be completely eliminated. In this respect, a recent meeting· of the Food and Drug Administration· advisory panel concluded that if the drug were to remain on the market, it would require a boxed warning, but some members recommended that the drug be withdrawn all together. Subsequently in October, Abbott Laboratories withdrew the drug from the US market. The European Medicine's Agency stated that the risks of the drug was greater than its benefits and advocated withdrawal of the drug.[4] In summary, it looks as though sibutramine is yet another drug designed to reduce weight but did not meet expectations.

B. J. Gersh, MB, ChB, DPhil, FRCP

References

1. International Obesity Taskforce. http://www.iotf.org/database/index.asp. Accessed August 2, 2010.
2. Wing RR, Hill JO. Successful weight loss maintenance. *Annu Rev Nutr.* 2001;21: 323-341.
3. Florentin M, Liberopoulos EN, Elisaf MS. Sibutramine-associated adverse effects: a practical guide for its safe use. *Obes Rev.* 2008;9:378-387.
4. European Medicine's Agency. Available at, http://www.ema.europa.eu/ema/index. jsp?curl=pages/news. Accessed January 21, 2010.

Statins and risk of incident diabetes: a collaborative meta-analysis of randomised statin trials
Sattar N, Preiss D, Murray HM, et al (Univ of Glasgow, UK; et al)
Lancet 375:735-742, 2010

Background.—Trials of statin therapy have had conflicting findings on the risk of development of diabetes mellitus in patients given statins. We aimed to establish by a meta-analysis of published and unpublished data whether any relation exists between statin use and development of diabetes.

Methods.—We searched Medline, Embase, and the Cochrane Central Register of Controlled Trials from 1994 to 2009, for randomised controlled endpoint trials of statins. We included only trials with more than 1000 patients, with identical follow-up in both groups and duration of more than 1 year. We excluded trials of patients with organ transplants or who needed haemodialysis. We used the I^2 statistic to measure heterogeneity between trials and calculated risk estimates for incident diabetes with random-effect meta-analysis.

Findings.—We identified 13 statin trials with 91 140 participants, of whom 4278 (2226 assigned statins and 2052 assigned control treatment) developed diabetes during a mean of 4 years. Statin therapy was associated with a 9% increased risk for incident diabetes (odds ratio [OR] 1·09; 95% CI 1·02—1·17), with little heterogeneity (I^2=11%) between trials. Meta-regression showed that risk of development of diabetes with statins was highest in trials with older participants, but neither baseline body-mass index nor change in LDL-cholesterol concentrations accounted for residual variation in risk. Treatment of 255 (95% CI 150—852) patients with statins for 4 years resulted in one extra case of diabetes.

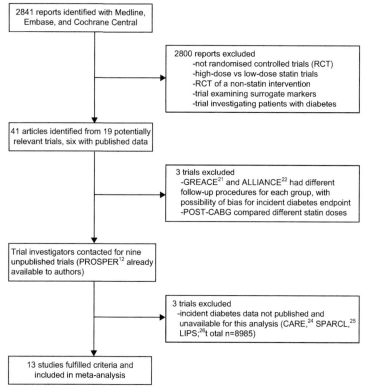

FIGURE 1.—Flow diagram of literature search to identify randomised placebo-controlled and standard care-controlled statin trials. (Reprinted from Sattar N, Preiss D, Murray HM, et al. Statins and risk of incident diabetes: a collaborative meta-analysis of randomised statin trials. *Lancet.* 2010;375:735-742, with permission from Elsevier.)

Interpretation.—Statin therapy is associated with a slightly increased risk of development of diabetes, but the risk is low both in absolute terms and when compared with the reduction in coronary events. Clinical practice in patients with moderate or high cardiovascular risk or existing cardiovascular disease should not change (Fig 1).

▶ This meta-analysis is useful and timely given the findings of a recent randomized trial of rosuvastatin, which demonstrated an increased risk of developing diabetes.[1] This meta-analysis based on 13 large placebo-controlled trials involving 91 000 individuals demonstrated a 9% increase in risk (odds ratio 1.09 and 95% confidence interval is 1.02-1.17). This appears to be present mainly in older patients over the age of 60 years and is likely a class effect of all statins.

So statins join the list of other cardiovascular drugs associated with an increased risk of developing diabetes, including thiazide diuretics, β-blockers, and niacin. All drugs and interventions for that matter have side effects, and it is simply a question of striking a balance between risk and benefits.

In this respect an excellent accompanying editorial really places this issue in perspective.[2] The meta-analysis shows that for every 255 patients treated with a statin for 4 years 1 additional patient would develop diabetes. In contrast the Cholesterol Treatment Trialist Collaboration estimated that over a 4-year period 5.4 deaths or myocardial infarctions would be avoided in addition to a similar number of strokes and coronary revascularization procedures .[3] Consequently, in the case of the statins, the benefits markedly outweigh the risks. Nonetheless, it is prudent to monitor patients and statins for the development of diabetes in addition to monitoring liver function and creatine kinase.

B. J. Gersh, MB, ChB, DPhil, FRCP

References

1. Ridker PM, Danielson E, Fonseca FA, et al. JUPITER Study Group. Rosuvastatin to prevent vascular events in men and women with elevated C-reactive protein. *N Engl J Med.* 2008;359:2195-2207.
2. Cannon CR. Balancing the benefits of statins versus a new risk-diabetes. *Lancet.* 2010;375:700-701.
3. Baigent C, Keech A, Kearney PM, et al. The Cholesterol Treatment Trialists' Collaborators. Efficacy and safety of cholesterol-lowering treatment: prospective meta-analysis of data from 90,056 participants in 14 randomized trials of statins. *Lancet.* 2005;366:1267-1278.

Don't worry, be happy: positive affect and reduced 10-year incident coronary heart disease: The Canadian Nova Scotia Health Survey
Davidson KW, Mostofsky E, Whang W (Columbia Univ Med Ctr, NY)
Eur Heart J 31:1065-1070, 2010

Aims.—Positive affect is believed to predict cardiovascular health independent of negative affect. We examined whether higher levels of positive affect are associated with a lower risk of coronary heart disease (CHD) in a large prospective study with 10 years of follow-up.

Methods and Results.—We examined the association between positive affect and cardiovascular events in 1739 adults (862 men and 877 women) in the 1995 Nova Scotia Health Survey. Trained nurses conducted Type A Structured Interviews, and coders rated the degree of outwardly displayed positive affect on a five-point scale. To test that positive affect predicts incident CHD when controlling for depressive symptoms and other negative affects, we used as covariates: Center for Epidemiological Studies Depressive Symptoms Scale, the Cook Medley Hostility scale, and the Spielberger Trait Anxiety Inventory. There were 145 (8.3%) acute non-fatal or fatal ischaemic heart disease events during the 14 916 person-years of observation. In a proportional hazards model controlling for age, sex, and cardiovascular risk factors, positive affect predicted CHD (adjusted HR, 0.78; 95% CI 0.63–0.96 per point; $P = 0.02$), the covariate depressive symptoms continued to predict CHD as had been published previously in the same patients (HR, 1.04; 95% CI 1.01–1.07 per point; $P = 0.004$) and hostility and anxiety did not (both $P > 0.05$).

Conclusion.—In this large, population-based study, increased positive affect was protective against 10-year incident CHD, suggesting that preventive strategies may be enhanced not only by reducing depressive symptoms but also by increasing positive affect.

▶ The relationship between cardiovascular disease (CVD) and depression is complex but well documented. Several studies have demonstrated an independent effect of early-onset depression and the development of CVD, even after correcting for major known cardiovascular risk factors and even in the absence of a diagnosis of major depression.[1] In some ways, depression is part of a vicious cycle in that patients with pre-existing cardiac conditions are at increased risk of developing depression, and the onset of depression is in itself a major adverse cardiovascular prognostic factor.[2]

Unfortunately, despite such a long association in addition to plausible mechanistic explanations consistent with a cause-and-effect relationship, the use of selective serotonin uptake inhibitors (SSRIs) and tricyclic antidepressants has not been shown to improve clinical outcomes. Moreover, in 1 study with congestive heart failure, cardiovascular-related mortality was actually increased by the use of both tricyclic antidepressants and SSRIs.[3]

This prospective population-based study from Nova Scotia points in a new direction. Positive affect as assessed by a variety of instruments was independently protective against the 10-year history of CVD, whereas the covariant depressive symptoms continue to predict coronary heart disease as noted previously in the same group of patients. So, to quote from the title of the article, "Don't worry, be happy" or from the editorial, "Have a happy day — just smile!" Potential interventions to augment positive affect (behavioral activation interventions) need to be tested in a controlled trial environment, and such trials are apparently underway.[4] Such approaches to improving a sense of well-being could provide a therapeutic breakthrough in an important and relatively under-appreciated area of concern.

B. J. Gersh, MB, ChB, DPhil, FRCP

References

1. Pitt B, Delvin PJ. Depression and cardiovascular disease: have a happy day—just smile! *Eur Heart J.* 2010;31:1036-1037.
2. Frasure-Smith N, Lespérance F, Habra M, et al. Elevated depression symptoms predict long-term cardiovascular mortality in patients with atrial fibrillation and heart failure. *Circulation.* 2009;120:134-140.
3. Fosbøl EL, Gislason GH, Paulsen HE, et al. Prognosis in heart failure and the value of {beta}-blockers are altered by the use of antidepressants and depend on the type of antidepressants used. *Circ Heart Fail.* 2009;2:582-590.
4. Charlson ME, Boutin-Foster C, Mancuso CA, et al. Randomized controlled trials of positive affect and self-affirmation to facilitate healthy behaviors in patients with cardiopulmonary diseases: rationale, trial design, and methods. *Contemp Clin Trials.* 2007;28:748-762.

Etiology of sudden death in the community: Results of anatomical, metabolic, and genetic evaluation

Adabag AS, Peterson G, Apple FS, et al (Univ of Minnesota, Minneapolis; Hennepin County Med Examiner's Office, Minneapolis, MN; et al)
Am Heart J 159:33-39, 2010

Background.—Identifying persons at risk for sudden cardiac death (SCD) is challenging. A comprehensive evaluation may reveal clues about the clinical, anatomical, genetic, and metabolic risk factors for SCD.

Methods.—Seventy-one patients who had SCD (25-60 years old) without an initially apparent cause of death were evaluated at the Hennepin County Medical Examiner's office (Minneapolis, MN) from August 2001 to July 2004. We reviewed their clinic records conducted next-of-kin interviews and performed autopsy, laboratory testing, and genetic analysis for mutations in genes associated with the long QT syndrome.

Results.—Mean age was 49.5 ± 7 years, 86% were male, and 2 subjects had history of coronary heart disease (CHD). Coronary risk factors were highly prevalent in comparison to individuals of the same age group in this community (eg, smoking 61%, hypertension 27%, hyperlipidemia 25%) but inadequately treated. On autopsy, 80% of the subjects had high-grade coronary stenoses. Acute coronary lesions and previous silent myocardial infarction (MI) were found in 27% and 34%, respectively. Furthermore, 32% of the subjects had recently smoked cigarettes, and 50% had ingested analgesics. Possible deleterious mutations of the ion channel genes were detected in 5 subjects (7%). Of these, 4 were in the sodium channel gene SCN5A.

Conclusions.—Most of the persons who had SCD in the community had severe subclinical CHD, including undetected previous MI. Traditional coronary risk factors were prevalent and undertreated. Mutations in the long QT syndrome genes were detected in a few subjects. These findings imply that improvements in the detection and treatment of subclinical CHD in the community are needed to prevent SCD (Table 2).

▶ Sudden cardiac death is responsible for about 50% of all deaths caused by cardiovascular disease and accounts for approximately 300 deaths annually in the United States.[1] There is strong evidence from epidemiological, pathological, and clinical sources that acute ischemia plays a major role in the pathophysiology of sudden cardiac death, in addition to the presence of a scar secondary to an old myocardial infarction. A classical paper by Myerburg pointed out that although the rate of sudden cardiac death is highest in high-risk individuals with reduced ejection fractions and prior myocardial infarction, the bulk of sudden cardiac death in the population is among patients without documented heart disease but with cardiovascular risk factors.[2]

This study of younger patients without an initially apparent cause of death in which autopsy data were combined with detailed reviews of clinical records, laboratory and genetic testing confirms the importance of coronary heart disease in the etiology. Over 80% had high-grade stenoses, and 44% had

TABLE 2.—Abnormalities Detected at Autopsy in the 71 Individuals Who Died Suddenly

CHD	
CHD (≥75% obstruction), n (%)	58 (82%)
Severely obstructed coronary arteries, n (%)	
1 vessel	18 (25%)
2 vessels	18 (25%)
3 vessels	22 (31%)
Left main coronary disease, n (%)	7 (10%)
Severity of the most significant lesion, n (%)	
<50%	5 (7%)
50%-74%	8 (11%)
75%-89%	12 (17%)
≥90%	46 (65%)
Acute thrombus or ruptured plaque, n (%)	19 (27%)
Acute MI, n (%)	4 (6%)
Recent MI (<4 wk), n (%)	8 (11%)
Old MI, n (%)	18 (25%)
Cardiac anatomical findings	
LV hypertrophy, n (%)	41 (58%)
Interstitial fibrosis, n (%)	39 (55%)
Cardiomegaly, n (%)	42 (59%)
Heart weight* (g)	497 ± 131
Range	255-960
LV thickness* (cm)	1.47 ± 0.2
Range	0.9-2.0
Other autopsy diagnoses	
Active lymphocytic myocarditis, n (%)	2 (3%)
Right ventricular cardiomyopathy, n (%)	2 (3%)
Anomalous coronary artery, n (%)	1 (1%)
Hypertrophic cardiomyopathy, n (%)	1 (1%)
Severe aortic valve stenosis, n (%)	1 (1%)
Acute aortic dissection, n (%)	1 (1%)
Coronary artery dissection, n (%)	1 (1%)
Pericardial tamponade, n (%)	1 (1%)

*Mean ± SD.

evidence of acute thrombus, plaque rupture, or a recent myocardial infarction. Regarding the primary prevention of sudden cardiac death, the direction is quite clear. Modification of risk factors and aggressive anti-ischemic therapies are likely to reduce the incidence of sudden cardiac death. However, in patients who have already survived an out-of-hospital cardiac arrest, anti-ischemic therapy alone will not suffice and the implantable cardioverter defibrillator is of proven value.

Regarding the toxicology data, there was quite a high incidence of the use of habitual substances and over-the-counter medications, and this was in recent proximity to the fatal events. It is difficult to know what to make of these data, but it does suggest that many patients may not have been feeling well shortly before death. It is also possible that smoking may have been a trigger in some cases.

The genetic data are also of interest in that potentially deleterious mutations in the genes encoding ion channels were found in 6%. Nonetheless, the identification of a genetic substrate or substrates in individuals with sudden cardiac death is a subject of ongoing investigation, and answers will not be forthcoming in the immediate future.[3]

B. J. Gersh, MB, ChB, DPhil, FRCP

References

1. Zheng Z, Croft JB, Giles WH, Mensah GA. Sudden cardiac death in the United States, 1989 to 1998. *Circulation.* 2001;104:2158-2163.
2. Myerburg RJ, Mitrani R, Interian A Jr, Castellanos A. Interpretation of outcomes of anti-arrhythmic clinical trials: design features and population impact. *Circulation.* 1998;97:1514-1521.
3. Jouven X, Desnos M, Guerot M, Ducimetière P. Predicting sudden death in the population: the Paris Prospective Study I. *Circulation.* 1999;99:1978-1983.

Exercise Capacity and Mortality in Older Men: A 20-Year Follow-Up Study
Kokkinos P, Myers J, Faselis C, et al (Veterans Affairs Med Ctr, Washington, DC; Veterans Affairs Palo Alto Health Care System, CA; et al)
Circulation 122:790-797, 2010

Background.—Epidemiological findings, based largely on middle-aged populations, support an inverse and independent association between exercise capacity and mortality risk. The information available in older individuals is limited.

Methods and Results.—Between 1986 and 2008, we assessed the association between exercise capacity and all-cause mortality in 5314 male veterans aged 65 to 92 years (mean ± SD, 71.4 ± 5.0 years) who completed an exercise test at the Veterans Affairs Medical Centers in Washington, DC, and Palo Alto, Calif. We established fitness categories based on peak metabolic equivalents (METs) achieved. During a median 8.1 years of follow-up (range, 0.1 to 25.3), there were 2137 deaths. Baseline exercise capacity was 6.3 ± 2.4 METs among survivors and 5.3 ± 2.0 METs in those who died ($P<0.001$) and emerged as a strong predictor of mortality. For each 1-MET increase in exercise capacity, the adjusted hazard for death was 12% lower (hazard ratio=0.88; confidence interval, 0.86 to 0.90). Compared with the least fit individuals (≤4 METs), the mortality risk was 38% lower for those who achieved 5.1 to 6.0 METs (hazard ratio=0.62; confidence interval, 0.54 to 0.71) and progressively declined to 61% (hazard ratio=0.39; confidence interval, 0.32 to 0.49) for those who achieved >9 METs, regardless of age. Unfit individuals who improved their fitness status with serial testing had a 35% lower mortality risk (hazard ratio=0.65; confidence interval, 0.46 to 0.93) compared with those who remained unfit.

Conclusions.—Exercise capacity is an independent predictor of all-cause mortality in older men. The relationship is inverse and graded, with most survival benefits achieved in those with an exercise capacity >5 METs. Survival improved significantly when unfit individuals became fit (Table 5).

▶ This large study on over 500 male veterans aged 65 to 92 years makes a strong statement that increasing levels of fitness, as judged by exercise capacity on stress testing, is strongly associated with mortality. The bulk of the benefit was evident at fitness levels reflected by an exercise capacity of 5 metabolic equivalents or more, which can be achieved by most individuals regardless of age by performing 20 to 40 minutes of moderate daily exercise, for example, brisk walking. Moreover, improvements in fitness status even among this older population appeared to result in a reduction in mortality risk. It should also be emphasized that multivariant analyses adjusted for age and that exercise capacity remained an independent predictor of mortality.

The strength of this study is the separate analyses that excluded patients who died within the initial 2 years of follow-up. This excludes bias caused by the

TABLE 5.—Adjusted* Hazard Ratios for Mortality Risk According to Fitness Categories (Conditional Exclusion of Study Participants)

MET Level Achieved	Excluding Deaths That Occurred During the First 2 y of Follow-Up (n=4889)	Excluding Those Who Did Not Achieve ≥85% of PMHR and Were Not Treated With β-Blockers (n=4624)	Excluding Those in the 2 Lowest Fitness Categories (≥5 METs) and BMI <20 (n=5186)	Excluding Those Who Met All 3 Conditions (n=4228)
≤4	1.0	1.0	1.0	1.0
4.1–5	0.93 (0.81−1.05)	0.88 (0.77−1.0)	0.92 (0.82−1.03)	0.86 (0.74−1.0)
5.1–6	0.67 (0.57−0.78)	0.54 (0.46−0.63)	0.62 (0.54−0.71)	0.58 (0.49−0.69)
6.1–7	0.60 (0.51−0.70)	0.51 (0.44−0.60)	0.54 (0.46−0.63)	0.57 (0.48−0.68)
7.1–8	0.55 (0.45−0.67)	0.51 (0.42−0.61)	0.53 (0.44−0.64)	0.52 (0.42−0.65)
8.1–9	0.52 (0.41−0.66)	0.45 (0.36−0.57)	0.48 (0.39−0.60)	0.49 (0.38−0.69)
>9	0.43 (0.34−0.54)	0.37 (0.30−0.46)	0.39 (0.31−0.48)	0.42 (0.33−0.54)

Values in parentheses represent 95% CIs. PMHR indicates predicted maximal HR.
*Adjusted for age (in years), peak METs achieved, resting systolic BP (mm Hg), BMI, ethnicity, CVD, cardiovascular medications (aspirin, angiotensin-converting enzyme inhibitors, calcium channel blockers, β-blockers, diuretics, vasodilators, and statins), and risk factors (hypertension, diabetes mellitus, dyslipidemia, and smoking).

inclusion of low fitness patients as a result of concomitant disease, for example, peripheral vascular disease or musculoskeletal diseases. In addition, another analysis excludes patients who were not on β-blockers but could not achieve 85% of their predicted heart rate in addition to an analysis that excluded patients in the lowest 2 fitness categories. In all of these analyses, the association of fitness level remained robust.

These data are consistent with other studies[1] and deliver a very important public health message, given that the proportion of Americans aged greater than 65 years will likely double by 2030.[2] Encouraging physical activity is both cheap and highly effective, and all health care professionals can play a major role in helping individuals to achieve a physically active lifestyle.

B. J. Gersh, MB, ChB, DPhil, FRCP

References

1. Goraya TY, Jacobsen SJ, Pellikka PA, et al. Prognostic value of treadmill exercise testing in elderly persons. *Ann Intern Med.* 2000;132:862-870.
2. Centers for Disease Control and Prevention and the Merck Company Foundation. The state of aging and health in America 2007. Available at, www.cdc.gov/aging. Accessed January 12, 2010.

Psychosocial and Economic Issues

Neighborhood Socioeconomic Context and Long-Term Survival After Myocardial Infarction

Gerber Y, for the Israel Study Group on First Acute Myocardial Infarction (Tel Aviv Univ, Israel)
Circulation 121:375-383, 2010

Background.—Neighborhood of residence has been suggested to affect cardiovascular risk above and beyond personal socioeconomic status (SES). However, such data are currently lacking for patients with myocardial infarction (MI). We examined all-cause and cardiac mortality according to neighborhood SES in a cohort of MI patients.

Methods and Results.—Consecutive patients ≤65 years of age discharged from 8 hospitals in central Israel after incident MI in 1992 to 1993 were followed up through 2005. Individual data were obtained at study entry, including education, income, and employment. Neighborhood SES was estimated through a composite census-derived index developed by the Israel Central Bureau of Statistics. During follow-up, 326 deaths occurred in 1179 patients. Patients residing in disadvantaged neighborhoods had higher mortality rates, with 13-year survival estimates of 61%, 74%, and 82% in increasing tertiles ($P_{trend}<0.001$). After adjustment for sociodemographic variables, traditional risk factors, MI severity indexes, and individual SES measures, the hazard ratios for death associated with neighborhood SES were 1.47 (95% confidence interval, 1.05 to 2.06) in the lower and 1.19 (95% confidence interval, 0.86 to 1.63) in the middle tertiles compared with the upper tertile ($P_{trend}=0.02$). The respective hazard ratios were even stronger for cardiac death (1.63; 95% confidence interval, 1.09 to 2.25; and 1.41; 95% confidence interval, 0.96 to 2.07). In the final models, neighborhood context and several individual SES measures were concurrently associated with all-cause and cardiac mortality.

Conclusions.—Neighborhood SES is strongly associated with long-term survival after MI. The association is partly, but not entirely, attributable to individual SES and clinical characteristics. These data support a multidimensional relationship between SES and MI outcome (Table 3).

▶ Socioeconomic status (SES) is a powerful independent predictor of many aspects of cardiovascular disease, including incidence, prevalence, and in many studies, late mortality, after a myocardial infarction.[1] The mechanisms, however, are poorly understood, including the individual's own SES, the impact of the neighborhood and the environment, comorbidities, access to health care and the quality of health care received, and compliance and affordability of drug therapy among other factors. The complexity of this issue was addressed in a recent review that emphasized that "one size does not fit all."[2] This study from Israel was designed to examine the long-term survival of patients younger than 65 years with incident myocardial infarction according to the SES level of their residential neighborhood, after taking into account individualized SES measures and other potential confounders.

The study demonstrated a strong relationship between neighborhood SES and long-term survival (particularly in regard to cardiac as opposed to all-cause mortality), but this was partly but not entirely attributable to individual SES and clinical characteristics.

TABLE 3.—Multivariable-Adjusted Associations With All-Cause Mortality and Cardiac Mortality for Various Socioeconomic Measures

	HR (95% CI)			
	All-Cause Death (n=326)		Cardiac Death (n=233)	
SES Characteristic	Model 1	Model 2	Model 1	Model 2
Education, 3 y	0.85 (0.78−0.92)	0.91 (0.84−0.99)	0.79 (0.72− 0.87)	0.86 (0.78−0.96)
Relative income				
Below average	1.59 (1.14−2.20)	1.07 (0.75−1.54)	1.84 (1.23−2.75)	1.15 (0.74−1.78)
Average	0.98 (0.67−1.42)	0.87 (0.59−1.27)	1.14 (0.72−1.79)	0.96 (0.60−1.53)
Above average	1 (Reference)	1 (Reference)	1 (Reference)	1 (Reference)
Pre-MI employment				
Unemployment	2.04 (1.56−2.68)	1.74 (1.31−2.31)	2.08 (1.51−2.87)	1.71 (1.22−2.39)
Part time	1.51 (0.98−2.32)	1.35 (0.87−2.09)	1.48 (0.87−2.50)	1.33 (0.78−2.26)
Full time	1 (Reference)	1 (Reference)	1 (Reference)	1 (Reference)
Living with a partner	0.59 (0.44−0.79)	0.66 (0.49−0.88)	0.61 (0.44−0.87)	0.70 (0.49−0.99)
Neighborhood SES tertile				
1 (Lower)	1.75 (1.28−2.40)	1.47 (1.05−2.06)	2.09 (1.42−3.05)	1.63 (1.09−2.45)
2	1.28 (0.93−1.75)	1.19 (0.86−1.63)	1.56 (1.07−2.28)	1.41 (0.96−2.07)
3	1 (Reference)	1 (Reference)	1 (Reference)	1 (Reference)

Model 1: adjusted for age, sex, origin, hypertension, diabetes, dyslipidemia, smoking, physical activity, ICU, anterior MI, comorbidity index, Killip class, coronary artery bypass graft within 45 days, percutaneous coronary angioplasty within 45 days, and self-rated health. Model 2: model 1 plus all other SES measures shown in the table.

These data are entirely consistent with other studies on populations in the United States, Canada, and Sweden. It would appear, therefore, that the neighborhood per se has less of an impact than the characteristics associated with the individual's own SES, although the results do demonstrate some additional independent contribution of residential neighborhood to mortality. It is interesting that the major impact is on cardiac death.

The multiplicity of mechanisms is thoroughly discussed by the authors and probably involves an interaction between the social and physical environments (including provision of health care) and individual characteristics, which in turn may include attitudes and behaviors. The implications though are quite profound including the provision or enhancement of secondary prevention and rehabilitation programs to deprived neighborhoods.

B. J. Gersh, MB, ChB, DPhil, FRCP

References

1. Rao SV, Schulman KA, Curtis LH, Gersh BJ, Jollis JG. Socioeconomic status and outcome following acute myocardial infarction in elderly patients. *Arch Intern Med.* 2004;164:1128-1133.
2. Braveman PA, Cubbin C, Egerter S, et al. Socioeconomic status in health research: one size does not fit all. *JAMA.* 2005;294:2879-2888.

Non-ST Elevation Acute Coronary Syndromes

Comparison of ticagrelor with clopidogrel in patients with a planned invasive strategy for acute coronary syndromes (PLATO): a randomized double-blind study

Cannon CP, for the PLATelet inhibition and patient Outcomes (PLATO) investigators (Brigham and Women's Hosp, Boston, MA; et al)
Lancet 375:283-293, 2010

Background.—Variation in and irreversibility of platelet inhibition with clopidogrel has led to controversy about its optimum dose and timing of administration in patients with acute coronary syndromes. We compared ticagrelor, a more potent reversible P2Y12 inhibitor with clopidogrel in such patients.

Methods.—At randomisation, an invasive strategy was planned for 13 408 (72·0%) of 18 624 patients hospitalised for acute coronary syndromes (with or without ST elevation). In a double-blind, double-dummy study, patients were randomly assigned in a one-to-one ratio to ticagrelor and placebo (180 mg loading dose followed by 90 mg twice a day), or to clopidogrel and placebo (300—600 mg loading dose or continuation with maintenance dose followed by 75 mg per day) for 6—12 months. All patients were given aspirin. The primary composite endpoint was cardiovascular death, myocardial infarction, or stroke. Analyses were by intention to treat. This trial is registered with ClinicalTrials.gov, number NCT00391872.

Findings.—6732 patients were assigned to ticagrelor and 6676 to clopidogrel. The primary composite endpoint occurred in fewer patients in the ticagrelor group than in the clopidogrel group (569 [event rate at 360 days 9·0%] *vs* 668 [10·7%], hazard ratio 0·84, 95% CI 0·75—0·94; p=0·0025). There was no diff erence between clopidogrel and ticagrelor groups in the rates of total major bleeding (691 [11·6%] *vs* 689 [11·5%], 0·99 [0·89—1·10]; p=0·8803) or severe bleeding, as defined according to the Global Use of Strategies To Open occluded coronary arteries, (198 [3·2%] *vs* 185 [2·9%], 0·91 [0·74—1·12]; p=0·3785).

Interpretation.—Ticagrelor seems to be a better option than clopidogrel for patients with acute coronary syndromes for whom an early invasive strategy is planned (Table 2).

▶ This emergence of expeditious coronary revascularization as the preferred approach versus conservative therapy in moderate to high-risk patients with

TABLE 2.—Efficacy of Ticagrelor Versus Clopidogrel

	Ticagrelor (n = 6732)	Clopidogrel (n = 6676)	Hazard ratio (95% CI)	p value
Primary efficacy endpoint				
Cardiovascular death + myocardial infarction* + stroke	569 (9·0%)	668 (10·7%)	0·84 (0·75—0·94)	0·0025
Secondary efficacy endpoint				
All-cause death + myocardial infarction* + stroke	595 (9·4%)	701 (11·2%)	0·84 (0·75—0·94)	0·0016
Cardiovascular death + myocardial infarction + stroke + severe recurrent cardiac ischaemia + recurrent cardiac ischaemia + transient ischaemic attack + other arterial thrombotic event	830 (13·1%)	964 (15·3%)	0·85 (0·77—0·93)	0·0005
Myocardial infarction*	328 (5·3%)	406 (6·6%)	0·80 (0·69—0·92)	0·0023
Cardiovascular death	221 (3·4%)	269 (4·3%)	0·82 (0·68—0·98)	0·0250
Stroke	75 (1·2%)	69 (1·1%)	1·08 (0·78—1·50)	0·6460
Ischaemic†	59 (0·9%)	59 (0·9%)	..	1·0000
Haemorrhagic†	12 (0·2%)	9 (0·1%)	..	0·6634
Unknown†	5 (0·07%)	1 (0·01%)	..	0·2187
All-cause death	252 (3·9%)	311 (5·0%)	0·81 (0·68—0·95)	0·0103
Stent thrombosis (n)	4949	4928	..	..
Definite	62 (1·3%)	97 (2·0%)	0·64 (0·46—0·88)	0·0054
Patients with a drug-eluting stent	17 (1·3%)	25 (1·8%)	0·69 (0·37—1·27)	0·2304
Patients with a bare-metal stent	45 (1·4%)	72 (2·1%)	0·62 (0·43—0·90)	0·0115
Definite or probable	104 (2·2%)	142 (3·0%)	0·73 (0·57—0·94)	0·0142
Patients with a drug-eluting stent	32 (2·3%)	36 (2·5%)	0·90 (0·56—1·45)	0·6581
Patients with a bare-metal stent	72 (2·2%)	106 (3·1%)	0·67 (0·50—0·91)	0·0092
Total (definite, probable, or possible)	132 (2·8%)	179 (3·8%)	0·73 (0·59—0·92)	0·0068
Patients with a drug-eluting stent	41 (3·1%)	53 (3·8%)	0·78 (0·52—1·17)	0·2349
Patients with a bare-metal stent	91 (2·7%)	126 (3·8%)	0·71 (0·55—0·94)	0·0142

Data are number (Kaplan-Meier estimated % at 360 days), unless otherwise indicated. p values calculated by use of univariate Cox model, unless otherwise indicated.

*Excludes silent myocardial infarction.

†Data are number (%), and p values calculated with Fisher's exact test.

acute coronary syndromes has emphasized the importance of defining the optimum antithrombotic regimen. The playing field is crowded, and there have been multiple trials over the last few years involving unfractionated heparin, low-molecular weight heparin, fondaparinux, bivalirudin, and the platelet inhibitors, namely, clopidogrel, aspirin, the IIB/IIIA platelet glycoprotein receptor inhibitors, prasugrel, and now ticagrelor.

The PLATO trial demonstrated a convincing benefit for ticagrelor over aspirin and clopidogrel,[1] and this is reaffirmed in this substudy of 13 000 patients managed with an early invasive approach. Both prasugrel and ticagrelor are more potent and rapid acting than clopidogrel. In general, however, drugs that increase efficacy for reducing ischemic complications do so at the price of an increase in bleeding. This certainly appears to have been the case with prasugrel in which the increased bleeding that was increased by coronary bypass surgery, all-cause bleeding and transfusions, as well as life-threatening and fatal bleeding largely offsets its expected benefits in reducing recurrent myocardial infarction and stent thrombosis. As a result, total mortality was no different at 15 months.[2]

In contrast, ticagrelor has not only demonstrated efficacy for the primary end point of cardiovascular death, myocardial infarction, or stroke, but there was a trend toward reduction in coronary bypass-related bleeding and no increase in major bleeding events, transfusions, or life-threatening or fatal bleeding. The net effect was a reduction in all-cause mortality at 12 months both in the trial overall and in those undergoing the invasive strategy. One explanation is that clopidogrel and prasugrel bind irreversibly to the platelet surface membrane receptors, whereas with ticagrelor, binding is reversible with platelet function returning to normal within 2-3 days as opposed to 5-10 days with the other agents. As a result, although bleeding unrelated to coronary bypass graft surgery could be increased with ticagrelor compared with clopidogrel because of its greater potency, such episodes might paradoxically be more manageable after discontinuation of ticagrelor than of clopidogrel.[3]

B. J. Gersh, MB, ChB, DPhil, FRCP

References

1. Wallentin L, Becker RC, Budaj A, et al. Ticagrelor versus clopidogrel in patients with acute coronary syndromes. *N Engl J Med.* 2009;361:1045-1057.
2. Wiviott SD, Braunwald E, McCabe CH, et al. Prasugrel versus clopidogrel in patients with acute coronary syndromes. *N Engl J Med.* 2007;357:2001-2015.
3. Stone GW. Ticagrelor in ACS: redefining a new standard of care? *Lancet.* 2010; 375:263-265.

Impact of Delay to Angioplasty in Patients With Acute Coronary Syndromes Undergoing Invasive Management: Analysis From the ACUITY (Acute Catheterization and Urgent Intervention Triage strategY) Trial

Sorajja P, Gersh BJ, Cox DA, et al (Mayo Clinic and Mayo Foundation, Rochester, MN; Mid Carolina Cardiology, Charlotte, NC; et al)
J Am Coll Cardiol 55:1416-1424, 2010

Objectives.—The aim of this study was to determine the impact of delay to angioplasty in patients with acute coronary syndromes (ACS).

Background.—There is a paucity of data on the impact of delays to percutaneous coronary intervention (PCI) in patients with non—ST-segment elevation acute coronary syndromes (NSTE-ACS) undergoing an invasive management strategy.

Methods.—Patients undergoing PCI in the ACUITY (Acute Catheterization and Urgent Intervention Triage strategY) trial were stratified according to timing of PCI after clinical presentation for outcome analysis.

Results.—Percutaneous coronary intervention was performed in 7,749 patients (median age 63 years; 73% male) with NSTE-ACS at a median of 19.5 h after presentation (<8 h [n = 2,197], 8 to 24 h [n = 2,740], and >24 h [n = 2,812]). Delay to PCI >24 h after clinical presentation was significantly associated with increased 30-day mortality, myocardial infarction (MI), and composite ischemia (death, MI, and unplanned revascularization). By multivariable analysis, delay to PCI of >24 h was a significant independent predictor of 30-day and 1-year mortality. The incremental risk of death attributable to PCI delay >24 h was greatest in those patients presenting with high-risk features.

Conclusions.—In this large-scale study, delaying revascularization with PCI >24 h in patients with NSTE-ACS was an independent predictor of early and late mortality and adverse ischemic outcomes. These findings suggest that urgent angiography and triage to revascularization should be a priority in NSTE-ACS patients.

▶ In the management of non-ST elevation acute coronary syndromes (NSTACSs), the role of an early aggressive invasive strategy versus a more conservative approach has been the subject of numerous randomized trials and an extraordinary number of meta-analyses. A confounding factor has been the differences in the definitions of early treatment in patients treated invasively. In addition, randomizing patients prior to angiography has also led to the inclusion of many low-risk patients.[1] I believe that we have come to the stage that there is now a general consensus that providing facilities are available, the most effective strategy is an early invasive approach.[2,3]

The remaining controversy revolves around the optimal timing of angiography, whether immediate, early (within 24 hours), or delayed (3-5 days or longer). A recent trial demonstrated that immediate or primary percutaneous coronary intervention is not necessary in the NSTEACS.[4] This article and 2 other trials strongly support a strategy of intervening within 8 to 24 hours following the clinical presentation.[5,6] Further delays beyond 24 hours resulted in a significant increase in both early and late mortality and recurrent events. One problem with an analysis of this type is the presence of confounders that might not be eliminated by statistical adjustments. For instance, in some situations, sicker patients might be treated invasively at an earlier stage, but in other situations, they could be treated later after a period of stabilization. A strength of this article is that the results hold up when stratified by thrombolysis in myocardial infarction risk score.

B. J. Gersh, MB, ChB, DPhil, FRCP

References

1. Antoniucci D. Do not put off until tomorrow what you can do today. *J Am Coll Cardiol.* 2010;55:1425-1426.
2. Fox KA, Clayton TC, Damman P, et al. Long-term outcome of a routine versus selective invasive strategy in patients with non-ST-segment elevation acute coronary syndrome: a meta-analysis of individual patient data. *J Am Coll Cardiol.* 2010;55:2435-2445.
3. O'Donoghue M, Boden WE, Braunwald E, et al. Early invasive vs conservative treatment strategies in women and men with unstable angina and non-ST-segment elevation myocardial infarction: a meta-analysis. *JAMA.* 2008;300:71-80.
4. Montalescot G, Cayla G, Collet JP, et al. Immediate vs delayed intervention for acute coronary syndromes: a randomized clinical trial. *JAMA.* 2009;302:947-954.
5. Neumann F-J, Kastrati A, Pogatsa-Murray G, et al. Evaluation of prolonged antithrombotic pre-treatment ("cooling-off" strategy) before intervention in patients with unstable coronary syndrome: a randomized controlled trial. *JAMA.* 2003;290:1593-1599.
6. Mehta SR, Granger CB, Boden WE, et al. Early versus delayed intervention in acute coronary syndromes. *N Engl J Med.* 2009;360:2165-2175.

Long-Term Outcome of a Routine Versus Selective Invasive Strategy in Patients With Non—ST-Segment Elevation Acute Coronary Syndrome A Meta-Analysis of Individual Patient Data

Fox KAA, for the FIR Collaboration (Univ and Royal Infirmary of Edinburgh, UK; et al)
J Am Coll Cardiol 55:2435-2445, 2010

Objectives.—This study was designed to determine: 1) whether a routine invasive (RI) strategy reduces the long-term frequency of cardiovascular death or nonfatal myocardial infarction (MI) using a meta-analysis of individual patient data from all randomized studies with 5-year outcomes; and 2) whether the results are influenced by baseline risk.

Background.—Pooled analyses of randomized trials show early benefit of routine intervention, but long-term results are inconsistent. The differences may reflect differing trial design, adjunctive therapies, and/or limited power. This meta-analysis (n = 5,467 patients) is designed to determine whether outcomes are improved despite trial differences.

Methods.—Individual patient data, with 5-year outcomes, were obtained from FRISC-II (Fragmin and Fast Revascularization During

Instability in Coronary Artery Disease), ICTUS (Invasive Versus Conservative Treatment in Unstable Coronary Syndromes), and RITA-3 (Randomized Trial of a Conservative Treatment Strategy Versus an Interventional Treatment Strategy in Patients with Unstable Angina) trials for a collaborative meta-analysis. A Cox regression analysis was used for a multivariable risk model, and a simplified integer model was derived.

Results.—Over 5 years, 14.7% (389 of 2,721) of patients randomized to an RI strategy experienced cardiovascular death or nonfatal MI versus 17.9% (475 of 2,746) in the selective invasive (SI) strategy (hazard ratio [HR]: 0.81, 95% confidence interval [CI]: 0.71 to 0.93; p = 0.002). The most marked treatment effect was on MI (10.0% RI strategy vs. 12.9% SI strategy), and there were consistent trends for cardiovascular deaths (HR: 0.83, 95% CI: 0.68 to 1.01; p = 0.068) and all deaths (HR: 0.90, 95% CI: 0.77 to 1.05). There were 2.0% to 3.8% absolute reductions in cardiovascular death or MI in the low- and intermediate-risk groups and an 11.1% absolute risk reduction in highest-risk patients.

Conclusions.—An RI strategy reduces long-term rates of cardiovascular death or MI and the largest absolute effect in seen in higher-risk patients.

▶ The issue of aggressive versus conservative strategies in patients with non-ST acute coronary syndromes has been subjected to multiple meta-analyses of both short- and long-term outcomes.[1] Although different trials have led to different conclusions, the overall trend has been in favor of a routine aggressive versus a selective invasive strategy, particularly when recent trials are taken into account, with the Invasive Versus Conservative Treatment in Unstable Coronary Syndromes trial being the exception.[2]

So one might ask what is the point of another meta-analysis? The strength of this collaborative analysis of 3 randomized trials is the length of follow-up, which provides 5-year outcomes. These data demonstrate that an aggressive approach (routine invasive) versus a selected invasive strategy reduces the rate of cardiovascular death and myocardial infarction over a 5-year period. The major impact is on myocardial infarction but with a consistent trend toward a reduction in cardiovascular mortality and overall death. What is quite striking are the outcomes according to baseline risk with a 2.0% to 3.8% absolute reduction in cardiovascular death and myocardial infarction and the lower- and intermediate-risk groups but an 11.1% absolute risk reduction in the highest risk patients. Moreover, the benefit was noted despite a substantial crossover to invasive therapy and the noninvasive arm in several trials. Another byproduct of this analysis is the development of a nomogram for estimating risk based upon 6 components namely: age, diabetes, prior myocardial infarction, ST-segment depression, hypertension, and the body mass index.

To my mind, this controversy has been put to rest. In regard to the timing of angiography and revascularization, several trials have addressed this and would suggest that immediate angiography is not necessary; that delaying for several days is detrimental; and that the optimal window for an aggressive approach is in the range of 24 hours, providing facilities are available.

B. J. Gersh, MB, ChB, DPhil, FRCP

References

1. Mehta SR, Cannon CP, Fox KA, et al. Routine vs selective invasive strategies in patients with acute coronary syndromes: a collaborative meta-analysis of randomized trials. *JAMA.* 2005;293:2908-2917.
2. de Winter RJ, Windhausen F, Cornel JH, et al. Early invasive versus selectively invasive management for acute coronary syndromes. *N Engl J Med.* 2005;353: 1095-1104.

Relationship between baseline hemoglobin and major bleeding complications in acute coronary syndromes
Bassand J-P, on the behalf of the OASIS 5 and OASIS 6 Investigators (Univ Hosp Jean Minjoz, France; et al)
Eur Heart J 31:50-58, 2010

Aims.—In patients with acute coronary syndromes (ACS), the negative impact of baseline haemoglobin levels on ischaemic events, particularly death, is well established, but the association with bleeding risk is less well studied. The aim of this study was to assess the impact of baseline haemoglobin levels on major bleeding complications.

Methods and results.—Pooled analysis of OASIS 5 and 6 data involving 32 170 patients with ACS with and without ST-segment elevation was performed. The association between baseline haemoglobin and major bleeding or ischaemic events was examined using multiple regression model. Main outcome measures were 30-day rates of major bleeding, death, and death/myocardial infarction (MI) analysed according to baseline haemoglobin levels. Baseline haemoglobin level independentlypredicted the risk of overall, procedure-related, and non-procedure-related major bleedings at 30 days [odds ratio (OR) 0.94, 95% CI 0.90–0.98; OR 0.94, 95% CI 0.90–0.99; and OR 0.89, 95% CI 0.83–0.95, respectively, per 1 g/dL haemoglobin increment above 10 g/dL]. In addition, a curvilinear relationship between baseline haemoglobin levels and death at 30 days was observed with a 6% decrease in the risk for every 1 g/dL haemoglobin increment above 10 g/dL up to 15.9 g/dL (OR 0.94, 95% CI 0.90–0.98) and a 19% increase above this value (OR 1.19, 95% CI, 0.98–1.43). A similar relationship for the composite outcome of death/MI was observed.

Conclusion.—A low baseline haemoglobin level is an independent predictor of the risk of major bleeding in ACS as well as of the risk of death and death and MI. Among other predictors of bleeding risk, baseline haemoglobin should be taken into account in patients presenting with ACS (Fig 1).

▶ Over the last few years, it has become clear that anemia is associated with increased early and late mortality in patients with acute coronary syndromes, chronic stable angina, heart failure, and in patients undergoing percutaneous coronary interventions (PCI).[1] In addition, the powerful independent impact of periprocedural bleeding on both the early and late outcomes of acute coronary

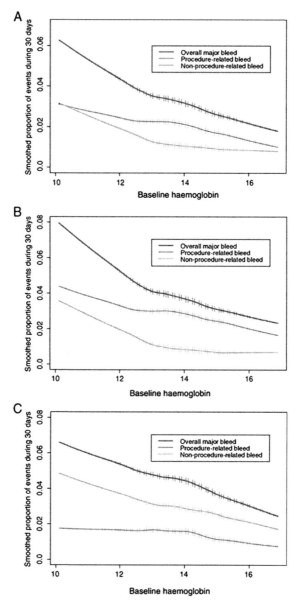

FIGURE 1.—Relationship between baseline haemoglobin and overall, procedure-related, and non-procedure-related bleedings at 30 days in the overall population (*A*), in non-ST-segment elevation acute coronary syndromes (*B*), and in ST-segment elevation myocardial infarction (*C*). (Reprinted from Bassand J-P, on the behalf of the OASIS 5 and OASIS 6 Investigators. Relationship between baseline hemoglobin and major bleeding complications in acute coronary syndromes. *Eur Heart J.* 2010;31:50-58, with permission from The European Society of Cardiology.)

syndromes is appropriately receiving increasing emphasis.[2] The deleterious impact of bleeding on early and late outcomes is likely the result of a number of interacting factors including increased comorbidities, withholding of anti-ischemic medications, and perhaps the adverse effects of blood transfusion.

This pooled analysis of non-ST-segment elevation acute coronary syndromes (NSTE-ACS) and ST-segment elevation myocardial infarction (STEMI) is subject to all the limitations of retrospective, post hoc analyses from large trials or registry databases. Nonetheless, the major finding is unequivocal. Anemia is associated with an increased major bleeding risk both in the overall cohort and in the subsets with STEMI and NSTE-ACS. The reasons are all likely multifactorial. First, patients with lower hemoglobin levels are older and have a greater prevalence of comorbidities, for example, diabetes, chronic renal failure, congestive heart failure, and malignancies, although the independent effect of anemia on bleeding is present after multivariant adjustments. Anemia can also be a marker of other conditions predisposing to bleeding, for example, occult gastrointestinal bleeding, inflammation, or a hemorrhagic diathesis. Increased hematocrit levels may in themselves play a protective role in regard to hemostasis by increasing platelet deposition to the arterial wall and activation of platelet function.[3]

The balance between the prevention of recurrent ischemic events and avoidance of bleeding is tricky. I agree with the authors that clinicians should encompass baseline hemoglobin levels in the initial risk assessment and development of risk scores for both bleeding and ischemia.

B. J. Gersh, MB, ChB, DPhil, FRCP

References

1. Sabatine MS, Morrow DA, Giugliano RP, et al. Association of hemoglobin levels with clinical outcomes in acute coronary syndromes. *Circulation*. 2005;111: 2042-2049.
2. Manoukian SV, Feit F, Mehran R, et al. Impact of major bleeding on 30-day mortality and clinical outcomes in patients with acute coronary syndromes: an analysis from the ACUITY trial. *J Am Coll Cardiol*. 2007;49:1362-1368.
3. Eugster M, Reinhart WH. The influence of the haematocrit on primary haemostasis in vitro. *Thromb Haemost*. 2005;94:1213-1218.

Timing of In-Hospital Coronary Artery Bypass Graft Surgery for Non–ST-Segment Elevation Myocardial Infarction Patients: Results From the National Cardiovascular Data Registry ACTION Registry–GWTG (Acute Coronary Treatment and Intervention Outcomes Network Registry–Get With The Guidelines)

Parikh SV, on behalf of the CRUSADE and ACTION Registry–GWTG Participants (Univ of Texas Southwestern Med Ctr, Dallas; et al)
J AM Coll Cardiol Intr 3:419-427, 2010

Objectives.—The aim of this study was to examine timing of in-hospital coronary artery bypass graft surgery (CABG) for non–ST-segment elevation myocardial infarction (NSTEMI) patients.

Background.—Although practice guidelines recommend delaying CABG for a few days after presentation for ST-segment elevation myocardial infarction patients, current guidelines for NSTEMI patients do not address optimal CABG timing.

Methods.—We evaluated rates and timing of in-hospital CABG among NSTEMI patients treated at U.S. hospitals from 2002 to 2008 with the CRUSADE (Can Rapid Risk Stratification of Unstable Angina Patients Suppress Adverse Outcomes with Early Implementation of the American College of Cardiology/American Heart Association Guidelines) (January 2002 to December 2006) and ACTION Registry—GWTG (Acute Coronary Treatment and Intervention Outcomes Network Registry—Get With The Guidelines) (January 2007 to June 2008) programs. Analyses designed to study the clinical characteristics and outcomes of early (≤48 h, n = 825) versus late (>48 h, n = 1,822) CABG focused upon more recent NSTEMI patients from the ACTION Registry—GWTG.

Results.—Both the rate (11% to 13%) and timing (30% early and 70% late) of in-hospital CABG remained consistent from 2002 to 2008. In the ACTION Registry—GWTG program, NSTEMI patients undergoing late CABG tended to have a higher risk profile than those undergoing early CABG. Inhospital mortality (3.6% vs. 3.8%, adjusted odds ratio: 1.12, 95% confidence interval: 0.71 to 1.78) and the composite outcome of death, myocardial infarction, congestive heart failure, or cardiogenic shock (12.6% vs. 12.4%, adjusted odds ratio: 0.94, 95% confidence interval: 0.69 to 1.28) were similar between patients undergoing early versus late CABG.

Conclusions.—Most NSTEMI patients undergo late CABG after hospital arrival. Although these patients have higher-risk clinical characteristics, they have the same risk of adverse clinical outcomes compared with patients who undergo early CABG. Thus, delaying CABG routinely after NSTEMI might increase resource use without improving outcomes. Additionally, the timing of CABG for NSTEMI patients might be appropriately determined by clinicians to minimize the risk of adverse clinical events.

▶ This is a difficult and somewhat contentious area without any randomized controlled trial data to support a position one way or another. Previous studies have not always distinguished between patients with non-ST-segment elevation myocardial infarction (NSTEMI) and STEMI.[1] This study using a large database adds to the literature by focusing on the timing of coronary artery bypass grafting (CABG) in patients with NSTEMI in the contemporary era of aggressive pharmacological and interventional therapy for NSTEMI. One problem with all studies addressing the timing of surgery is the issue of confounding variables, and in this respect, some patients treated earlier may be sicker requiring emergency revascularization. On the other hand, in other situations, it may be the sicker patients who are treated later because they require a period of stabilization.

This study does not eliminate these biases but does attempt to adjust for them and suggests that patients undergoing delayed surgery are a sicker group. Moreover, much of the delay is upstream because of delays in performing angiography or the use of clopidogrel and low-molecular-weight heparin. The fact that outcomes are no different between the 2 groups (using a cutoff for 48 hours) is helpful in that it supports a policy of individualization based upon clinical risk and patient stability. Nonetheless, delaying bypass surgery routinely for at least 48 hours also does not appear to be necessary and may increase resource utilization without improving outcomes.

It is interesting that rates of CABG have not changed much with time. It is likely that this is the result of more liberal indications for cardiac catheterization and consequently the identification of more patients with severe multivessel disease, particularly in the era of diabetes.

This study does not address the issue of CABG after STEMI. Previous studies have shown a higher mortality early after MI, which is probably a reflection of urgent surgery in decompensated patients.[2] Moreover, there is certainly an increased bleeding risk and mortality in patients who undergo CABG after thrombolytic therapy.[3] In general, most recommend delaying surgery for approximately 7 days after a STEMI if possible, and this seems reasonable given the potential for stunned myocardium to improve and the arrhythmogenic milieu of acute STEMI.

B. J. Gersh, MB, ChB, DPhil, FRCP

References

1. Weiss ES, Chang DD, Joyce DL, Nwakanma LU, Yuh DD. Optimal timing of coronary artery bypass after acute myocardial infarction: a review of California discharge data. *J Thorac Cardiovasc Surg.* 2008;135:503-511. 511.e1-511.e3.
2. Raghavan R, Benzaquen BS, Rudski L. Timing of bypass surgery in stable patients after acute myocardial infarction. *Can J Cardiol.* 2007;23:976-982.
3. Gersh BJ, Chesebro JH, Braunwald E, et al. Coronary artery bypass graft surgery after thrombolytic therapy in the Thrombolysis Myocardial Infarction Trial, Phase II (TIMI II). *J Am Coll Cardiol.* 1995;25:395-402.

Pathophysiology

Relationship of Thrombus Healing to Underlying Plaque Morphology in Sudden Coronary Death

Kramer MCA, Rittersma SZH, de Winter RJ, et al (Univ of Amsterdam, The Netherlands; et al)
J Am Coll Cardiol 55:122-132, 2010

Objectives.—The aim of this study was to assess differences in thrombus healing between ruptured and eroded plaques, given the natural difference in lesion substrate and that thrombi might exist days to weeks before the presentation of sudden coronary death.

Background.—Although the ability to distinguish ruptures and erosions remains a major clinical challenge, in-hospital patients dying with acute myocardial infarction establish that erosions account for 25% of all deaths, where women experience a higher incidence compared with men.

Methods.—Coronary lesions with thrombi (ruptures, n = 65; erosions, n = 50) received in consultation from the Medical Examiner's Office from 111 sudden death victims were studied. Thrombus healing was classified as early (<1 day) or late stage characterized in phases of lytic (1 to 3 days), infiltrating (4 to 7 days), or healing (>7 days). Morphometric analysis included vessel dimensions, necrotic core size, and macrophage density.

Results.—Late-stage thrombi were identified in 79 of 115 (69%) culprit plaques. Women more frequently had erosion with a greater prevalence of late-stage thrombi (44 of 50, 88%) than ruptures (35 of 65, 54%, p < 0.0001). The internal elastic lamina area and percent stenosis were significantly smaller in erosions compared with ruptures (p < 0.0001 and p = 0.02), where plaque burden was greater (p = 0.008). Although macrophage infiltration in erosions was significantly less than ruptures (p = 0.03), there was no established relationship with thrombus organization. Other parameters of thrombus length and occlusive versus nonocclusive showed no association with healing.

Conclusions.—Approximately two-thirds of coronary thrombi in sudden coronary deaths are organizing, particularly in young individuals—especially women, who perhaps might require a different strategy of treatment (Fig 1).

▶ There is abundant evidence from multiple sources that ischemia plays a key role in sudden cardiac death. This has been documented in epidemiologic and morphological studies and in clinical reports of patients dying while undergoing Holter monitoring or stress testing. Nonetheless, although an acute coronary event may underlay many episodes of sudden cardiac death, in other situations the etiology is probably an electrical interaction with a fixed substrate, for example, scar and viable tissue.

Much is known about the presence of plaque rupture or erosions causing coronary thrombosis leading to sudden cardiac death and myocardial infarction. Less is known, however, about the temporal relationships between the onset of coronary events and thrombus maturation. There is evidence that sudden cardiac death may not be related to an acute event such as plaque rupture, but that this occurs when plaques are in various stages of the process of healing.[1] Thus, acute coronary occlusion might represent the age of final phase in a series of non-occlusive atheromatous events. In addition, there is evidence that the thrombus and in this respect older thrombi, are an independent predictor of an adverse long-term mortality.[2]

This study from a group who have a long track record of seminal work on the pathophysiology of sudden cardiac death shows quite strikingly that two-thirds of coronary thrombi in sudden cardiac death are organizing—particularly in young individuals and women and that in these subjects, plaque erosions are more common than plaque rupture.

The therapeutic implications are less clear, but it does appear that erosions and not rupture are the major causes in young men and women and that they both have a greater propensity for distal embolization. This also suggests that we need to pay attention to premonitory symptoms suggestive of non-occlusive

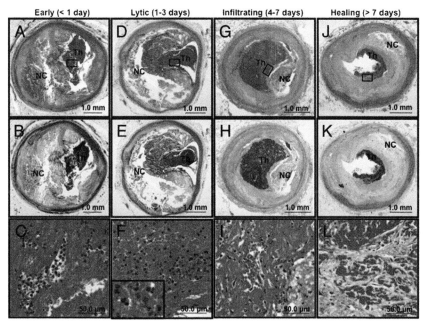

FIGURE 1.—Morphology of coronary thrombi with early, late (lytic), infiltrating, and healing maturation in plaque rupture. (**A and B**) Corresponding low-power views of a human ruptured coronary lesion showing a relatively large necrotic core with an acute superimposed thrombus (<1 day in age). (**C**) Higher magnification showing platelets and fibrin, and focal collections of neutrophils without inflammatory cells lysis. (**D and E**) Rupture with a superimposed lytic thrombus (1 to 3 days in age). (**F**) Higher-power views of the thrombus with degrading inflammatory cells (see **inset** ×1,000 magnification). (**G and H**) Rupture with an occlusive infiltrative thrombus (4 to 7 days in age). (**I**) Corresponding higher-power view of an infiltrative thrombus demonstrating invading mesenchymal cells resembling smooth muscle cells (SMCs) and endothelial cells. (**J and K**) Rupture with a healing thrombus (>7 days in age). (**L**) Higher-power view of a healing thrombus characterized by organized layers of SMCs and proteoglycan-collagen matrix. **A, D, G, J:** ×20 magnification, hematoxylin and eosin (H&E) staining; **B, E, J, K:** ×20 magnification, Movat Pentachrome staining; and **C, F, I, L:** ×400 magnification; image fields represent the areas within the **black boxes of A, D, G, J,** respectively. H&E staining. NC = necrotic core; Th = thrombus. (Reprinted from Kramer MCA, Rittersma SZH, de Winter RJ, et al. Relationship of thrombus healing to underlying plaque morphology in sudden coronary death. *J Am Coll Cardiol.* 2010;55:122-132, with permission from the American College of Cardiology Foundation.)

atheromatous events. This is a highly selective population and probably not representative of the wider population experiencing who have died of sudden cardiac death. The differences are quite significant, and I agree with the authors that we should start thinking about the possibility that as we understand these different pathophysiological processes this will lead to changes in therapy. One can think of this as another developing principal of personalized medicine based on better pathophysiological understanding.[3]

B. J. Gersh, MB, ChB, DPhil, FRCP

References

1. Mann J, Davies MJ. Mechanisms of progression in native coronary artery disease: the role of healed plaque disruption. *Heart.* 1999;82:265-268.

2. Kramer MC, van der Wal AC, Koch KT, et al. Presence of older thrombus is an independent predictor of long-term mortality in patients with ST-elevation myocardial infarction treated with thrombus aspiration during primary percutaneous coronary intervention. *Circulation.* 2008;118:1810-1816.
3. Levin RI. Plaque vulnerability pathologic form and patient fate [editorial]. *J Am Coll Cardiol.* 2010;55:133-134.

5 Non-Coronary Heart Disease in Adults

Introduction

Articles on congestive heart failure continue to dominate this section of the YEAR BOOK. Interest in cardiac resynchronization therapy (CRT), especially on identifying criteria that are predictive of a beneficial effect in regard to exercise capacity, ventricular remodeling, and survival, continues with 6 articles in this chapter. Also of interest is a report from the European Society of Cardiology (ESC) on guidelines for the use of cardiac devices in patients with late-stage heart failure. There are a number of articles on management of patients with congestive heart failure, especially on means of diuresis in patients refractory to the usual therapy. Several studies address the use of B-type natriuretic peptides in managing heart failure patients to prevent early hospital readmission for heart failure. The best therapy for patients with heart failure with preserved systolic function (diastolic heart failure) is still undetermined. Kapur et al report that soluble endoglin is a serum marker for diastolic dysfunction that will help identify patients with diastolic heart failure. And in a review, Paulus explores several novel strategies for the treatment of diastolic heart failure.

The study by Gujja et al on iron overload cardiomyopathy is important because this is one of only a few cardiomyopathies that, when diagnosed early, is reversible. Another important article demonstrates that a PDE5 inhibitor, tadalafil, can attenuate doxorubicin cardiomyopathy without interfering with its chemotherapeutic effects. Studies on infective endocarditis (IE) are again featured this year. There are several papers presenting evidence that supports early surgery in patients with IE, especially with vegetations to prevent systemic emboli and strokes. There are excellent studies supporting the class I recommendation for surgical replacement in patients with symptomatic aortic stenosis. There are an increasing number of studies of asymptomatic patients with severe aortic stenosis providing evidence that early surgery in these patients is attended by a better outcome, including survival, than is seen with close monitoring and surgery at the time of symptom onset. Another extremely important development has been that of transcatheter aortic valve implantation. The early studies are in those with high-risk aortic stenosis, those with decreased left ventricular ejection fractions, or with comorbidities, making such patients poor candidates for surgery. Shortly there will be studies reported that explore the possibility that transcatheter implantation will be as safe or safer than surgical aortic valve replacement in aortic stenosis patients who are good risk candidates for valve surgery.

Finally, there are articles on identifying patients with pulmonary embolism who are not hypotensive and who benefit from thrombolysis, reports on the value of colchicine in preventing pericarditis, and studies of patients with recurrent pericarditis. An intriguing paper on patients with syndrome X, patients with angina and evidence of myocardial ischemia who have normal coronary arteriograms, finds that a significant proportion of these patients have evidence of intramural coronary artery viral infection as a possible stimulus for coronary artery spasm. Obviously, limitations of space have prevented the inclusion of many other studies of interest and importance. To find these, it is still important to scan the medical literature as the journals are published.

Melvin D. Cheitlin, MD, MACC

Congestive Heart Failure Therapy and Technology

2010 Focused Update of ESC Guidelines on device therapy in heart failure: An update of the 2008 ESC Guidelines for the diagnosis and treatment of acute and chronic heart failure and the 2007 ESC guidelines for cardiac and resynchronization therapy: Developed with the special contribution of the Heart Failure Association and the European Heart Rhythm Association
Dickstein K, Vardas PE, Auricchio A, et al (Stavanger Univ Hosp, Stavanger, Norway)
Eur Heart J 31:2677-2687, 2010

The Committee for Practice Guidelines (CPG) of the European Society of Cardiology recognizes that new evidence from clinical research trials may impact on current recommendations. The current heart failure (HF) guidelines were published in 2008 and the cardiac pacing guidelines in 2007. In order to keep these guidelines up to date, it would be appropriate to modify the recommendations and levels of evidence according to the most recent clinical trial evidence. This Focused Update on the use of devices in heart failure 2010 is the first publication of its kind from the CPG.

Practice Guideline recommendations should represent evidence-based medicine. Traditionally, these recommendations are based on the outcomes in the cohort of patients described by the inclusion criteria in the protocols of randomized clinical trials (RCTs). More recently, based on the fact that the characteristics of the patients actually included in a trial may differ substantially from the eligibility criteria, Guideline Task Force members frequently favour restricting the applicability of these recommendations to the clinical profile and outcomes of the enrolled cohort, representing a more accurate interpretation of the evidence provided by a trial's result.

In contrast to previous guidelines, this focused update considers the characteristics of the patients included in the trials and contains several examples. In MADIT-CRT, although the protocol permitted inclusion of patients in both New York Heart Association (NYHA) I and II function class, only 15% of the patients included in this trial were classified as NYHA I, many of whom had been previously symptomatic. Similarly, although the inclusion criteria permitted randomization of patients with a QRS width of ≥ 130 m, the favourable effect on the primary endpoint was limited to patients with a QRS width of ≥ 150 ms, a prospective, pre-specified cut-off. The text accompanying these recommendations explains and justifies the decisions to diverge from a traditional recommendation based strictly on the protocol inclusion criteria. The Task Force hopes that the users of the Guidelines will appreciate that this adjustment provides a more realistic application of the trial evidence to daily clinical practice.

▶ There is a plethora of articles concerning the use of devices in the therapy of heart failure, with a sometimes confusing set of recommendations about what the criteria are for the successful use of cardiac resynchronization therapy with and without pacemakers or defibrillators and in patients with atrial fibrillation. The other devices that are becoming more useful in patients with end-stage heart failure are left ventricular assist devices, even as destination therapy. This article is a focused update of previous guidelines for the treatment of acute and chronic heart failure and the use of cardiac resynchronization therapy. In this guideline from the European Society of Cardiology with contributions from the Heart Failure Association and the European Heart Rhythm Association, the subject is reviewed in detail and the literature and evidence tables supporting the recommendations are presented, with special attention paid to the characteristics of the patients with heart failure included in the trials. This is a valuable resource for those dealing with heart failure patients.

M. D. Cheitlin, MD

A randomized double-blind comparison of biventricular versus left ventricular stimulation for cardiac resynchronization therapy: The Biventricular versus Left Univentricular Pacing with ICD Back-up in Heart Failure Patients (B-LEFT HF) trial

Boriani G, for the B-LEFT HF study group (Univ of Bologna, Rome, Italy; et al)
Am Heart J 159:1052-1058.e1, 2010

Background.—Biventricular (BiV) stimulation is the preferred means of delivering cardiac resynchronization therapy (CRT), although left ventricular (LV)—only stimulation might be as safe and effective. B-LEFT HF is a prospective, multicenter, randomized, double-blind study aimed to examine whether LV-only is noninferior to BiV pacing regarding clinical and echocardiographic responses.

Methods.—B-LEFT HF randomly assigned 176 CRT-D recipients, in New York Heart Association class III or IV, with an LV ejection fraction

≤35% and QRS ≥130 milliseconds, to a BiV (n = 90) versus LV (n = 86) stimulation group. Clinical status and echocardiograms were analyzed at baseline and 6 months after CRT-D implant to test the noninferiority of LV-only compared with BiV stimulation.

Results.—The proportion of responders was in line with current literature on CRT, with improvement in heart failure composite score in 76.2% and 74.7% of patients in BiV and LV groups, respectively. Comparing LV versus BiV pacing, the small differences in response rates and corresponding 95% CI indicated that LV pacing was noninferior to BiV pacing for a series of response criteria (combination of improvement in New York Heart Association and reverse remodeling, improvement in heart failure composite score, reduction in LV end-systolic volume of at least 10%), both at intention-to-treat and at per-protocol analysis.

Conclusions.—Left ventricular only pacing is noninferior to BiV pacing in a 6-month follow-up with regard to clinical and echocardiographic responses. Left ventricular pacing may be considered as a clinical alternative option to BiV pacing (Figs 2 and 3).

▶ Cardiac resynchronization therapy (CRT) has been shown to improve left ventricular (LV) function, clinical outcome, and survival in patients with advanced heart failure on maximal medical management, an LV ejection fraction

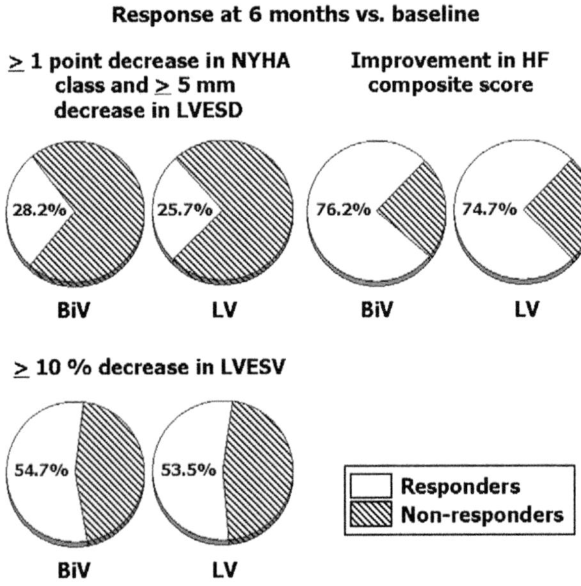

FIGURE 2.—Proportions of patients who did (responders) versus patients who did not (nonresponders) reach (*a*) the decrease in NYHA functional class + ≥5-mm decrease in LVESD (top left), (*b*) the improvement in HF composite score (top right), and (*c*) the ≥10% decrease in LVESV (bottom left) end points. (Reprinted from Boriani G, for the B-LEFT HF study group. A randomized double-blind comparison of biventricular versus left ventricular stimulation for cardiac resynchronization therapy: the Biventricular versus Left Univentricular Pacing with ICD Back-up in Heart Failure Patients (B-LEFT HF) trial. *Am Heart J.* 2010;159:1052-1058.e1, with permission from Elsevier.)

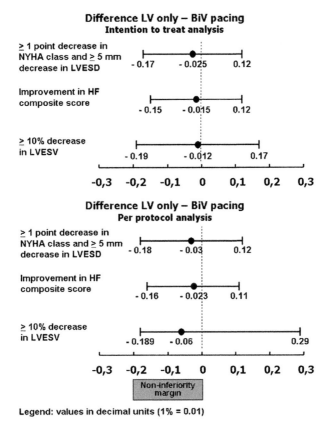

Legend: values in decimal units (1% = 0.01)

FIGURE 3.—Absolute differences between BiV and LV stimulation groups in (*a*) the decrease in NYHA functional class and in LVESD, (*b*) the improvement in HF composite score, and (*c*) LV reverse remodeling (≥10% decrease in LVESV) by intention-to-treat (top) and per-protocol (bottom) analysis. Values in decimal units (1% = 0.01). (Reprinted from Boriani G, for the B-LEFT HF study group. A randomized double-blind comparison of biventricular versus left ventricular stimulation for cardiac resynchronization therapy: the Biventricular versus Left Univentricular Pacing with ICD Back-up in Heart Failure Patients (B-LEFT HF) trial. *Am Heart J.* 2010;159:1052-1058.e1, with permission from Elsevier.)

of < 35% and a QRS duration of ≥120 ms.[1] In most controlled studies, CRT is delivered sequentially or simultaneously through 2 electrodes, 1 in the LV lateral wall through a branch of the coronary sinus and 1 in the right ventricle. However, Leclercq and colleagues[2] have shown that stimulation of the LV alone in such patients improves LV mechanical dyssynchrony. Small, short-term, hemodynamic studies and other small, uncontrolled, long-term studies have reported LV stimulation to be as effective as biventricular stimulation.[3-5] This randomized double-blind trial comparing the clinical response with LV-only versus biventricular stimulation in candidates for CRT has shown that LV-only stimulation is as safe and effective as biventricular stimulation in clinical and hemodynamic outcomes at 6 months as well as quality of life outcomes. Although there have been clinical trials showing equivalence of

LV-alone versus biventricular pacing,[6-8] they have included New York Heart Association Class II patients and were underpowered to compare the 2 forms of ventricular stimulation. The importance of these studies is that a DDD pacemaker using only an atrial and LV lead can be used for CRT, which would be simpler and cost-effective compared with biventricular pacing requiring 3 leads. Also, a CRT-pacemaker system programmed for only LV stimulation would lengthen battery life for up to 1.5 years.

M. D. Cheitlin, MD

References

1. Epstein AE, Dimarco JP, Ellenbogen KA, et al. ACC/AHA/HRS 2008 guidelines for device-based therapy of cardiac rhythm abnormalities. *Heart Rhythm.* 2008; 5:e1-e62.
2. Leclercq C, Faris O, Tunin R, et al. Systolic improvement and mechanical resynchronization does not require electrical synchrony in the dilated failing heart with left bundle-branch block. *Circulation.* 2002;106:1760-1763.
3. Kass DA, Chen CH, Curry C, et al. Improved left ventricular mechanics from acute VDD pacing in patients with dilated cardiomyopathy and ventricular conduction delay. *Circulation.* 1999;99:1567-1573.
4. Lieberman R, Padeletti L, Schreuder J, et al. Ventricular pacing lead location alters systemic hemodynamics and left ventricular function in patients with and without reduced ejection fraction. *J Am Coll Cardiol.* 2006;48:1634-1641.
5. Gasparini M, Bocchiardo M, Lunati M, et al. Comparison of 1-year effects of left ventricular and biventricular pacing in patients with heart failure who have ventricular arrhythmias and left bundle-branch block: the Bi vs Left Ventricular Pacing: an International Pilot Evaluation on Heart Failure Patients with Ventricular Arrhythmias (BELIEVE) multicenter prospective randomized pilot study. *Am Heart J.* 2006;152:155.e1-155.e7.
6. Touiza A, Etienne Y, Gilard M, Fatemi M, Mansourati J, Blanc JJ. Long-term left ventricular pacing: assessment and comparison with biventricular pacing in patients with severe congestive heart failure. *J Am Coll Cardiol.* 2001;38: 1966-1970.
7. Blanc JJ, Bertault-Valls V, Fatemi M, Gilard M, Pennec PY, Etienne Y. Midterm benefits of left univentricular pacing in patients with congestive heart failure. *Circulation.* 2004;109:1741-1744.
8. Valzania C, Rocchi G, Biffi M, et al. Left ventricular versus biventricular pacing: a randomized comparative study evaluating mid-term electromechanical and clinical effects. *Echocardiography.* 2008;25:141-148.

Cardiac Resynchronization Induces Major Structural and Functional Reverse Remodeling in Patients With New York Heart Association Class I/II Heart Failure

St John Sutton M, on Behalf of the REsynchronization reVErses Remodeling in Systolic left vEntricular dysfunction (REVERSE) Study Group (Univ of Pennsylvania Med Ctr, Philadelphia; et al)

Circulation 120:1858-1865, 2009

Background.—Cardiac resynchronization therapy (CRT) improves LV structure, function, and clinical outcomes in New York Heart Association class III/IV heart failure with prolonged QRS. It is not known whether patients with New York Heart Association class I/II systolic heart failure exhibit left ventricular (LV) reverse remodeling with CRT or whether reverse remodeling is modified by the cause of heart failure.

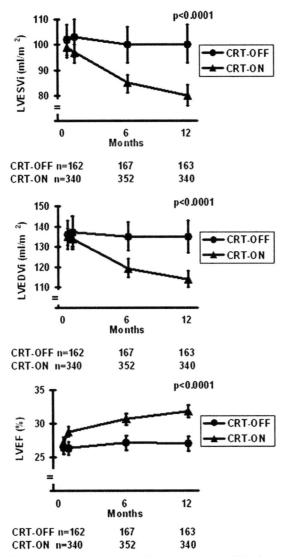

FIGURE 1.—Time course of changes in echocardiographic estimates of LV volumes, dimensions, and ejection fraction in the CRT-ON and CRT-OFF groups. Baseline values were obtained before device implantation, after which CRT was either on at all subsequent time points or off at all subsequent time points. Means and 95% confidence intervals. P-values compare changes from baseline to 12 months between CRT-ON and CRT-OFF. n is the number of paired data (with baseline) available at PHD, 6 and 12 months. (Reprinted from St John Sutton M, on Behalf of the REsynchronization reVErses Remodeling in Systolic left vEntricular dysfunction (REVERSE) Study Group. Cardiac resynchronization induces major structural and functional reverse remodeling in patients with New York Heart Association class I/II heart failure. *Circulation.* 2009;120:1858-1865.)

Methods and Results.—Six hundred ten patients with New York Heart Association class I/II heart failure, QRS duration ≥120 ms, LV end-diastolic dimension ≥55 mm, and LV ejection fraction ≤40% were randomized to active therapy (CRT on; n = 419) or control (CRT off; n = 191) for 12 months. Doppler echocardiograms were recorded at baseline, before hospital discharge, and at 6 and 12 months. When CRT was turned on initially, immediate changes occurred in LV volumes and ejection fraction; however, these changes did not correlate with the long-term changes (12 months) in LV end-systolic ($r = 0.11$, $P = 0.31$) or end-diastolic ($r = 0.10$, $P = 0.38$) volume indexes or LV ejection fraction ($r = 0.07$, $P = 0.72$). LV end-diastolic and end-systolic volume indexes decreased in patients with CRT turned on (both $P < 0.001$ compared

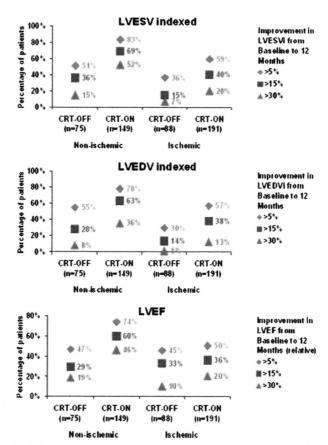

FIGURE 2.—Effect of HF origin on LVESVi, LVEDVi, and LVEF; relative changes from baseline to 12 months. The percent of patients who improved with CRT and the magnitude of improvement at 3 arbitrarily chosen levels (5%, 15%, and 30%) are shown. (Reprinted from St John Sutton M, on Behalf of the REsynchronization reVErses Remodeling in Systolic left vEntricular dysfunction (REVERSE) Study Group. Cardiac resynchronization induces major structural and functional reverse remodeling in patients with New York Association Class I/II heart failure. *Circulation.* 2009;120:1858-1865.)

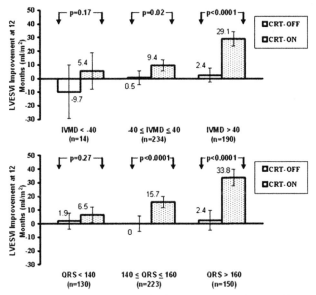

FIGURE 3.—Relationship between IVMD and reduction in LVESVi (above) and between QRS duration and reduction in LVESVi (below) between CRT-ON and CRT-OFF groups. Mean ± SD values are presented. *P* values are between groups (CRT-ON vs CRT-OFF) and are not adjusted for multiple comparisons. With Bonferroni correction for multiple comparisons, *P* values should be $<0.05/3 = 0.0167$ to be considered statistically significant. (Reprinted from St John Sutton M, on Behalf of the REsynchronization reVErses Remodeling in Systolic left vEntricular dysfunction (REVERSE) Study Group. Cardiac resynchronization induces major structural and functional reverse remodeling in patients with New York Heart Association class I/II heart failure. *Circulation.* 2009;120:1858-1865.)

with CRT off), whereas LV ejection fraction in CRT-on patients increased ($P < 0.0001$ compared with CRT off) from baseline through 12 months. LV mass, mitral regurgitation, and LV diastolic function did not change in either group by 12 months; however, there was a 3-fold greater reduction in LV end-diastolic and end-systolic volume indexes and a 3-fold greater increase in LV ejection fraction in patients with nonischemic causes of heart failure.

Conclusions.—CRT in patients with New York Heart Association I/II resulted in major structural and functional reverse remodeling at 1 year, with the greatest changes occurring in patients with a nonischemic cause of heart failure. CRT may interrupt the natural disease progression in these patients.

Clinical Trial Registration.—Clinicaltrials.gov Identifier: NCT00271154 (Figs 1-3).

▶ Cardiac resynchronization therapy (CRT) is well recognized as being effective in patients with heart failure (HF) New York Heart Association (NYHA) class III/IV, QRS ≥120 ms, and a left ventricular ejection fraction (LVEF) ≤40%, refractory to optimal medical management. CRT improves clinical symptoms, LV function, and is associated with beneficial LV remodeling and survival.[1] Less is known or certain about similar patients with HF who are less symptomatic, NYHA I/II.[2] Whether reverse LV remodeling occurs long term and whether the etiology of the HF, ischemic or nonischemic, affects LV remodeling are also not known. This study has shown that patients on optimal medical management and with minimal symptoms of HF, a wide QRS, and a reduced LVEF can have an additive reverse remodeling with CRT and that the reduction in end-systolic and end-diastolic volume and increase in LVEF persists for at least 1 year. If this long-term effect continues, the implication is that CRT may not only delay but may stop the natural disease progression in patients with HF with NYHA class I/II. Another important finding is that the reverse remodeling was more dramatic, causing a 3-fold decrease in LV volumes in those patients with nonischemic cardiomyopathy than in those with HF due to coronary artery disease. The fact that at the end of 1 year of CRT, the LV volumes decreased without a change in systolic pressure or LV mass means that there was a decrease in end-systolic wall stress, a major determinant of LV structure and function. Finally, the study showed that at 1 year of CRT, there was a decrease in interventricular mechanical delay (IVMD) as a measure of interventricular dyssynchrony. The greater the IVMD, the greater the extent of LV reverse remodeling and the potential for clinical benefit.[3,4] This study certainly supports the idea that patients with a wide QRS and decreased LVEF on optimal medical therapy might benefit from early use of CRT while the patient is still only in NYHA class I/II, especially those with nonischemic etiology for their HF.

M. D. Cheitlin, MD

References

1. Yu CM, Bleeker GB, Fung JW, et al. Left ventricular reverse remodeling but not clinical improvement predicts long-term survival after cardiac resynchronization therapy. *Circulation.* 2005;112:1580-1586.
2. Linde C, Gold M, Abraham WT, Daubert JC. Rationale and design of a randomized controlled trial to assess the safety and efficacy of cardiac resynchronization therapy in patients with asymptomatic left ventricular dysfunction with previous symptoms or mild heart failure: the REsynchronization reVErses Remodeling in Systolic left vEntricular dysfunction (REVERSE) study. *Am Heart J.* 2006;151:288-294.
3. Cleland JG, Daubert JC, Erdmann E, et al. The effect of cardiac resynchronization on morbidity and mortality in heart failure. *N Engl J Med.* 2005;352:1539-1549.
4. Linde C, Gold M, Abraham WT, Daubert JC. Baseline characteristics of patients randomized in The Resynchronization Reverses Remodeling in Systolic Left Ventricular Dysfunction (REVERSE) study. *Congest Heart Fail.* 2008;14:66-74.

Characteristics of heart failure patients associated with good and poor response to cardiac resynchronization therapy: a PROSPECT (Predictors of Response to CRT) sub-analysis
van Bommel RJ, Bax JJ, Abraham WT, et al (Leiden Univ Med Ctr, The Netherlands; The Ohio State Univ Heart Ctr, Columbus; et al)
Eur Heart J 30:2470-2477, 2009

Aims.—Predictors of Response to Cardiac Resynchronization Therapy (CRT) (PROSPECT) was the first large-scale, multicentre clinical trial that evaluated the ability of several echocardiographic measures of mechanical dyssynchrony to predict response to CRT. Since response to CRT may be defined as a spectrum and likely influenced by many factors, this sub-analysis aimed to investigate the relationship between baseline characteristics and measures of response to CRT.

Methods and Results.—A total of 286 patients were grouped according to relative reduction in left ventricular end-systolic volume (LVESV) after 6 months of CRT: super-responders (reduction in LVESV ≥ 30%), responders (reduction in LVESV 15−29%), non-responders (reduction in LVESV 0−14%), and negative responders (increase in LVESV). In addition, three subgroups were formed according to clinical and/or echocardiographic response: +/+ responders (clinical improvement and a reduction in LVESV ≥ 15%), +/− responders (clinical improvement or a reduction in LVESV ≥ 15%), and −/− responders (no clinical improvement and no reduction in LVESV ≥ 15%). Differences in clinical and echocardiographic baseline characteristics between these subgroups were analysed. Super-responders were more frequently females, had non-ischaemic heart failure (HF), and had a wider QRS complex and more extensive mechanical dyssynchrony at baseline. Conversely, negative responders were more frequently in New York Heart Association class IV and had a history of ventricular tachycardia (VT). Combined positive responders after CRT (+/+ responders) had more non-ischaemic aetiology, more extensive mechanical dyssynchrony at baseline, and no history of VT.

Conclusion.—Sub-analysis of data from PROSPECT showed that gender, aetiology of HF, QRS duration, severity of HF, a history of VT, and the presence of baseline mechanical dyssynchrony influence clinical and/or LV reverse remodelling after CRT. Although integration of information about these characteristics would improve patient selection and counselling for CRT, further randomized controlled trials are necessary prior to changing the current guidelines regarding patient selection for CRT (Figs 1 and 2).

▶ Cardiac resynchronization therapy (CRT) in patients with appropriate indications improves the clinical status of patients with heart failure in about 70% of

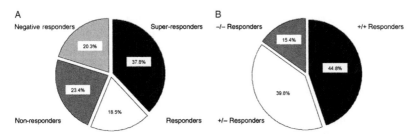

FIGURE 1.—Percentage of responders, according to the extent of reduction in left ventricular end-systolic volume (*A*) and the combination of clinical response and a reduction in left ventricular end-systolic volume ≥15% (*B*). (Reprinted from van Bommel RJ, Bax JJ, Abraham WT, et al. Characteristics of heart failure patients associated with good and poor response to cardiac resynchronization therapy: a PROSPECT (Predictors of Response to CRT) sub-analysis. *Eur Heart J.* 2009;30:2470-2477, with permission from The Author.)

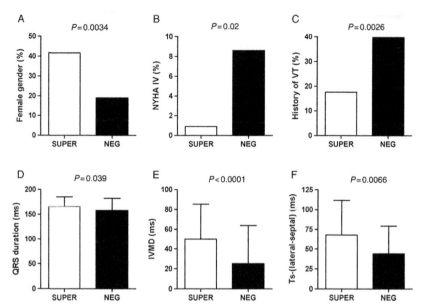

FIGURE 2.—Differences in clinical (*A−D*) and echocardiographic (*E−F*) baseline characteristics between left ventricular end-systolic volume super-responders (SUPER) and negative responders (NEG). (*D−F*) mean and 1 standard deviation. IVMD, inter-ventricular mechanical delay; NYHA, New York Heart Association; Ts, time to peak systolic velocity; VT, ventricular tachycardia. (Reprinted from van Bommel RJ, Bax JJ, Abraham WT, et al. Characteristics of heart failure patients associated with good and poor response to cardiac resynchronization therapy: a PROSPECT (Predictors of Response to CRT) sub-analysis. *Eur Heart J.* 2009;30:2470-2477, with permission from The Author.)

cases. The prospective multicenter Predictors of Response to Cardiac Resynchronization Therapy (PROSPECT) study in 498 patients with standard CRT indications (New York Heart Association [NYHA] class III-IV heart failure, left ventricular ejection fraction ≤35%, QRS ≥130 ms, and stable medical regimen) evaluated the effectiveness of 12 echocardiographic parameters in predicting response to CRT.[1] They found that there was no single echocardiographic measure of dyssynchrony that improved the patient selection for CRT beyond the standard guidelines.

This report is a substudy of the PROSPECT study that looked at the response to CRT by the extent of left ventricular remodeling at 6 months' follow-up as measured by the percent decrease in left ventricular end-systolic volume and a combination of clinical and echocardiographic improvements after CRT. Clinical improvement at 6 months' follow-up, defined as patient survival without hospitalization for heart failure, demonstrated improvement in NYHA class or moderate-marked improvement in patient global assessment score. The findings in this study that gender, NYHA class, the etiology of the heart failure, QRS duration, the severity of the asynchrony, and a history of ventricular tachycardia are variables that help predict the response to CRT are consistent with the need to integrate these factors into the selection of patients for CRT.

Together with the findings of the parent study that found that no 1 echocardiographic predictor was better than the standard CRT indications, this study is consistent with the probability that there are factors other than reducing ventricular asynchrony, such as abnormally high regional wall stress, extent of myocardial scar, or exact position of the left ventricular lead, involved in the good or poor CRT response.

M. D. Cheitlin, MD

Reference

1. Chung ES, Leon AR, Tavazzi L, et al. Results of the Predictors of Response to CRT (PROSPECT) trial. *Circulation.* 2008;117:2608-2616.

Impact of reduction in early- and late-systolic functional mitral regurgitation on reverse remodelling after cardiac resynchronization therapy
Liang Y-J, Zhang Q, Fung JW-H, et al (The Chinese Univ of Hong Kong, Shatin, N.T; et al)
Eur Heart J 31:2359-2368, 2010

Aims.—To examine whether the presence of pre-pacing functional mitral regurgitation (MR) and its improvement would affect the extent of left ventricular (LV) reverse remodelling after cardiac resynchronization therapy (CRT).

Methods and Results.—Echocardiographic assessment was performed in 83 patients before and 3 months after CRT. Total MR volume and the early- and late-systolic MR flow rate were assessed. At 3 months, there was reduction in total MR volume (38 ± 20 vs. 33 ± 21 mL) with decrease in both early- (71 ± 52 vs. 60 ± 51 mL/s) and late-systolic (49 ± 46 vs. 42 ± 46 mL/s) MR flow rate (all $P < 0.05$). Receiver-operating characteristic curve found that an 11% decrease in total MR volume was associated with LV reverse remodelling [defined by the reduction in LV end-systolic volume (LVESV) of ≥15%] [sensitivity, 90%; specificity, 80%; area under the curve (AUC), 0.85; $P < 0.001$]. The improvement in early- and late-systolic MR was also associated with LV reverse remodelling, in which improvement in early-systolic MR had higher sensitivity, specificity, and AUC than late-systolic MR. The extent of reverse remodelling with gain in LV ejection fraction and forward stroke volume was greatest in patients with improvement in total MR, intermediate in those with mild or no MR at baseline, and the least in those without improvement in total MR (LVESV, −29.8 ± 12.0 vs. −18.6 ± 16.6 vs. −5.5 ± 8.6%; ejection fraction, 11.8 ± 6.2 vs. 7.0 ± 6.8 vs. 3.0 ± 5.0%; forward stroke volume, 43.1 ± 37.9 vs. 21.1 ± 26.1 vs. 6.8 ± 34.6%; all $P < 0.05$).

Conclusion.—Improvement of functional MR contributes to LV reverse remodelling after CRT, whereas reduction of early-systolic MR is more powerful than late-systolic MR (Figs 1 and 2).

▶ Cardiac resynchronization therapy (CRT) in patients with heart failure (HF) and appropriate criteria (New York Heart Association class III-IV, left ventricular

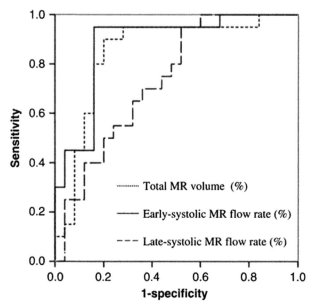

FIGURE 1.—Receiver-operating characteristic curves showing the associations between the percentage change in total mitral regurgitation volume (dotted line) and early- (solid line) and late-systolic (dashed line) mitral regurgitation flow rate and left ventricular reverse remodelling after cardiac resynchronization therapy. (Reprinted from Liang Y-J, Zhang Q, Fung JW-H, et al. Impact of reduction in early- and late-systolic functional mitral regurgitation on reverse remodelling after cardiac resynchronization therapy. *Eur Heart J.* 2010;31:2359-2368, with permission of The European Society of Cardiology.)

[LV] ejection fraction ≤0.35, and QRS ≥ 120 msec) has been shown to reverse remodeling, improve symptoms, increase functional capacity, and even improve prognosis.[1-5] HF can cause functional mitral regurgitation (MR) through LV dilatation by failure of mitral leaflets to coapt, by displacement of the papillary muscles, resulting in unfavorable changes in the direction of pull on the leaflets resulting in poor coaptation force, and in those with wide QRS complexes, by dyssynchrony of LV papillary muscle or LV contraction, thereby distorting the geometry of valve closure. Functional MR has also been reported to decrease.[6] Since MR increases LV end-diastolic volume, eventually this could accelerate LV remodeling and worsen systolic LV function. The role that decreasing MR plays in improving LV function and remodeling is unclear. Theoretically, reducing functional MR in patients with HF should be beneficial since it decreases LV end-diastolic volume and geometrically becomes less globular in shape, thereby decreasing LV wall tension and decreasing both volume and pressure load on the left atrium. This study showed that CRT reduced the volume of MR, increased LV reverse remodeling, and increased LV ejection fraction, and forward stroke volume. The patients with more than mild MR had the most reverse remodeling, measured by reduction in LV end-systolic volume (LVESV), most from reduction in early-systolic MR, and decrease in LVESV was more than 5-fold different in patients with and without significant improvement of pre-pacing MR. Those with no decrease in functional MR had the least

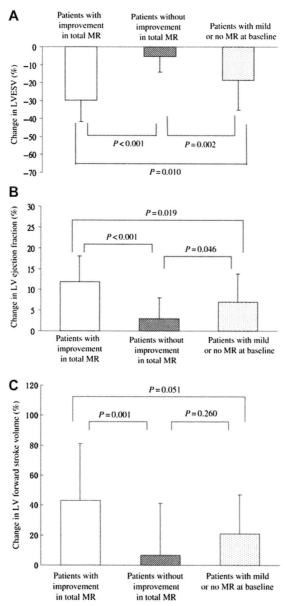

FIGURE 2.—Bar charts comparing the extent of reduction in left ventricular end-systolic volume (*A*), gain in left ventricular ejection fraction (*B*), and gain in left ventricular forward stroke volume (*C*) among the three groups, namely patients with improvement in total mitral regurgitation, patients without improvement in total mitral regurgitation, and patients with mild or no mitral regurgitation at baseline. (Reprinted from Liang Y-J, Zhang Q, Fung JW-H, et al. Impact of reduction in early-and late-systolic functional mitral regurgitation on reverse remodelling after cardiac resynchronization therapy. *Eur Heart J.* 2010;31:2359-2368, with permission of The European Society of Cardiology.)

decrease in LVESV. Since the response to CRT was measured at 3 months, it is unknown whether with longer time, there would be further improvement in reverse remodeling. This study demonstrates that the status of functional MR plays a role in determining response to CRT.

M. D. Cheitlin, MD

References

1. Cazeau S, Leclercq C, Lavergne T, et al. Effects of multisite biventricular pacing in patients with heart failure and intraventricular conduction delay. *N Engl J Med.* 2001;344:873-880.
2. Abraham WT, Fisher WG, Smith AL, et al. Cardiac resynchronization in chronic heart failure. *N Engl J Med.* 2002;346:1845-1853.
3. St John Sutton MG, Plappert T, Abraham WT, et al. Effect of cardiac resynchronization therapy on left ventricular size and function in chronic heart failure. *Circulation.* 2003;107:1985-1990.
4. Bradley DJ, Bradley EA, Baughman KL, et al. Cardiac resynchronization and death from progressive heart failure: a meta-analysis of randomized controlled trials. *JAMA.* 2003;289:730-740.
5. Cleland JG, Daubert JC, Erdmann E, et al. The effect of cardiac resynchronization on morbidity and mortality in heart failure. *N Engl J Med.* 2005;352:1539-1549.
6. Ypenburg C, Lancellotti P, Tops LF, et al. Mechanism of improvement in mitral regurgitation after cardiac resynchronization therapy. *Eur Heart J.* 2008;29: 757-765.

Presence of left ventricular contractile reserve predicts midterm response to cardiac resynchronization therapy—results from the LOw dose DObutamine Stress-Echo Test in Cardiac Resynchronization Therapy (LODO-CRT) Trial

Muto C, Gasparini M, Neja CP, et al (Ospedale Santa Maria di Loreto Mare, Napoli, Italia; IRCCS Istituto Clinico Humanitas, Rozzano, Milano, Italia; Ospedale Fatebenefratelli, San Giovanni Calibita, Roma, Italia; et al)

Heart Rhythm 7:1600-1605, 2010

Background.—Cardiac resynchronization therapy (CRT) is effective in selected patients with heart failure (HF). Nevertheless, the nonresponder rate remains high. The low-dose dobutamine stress-echo (DSE) test detects the presence of left ventricular (LV) contractile reserve (LVCR) in HF patients of any etiology and may be useful in predicting response to resynchronization.

Objective.—The purpose of this study was to present the results of the LODO-CRT trial, which evaluated whether LVCR presence at baseline increases the chances of response to CRT.

Methods.—LODO-CRT is a multicenter prospective study that enrolled CRT candidates according to guidelines. LVCR presence was defined as an LV ejection fraction increase >5 units during DSE test. CRT response is assessed at 6-month follow-up as an LV end-systolic volume reduction ≥10%.

Results.—Two hundred seventy-one patients were enrolled. The DSE test was feasible without complications in 99% of patients. Nine patients died from noncardiac disease, and 31 presented inadequate data. Two hundred thirty-one patients were included in the analysis. Mean patient age was 67 ± 10 years; 95% were in New York Heart Association class III, and 42% had HF of ischemic etiology. Mean QRS and LV ejection fraction were 147 ± 25 ms and 27% ± 6%, respectively. LVCR presence was found in 185 subjects (80%). At follow-up, 170 (74%) patients responded to CRT, 145/185 in the group with LVCR (78%) and 25/46 (54%) in the group without LVCR. Difference in responder proportion to CRT was 24% (*P* <.001). Reported test sensitivity is 85%.

Conclusion.—The DSE test in CRT candidates is safe and feasible. LVCR presence at baseline increases the chances of response to CRT (Fig 2, Table 2).

▶ Cardiac resynchronization therapy (CRT) in patients with New York Heart Association class III to IV systolic heart failure (HF) symptoms and electrocardiographic evidence of ventricular dyssynchrony have shown improvement in symptoms and physical capacity, left ventricular function, and even overall mortality.[1-4] Although the majority of appropriate patients improve with CRT, in randomized trials 30% to as many as 50% are classified as nonresponders according to a variety of definitions of nonresponse. Therefore, other means of identifying potential responders to CRT are still desirable. A few small studies have reported that left ventricular contractile reserve (LVCR) by low-dose dopamine stress echocardiography (DSE) was predictive of a positive response on follow-up to CRT.[5-7] A positive response to DSE was defined as an increase of 5 left ventricular ejection fraction (LVEF) points to dobutamine infusion.[8] This multicenter, prospective, observational study was designed to detect the presence of LVCR in HF patients with HF who are highly symptomatic with appropriate criteria for ventricular dyssynchrony by DSE and assess the

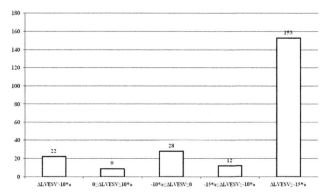

FIGURE 2.—LVESV modifications after CRT. (Reprinted from Muto C, Gasparini M, Neja CP, et al. Presence of left ventricular contractile reserve predicts midterm response to cardiac resynchronization therapy—results from the LOw dose DObutamine Stress-Echo Test in Cardiac Resynchronization Therapy (LODO-CRT) Trial. *Heart Rhythm.* 2010;7:1600-1605, with permission from Heart Rhythm Society.)

TABLE 2.—Distribution of CRT Response in the Groups With and Without LVCR
(N = 231)

	CRT Responders	CRT Nonresponders
LVCR yes	145	40
LVCR no	25	21

presence of LVCR at baseline with a positive response to the CRT as manifested by a left ventricular end-systolic volume reduction of 10% at a 6-month follow-up. Using the criteria of an increase in LVEF of 5 points, the sensitivity of a positive test was 85% and the positive predictive value was 78%. Using any increase in LVEF points as criteria for a positive test, the sensitivity rose to 95% and the positive predictive value to 80%. Impressively, the outcome of a multivariable logistic regression analysis, including demographics, disease etiology, and echocardiographic variables, confirmed the independent power of LVCR at baseline in predicting response to CRT (odds ratio, 5.59; $P = .001$). On the other hand, a lack of finding LVCR does not exclude the possibility of a positive response to treatment with CRT. Of 46 patients without LVCR at baseline, 25 (54%) eventually met the criteria for a positive response to CRT. The previous smaller studies reported that DSE was able to detect nonresponders to CRT with high specificity.[5-7] The possible explanations for the differences are the different arbitrary criteria for a positive LVCR test and different criteria for CRT responsiveness. This is the first multicenter large clinical trial that shows a strong association with the presence of viable myocardium as detected by a low-dose DSE and a positive response to CRT. Further studies, including those with less advanced disease, are necessary to determine the minimum baseline conditions to be assessed to accurately identify patients who will respond to CRT.

M. D. Cheitlin, MD

References

1. Cazeau S, Leclercq C, Lavergne T, et al. Multisite Stimulation in Cardiomyopathies (MUSTIC) Study Investigators. Effects of multisite biventricular pacing in patients with heart failure and intraventricular conduction delay. *N Engl J Med.* 2001;344:873-880.
2. Cleland JG, Daubert JC, Erdmann E, et al. Cardiac Resynchronization-Heart Failure (CARE-HF) Study Investigators. The effect of cardiac resynchronization on morbidity and mortality in heart failure. *N Engl J Med.* 2005;352:1539-1549.
3. Bristow MR, Saxon LA, Boehmer J, et al. Comparison of Medical Therapy, Pacing, and Defibrillation in Heart Failure (COMPANION) Investigators. Cardiac resynchronization therapy with or without an implantable defibrillator in advanced chronic heart failure. *N Engl J Med.* 2004;350:2140-2150.
4. Abraham WT, Fisher WG, Smith AL, et al. MIRACLE Study Group. Multicenter InSync Randomized Clinical Evaluation. Cardiac resynchronization in chronic heart failure. *N Engl J Med.* 2002;346:1845-1853.
5. Da Costa A, Thévenin J, Roche F, et al. Prospective validation of stress echocardiography as an identifier of cardiac resynchronization therapy responders. *Heart Rhythm.* 2006;3:406-413.

6. Ypenburg C, Sieders A, Bleeker GB, et al. Myocardial contractile reserve predicts improvement in left ventricular function after cardiac resynchronization therapy. *Am Heart J.* 2007;154:1160-1165.

7. Tuccillo B, Muto C, Iengo R, et al. Presence of left ventricular contractile reserve, evaluated by means of dobutamine stress-echo test, is able to predict response to cardiac resynchronization therapy. *J Interv Card Electrophysiol.* 2008;23: 121-126.

8. Agricola E, Oppizzi M, Pisani M, Margonato A. Stress echocardiography in heart failure. *Cardiovasc Ultrasound.* 2004;30:2-11.

Relationship of Echocardiographic Dyssynchrony to Long-Term Survival After Cardiac Resynchronization Therapy

Gorcsan J III, Oyenuga O, Habib PJ, et al (Univ of Pittsburgh, PA)
Circulation 122:1910-1918, 2010

Background.—The ability of echocardiographic dyssynchrony to predict response to cardiac resynchronization therapy (CRT) has been unclear.

Methods and Results.—A prospective, longitudinal study was designed with predefined dyssynchrony indexes and outcome variables to test the hypothesis that baseline dyssynchrony is associated with long-term survival after CRT. We studied 229 consecutive class III to IV heart failure patients with ejection fraction ≤35% and QRS duration ≥120 milliseconds for CRT. Dyssynchrony before CRT was defined as tissue Doppler velocity opposing-wall delay ≥65 milliseconds, 12-site SD (Yu Index) ≥32 milliseconds, speckle tracking radial strain anteroseptal-to-posterior wall delay ≥130 milliseconds, or pulsed Doppler interventricular mechanical delay ≥40 milliseconds. Outcome was defined as freedom from death, heart transplantation, or left ventricular assist device implantation. Of 210 patients (89%) with dyssynchrony data available, there were 62 events: 47 deaths, 9 transplantations, and 6 left ventricular assist device implantations over 4 years. Event-free survival was associated with Yu Index (P=0.003), speckle tracking radial strain (P=0.003), and interventricular mechanical delay (P=0.019). When adjusted for confounding baseline variables of ischemic origin and QRS duration, Yu Index and radial strain dyssynchrony remained independently associated with outcome (P<0.05). Lack of radial dyssynchrony was particularly associated with unfavorable outcome in those with QRS duration of 120 to 150 milliseconds (P=0.002).

Conclusions.—The absence of echocardiographic dyssynchrony was associated with significantly less favorable event-free survival after CRT. Patients with narrower QRS duration who lacked dyssynchrony had the least favorable long-term outcome. These observations support the relationship of dyssynchrony and CRT response.

▶ Cardiac resynchronization therapy (CRT) has been shown to have important clinical benefits in terms of morbidity and mortality in patients with heart failure, a left ventricular ejection fraction $\leq$ 0.35, and a QRS $\geq$ 120 milliseconds.[1,2] However, about one-third of such patients do not appear to benefit from CRT. The prevailing concept for the mechanism for the benefit of CRT is that the correction of ventricular dyssynchrony improves ventricular function and in patients without ventricular dyssynchrony, in spite of a wide QRS, CRT is of less or no benefit.[3,4] At present, the wide QRS is taken as a surrogate for ventricular dyssynchrony. A large number of single-center, usually small studies support the mechanism of success of CRT as being ventricular dyssynchrony, defined by a variety of echocardiographic parameters. Unfortunately, the largest prospective multicenter trial of almost 500 patients, the Predictors of Response to Cardiac Resynchronization Therapy (PROSPECT), failed to define the optimal echocardiographic dyssynchrony parameters[5] and raised concerns about the feasibility and reproducibility of echocardiographic methods.[6] There were admittedly a number of problems with the PROSPECT trial, including use of 3 different echocardiographic systems and software, poor image quality in about one-third of patients, and a short follow-up of 6 months that may have been too short to demonstrate the relationship of dyssynchrony to outcome.[6]

In the present study, a group of echocardiographic measurements of dyssynchrony were prospectively collected in patients receiving CRT and followed up for a period of 4 years with a predetermined outcome defined as freedom from death, heart transplantation, or left ventricular assist device (LVAD) implantation. The echocardiographic parameters defining dyssynchrony were prospectively designated as tissue Doppler velocity of opposing wall delay of 65 milliseconds, speckle tracking radial strain anteroseptal-to-posterior wall delay of 130 milliseconds, pulsed Doppler interventricular mechanical delay of 40 milliseconds, and 12-site systolic dyssynchrony Yu index (difference in time to peak myocardial systolic contraction of 12 left ventricular segments) $\geq$ 32 milliseconds. These echocardiographic measurements require high-quality images and user experience to be reproducible and therefore may not be as useful when outside a strictly controlled trial. Although the patients who had echocardiographic ventricular dyssynchrony as defined above had a more favorable outcome on CRT, the most interesting finding was that the absence of dyssynchrony predicts a comparatively higher risk for death, transplantation, or LVAD implantation after CRT. This study establishes the positive effect of CRT in its reversal of ventricular dyssynchrony and gives some echocardiographic parameters for defining ventricular dyssynchrony even in the absence of a prolonged QRS.

M. D. Cheitlin, MD

References

1. Cleland JG, Daubert JC, Erdmann E, et al. The effect of cardiac resynchronization on morbidity and mortality in heart failure. *N Engl J Med.* 2005;352:1539-1549.
2. Abraham WT, Fisher WG, Smith AL, et al. Cardiac resynchronization in chronic heart failure. *N Engl J Med.* 2002;346:1845-1853.
3. Bax JJ, Abraham T, Barold SS, et al. Cardiac resynchronization therapy: part 1—issues before device implantation. *J Am Coll Cardiol.* 2005;46:2153-2167.
4. Yu CM, Fung WH, Lin H, et al. Predictors of left ventricular reverse remodeling after cardiac resynchronization therapy for heart failure secondary to idiopathic dilated or ischemic cardiomyopathy. *Am J Cardiol.* 2003;91:684-688.

5. Chung ES, Leon AR, Tavazzi L, et al. Results of the Predictors of Response to CRT (PROSPECT) trial. *Circulation.* 2008;117:2608-2616.
6. Yu CM, Bax JJ, Gorcsan J III. Critical appraisal of methods to assess mechanical dyssynchrony. *Curr Opin Cardiol.* 2009;24:18-28.

Ultrafiltration is Associated With Fewer Rehospitalizations than Continuous Diuretic Infusion in Patients With Decompensated Heart Failure: Results From UNLOAD

Costanzo MR, Ultrafiltration Versus Intravenous Diuretics for Patients Hospitalized for Acute Decompensated Heart Failure (UNLOAD) Investigators (Midwest Heart Foundation, Lombard, IL; et al)
J Cardiac Fail 16:277-284, 2010

Background.—Compare outcomes of ultrafiltration (UF) versus standard intravenous (IV) diuretics by continuous infusion or bolus injection in volume overloaded heart failure (HF) patients. In the Ultrafiltration versus Intravenous Diuretics for Patients Hospitalized for Acute Decompensated heart Failure (UNLOAD) study, UF produced greater fluid reduction and fewer HF rehospitalizations than IV diuretics in 200 hospitalized HF patients. Outcomes may be due to greater fluid removal, but UF removes more sodium/unit volume than diuretics.

Methods and Results.—Outcomes of 100 patients randomized to UF were compared with those of patients randomized to standard IV diuretic therapy with continuous infusion (32) or bolus injections (68). Choice of diuretic therapy was by the treating physician. Forty-eight hour weight loss (kg): 5.0 ± 3.1 UF, 3.6 ± 3.5 continuous infusion, and 2.9 ± 3.5 bolus diuretics ($P = .001$ UF versus bolus diuretic; $P > .05$ for the other comparisons). Net fluid loss (L): 4.6 ± 2.6 UF, 3.9 ± 2.7 continuous infusion, and 3.1 ± 2.6 bolus diuretics ($P < .001$ UF versus bolus diuretic; $P > .05$ for the other comparisons). At 90 days, rehospitalizations plus unscheduled visits for HF/patient (rehospitalization equivalents) were fewer in UF group (0.65 ± 1.36) than in continuous infusion (2.29 ± 3.23; $P = .016$ versus UF) and bolus diuretics (1.31 ± 1.87; $P = .050$ versus UF) groups. No serum creatinine differences occurred between groups up to 90 days.

Conclusions.—Despite similar fluid loss with UF and continuous diuretic infusion, fewer HF rehospitalizations equivalents occurred only with UF. Removal of isotonic fluid by UF compared with hypotonic urine by diuretics more effectively reduces total body sodium in congested HF patients (Figs 1, 3 and 4).

▶ From prospective trials and registries, hospitalization of 90% of patients with heart failure (HF) is related to fluid overload because of sodium and water retention.[1-3] The primary therapy in patients with decompensated HF and signs of fluid overload that results in decrease in symptoms, especially shortness of breath, is diuretics. The diuretic, usually furosemide, is given either orally, by bolus

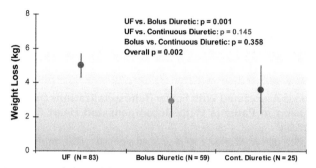

FIGURE 1.—Mean weight loss in kilograms at 48 hours after randomization in the ultrafiltration (red circle), intravenous (IV) bolus diuretic (green circle), and IV continuous diuretic (blue circle) groups; *P* values are for the comparison between ultrafiltration and IV bolus diuretic, ultrafiltration, and IV continuous diuretic, IV bolus diuretic, and IV continuous diuretic. Error bars indicate 95% CI. For interpretation of the references to color in this figure legend, the reader is referred to web version of this article. (Reprinted from Costanzo MR, Ultrafiltration Versus Intravenous Diuretics for Patients Hospitalized for Acute Decompensated Heart Failure (UNLOAD) Investigators, Ultrafiltration is associated with fewer rehospitalizations than continuous diuretic infusion in patients with decompensated heart failure: results from UNLOAD. *J Card Fail.* 2010;16:277-284, copyright 2010, with permission from Elsevier.)

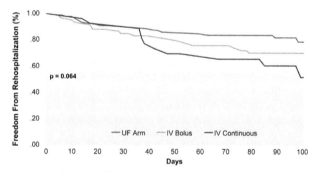

FIGURE 3.—Freedom from heart failure rehospitalization. Kaplan-Meier estimate of freedom from rehospitalization for heart failure within 90 days after discharge in the ultrafiltration (red line), intravenous (IV) bolus diuretic (green line), and IV continuous diuretic (blue line) groups. For interpretation of the references to color in this figure legend, the reader is referred to web version of this article. (Reprinted from Costanzo MR, Ultrafiltration Versus Intravenous Diuretics for Patients Hospitalized for Acute Decompensated Heart Failure (UNLOAD) Investigators, Ultrafiltration is associated with fewer rehospitalizations than continuous diuretic infusion in patients with decompensated heart failure: results from UNLOAD. *J Card Fail.* 2010;16:277-284, copyright 2010, with permission from Elsevier.)

injection, or by continuous infusion. However, many patients are discharged with minimal fluid loss, still having symptoms, and up to 50% are rehospitalized within 6 months.[1,4] Studies in patients with acute decompensated HF showing greater urine output, fewer rehospitalizations, and reduced mortality on follow-up in patients with continuous infusion versus bolus diuretics[5] suggest that the difference is because of better decongestion because of the increased fluid removed. This study further analyzes data from the Ultrafiltration versus Intravenous Diuretics for Patients Hospitalized for Acute Decompensated Heart Failure (UNLOAD) clinical trial[6] that showed that ultrafiltration (UF) produced greater fluid and weight loss than intravenous (IV) diuretics and reduced the number of rehospitalization equivalents (hospitalizations, unscheduled office visits and

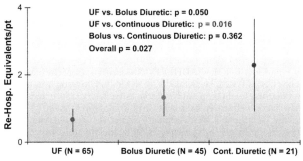

FIGURE 4.—Mean rehospitalization equivalents (rehospitalization + unscheduled office and emergency department visits for heart failure) in the ultrafiltration (red circle), intravenous (IV) bolus diuretic (green circle), and IV continuous diuretic (blue circle) groups; *P* values are for the comparison between ultrafiltration and IV bolus diuretic, ultrafiltration and IV continuous diuretic, IV bolus diuretic, and IV continuous diuretic. Error bars indicate 95% CI. For interpretation of the references to color in this figure legend, the reader is referred to web version of this article. (Reprinted from Costanzo MR, Ultrafiltration Versus Intravenous Diuretics for Patients Hospitalized for Acute Decompensated Heart Failure (UNLOAD) Investigators, Ultrafiltration is associated with fewer rehospitalizations than continuous diuretic infusion in patients with decompensated heart failure: results from UNLOAD. *J Card Fail*. 2010;16:277-284, copyright 2010, with permission from Elsevier.)

visits to the emergency department in 90 days after discharge). This analysis of the UNLOAD trial showed that despite similar weight and fluid loss by UF and continuous diuretic infusion, patients treated with UF had better clinical benefit in terms of functional capacity and fewer rehospitalization equivalents because of sustained clinical benefit. The possible explanation is that UF removes fluid with the same sodium concentration as plasma (isotonic urine), whereas diuretics produce an excess of water over sodium (hypotonic urine) and the composition of the fluid lost is the important factor that influences postdischarge outcomes.[6,7] Since decompensated HF fluid overload is isotonic, in edematous patients with normal serum sodium, there is appreciable body sodium excess. Loop diuretics produce hypotonic fluid reducing the excess body water but not the excess body sodium. Another advantage of UF over diuretics was the less frequent occurrence of hypokalemia, and although not measured in this study, UF-treated patients compared with diuretic-treated patients have lower plasma renin activity and norepinephrine and aldosterone levels up to 90 days after treatment. The study has significant limitations in that it was not blinded so that investigator bias cannot be excluded, the patients randomized to diuretics might have been the sicker patients treated with continuous infusion of IV loop diuretics, the total amount of sodium removed was not measured, and there were no measurements of plasma renin, norepinephrine, and aldosterone levels. Finally, the economic impact of using UF as an initial therapy over diuretics was not addressed, although the fewer rehospitalization equivalents on near-term follow-up markedly favor UF. Other studies will be needed to fill in the gaps of knowledge, but this study favors UF over diuretics, at least in the sickest fluid overloaded HF patients.[8,9]

M. D. Cheitlin, MD

References

1. Adams KF Jr, Fonarow GC, Emerman CL, et al. Characteristics and outcomes of patients hospitalized for heart failure in the United States: rationale, design, and preliminary observations from 100,000 cases in the Acute Decompensated Heart failure national Registry (ADHERE). *Am Heart J.* 2005;149:209-216.
2. Binanay C, Califf RM, Hasselblad V, et al. ESCAPE Investigators and ESCAPE Study Coordinators. Evaluation study of congestive heart failure and pulmonary artery catheterization effectiveness: the ESCAPE trial. *JAMA.* 2005;294:1625-1633.
3. Fonarow GC, Stough WG, Abraham WT, et al. Characteristics, treatments, and outcomes of patients with preserved systolic function hospitalized for heart failure. a report from the OPTIMIZE-HF registry. *J Am Coll Cardiol.* 2007;50:768-777.
4. Salvador DRK, Punzalan FE, Ramos GC. Continuous infusion versus bolus injection of loop diuretics in congestive heart failure. *Cochrane Database Syst Rev.* 2005;(3). CD003178.
5. Costanzo MR, Guglin ME, Saltzberg MT, et al. Ultrafiltration versus intravenous diuretics for patients hospitalized for acute decompensated heart failure. *J Am Coll Cardiol.* 2007;49:675-683.
6. Ellison DH. Diuretic therapy and resistance in congestive heart failure. *Cardiology.* 2001;96:132-143.
7. Schrier RW. Role of diminished renal function in cardiovascular mortality. Marker or pathogenic factor? *J Am Coll Cardiol.* 2006;47:1-8.
8. Verbalis JG. Disorders of body water homeostasis. *Best Pract Res Clin Endocrinol Metab.* 2003;17:471-503.
9. Agostoni PG, Marenzi GC, Lauri G, et al. Sustained improvement in functional capacity after removal of body fluid with isolated ultrafiltration in chronic cardiac insufficiency: failure of furosemide to provide the same result. *Am J Med.* 1994;96:191-199.

Medical Treatment of Congestive Heart Failure

Combination of Loop Diuretics With Thiazide-Type Diuretics in Heart Failure

Jentzer JC, DeWald TA, Hernandez AF (Duke Univ School of Medicine, Durham, NC)

J Am Coll Cardiol 56:1527-1534, 2010

Volume overload is an important clinical target in heart failure management, typically addressed using loop diuretics. An important and challenging subset of heart failure patients exhibit fluid overload despite significant doses of loop diuretics. One approach to overcome loop diuretic resistance is the addition of a thiazide-type diuretic to produce diuretic synergy via "sequential nephron blockade," first described more than 40 years ago. Although potentially able to induce diuresis in patients otherwise resistant to high doses of loop diuretics, this strategy has not been subjected to large-scale clinical trials to establish safety and clinical efficacy. We summarize the existing literature evaluating the combination of loop and thiazide diuretics in patients with heart failure in order to describe the possible benefits and hazards associated with this therapy. Combination diuretic therapy using any of several thiazide-type diuretics can more than double daily urine sodium excretion to induce weight loss and edema resolution, at the risk of inducing severe hypokalemia in addition to hyponatremia, hypotension, and worsening renal function. We provide considerations about prudent use of this therapy and review potential misconceptions about this long-used diuretic approach. Finally, we seek to highlight the need for pragmatic clinical trials for this commonly used therapy (Fig 1, Tables 3 and 4).

▶ Patients with severe heart failure frequently present with fluid overload and first-line therapy with diuretics results in marked symptom relief. With chronic diuretic use, diuretic resistance occurs from an interaction between the pathophysiology of sodium retention in heart failure and the renal response to diuretic therapy.[1] For 40 years, the use of a combination of a thiazide and a loop diuretic, each working at different levels of the nephron has increased diuresis in these diuretic-resistant patients. A review of the literature reveals the fact that

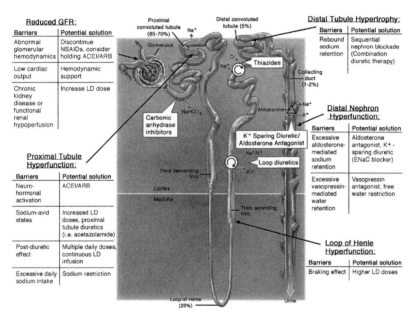

FIGURE 1.—Diuretic Resistance and the Nephron. Sites of diuretic action and sodium retention with suggested strategies to overcome diuretic resistance. Sodium delivery into tubular fluid is determined by glomerular filtration rate (GFR). Percentage of filtered sodium reabsorbed in each nephron segment is denoted in parentheses. Proximal convoluted tubule reabsorbs the majority of filtered sodium and proximal reabsorption is increased in sodium-retaining states under the control of neurohormones (alpha-1 adrenergic, angiotensin-II), producing the post-diuretic effect. Loop of Henle is the site of action of loop diuretics (LD) and absorbs most of the sodium that escapes the proximal tubule; braking effect appears to occur here due to up-regulation of the Na/K/Cl cotransporter after exposure to LD. Distal convoluted tubule reabsorbs a lesser amount of filtered sodium via NaCl cotransporter (inhibited by thiazide-type diuretics [TD]) but size and function may increase dramatically after chronic LD exposure, accounting for rebound sodium retention. Distal nephron collecting duct is the site of regulated sodium and water reabsorption under control of aldosterone and vasopressin via epithelial sodium channels (ENaC) and aquaporins, respectively. Multiple mechanisms of diuretic resistance may occur in a single patient, requiring a systematic approach to diuretic therapy. Figure illustration by Craig Skaggs based on the author's description and an example nephron from Ernst ME, Moser M. Use of diuretics in patients with hypertension. N Engl J Med 2009;36:2153−64. ACEI = angiotensin-converting enzyme inhibitor; ARB = angiotensin-receptor blocker. (Reprinted from Jentzer JC, DeWald TA, Hernandez AF. Combination of loop diuretics with thiazide-type diuretics in heart failure. *J Am Coll Cardiol.* 2010;56:1527-1534, copyright © 2010, with permission from the American College of Cardiology Foundation.)

TABLE 3.—Potential Benefits and Adverse Effects of CDT

Potential Benefits	Potential Adverse Effects
Overcoming diuretic resistance	Hypokalemia
Relief of fluid overload + edema	Worsening renal function/azotemia
Weight loss	Hyponatremia
Low drug cost	Hypochloremic metabolic alkalosis
Symptomatic improvement	Hypotension
Decrease in systemic congestion	Hypovolemia/dehydration
Diuresis in chronic renal failure	Worsening hepatic encephalopathy
Improved ventricular function	Cardiac arrhythmias/ectopy
Hospital discharge	Hypomagnesemia
Prevention of readmission	Hyperuricemia

CDT = combination diuretic therapy.

TABLE 4.—Important Considerations Regarding CDT

- Addition of thiazide-type diuretics can induce diuresis in patients refractory to massive loop diuretic doses
- Combination of loop + thiazide-type diuretics can be effective in patients with advanced chronic kidney disease
- Synergistic effects of thiazide-type diuretics on diuresis appear to be a class effect seen with all drugs studied
- Potentially dangerous hypokalemia can develop with CDT, warranting close laboratory monitoring
- Reversible increases in serum creatinine may be seen but are not the rule; reductions in creatinine can occur as well
- Safety and effects on morbidity and mortality with CDT are unknown

CDT = combination diuretic therapy.

most of the studies involving combined diuretic use are small and nonplacebo controlled. This article is a very good summary of the history of diuretic resistance and the safety and effectiveness of combined diuretic therapy in patients with severe diuretic-resistant congestive heart failure.

M. D. Cheitlin, MD

Reference

1. Ellison DH. Diuretic therapy and resistance in congestive heart failure. *Cardiology.* 2001;96:132-143.

Coenzyme Q$_{10}$, Rosuvastatin, and Clinical Outcomes in Heart Failure: A Pre-Specified Substudy of CORONA (Controlled Rosuvastatin Multinational Study in Heart Failure)
McMurray JJV, on behalf of the CORONA Study Group (Univ of Glasgow, UK; et al)
J Am Coll Cardiol 56:1196-1204, 2010

Objectives.—The purpose of this study was to determine whether coenzyme Q$_{10}$ is an independent predictor of prognosis in heart failure.

Background.—Blood and tissue concentrations of the essential cofactor coenzyme Q_{10} are decreased by statins, and this could be harmful in patients with heart failure.

Methods.—We measured serum coenzyme Q_{10} in 1,191 patients with ischemic systolic heart failure enrolled in CORONA (Controlled Rosuvastatin Multinational Study in Heart Failure) and related this to clinical outcomes.

Results.—Patients with lower coenzyme Q_{10} concentrations were older and had more advanced heart failure. Mortality was significantly higher among patients in the lowest compared to the highest coenzyme Q_{10} tertile in a univariate analysis (hazard ratio: 1.50, 95% confidence interval: 1.04 to 2.6, p = 0.03) but not in a multivariable analysis. Coenzyme Q_{10} was not an independent predictor of any other clinical outcome. Rosuvastatin reduced coenzyme Q_{10} but there was no interaction between coenzyme Q_{10} and the effect of rosuvastatin.

Conclusions.—Coenzyme Q_{10} is not an independent prognostic variable in heart failure. Rosuvastatin reduced coenzyme Q_{10}, but even in patients with a low baseline coenzyme Q_{10}, rosuvastatin treatment was not associated with a significantly worse outcome. (Controlled Rosuvastatin Multinational Study in Heart Failure [CORONA]; NCT00206310).

► For years, there have been hundreds of articles examining the significance of low levels of coenzyme Q_{10} (ubiquinone) in patients with heart failure (HF). Q_{10} acts as an electron transporter and is a lipid-soluble essential cofactor in mitochondrial oxidative phosphorylation and generation of adenosine triphosphate.[1,2] Another possible action is as a lipophilic antioxidant protecting cell membranes and lipoproteins from oxidation.[1-3] Because the synthesis of Q_{10} is through the mevalonate pathway that is blocked by statins,[1-3] theoretically, Q_{10} depletion could lead to muscle dysfunction, both peripheral and myocardial, of especial concern in patients with HF. In an article by Molyneux and colleagues,[4] low Q_{10} serum levels were found to be an independent predictor of mortality in patients with HF. These facts have resulted in some physicians recommending Q_{10} supplements and avoiding indicated statins in patients with HF, causing the Food and Drug Administration to request that this study be done to examine the relationship of Q_{10} to adverse events in patients with HF. Compared with the previously mentioned study, this study is 5 times as large with 350 versus 76 deaths. Although this study also found that a low serum Q_{10} level was associated with worse outcomes in patients with HF, the low serum Q_{10} level served as a marker for advanced disease and was not independent of a low left ventricular ejection fraction, reduced glomerular filtration rate, higher New York Heart Association class, or increased N-terminal pro—B-type natriuretic peptide concentration as a predictor of mortality in patients with HF. Finally, in the study by Molyneux and colleagues, multivariable analysis adjusted for only 5 baseline variables in addition to Q_{10} levels, whereas in this study, 14 independent variables previously shown to be predictors of outcome were used. All these differences make this study more robust and its conclusions more likely to be correct. Additionally, there was evidence that statins increased muscle symptoms or creatine kinase in patients with low Q_{10} serum levels. Hopefully, this article will dampen the enthusiasm for prescribing Q_{10} to patients with HF and eliminate the hesitation for giving statins to patients where they are indicated.

M. D. Cheitlin, MD

References

1. Crane FL. Discovery of ubiquinone (coenzyme Q) and an overview of function. *Mitochondrion.* 2007;7:S2-S7.
2. Bentinger M, Brismar K, Dallner G. The antioxidant role of coenzyme Q. *Mitochondrion.* 2007;7:S41-S50.
3. Rustin P, Munnich A, Rötig A. Mitochondrial respiratory chain dysfunction caused by coenzyme Q deficiency. *Methods Enzymol.* 2004;382:81-88.
4. Molyneux SL, Florkowski CM, George PM, et al. Coenzyme Q10: an independent predictor of mortality in chronic heart failure. *J Am Coll Cardiol.* 2008;52:1435-1441.

Effects of Telmisartan Added to Angiotensin-Converting Enzyme Inhibitors on Mortality and Morbidity in Hemodialysis Patients With Chronic Heart Failure: A Double-Blind, Placebo-Controlled Trial

Cice G, Di Benedetto A, D'Isa S, et al (Second Univ of Naples, Italy; NephroCare Italy, Naples; IRCCS San Raffaele Pisana, Rome, Italy; et al)

J Am Coll Cardiol 56:1701-1708, 2010

Objectives.—The aim of this study was to determine whether telmisartan decreases all-cause and cardiovascular mortality and morbidity in hemodialysis patients with chronic heart failure (CHF) and impaired left ventricular ejection fraction (LVEF) when added to standard therapies with angiotensin-converting enzyme inhibitors.

Background.—In hemodialysis patients, CHF is responsible for a high mortality rate, but presently very few data are available with regard to this population.

Methods.—A 3-year randomized, double-blind, placebo-controlled, multicenter trial was performed involving 30 Italian clinics. Hemodialysis patients with CHF (New York Heart Association functional class II to III; LVEF ≤40%) were randomized to telmisartan or placebo in addition to angiotensin-converting enzyme inhibitor therapy. A total of 332 patients were enrolled (165 telmisartan, 167 placebo). Drug dosage was titrated to a target dose of telmisartan of 80 mg or placebo. Mean follow-up period was 35.5 ± 8.5 months (median: 36 months; range: 2 to 40 months). Primary outcomes were: 1) all-cause mortality; 2) cardiovascular mortality; and 3) CHF hospital stay.

Results.—At 3 years, telmisartan significantly reduced all-cause mortality (35.1% vs. 54.4%; p < 0.001), cardiovascular death (30.3% vs. 43.7%; p < 0.001), and hospital admission for CHF (33.9% vs. 55.1%; p < 0.0001). With Cox proportional hazards analysis, telmisartan was an independent determinant of all-cause mortality (hazard ratio [HR]:

0.51; 95% confidence interval [CI]: 0.32 to 0.82; p < 0.01), cardiovascular mortality (HR: 0.42; 95% CI: 0.38 to 0.61; p < 0.0001), and hospital stay for deterioration of heart failure (HR: 0.38; 95% CI: 0.19 to 0.51; p < 0.0001). Adverse effects, mainly hypotension, occurred in 16.3% of the telmisartan group versus 10.7% in the placebo group.

Conclusions.—Addition of telmisartan to standard therapies significantly reduces all-cause mortality, cardiovascular death, and heart failure hospital stays in hemodialysis patients with CHF and LVEF ≤40%. (Effects Of Telmisartan Added To Angiotensin Converting Enzyme Inhibitors On Mortality And Morbidity In Haemodialysed Patients With Chronic Heart Failure: A Double-Blind Placebo-Controlled Trial; NCT00490958) (Figs 2 and 3).

▶ Patients with end-stage renal disease (ESRD) on hemodialysis who have heart failure (HF) have a very poor prognosis.[1] Among those with ESRD starting dialysis, 36% have HF, and an additional 7% develop HF while on dialysis.[2] The mortality of patients on dialysis is doubled in those with concomitant HF.[3] Although angiotensin converting enzyme inhibitors (ACEIs) and angiotensin II type 1 receptor blockers (ARBs) have been shown to improve hemodynamics, neurohumoral activation, ventricular remodeling, mortality, and morbidity of patients with HF when added to ACEI, there are no studies showing benefit of these drugs when added to standard therapy in patients with ESRD on

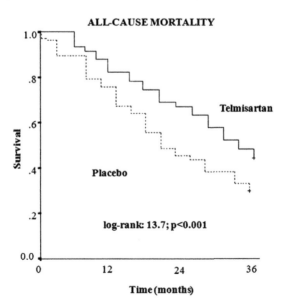

FIGURE 2.—Kaplan-Meier Life-Table Analysis for All-Cause Mortality. The cumulative 3-year mean survival time was 30.6 months in the telmisartan group (**solid line**) and 24.2 months in the placebo group (**dotted line**). (Reprinted from the Journal of the American College of Cardiology, Cice G, Di Benedetto A, D'Isa S, et al. Effects of telmisartan added to angiotensin-converting enzyme inhibitors on mortality and morbidity in hemodialysis patients with chronic heart failure: a double-blind, placebo-controlled trial. *J Am Coll Cardiol.* 2010;56:1701-1708. Copyright 2010, with permission from the American College of Cardiology Foundation.)

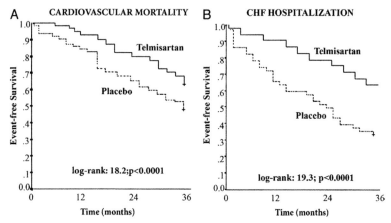

FIGURE 3.—Kaplan-Meier Life-Table Analysis for Cardiovascular Mortality and CHF Hospital Stay. Cumulative 3-year survival time free of cardiovascular deaths (**A**) and hospital admissions (**B**) in patients treated with telmisartan (**solid line**) or placebo (**dotted line**). CHF = chronic heart failure. (Reprinted from the Journal of the American College of Cardiology, Cice G, Di Benedetto A, D'Isa S, et al. Effects of telmisartan added to angiotensin-converting enzyme inhibitors on mortality and morbidity in hemodialysis patients with chronic heart failure: a double-blind, placebo-controlled trial. *J Am Coll Cardiol*. 2010;56:1701-1708. Copyright 2010, with permission from the American College of Cardiology Foundation.)

hemodialysis with HF.[4,5] This is the first randomized double-blind study in this population on hemodialysis with systolic HF and a reduced ejection fraction that has shown a remarkable reduction in all-cause mortality, cardiovascular mortality, hospitalization for worsening HF, improvement in ejection fraction, and ventricular remodeling. The decrease in mortality was due to a decrease in noncardiovascular mortality, sudden death, and pump failure. In spite of almost half the patients having known coronary disease, there were few myocardial infarctions or strokes overall. The mechanism that accounts for this remarkable benefit is unclear but must involve a reduction in the activated sympathetic and renin-angiotensin-aldosterone system (RAAS) present in HF. One possibility is that hemodialysis largely removes ACEI, so that levels that are effective in improving outcome in patients who are nonuremic cannot be achieved in dialysis.[6,7] With the addition of an ARB, there is more effective blockade of the RAAS with its attending benefits. Whether a greater decrease in blood pressure was also a factor in the improvement seen is questionable. The major side effect was a drop in blood pressure to hypotensive levels that might limit the use of combined ACEI and ARB treatment in these patients. There is an interesting editorial that accompanies this article that raises questions that might decrease the certainty that this combined ACEI and ARB blockade together with β-blockers should be the standard of care in these patients.[8]

M. D. Cheitlin, MD

References

1. Schreiber BD. Congestive heart failure in patients with chronic kidney disease and on dialysis. *Am J Med Sci*. 2003;325:179-193.

2. Stack AG, Bloembergen WE. A cross-sectional study of the prevalence and clinical correlates of congestive heart failure among incident US dialysis patients. *Am J Kidney Dis.* 2001;38:992-1000.

3. Harnett JD, Foley RN, Kent GM, Barre PE, Murray D, Parfrey PS. Congestive heart failure in dialysis patients: prevalence, incidence, prognosis and risk factors. *Kidney Int.* 1995;47:884-890.

4. Cohn JN, Tognoni G, Valsartan Heart Failure Trial Investigators. A randomized trial of the angiotensin-receptor blocker valsartan in chronic heart failure. *N Engl J Med.* 2001;345:1667-1675.

5. Pfeffer MA, Swedberg K, Granger CB, et al. Effects of candesartan on mortality and morbidity in patients with chronic heart failure: the CHARM-Overall programme. *Lancet.* 2003;362:759-766.

6. Brenner BM. *Brenner and Rector's The Kidney.* 8th ed. Philadelphia, PA: Saunders Book Company; 2007.

7. Kelly JG, Doyle GD, Carmody M, Glover DR, Cooper WD. Pharmacokinetics of lisinopril, enalapril and enalaprilat in renal failure: effects of haemodialysis. *Br J Clin Pharmacol.* 1988;26:781-786.

8. Sipahi I, Fang JC. Treating heart failure on dialysis. Finally getting some evidence. *J Am Coll Cardiol.* 2010;56:1709-1711.

Ivabradine and outcomes in chronic heart failure (SHIFT): a randomised placebo-controlled study

Swedberg K, on behalf of the SHIFT Investigators (Univ of Gothenburg, Göteborg, Sweden; et al)
Lancet 376:875-885, 2010

Background.—Chronic heart failure is associated with high mortality and morbidity. Raised resting heart rate is a risk factor for adverse outcomes. We aimed to assess the effect of heart-rate reduction by the selective sinus-node inhibitor ivabradine on outcomes in heart failure.

Methods.—Patients were eligible for participation in this randomised, double-blind, placebo-controlled, parallel-group study if they had symptomatic heart failure and a left-ventricular ejection fraction of 35% or lower, were in sinus rhythm with heart rate 70 beats per min or higher, had been admitted to hospital for heart failure within the previous year, and were on stable background treatment including a β blocker if tolerated. Patients were randomly assigned by computer-generated allocation schedule to ivabradine titrated to a maximum of 7·5 mg twice daily or matching placebo. Patients and investigators were masked to treatment allocation. The primary endpoint was the composite of cardiovascular death or hospital admission for worsening heart failure. Analysis was by intention to treat. This trial is registered, number ISRCTN70429960.

Findings.—6558 patients were randomly assigned to treatment groups (3268 ivabradine, 3290 placebo). Data were available for analysis for 3241 patients in the ivabradine group and 3264 patients allocated placebo. Median follow-up was 22·9 (IQR 18—28) months. 793 (24%) patients in the ivabradine group and 937 (29%) of those taking placebo had a primary endpoint event (HR 0·82, 95% CI 0·75—0·90, p<0·0001). The effects were driven mainly by hospital admissions for worsening heart failure (672 [21%] placebo vs 514 [16%] ivabradine; HR 0·74, 0·66−0·83; p<0·0001) and deaths due to heart failure (151 [5%] vs 113 [3%]; HR 0·74, 0·58−0·94, p=0·014). Fewer serious adverse events occurred in the ivabradine group (3388 events) than in the placebo group (3847; p=0·025). 150 (5%) of ivabradine patients had symptomatic bradycardia compared with 32 (1%) of the placebo group (p<0·0001). Visual side-effects (phosphenes) were reported by 89 (3%) of patients on ivabradine and 17 (1%) on placebo (p<0·0001).

Interpretation.—Our results support the importance of heart-rate reduction with ivabradine for improvement of clinical outcomes in heart failure and confirm the important role of heart rate in the pathophysiology of this disorder.

▶ The treatment of heart failure (HF) has improved substantially over the last 20 years with the use of β-blockers and antagonists of the renin-angiotensin-aldosterone (RAAS) system. β-blockers reduce mortality and morbidity beyond that of RAAS blockade alone.[1] The effect of these drugs in improving left ventricular remodeling[2] and sudden death[3] may be in part associated with their effect on lowering the heart rate.[4,5] The heart rate−lowering effect of β-blockers attenuates the effect of energy depletion of the myocardium in HF[6] but has other undesirable effects such as a depressing effect on myocardial contractility. It is known that raised heart rate is a risk factor for mortality and cardiovascular outcomes in epidemiological and observational studies.[7,8] Patients with HF treated with β-blockers frequently still have an elevated heart rate,[9] so additional therapies to further reduce heart rate might be useful. This study is the first to specifically test the hypothesis that isolated heart rate reduction will decrease the incidence of adverse outcomes in a population of patients with HF. Ivabradine is a specific inhibitor of the I_f current in the sino-atrial node[10] and has no effect on myocardial contractility and intracardiac conduction. Patients with chronic systolic HF, an ejection fraction ≤35% on optimal medical management including β-blockers with a persistent heart rate ≥70 beats/min showed a significant decrease of 18% in the composite of cardiovascular deaths or hospital admissions for worsening HF in those taking ivabradine. Although there was no reduction in cardiovascular deaths or sudden deaths, there was a significant drop in deaths caused by HF and all-cause hospital admissions, all of which became apparent within 3 months of initiation of treatment. The effects were consistent across all prespecified subgroups, but were most striking in those with baseline higher heart rates. Before the authors concluded that ivabradine should be a part of optimal therapy for patients with HF with residual heart rate ≥70 beats/min, in this study, the minority of patients on β-blockers were at the recommended target dose, so the same result might have been found with higher doses of β-blockers. Also, the mechanism by which the reduction in the outcome end points was achieved by ivabradine is still unclear. However, any advance in therapy for patients with severe HF is important since the mortality and morbidity are still high.

M. D. Cheitlin, MD

References

1. Gheorghiade M, Colucci WS, Swedberg K. Beta-blockers in chronic heart failure. *Circulation*. 2003;107:1570-1575.
2. Udelson JE. Ventricular remodeling in heart failure and the effect of beta-blockade. *Am J Cardiol*. 2004;93:43B-48B.
3. MERIT-HF Study Group. Effect of metoprolol CR/XL in chronic heart failure: Metoprolol CR/XL Randomised Intervention Trial in Congestive Heart Failure (MERIT-HF). *Lancet*. 1999;353:2001-2007.
4. Lechat P, Hulot JS, Escolano S, et al. Heart rate and cardiac rhythm relationships with bisoprolol benefit in chronic heart failure in CIBIS II Trial. *Circulation*. 2001;103:1428-1433.
5. McAlister FA, Wiebe N, Ezekowitz JA, Leung AA, Armstrong PW. Meta-analysis: beta-blocker dose, heart rate reduction, and death in patients with heart failure. *Ann Intern Med*. 2009;150:784-794.
6. Katz AM. The myocardium in congestive heart failure. *Am J Cardiol*. 1989;63:12A-16A.
7. Diaz A, Bourassa MG, Guertin MC, Tardif JC. Long-term prognostic value of resting heart rate in patients with suspected or proven coronary artery disease. *Eur Heart J*. 2005;26:967-974.
8. Wilhelmsen L, Berglund G, Elmfeldt D, et al. The multifactor primary prevention trial in Göteborg Sweden. *Eur Heart J*. 1986;7:279-288.
9. Komajda M, Follath F, Swedberg K, et al. The EuroHeart Failure Survey programme—a survey on the quality of care among patients with heart failure in Europe. Part 2: treatment. *Eur Heart J*. 2003;24:464-474.
10. DiFrancesco D. Funny channels in the control of cardiac rhythm and mode of action of selective blockers. *Pharmacol Res*. 2006;53:399-406.

PDE5 Inhibition With Sildenafil Improves Left Ventricular Diastolic Function, Cardiac Geometry, and Clinical Status in Patients With Stable Systolic Heart Failure: Results of a 1-Year, Prospective, Randomized, Placebo-Controlled Study

Guazzi M, Vicenzi M, Arena R, et al (Univ of Milano, Milan, Italy; Virginia Commonwealth Univ, Richmond)
Circ Heart Fail 4:8-17, 2011

Background.—In heart failure (HF), a defective nitric oxide signaling is involved in left ventricular (LV) diastolic abnormalities and remodeling. PDE5 inhibition, by blocking degradation of nitric oxide second-messenger cyclic guanosine monophosphate, might be beneficial. In a cohort of systolic HF patients, we tested the effects of PDE5 inhibition (sildenafil) on LV ejection fraction, diastolic function, cardiac geometry, and clinical status.

Methods and Results.—Forty-five HF patients (New York Heart Association class II-III) were randomly assigned to placebo or sildenafil (50 mg three times per day) for 1 year, with assessment (6 months and 1 year) of LV ejection fraction, diastolic function, geometry, cardiopulmonary exercise performance, and quality of life. In the sildenafil group only, at 6 months and 1 year, LV ejection fraction, early diastolic tissue Doppler velocities (E') at the mitral lateral (from 4.62 to 5.20

and 5.19 m/s) and septal (from 4.71 to 5.23 and 5.24 m/s) annuli significantly increased, whereas the ratio of early transmitral (E) to E' lateral decreased (from 13.1 to 9.8 to 9.4) ($P<0.01$). Changes were accompanied by a reverse remodeling of left atrial volume index (from 32.0 to 29.0 and 29.1 mL/m^2; $P<0.01$) and LV mass index (from 148.0 to 130.0 and 128.0 g/m^2; $P<0.01$). Furthermore, sildenafil improved exercise performance (peak Vo_2), ventilation efficiency (ventilation to CO_2 production slope), and quality of life ($P<0.01$). Minor adverse effects were noted: flushing in 4 and headache in 2 treated patients.

Conclusions.—Findings confirm that in HF, sildenafil improves functional capacity and clinical status and provide the first human evidence that LV diastolic function and cardiac geometry are additional targets of benefits related to chronic PDE5 inhibition.

▶ Patients with congestive heart failure (HF) have neurohormonal activation and frequently fluid retention, and pharmacotherapy is directed at these targets. There is growing evidence that an abnormal nitric oxide (NO) pathway is involved in a number of pathophysiologic abnormalities in HF,[1] and therefore, overexpressing NO may be a novel therapy. Phosphodiesterase-5 (PDE5) inhibition enhances NO signaling by increasing the cyclic guanosine monophosphate (cGMP) availability, and there are recent clinical studies that tested the possibility that PDE5 inhibitors would be useful in patients with HF.[2] In HF and left-sided pulmonary hypertension, PDE5 is highly expressed in the pulmonary circulation,[3-7] and positive effects of PDE5 inhibition have been demonstrated clinically on functional capacity, exercise ventilation efficiency,[3-7] systemic endothelial function,[8] and quality of life.[5,9] In this randomized, double-blinded, placebo-controlled trial in stable New York Heart Association class II-III patients with systolic HF, year-long treatment with the PDE5 inhibitor sildenafil 50 mg thrice a day significantly improved diastolic function, improved left atrial and ventricular geometry and improved clinical status in patients who were already treated with optimal guideline-recommended medical management.

This study showed for the first time in humans a beneficial effect of chronic PDE5 inhibition on left ventricular diastolic function and left-sided chamber remodeling in patients with HF. The mechanism by which PDE5 inhibition acts in failing hearts is unknown, but certain possibilities are discussed, such as reversing ventricular hypertrophy and fibrosis,[10,11] protecting myocardium from reperfusion injury and apoptosis,[12] and correcting defective cGMP-induced phosphorylation of troponin I that facilitates calcium-independent diastolic cross-bridge cycling and myocardial diastolic stiffening.[13] A number of experimental studies suggest that increasing intracellular cGMP by PDE5 inhibitors affects the biologic properties of myocytes that may block adrenergic, hypertrophic, and proapoptotic signaling.[14] The study was well designed but small, with only 45 HF male patients without diabetes. Further studies are necessary before PDE5 inhibition becomes a class 1 indication in patients with HF.

M. D. Cheitlin, MD

References

1. Saraiva RM, Hare JM. Nitric oxide signaling in the cardiovascular system: implications for heart failure. *Curr Opin Cardiol.* 2006;21:221-228.
2. Guazzi M. Clinical use of phosphodiesterase-5 inhibitors in chronic heart failure. *Circ Heart Fail.* 2008;1:272-280.
3. Guazzi M, Tumminello G, Di Marco F, et al. The effects of phosphodiesterase-5 inhibition with sildenafil on pulmonary hemodynamics and diffusion capacity, exercise ventilatory efficiency, and oxygen uptake kinetics in chronic heart failure. *J Am Coll Cardiol.* 2004;44:2339-2348.
4. Lewis GD, Lachmann J, Camuso J, et al. Sildenafil improves exercise hemodynamics and oxygen uptake in patients with systolic heart failure. *Circulation.* 2007;115:59-66.
5. Guazzi M, Samaja M, Arena R, Vicenzi M, Guazzi MD. Long-term use of sildenafil in the therapeutic management of heart failure. *J Am Coll Cardiol.* 2007;50: 2136-2144.
6. Lewis GD, Shah R, Shahzad K, et al. Sildenafil improves exercise capacity and quality of life in patients with systolic heart failure and secondary pulmonary hypertension. *Circulation.* 2007;116:1555-1562.
7. Behling A, Rohde LE, Colombo FC, Goldraich LA, Stein R, Clausell N. Effects of 5'-phosphodiesterase four-week long inhibition with sildenafil in patients with chronic heart failure: a double-blind, placebo-controlled clinical trial. *J Card Fail.* 2008;14:189-197.
8. Guazzi M, Casali M, Berti F, Rossoni G, Colonna VD, Guazzi MD. Endothelium-mediated modulation of ergoreflex and improvement in exercise ventilation by acute sildenafil in heart failure patients. *Clin Pharmacol Ther.* 2008;83:336-341.
9. Webster LJ, Michelakis ED, Davis T, Archer SL. Use of sildenafil for safe improvement of erectile function and quality of life in men with New York Heart Association classes II and III congestive heart failure: a prospective, placebo-controlled, double-blind crossover trial. *Arch Intern Med.* 2004;164:514-520.
10. Takimoto E, Champion HC, Li M, et al. Chronic inhibition of cyclic GMP phosphodiesterase 5A prevents and reverses cardiac hypertrophy. *Nat Med.* 2005;11: 214-222.
11. Nagayama T, Hsu S, Zhang M, et al. Sildenafil stops progressive chamber, cellular, and molecular remodeling and improves calcium handling and function in hearts with pre-existing advanced hypertrophy caused by pressure overload. *J Am Coll Cardiol.* 2009;53:207-215.
12. Fisher PW, Salloum F, Das A, Hyder H, Kukreja RC. Phosphodiesterase-5 inhibition with sildenafil attenuates cardiomyocyte apoptosis and left ventricular dysfunction in a chronic model of doxorubicin cardiotoxicity. *Circulation.* 2005;111:1601-1610.
13. Paulus WJ, Vantrimpont PJ, Shah AM. Acute effects of nitric oxide on left ventricular relaxation and diastolic distensibility in humans: Assessment by bicoronary sodium nitroprusside infusion. *Circulation.* 1994;89:2070-2078.
14. Kass DA, Champion HC, Beavo JA. Phosphodiesterase type 5: expanding roles in cardiovascular regulation. *Circ Res.* 2007;101:1084-1095.

Spironolactone use at discharge was associated with improved survival in hospitalized patients with systolic heart failure

Hamaguchi S, Kinugawa S, Tsuchihashi-Makaya M, et al (Hokkaido Univ Graduate School of Medicine, Sapporo, Japan)
Am Heart J 160:1156-1162, 2010

Background.—The RALES trial demonstrated that spironolactone improved the prognosis of patients with heart failure (HF). However, it is unknown whether the discharge use of spironolactone is associated with better long-term outcomes among hospitalized systolic HF patients in routine clinical practice. We examined the effects of spironolactone use at discharge on mortality and rehospitalization by comparing with outcomes in patients who did not receive spironolactone.

Methods.—The JCARE-CARD studied prospectively the characteristics and treatments in a broad sample of patients hospitalized with worsening HF and the outcomes were followed with an average of 2.2 years of follow-up.

Results.—A total of 946 patients had HF with reduced left ventricular ejection fraction (LVEF) (<40%), among whom spironolactone was prescribed at discharge in 435 patients (46%), but not in 511 patients (54%). The mean age was 66.3 years and 72.2% were male. Etiology was ischemic in 39.7% and mean LVEF was 27.1%. After adjustment for covariates, discharge use of spironolactone was associated with a significant reduction in all-cause death (adjusted hazard ratio 0.612, $P = .020$) and cardiac death (adjusted hazard ratio 0.524, $P = .013$).

Conclusions.—Among patients with HF hospitalized for systolic dysfunction, spironolactone use at the time of discharge was associated with long-term survival benefit. These findings provide further support for the idea that spironolactone may be useful in patients hospitalized with HF and reduced LVEF (Fig 1).

▶ The treatment of patients with congestive heart failure (CHF) has markedly improved survival with the addition of β-blockers, angiotensin-converting enzyme inhibitors (ACEI), and angiotensin II receptor blockers and the addition of aldosterone blockade. Because aldosterone plays an important role in the progression of CHF by inducing vascular damage, myocardial hypertrophy, and fibrosis,[1-3] aldosterone antagonism by spironolactone and eplerenone, a selective aldosterone antagonist with fewer side effects than spironolactone, was an important advance in that both the Randomized Aldosterone Evaluation Study (RALES) and Eplerenone Post-Acute Myocardial Infarction Heart Failure Efficacy and Survival Study (EPHESUS) showed a significant decrease in mortality and morbidity in patients with systolic dysfunction CHF when added to β-blockers and ACEI.[4,5] Both the current American College of Cardiology/American Heart Association and European Society of Cardiology guidelines recommend spironolactone in patients with CHF, a reduced left ventricular ejection fraction (LVEF), and symptoms in spite of β-blockers, ACEI, and diuretics.[6,7] However, both these trials, like most randomized placebo-controlled trials, had a strictly limited inclusion population. The RALES trial included patients with New York Heart Association class III to IV symptoms with LVEF ≤ 35%. Further, they excluded patients with serum creatinine > 2.5 mg/dL and only 10% were taking a β-blocker. The CHF population taking aldosterone antagonists at present are older, are less symptomatic, and some have serum creatinine > 2.5 mg/dL. Therefore, it is not clear that spironolactone will have the same beneficial effect in these patients as in those in the controlled trials. The importance of this study is that unselected patients with CHF and an LVEF < 40% were divided into those taking

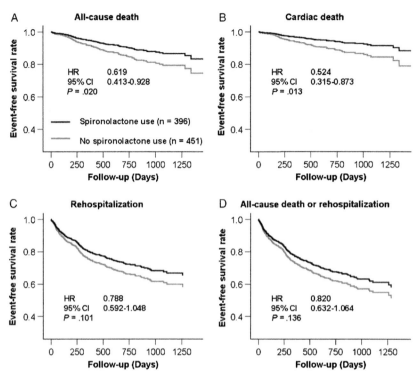

FIGURE 1.—Kaplan-Meier survival curves free from all-cause death (**A**), cardiac death (**B**), rehospitalization due to worsening HF (**C**), and all-cause death or rehospitalization (**D**) in hospitalized patients with spironolactone use (black lines, n = 396) versus no spironolactone use (red lines, n = 451) at discharge. For interpretation of the references to color in this figure legend, the reader is referred to web version of this article. (Reprinted from Hamaguchi S, Kinugawa S, Tsuchihashi-Makaya M, et al. Spironolactone use at discharge was associated with improved survival in hospitalized patients with systolic heart failure. *Am Heart J*. 2010;160:1156-1162, with permission from Mosby, Inc.)

and not taking spironolactone on hospital discharge, and it was found that spironolactone was associated with a 48% reduction in the risk for cardiac death when followed up for 2.2 years. There are a number of possible reasons that aldosterone antagonists could be beneficial. Spironolactone could induce reversed left ventricular (LV) remodeling,[8] improving LV function and exercise tolerance,[9] decrease cardiac fibrosis,[10] and improve endothelial function in asymptomatic or mildly symptomatic patients when added to optimal treatment including β-blockers.[11] This study therefore suggests that the beneficial effects of aldosterone antagonists seen in the RALES and EMPHSUS trials extend to a more unselected population of patients with systolic dysfunction CHF.

M. D. Cheitlin, MD

References

1. Rocha R, Rudolph AE, Frierdich GE, et al. Aldosterone induces a vascular inflammatory phenotype in the rat heart. *Am J Physiol Heart Circ Physiol*. 2002;283:H1802-H1810.

2. Schunkert H, Hense HW, Muscholl M, et al. Associations between circulating components of the renin-angiotensin-aldosterone system and left ventricular mass. *Heart.* 1997;77:24-31.

3. Weber KT, Brilla CG. Pathological hypertrophy and cardiac interstitium. Fibrosis and renin-angiotensin-aldosterone system. *Circulation.* 1991;83:1849-1865.

4. Pitt B, Zannad F, Remme WJ, et al. The effect of spironolactone on morbidity and mortality in patients with severe heart failure. Randomized Aldactone Evaluation Study Investigators. *N Engl J Med.* 1999;341:709-717.

5. Pitt B, Remme W, Zannad F, et al. Eplerenone, a selective aldosterone blocker, in patients with left ventricular dysfunction after myocardial infarction. *N Engl J Med.* 2003;348:1309-1321.

6. Hunt SA, Abraham WT, Chin MH, et al. ACC/AHA 2005 Guideline Update for the Diagnosis and Management of Chronic Heart Failure in the Adult: a report of the American College of Cardiology/American Heart Association Task Force on Practice Guidelines (Writing Committee to Update the 2001 Guidelines for the Evaluation and Management of Heart Failure): developed in collaboration with the American College of Chest Physicians and the International Society for Heart and Lung Transplantation: endorsed by the Heart Rhythm Society. *Circulation.* 2005;112:e154-235.

7. Dickstein K, Cohen-Solal A, Filippatos G, et al. ESC guidelines for the diagnosis and treatment of acute and chronic heart failure 2008: the Task Force for the Diagnosis and Treatment of Acute and Chronic Heart Failure 2008 of the European Society of Cardiology. Developed in collaboration with the Heart Failure Association of the ESC (HFA) and endorsed by the European Society of Intensive Care Medicine (ESICM). *Eur Heart J.* 2008;29:2388-2442.

8. Chan AK, Sanderson JE, Wang T, et al. Aldosterone receptor antagonism induces reverse remodeling when added to angiotensin receptor blockade in chronic heart failure. *J Am Coll Cardiol.* 2007;50:591-596.

9. Cicoira M, Zanolla L, Rossi A, et al. Long-term, dose-dependent effects of spironolactone on left ventricular function and exercise tolerance in patients with chronic heart failure. *J Am Coll Cardiol.* 2002;40:304-310.

10. Zannad F, Alla F, Dousset B, Perez A, Pitt B. Limitation of excessive extracellular matrix turnover may contribute to survival benefit of spironolactone therapy in patients with congestive heart failure: insights from the randomized aldactone evaluation study (RALES). Rales Investigators. *Circulation.* 2000;102:2700-2706.

11. Macdonald JE, Kennedy N, Struthers AD. Effects of spironolactone on endothelial function, vascular angiotensin converting enzyme activity, and other prognostic markers in patients with mild heart failure already taking optimal treatment. *Heart.* 2004;90:765-770.

How often we need to measure brain natriuretic peptide (BNP) blood levels in patients admitted to the hospital for acute severe heart failure? Role of serial measurements to improve short-term prognostic stratification

Faggiano P, Valle R, Aspromonte N, et al (Spedali Civili and Univ of Brescia, Italy; Ospedale Civile, San Donà di Piave, Italy; Ospedale Santo Spirito, Rome, Italy; et al)
Int J Cardiol 140:88-94, 2010

Background.—Brain natriuretic peptide (BNP) is increasingly used in the management of patients with heart failure (HF). It is still unclear how to use serial BNP measurement in HF.

Aim.—To evaluate the usefulness of three consecutive measurements of BNP in patients (pts) hospitalized for acute HF.

Methods.—Clinical evaluation, BNP levels and echocardiography were assessed in 150 pts (67% males, age: 69 ± 12 years; left ventricular ejection fraction: 34 ± 14%) admitted for severe HF (NYHA class III—IV: 146/150). BNP measurements were obtained: at admission (basal, T0), at discharge (T1) and at first ambulatory control (T2), after optimization of medical therapy in those with discharge BNP level >250 pg/mL. Endpoints were death and hospital readmission during 6-month follow-up.

Results.—According to BNP levels 3 groups of patients were identified: Group 1 (62 pts, 41%), in whom discharge (T1) BNP was high and persisted elevated at T2 despite aggressive medical therapy; at 6-month follow-up 72% died or were hospitalized for HF. Group 2 (36 pts, 24%), in whom discharge (T1) BNP was high but decreased after medical therapy (T2); death and HF-readmission were observed in 8 pts (26%). Group 3 (52 pts, 35%), in whom discharge (T1) BNP levels were <250 pg/mL and persisted below this value at T2; death and HF-hospital readmission were observed in 6 pts (12%). Event rate differences among groups were statistically significant ($p<0.001$). At Cox-analysis discharge BNP cutoff of 250 pg/mL was the only parameter predictive of a worse outcome.

Conclusion.—These data suggest that 3 BNP measurements, at admission, at discharge and few weeks later can allow to identify HF pts whom, despite a further potentiation of medical therapy, will present a worsening or even will die during short-term follow-up (Figs 1 and 2, Table 2).

▶ Patients admitted with worsening severe heart failure (HF) continue to have a high mortality in the range of 50% and a high readmission rate of 30%.[1] B-type natriuretic peptide (BNP), a cardiac hormone released primarily from the left ventricle (LV) in response to a pressure or volume overload, is known to reflect the level of neurohormonal activation, with a lower BNP predicting

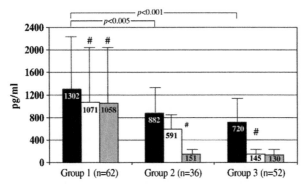

FIGURE 1.—Behaviour of BNP serum levels at hospital admission (T0), hospital discharge (T1) and first ambulatory visit (T2) in the three groups. *p* refers to Oneway ANOVA and post-hoc Tukey test. #*p*<0.001 Kruskall—Wallis ANOVA for repeated measures. (Reprinted from Faggiano P, Valle R, Aspromonte N, et al. How often we need to measure brain natriuretic peptide (BNP) blood levels in patients admitted to the hospital for acute severe heart failure? Role of serial measurements to improve short-term prognostic stratification. *Int J Cardiol.* 2010;140:88-94, with permission from Elsevier Ireland Ltd.)

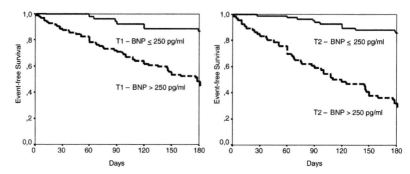

FIGURE 2.—Kaplan—Meier curves showing the cumulative incidence of death and readmission according to BNP levels in the study population. *Left*, BNP values obtained at discharge (T1); *right*, BNP values obtained at the first ambulatory control (T2). Tarone—Ware's test <0.001 for all the comparisons. (Reprinted from Faggiano P, Valle R, Aspromonte N, et al. How often we need to measure brain natriuretic peptide (BNP) blood levels in patients admitted to the hospital for acute severe heart failure? Role of serial measurements to improve short-term prognostic stratification. *Int J Cardiol.* 2010;140: 88-94, with permission from Elsevier Ireland Ltd.)

TABLE 2.—Six-Month Outcome in the Three Groups of Patients Identified According to the Behaviour of Serum BNP Levels

	Hospitalization	Mortality
Group 1 (n=62)	15 (24%)*	30 (48%)*
Group 2 (n=36)	3 (8%)	5 (18%)
Group 3 (n=52)	1 (2%)	5 (10%)

*p<0.001 versus Group 2 and Group 3. Pearson Chi Square test.

a better short- and long-term outcome.[2,3] Although there have been a number of reports of the prognostic value of serial measurements of BNP in patients with HF,[4-6] the ideal number and timing of BNP measurements have not been well defined. This study prospectively defined 3 measurements of BNP in patients admitted with severe HF (New York Heart Association [NYHA] class III-IV). The first measurement was at the time of admission, the second at the time of discharge when the patient has clinically improved after optimal medical management, and the third at the first ambulatory visit at a mean of 20±5 days. The etiology of the HF was chronic ischemic heart disease in half, dilated cardiomyopathy in a quarter, and hypertension in another quarter. With optimal medical management, the authors were able to achieve a reduction in BNP to <250 pg/mL in 35% at the time of discharge and another 24% at the first ambulatory visit. In a Cox regression analysis using a discharge BNP cutoff of 250 pg/mL, the hazard ratio of a BNP greater than or equal to 250 pg/mL was 4.5 compared with 1.8 for NYHA class. These were the only statistically significant predictors of death or rehospitalization for worsening HF at 6 months, including echocardiographic restrictive pattern, LV ejection fraction, and serum creatinine. Recently, Jourdain and colleagues[7] reported that in patients with stable HF, the strategy of medical management to a BNP of

<100 pg/mL was associated with a low death and rehospitalization rate compared with conventional management. Because all the patients were discharged at the time when clinical improvement had occurred on optimal medical management, these data support the concept that medical management pushed to achieve a BNP <250 pg/mL before discharge would be preferable to discharge on the basis of symptom improvement alone.

M. D. Cheitlin, MD

References

1. Cleland JG, Swedberg K, Follath F, et al. The EuroHeart Failure survey programme— a survey on the quality of care among patients with heart failure in Europe. Part 1: patient characteristics and diagnosis. *Eur Heart J.* 2003;24:442-463.
2. Kazanegra R, Cheng V, Garcia A, et al. A rapid test for B-type natriuretic peptide correlates with falling wedge pressures in patients treated for decompensated heart failure: a pilot study. *J Card Fail.* 2001;7:21-29.
3. Feola M, Aspromonte N, Canali C, et al. Prognostic value of plasma brain natriuretic peptide, urea nitrogen and creatinine in outpatients > 70 years of age with heart failure. *Am J Cardiol.* 2005;96:705-709.
4. Logeart D, Thabut G, Jourdain P, et al. Predischarge B-type natriuretic peptide assay for identifying patients at high risk of re-admission after decompensated heart failure. *J Am Coll Card.* 2004;43:635-641.
5. O'Brien RJ, Squire IB, Demme B, Davies JE, Ng LL. Pre-discharge, but not admission, levels of NT-proBNP predict adverse prognosis following acute LVF. *Eur J Heart Fail.* 2003;5:499-506.
6. Bettencourt P, Azevedo A, Pimenta J, Friões F, Ferreira S, Ferreira A. N-terminal-pro-brain natriuretic peptide predicts outcome after hospital discharge in heart failure patients. *Circulation.* 2004;110:2168-2174.
7. Jourdain P, Jondeau G, Fucnk F, et al. Plasma natriuretic peptide-guided therapy to improve outcome in heart failure: the STARS-BNP Multicenter Study. *J Am Coll Cardiol.* 2007;49:1733-1739.

N-Terminal Pro–B-Type Natriuretic Peptide–Guided, Intensive Patient Management in Addition to Multidisciplinary Care in Chronic Heart Failure: A 3-Arm, Prospective, Randomized Pilot Study

Berger R, Moertl D, Peter S, et al (Med Univ of Vienna, Austria; et al)
J Am Coll Cardiol 55:645-653, 2010

Objectives.—This study was designed to investigate whether the addition of N-terminal pro–B-type natriuretic peptide–guided, intensive patient management (BM) to multidisciplinary care (MC) improves outcome in patients following hospitalization due to heart failure (HF).

Background.—Patients hospitalized due to HF experience frequent rehospitalizations and high mortality.

Methods.—Patients hospitalized due to HF were randomized to BM, MC, or usual care (UC). Multidisciplinary care included 2 consultations from an HF specialist who provided therapeutic recommendations and home care by a specialized HF nurse. In addition, BM included intensified up-titration of medication by HF specialists in high-risk patients. NT-proBNP was used to define the level of risk and to monitor wall stress.

This monitoring allowed for anticipation of cardiac decompensation and adjustment of medication in advance.

Results.—A total of 278 patients were randomized in 8 Viennese hospitals. After 12 months, the BM group had the highest proportion of antineurohormonal triple-therapy (difference among all groups). Accordingly, BM reduced days of HF hospitalization (488 days) compared with the hospitalization for the MC (1,254 days) and UC (1,588 days) groups ($p < 0.0001$; significant differences among all groups). Using Kaplan-Meier analysis, the first HF rehospitalization (28%) was lower in the BM versus MC groups (40%; $p = 0.06$) and the MC versus UC groups (61%; $p = 0.01$). Moreover, the combined end point of death or HF rehospitalization was lower in the BM (37%) than in the MC group (50%; $p < 0.05$) and in the MC than in the UC group (65%; $p = 0.04$). Death rate was similar between the BM (22%) and MC groups (22%), but was lower compared with the UC group (39%; vs. BM: $p < 0.02$; vs. MC: $p < 0.02$).

Conclusions.—Compared with MC alone, additional BM improves clinical outcome in patients after HF hospitalization. (BNP Guided Care in Addition to Multidisciplinary Care; NCT00355017) (Figs 3 and 4).

▶ Hospitalized patients with congestive heart failure (CHF) after discharge in spite of advances in management have a rehospitalization rate of about 30% within 1 to 2 months and mortality within this time of about 10%.[1] Various attempts to improve these statistics have been tried, such as development of heart failure clinics, involvement of specialized CHF nurses, computer programs that provide 2-way frequent communication between health care workers and individual patients, and concentration of specialized care on patients at the highest risk as determined by monitoring natriuretic peptides (NPs).[2-5] The

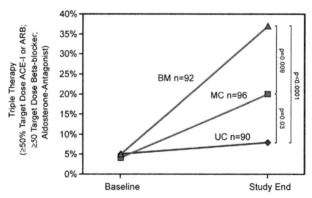

FIGURE 3.—Effect of UC, MC, and BM on Heart Failure Therapy. The proportion of triple therapy (spironolactone and ≥50% of the target dose of an angiotensin-converting enzyme inhibitor/angiotensin receptor blocker and of a beta-blocker) was similar among groups at baseline, but was higher in the BM group versus the MC group, and higher in the MC versus the usual care (UC) group at follow-up. Abbreviations as in Figure 1. (Reprinted from Berger R, Moertl D, Peter S, et al. N-terminal pro–B-type natriuretic peptide–guided, intensive patient management in addition to multidisciplinary care in chronic heart failure: a 3-arm, prospective, randomized pilot study. *J Am Coll Cardiol.* 2010;55:645-653, with permission from the American College of Cardiology Foundation.)

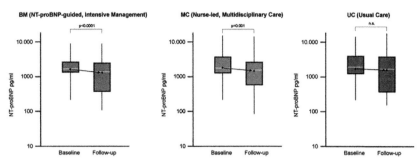

FIGURE 4.—Baseline and Follow-Up Values of NT-ProBNP. Box plot with mean [+], median, lower and upper quartiles, and 95% confidence intervals: the decrease of NT-proBNP levels from discharge to follow-up was more pronounced in the BM group than in the MC group. No decrease was observed in the UC group. Abbreviations as in Figures 1 and 3. (Reprinted from Berger R, Moertl D, Peter S, et al. N-terminal pro—B-type natriuretic peptide—guided, intensive patient management in addition to multidisciplinary care in chronic heart failure: a 3-arm, prospective, randomized pilot study. *J Am Coll Cardiol.* 2010;55:645-653, with permission from the American College of Cardiology Foundation.)

concept is that with periodic outpatient monitoring, clinical deterioration such as increasing symptoms or weight gain can be detected early and appropriate response made, such as increasing diuretics and adding or titrating upward neurohormonal antagonists, either with or without a physician visit. In contrast to monitoring the patient for increasing symptoms, *N*-terminal pro-B-type natriuretic peptide (NTproBNP) is an objective prognostic biomarker that predicts survival better than traditional prognostic indicators in CHF.[6] Studies show that patients with a high risk for rehospitalization for and death from CHF can be identified by assessing levels of serum NP at discharge.[7,8] NPs have also been shown to detect short-term improvement or deterioration in high-risk patients being followed for CHF[9] in that changes in serum levels parallel changes in left ventricular wall stress. This study is the first to use the prognostic power of measuring discharged NP for individualized postdischarge management. The end points in this study were rehospitalization, time to reach the combined end point of death and CHF rehospitalization, and death. Patients managed by nurse-led multidisciplinary care (MC) guided by NTproBNP levels when compared with MC alone had a higher proportion of patients on antineurohormonal triple therapy, more frequent diuretic adjustments, a more pronounced decrease in BNP levels, and an improved clinical outcome. The MC group did better than the usual care patients. This is the first study showing the incremental value of adding NP level monitoring to MC in identifying high-risk patients with CHF and customizing the frequency and intensity of appropriate therapy.

M. D. Cheitlin, MD

References

1. Fonarow GC, Abraham WT, Albert NM, et al. Association between performance measures and clinical outcomes for patients hospitalized with heart failure. *JAMA.* 2007;297:61-70.

2. McAlister FA, Stewart S, Ferrua S, McMurray JJV. Multidisciplinary strategies for the management of heart failure patients at high risk for admission: a systematic review of randomized trials. *J Am Coll Cardiol.* 2004;44:810-819.
3. Blue L, McMurray J. How much responsibility should heart failure nurses take? *Eur J Heart Fail.* 2005;7:351-361.
4. West JA, Miller NH, Parker KM, et al. A comprehensive management system for heart failure improves clinical outcomes and reduces medical resource utilization. *Am J Cardiol.* 1997;79:58-63.
5. Klersy C, De Silvestri A, Gabutti G, Regoli F, Auricchio A. A meta-analysis of remote monitoring of heart failure patients. *J Am Coll Cardiol.* 2009;54: 1683-1694.
6. Berger R, Huelsman M, Strecker K, et al. B-type natriuretic peptide predicts sudden death in patients with chronic heart failure. *Circulation.* 2002;105: 2392-2397.
7. Logeart D, Thabut G, Jourdain P, et al. Predischarge B-type natriuretic peptide assay for identifying patients at high risk of re-admission after decompensated heart failure. *J Am Coll Cardiol.* 2004;43:635-641.
8. Cheng V, Kazanagra R, Garcia A, et al. A rapid bedside test for B-type peptide predicts treatment outcomes in patients admitted for decompensated heart failure: a pilot study. *J Am Coll Cardiol.* 2001;37:386-391.
9. Moertl D, Hammer A, Huelsmann M, Pacher R, Berger R. Prognostic value of sequential measurements of amino-terminal prohormone of B-type natriuretic peptide in ambulatory heart failure patients. *Eur J Heart Fail.* 2008;10:404-411.

Improved Outcomes With Early Collaborative Care of Ambulatory Heart Failure Patients Discharged From the Emergency Department

Lee DS, Stukel TA, Austin PC, et al (Inst for Clinical Evaluative Sciences, Toronto, Ontario, Canada)
Circulation 122:1806-1814, 2010

Background.—The type of outpatient physician care after an emergency department visit for heart failure may affect patients' outcomes.

Methods and Results.—Using the National Ambulatory Care Reporting System, we examined the care and outcomes of heart failure patients who visited and were discharged from the emergency department in Ontario, Canada (April 2004 to March 2007). Early collaborative care by a cardiologist and primary care (PC) physician within 30 days after discharge was compared with PC alone. Care for 10 599 patients (age, 74.9 ± 11.9 years; 50.2% male) was provided by PC alone (n=6596), cardiologist alone (n=535), or concurrently by both cardiologist and PC (n=1478); 1990 did not visit a physician. Collaborative care patients were more likely to undergo assessment of left ventricular function (57.4% versus 28.7%), noninvasive stress testing (20.1% versus 7.8%), and cardiac catheterization (11.6% versus 2.7%) compared with PC. Drug prescriptions (patients ≥65 years of age) demonstrated higher use of angiotensin-converting enzyme inhibitors (58.8% versus 54.6%), angiotensin receptor blockers (22.7% versus 18.1%), β-adrenoceptor antagonists (63.4% versus 48.0%), loop diuretics (84.2% versus 79.6%), metolazone (4.8% versus 3.4%), and spironolactone (19.8% versus 12.7%) within 100 days after emergency department discharge for collaborative care compared with

PC. In a propensity-matched model, mortality was lower with PC compared with no physician visit (hazard ratio, 0.75; 95% confidence interval, 0.64 to 0.87; *P*<0.001). Collaborative care reduced mortality compared with PC (hazard ratio, 0.79; 95% confidence interval, 0.63 to 1.00; *P*=0.045). Sole cardiology care conferred a trend to increased mortality (hazard ratio, 1.41 versus collaborative care; 95% confidence interval, 0.98 to 2.03; *P*=0.067).

Conclusions.—Early collaborative heart failure care was associated with increased use of drug therapies and cardiovascular diagnostic tests and better outcomes compared with PC alone.

▶ Heart failure (HF) is a major contributor to the rising cost of health care with most costs attributable to care in the emergency department (ED) and hospitalizations.[1] Patients with HF are frequently seen first in the ED. If they are hospitalized, they receive rapid treatment, and on discharge, arrangements are made for follow-up. If ambulatory patients are deemed low risk and discharged home from the ED, the care they receive as an outpatient is decided largely by the primary care physician (PCP), who is the gatekeeper of referral to specialists. Follow-up may be by a PCP, a cardiologist, or both concurrently. However, some receive no early physician follow-up at all. The impact of shared care in patients with HF is a source of debate, with some studies finding that patients receiving concurrent care by PCP and cardiologist after an acute myocardial infarction have lower mortality rates than those treated by either alone.[2] Others find that shared care in patients with HF involves a trade-off between lower mortality and higher hospitalization rates[3] or that there is no advantage to being followed by a cardiologist over a PCP.[4]

This study is a population-based study of patients with HF, who were seen in and discharged from the ED, examining the type of physician care received within a month after discharge. Those receiving collaborative care of a PCP and cardiologist within 30 days of discharge had a lower death rate, had lower repeat ED visits and rehospitalizations, were more likely to have important diagnostic tests (both for cardiac functional assessment and evaluation of the extent of myocardial ischemia), were more likely to have coronary revascularization, and received more evidence-based drugs than those followed by a PCP alone.

These improved outcomes are likely at least in part because of improved care resulting from knowledge of the importance of pathophysiology, targeted diagnostic tests, and pharmacotherapy for patients with HF among cardiologists.[5] Unfortunately, a large proportion of patients with HF discharged from the ED received no physician follow-up, and these patients had the greatest risk of death and adverse events. The study cohort by design had not been hospitalized, had survived the initial month(s) after discharge when the increased risk of adverse events occurs,[6,7] and therefore represented a milder spectrum of patients with HF.

The implications of the study are that patients with HF, considered to be low risk enough to be discharged from the ED, are at risk of death and serious morbidity and should require early follow-up. Furthermore, early collaborative physician involvement can lead to improved outcomes and a substantial decrease in morbidity and mortality.

M. D. Cheitlin, MD

References

1. Rydén-Bergsten T, Andersson F. The health care costs of heart failure in Sweden. *J Intern Med.* 1999;246:275-284.
2. Ayanian JZ, Landrum MB, Guadagnoli E, Gaccione P. Specialty of ambulatory care physicians and mortality among elderly patients after myocardial infarction. *N Engl J Med.* 2002;347:1678-1686.
3. Ezekowitz JA, van Walraven C, McAlister FA, Armstrong PW, Kaul P. Impact of specialist follow-up in outpatients with congestive heart failure. *CMAJ.* 2005; 172:189-194.
4. Franciosa JA, Massie BM, Lukas MA, et al. Beta-blocker therapy for heart failure outside the clinical trial setting: findings of a community-based registry. *Am Heart J.* 2004;148:718-726.
5. Baker DW, Hayes RP, Massie BM, Craig CA. Variations in family physicians' and cardiologists' care for patients with heart failure. *Am Heart J.* 1999;138:826-834.
6. Solomon SD, Dobson J, Pocock S, et al. Influence of nonfatal hospitalization for heart failure on subsequent mortality in patients with chronic heart failure. *Circulation.* 2007;116:1482-1487.
7. Lee DS, Schull MJ, Alter DA, et al. Early deaths in patients with heart failure discharged from the emergency department: a population-based analysis. *Circ Heart Fail.* 2010;3:228-235.

Novel strategies in diastolic heart failure

Paulus WJ (VU Univ Med Ctr Amsterdam, The Netherlands)
Heart 96:1147-1153, 2010

The diagnosis of diastolic heart failure (DHF) is based on the presence of a triad consisting of signs or symptoms of congestive heart failure, a normal left ventricular (LV) systolic function, and evidence of diastolic LV dysfunction. As diastolic LV dysfunction is not unique to DHF but also occurs in patients with heart failure and reduced LV systolic function (ie, systolic heart failure), DHF is often referred to as heart failure with normal LV ejection fraction (EF) (HFNEF)[w1] or heart failure with preserved LVEF (HFPEF).[w2] DHF currently accounts for more than 50% of all heart failure cases in western societies. Although prognosis of patients with DHF was initially perceived as superior to patients with systolic heart failure (SHF), recent evidence shows prognosis to be equally poor in both conditions. Furthermore, whereas the prognosis of patients with SHF has improved over the last two decades as a result of modern heart failure treatment, the prognosis of patients with DHF has not improved notably over the same time period. This review will focus on current diagnostic and therapeutic strategies for DHF (Figs 1 and 3).

▶ This article is a scholarly extensive review of the numerous therapeutic trials of patients with diastolic heart failure (DHF). Paulus reviews the diagnostic

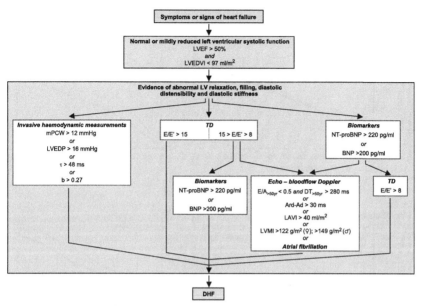

FIGURE 1.—Flowchart for the diagnosis of diastolic heart failure (DHF). LVEDVI, left ventricular end-diastolic volume index; mPCW, mean pulmonary capillary wedge pressure; LVEDP, left ventricular end-diastolic pressure; τ, time constant of left ventricular relaxation; b, constant of left ventricular chamber stiffness; TD, tissue Doppler; E, early mitral valve flow velocity; E', early TD lengthening velocity; NT-proBNP, N-terminal pro-brain natriuretic peptide; BNP, brain natriuretic peptide; E/A, ratio of early (E) to late (A) mitral valve flow velocity; DT, deceleration time; LVMI, left ventricular mass index; LAVI, left atrial volume index; Ard, duration of reverse pulmonary vein atrial systole flow; Ad, duration of mitral valve atrial wave flow. Reproduced with permission from Paulus *et al.*[1] *Editor's Note:* Please refer to original journal article for full references. (Reprinted from Paulus WJ. Novel strategies in diastolic heart failure. *Heart.* 2010;96:1147-1153, with permission from the BMJ Publishing Group Ltd.)

criteria in each of the randomized placebo-controlled trials that involved angiotensin converting enzyme inhibitors, angiotensin II type 1 receptor blockers, β-blockers, aldosterone antagonists, and statins. Almost without exception, there was no survival benefit in patients with DHF with any of these agents, except in 1 trial with statins.[1]

Many of these trials did not have as part of the diagnostic criteria for DHF any evidence for diastolic dysfunction, only requiring heart failure symptoms, and a normal left ventricular ejection fraction (LVEF). In many of the trials, a symptomatic patient with an LVEF > 35% or 40% was accepted as a criterion for DHF, when others would call him/her a patient with systolic heart failure (SHF). These differences could account for the discrepant findings concerning the effectiveness of drug therapy in patients with DHF. Also reviewed are the pathophysiologic differences between SHF and DHF, with SHF having eccentric hypertrophy and reduced systolic function, whereas patients with DHF have concentric hypertrophy, frequently with hypertension, diabetes, and/or obesity, as well as a normal LVEF and echocardiographic evidence of diastolic dysfunction. The author concludes that because of the discordant outcome of similar drug therapy in SHF and DHF, the evidence is consistent with different signal

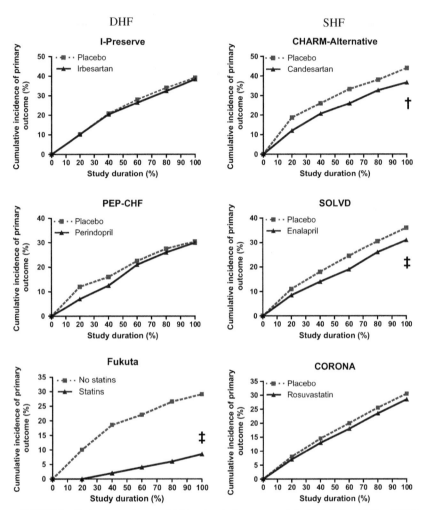

FIGURE 3.—Contrasting outcomes of trials using similar compounds in diastolic heart failure (DHF) and systolic heart failure (SHF). For both angiotensin II receptor blocker (ARB) and angiotensin converting enzyme inhibitor (ACEI), a neutral outcome is observed in DHF[11][14] but a positive outcome in SHF.[10][w31] Conversely, for statins, a positive outcome is observed in DHF[19] but a neutral outcome in SHF.[w30] †p<0.0001; ‡p<0.01. *Editor's Note:* Please refer to original journal article for full references. (Reprinted from Paulus WJ. Novel strategies in diastolic heart failure. *Heart.* 2010;96:1147-1153, with permission from the BMJ Publishing Group Ltd.)

transduction cascades promoting myocardial remodeling in both conditions and that specific DHF therapy should be designed to address the structural and functional abnormalities[2] characteristically seen in DHF, including cardiomyocyte hypertrophy, cardiomyocyte stiffness, and a shift in myocardial metabolism from glucose to free fatty acids because of frequent comorbidities, such as type 2 diabetes and metabolic syndrome. Finally, the same author has written a similar article[3] describing in more detail the pathophysiologic differences between SHF and DHF that result in the positive outcomes in SHF and the neutral responses in DHF to drug therapy.

M. D. Cheitlin, MD

References

1. Fukata H, Sane DC, Brucks S, Little WC. Statin therapy may be associated with lower mortality in patients with diastolic heart failure: a preliminary report. *Circulation.* 2005;112:357-363.
2. van Heerebeek L, Borbély A, Niessen HW, et al. Myocardial structure and function differ in systolic and diastolic heart failure. *Circulation.* 2006;113:1966-1973.
3. Paulus WJ, van Ballegoij JJ. Treatment of heart failure with normal ejection fraction: an inconvenient truth. *J Am Coll Cardiol.* 2010;55:526-537.

Pathogenesis and Prognosis

Concordant Versus Discordant Left Bundle Branch Block in Heart Failure Patients: Novel Clinical Value of an Old Electrocardiographic Diagnosis

Padeletti L, Valleggi A, Vergaro G, et al (Univ of Florence, Italy; Fondazione Gabriele Monasterio CNR-Regione Toscana, Pisa, Italy; et al)

J Card Fail 16:320-326, 2010

Background.—Over the last 50 years left bundle branch block (LBBB) has been defined as homophasic (concordant: cLBBB) or heterophasic (discordant: dLBBB) when associated with a positive or negative T wave in leads I and V5-V6, respectively. LBBB is recognized as an adverse prognostic factor in heart failure (HF). The prevalence and clinical significance of cLBBB and dLBBB in HF patients are unknown.

Methods and Results.—A total of 897 consecutive systolic HF patients (age 65 ± 13 years, left ventricular ejection fraction [LVEF], $34 \pm 10\%$) underwent clinical characterization, electrocardiographic evaluation for LBBB diagnosis and classification, and follow-up for cardiac events (median 37 months, range 1-84). LBBB was diagnosed in 232 patients (26%), cLBBB in 71 (31%), and dLBBB in 161 (69%). The dLBBB patients were older than those with cLBBB, and presented with lower LVEF, greater left ventricular telediastolic diameter and left ventricular mass index, higher level of brain natriuretic peptide, N-terminal probrain natriuretic peptide, renin activity, and norepinephrine (all $P < .05$). At Kaplan-Meier analysis, LBBB ($P = .003$) and dLBBB ($P = .036$) were associated with a worse prognosis when the composite end point of sudden death and implantable cardioverter defibrillator shock was considered.

Conclusions.—In systolic HF, dLBBB is associated with a worse clinical, neurohormonal, and prognostic profile. LBBB classification could represent a useful tool in routine clinical evaluation (Figs 2 and 3).

▶ It is always interesting to find new value in old noninvasive technology. Left bundle branch block (LBBB) is known to predict an adverse prognosis in patients with heart failure (HF).[1,2] This study explored whether an observation

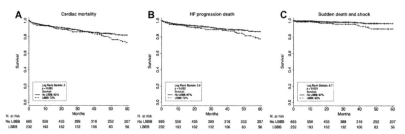

FIGURE 2.—Left bundle branch block (LBBB) and survival. Kaplan-Meier survival plot in heart failure (HF) patients with LBBB compared with patients without LBBB, as concerns the end point of cardiac death (A), of death from HF progression (B), and the composite end point of sudden death and life-threatening ventricular tachyarrhythmia requiring cardioverter-defibrillator shock (C). (Reprinted from Padeletti L, Valleggi A, Vergaro G, et al. Concordant versus discordant left bundle branch block in heart failure patients: novel clinical value of an old electrocardiographic diagnosis. *J Card Fail.* 2010;16:320-326, with permission from Elsevier.)

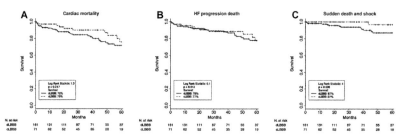

FIGURE 3.—Discordant versus concordant left bundle branch block (LBBB) and survival in heart failure. Kaplan-Meier survival plot in heart failure (HF) patients with discordant left bundle branch block compared with patients without concordant LBBB (cLBBB), as concerns the end point of cardiac death (A), of death from HF progression (B), and the composite end point of sudden death and life-threatening ventricular tachyarrhythmia requiring cardioverter-defibrillator shock (C). dLBBB = discordant LBBB; cLBBB = concordant LBBB. (Reprinted from Padeletti L, Valleggi A, Vergaro G, et al. Concordant versus discordant left bundle branch block in heart failure patients: novel clinical value of an old electrocardiographic diagnosis. *J Card Fail.* 2010;16:320-326, with permission from Elsevier.)

made years ago, that (LBBB) had 2 variations depending on whether the T waves in leads I and V5 or V6 are positive, called concordant LBBB (cLBBB), or negative, called discordant LBBB (dLBBB), had any prognostic significance in patients with HF. The authors found that patients with systolic HF and dLBBB had a higher incidence than those with cLBBB of the composite end point of sudden death and implantable cardioverter defibrillator shock. LBBB-related dyssynchrony in patients with HF promotes neurohormonal activation and left ventricular (LV) remodeling and dysfunction, and in some patients with depressed LV ejection fraction, cardiac resynchronization therapy (CRT) has proven effective in decreasing symptoms, reversing the structural and functional deterioration, and even improving survival.[3,4] Whether this new information about the worse prognosis for what are probably malignant ventricular arrhythmias in patients with systolic HF with dLBBB will be helpful in selecting patients who will benefit from CRT needs to be investigated.

M. D. Cheitlin, MD

References

1. Baldasseroni S, Opasich C, Gorin M, et al. on behalf of the Italian Network on Congestive Heart Failure Investigators. Left bundle-branch block is associated with increased 1-year sudden and total mortality rate in 5517 outpatients with congestive heart failure: a report from the Italian network on congestive heart failure. *Am Heart J.* 2002;143:398-405.
2. Grigioni F, Barbieri A, Magnani G, et al. Serial versus isolated assessment of clinical and instrumental parameters in heart failure: prognostic and therapeutic implications. *Am Heart J.* 2003;146:298-303.
3. Ghio S, Freemantle N, Scelsi L, et al. Long-term left ventricular reverse remodelling with cardiac resynchronization therapy: results from the CARE-HF trial. *Eur J Heart Fail.* 2009;11:480-488.
4. Ypenburg C, van Bommel RJ, Borleffs CJ, et al. Long-term prognosis after cardiac resynchronization therapy is related to the extent of left ventricular reverse remodeling at midterm follow-up. *J Am Coll Cardiol.* 2009;53:483-490.

Obesity and survival in patients with heart failure and preserved systolic function: A U-shaped relationship

Kapoor JR, Heidenreich PA (Stanford Univ, Palo Alto, CA; VA Palo Alto Health Care System, CA)
Am Heart J 159:75-80, 2010

Background.—Studies document better survival in heart failure patients with decreased left ventricular ejection fraction (EF) and higher body mass index (BMI; kg/m^2) compared to those with a lower BMI. However, it is unknown if this "obesity paradox" applies to heart failure patients with preserved EF or if it extends to the very obese (BMI >35).

Methods.—We determined all-cause mortality for 1,236 consecutive patients with a prior diagnosis of heart failure and a preserved EF ($\geq$50%).

Results.—Obesity (BMI>30) was noted in 542 patients (44%). The mean age was 71 ± 12 years, but this varied depending on BMI. One-year all-cause mortality decreased with increasing BMI, except at BMI >45 where mortality began to increase (55% if BMI <20, 38% if BMI 20-25, 26% if BMI 26-30, 25% if BMI 31-35, 17% if BMI 36-40, 18% if BMI 41-45, and 25% if BMI>45, P < .001). After adjustment for patient age, history, medications, and laboratory and echocardiographic parameters, the hazard ratios for total mortality (relative to BMI 26-30) were 1.68 (95% CI, 1.04-2.69) for BMI <20, 1.25 (95% CI, 0.92-1.68) for BMI 20 to 25, 0.99 (95% CI, 0.71-1.36) for BMI 31-35, 0.58 (95% CI, 0.35-0.97) for BMI 36 to 40, 0.79 (95% CI, 0.44-1.4) for BMI 41 to 45, and 1.38 (95% CI 0.74-2.6) for BMI >45 (P < .0001).

Conclusions.—Low BMI is associated with increased mortality in patients with heart failure and preserved systolic function. However, with a BMI of >45, mortality increased, raising the possibility of a U-shaped relationship between BMI and survival (Figs 1 and 2).

▶ There is an epidemic in the United States with 61% of Americans overweight (body mass index [BMI] $\geq$25 kg/m^2) or obese (BMI $\geq$30 Kg/m^2).[1] Because

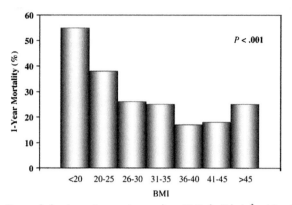

FIGURE 1.—Bar graph showing an increase in mortality a BMI of >45 kg/m², raising the possibility of a U-shaped relationship between unadjusted all-cause mortality and BMI. (Reprinted from the American Heart Journal, Kapoor JR, Heidenreich PA. Obesity and survival in patients with heart failure and preserved systolic function: a U-shaped relationship. *Am Heart J.* 2010;159:75-80, with permission from Elsevier Inc.)

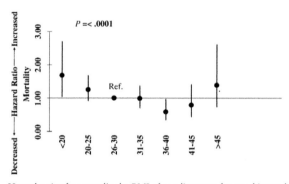

FIGURE 2.—Hazard ratios for mortality by BMI after adjustment for age, history, labs, medications and echocardiographic findings (all *P* < .0001). A U-shape relationship persists between BMI and mortality. (Reprinted from the American Heart Journal, Kapoor JR, Heidenreich PA. Obesity and survival in patients with heart failure and preserved systolic function: a U-shaped relationship. *Am Heart J.* 2010;159:75-80, with permission from Elsevier Inc.)

obesity is associated with increased incidence of hypertension, diabetes, and dyslipidemia, it is reasonable to expect that obesity would increase the mortality of patients with congestive heart failure (CHF). Although there are some small studies that support this view, on the contrary, many studies have shown that among patients with CHF and decreased left ventricular function, patients with an increased BMI have a decreased incidence of adverse outcomes than patients with normal or low BMIs regardless of age, the so-called obesity paradox.[2-4] Many of these studies did not address the prognostic utility of an increased BMI and most did not include CHF patients with preserved left ventricular function. In addition, there were too few patients with BMI ≥35 kg/m² to know whether the paradox applies to the very obese. This study addresses both these areas and shows that the paradox of the inverse relationship between

BMI and all-cause mortality is operative in patients with CHF and preserved left ventricular function and that with BMI above 45 kg/m^2, the mortality increases, forming a U-shaped curve. This U-shaped relationship remained after adjusting for multiple factors, including age, hypertension, malignancy, and diabetes.

The mechanism by which this paradox occurs is unknown, and it is not known whether patients with CHF who gain real weight (as opposed to edematous fluid) would have a survival benefit. The American Heart Association/ American College of Cardiology Guidelines do address the management of obese patients with CHF,[5] and the European Society of Cardiology recommends weight loss in such patients.[6] There is no evidence supporting the recommendation for losing weight in patients with CHF. One possibility is that the maintenance of weight is an indication of a favorable inflammatory, hormonal, and metabolic state.

In this era, stressing the many health problems associated with being overweight, there seems to be 1 group, those already with heart failure, where being overweight or even obese confers an advantage.

M. D. Cheitlin, MD

References

1. US Department of Health and Human Services. *The Surgeon General's Call to Action to Prevent and Decrease Overweight and Obesity.* Rockville, MD: U.S. Department of Health and Human Services, Public Health Service, Office of the Surgeon General; 2001.
2. Horwich TB, Fonarow GC, Hamilton MA, MacLellan WR, Woo MA, Tillisch JH. The relationship between obesity and mortality in patients with heart failure. *J Am Coll Cardiol.* 2001;38:789-795.
3. Davos CH, Doehner W, Rauchhaus M, et al. Body mass and survival in patients with chronic heart failure without cachexia: the importance of obesity. *J Card Fail.* 2003;9:29-35.
4. Lavie CJ, Osman AF, Milani RV, Mehra MR. Body composition and prognosis in chronic systolic heart failure: the obesity paradox. *Am J Cardiol.* 2003;91:891-894.
5. Hunt SA, Abraham WT, Chin MH, et al. ACC/AHA 2005 guideline update for diagnosis and management of heart failure in the adult. *J Am Coll Cardiol.* 2005;46:1116-1143.
6. Remme WJ, Swedberg K. Guidelines for the diagnosis and treatment of chronic heart failure. *Eur Heart J.* 2001;22:1527-1560.

Relation of Left Ventricular Ejection Fraction and Functional Capacity With Metabolism and Inflammation in Chronic Heart Failure With Reduced Ejection Fraction (from the MIMICA Study)

Thierer J, Acosta A, Vainstein N, et al (Instituto Cardiovascular de Buenos Aires, Argentina; et al)

Am J Cardiol 105:977-983, 2010

Catabolism and inflammation play a role in the physiopathology of heart failure with reduced ejection fraction and are more pronounced in the advanced stages of the disease. Our aim was to demonstrate that in patients with stable heart failure with reduced ejection fraction adequately treated, a direct relation exists between functional impairment, as evaluated by left ventricular ejection fraction (LVEF) and the 6-minute walking distance (6MWD), and catabolic and inflammatory markers. In 151 outpatients with heart failure and a LVEF of ≤40% (median age 64 years, LVEF 29%, and 6MWD 290 m) we measured the laboratory and body composition parameters that indicate directly or indirectly inflammatory activation, anabolic-catabolic balance, and nutritional status. We performed an analysis stratified by quartiles of LVEF and 6MWD and linear regression analysis to explore our hypothesis. In the linear regression analysis, after adjusting for age, gender, and etiology, LVEF was not related to the metabolic, inflammatory, or nutritional parameters. The 6MWD was directly related to albumin (p = 0.002) and log transformation of dehydroepiandrosterone (p = 0.013) and inversely to adiponectin (p − 0.001) and the log-transformation of high-sensitivity C-reactive protein (p = 0.037). In conclusion, in a population with stable heart failure with reduced ejection fraction, the 6MWD was related to the degree of inflammatory activity and catabolism, but LVEF was not. Even a slightly diminished functional capacity implies underlying inflammation and catabolic activation (Figs 1 and 2, Table 5).

▶ Patients with systolic dysfunction and congestive heart failure have neurohormonal activation that progressively increases the severity of the heart failure.

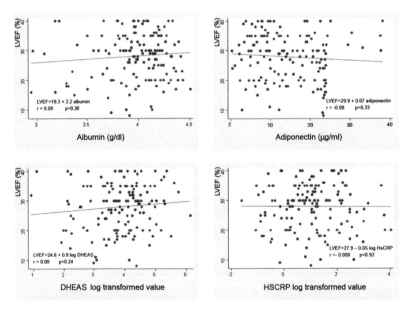

FIGURE 1.—Relation of LVEF to inflammatory and catabolic parameters. (Reprinted from Thierer J, Acosta A, Vainstein N, et al. Relation of left ventricular ejection fraction and functional capacity with metabolism and inflammation in chronic heart failure with reduced ejection fraction (from the MIMICA study). *Am J Cardiol.* 2010;105:977-983, with permission from Elsevier.)

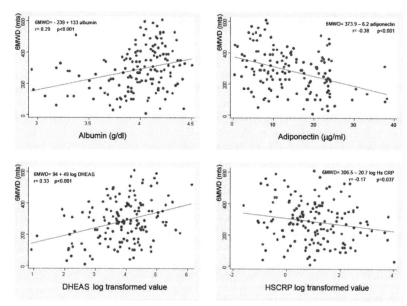

FIGURE 2.—Relation of 6MWD to inflammatory and catabolic parameters. (Reprinted from Thierer J, Acosta A, Vainstein N, et al. Relation of left ventricular ejection fraction and functional capacity with metabolism and inflammation in chronic heart failure with reduced ejection fraction (from the MIMICA study). *Am J Cardiol.* 2010;105:977-983, with permission from Elsevier.)

TABLE 5.—Linear Regression Analysis for 6-minute Walking Distance (6MWD)

Variable	Simple Linear Regression Analysis			Adjusted Linear Regression Analysis		
	β Coefficient	SE	p Value	β Coefficient	SE	p Value
Age (years)	−5.40	0.88	<0.001			
Hemoglobin (g/dl)	19.6	6.8	0.005	6.8	6.8	0.32
Globular sedimentation rate (mm/s)	−1.17	0.7	0.10	−0.28	0.66	0.67
Albumin (g/dl)	133	35	<0.001	94.3	34	0.003
Log dehydroepiandrosterone sulphate	49	11	<0.001	30.6	11	0.011
Log high-sensitivity C-reactive protein	−21.7	10	0.03	−19.3	9	0.030
log N-terminal pro-brain natriuretic peptide (pg/ml)	−93.3	18.1	<0.001	−56.4	19	0.003
Adiponectin (μg/ml)	−6.2	1.2	<0.001	−3.8	1.3	0.002
Muscle mass (%)	600	282	0.03	386	409	0.35

Variables significant at p ≤0.15 on simple linear regression analysis are displayed.

There is evidence that inflammatory and metabolic changes play a pathophysiologic role in the progression of heart failure in patients with a reduced ejection fraction.[1] This study of patients with stable congestive heart failure and an ejection fraction of ≤40% on optimum medical management had a direct relationship by adjusted linear regression analysis between ventricular functional impairment as expressed by the 6-minute walking distance (6MWD) and catabolic (albumin, the anabolic hormone dehydroepiandrosterone, and adiponectin) and inflammatory markers (high-sensitive C-reactive protein). Possibly because of the high rate of neurohormonal antagonist use and because only patients with reduced ejection fractions were studied, there was no relation between progressively reduced ejection fraction and either the metabolic or inflammatory markers. Although other studies have correlated inflammatory and metabolic markers with the severity of heart failure and decrease in functional capacity,[2,3] this study is the first to comprehensively study and show the relationship of these inflammatory and metabolic markers to functional capacity as expressed by the continuous variable 6MWD in a wide range of patients with reduced ejection fractions who were mostly in New York Heart Association class I and II, were well nourished, and were receiving recommended medical therapy. Therefore, the relations they found were maintained despite the antiinflammatory and anticatabolic effects of the neurohormonal antagonists. Whether decreasing the inflammatory cytokines and improving the catabolic state can improve functional capacity or increase survival is unknown.

M. D. Cheitlin, MD

References

1. Anker SD, von Haehling S. Inflammatory mediators in chronic heart failure: an overview. *Heart.* 2004;90:464-470.
2. Horwich TB, Kalantar-Zadeh K, MacLellan RW, Fonarow GC. Albumin levels predict survival in patients with systolic heart failure. *Am Heart J.* 2008;155: 883-889.
3. Windram JD, Loh PH, Rigby AS, Hanning I, Clark AL, Cleland JG. Relationship of high-sensitivity C-reactive protein to prognosis and other prognostic markers in outpatients with heart failure. *Am Heart J.* 2007;153:1048-1055.

Usefulness of Soluble Endoglin as a Noninvasive Measure of Left Ventricular Filling Pressure in Heart Failure

Kapur NK, Heffernan KS, Yunis AA, et al (Tufts Med Ctr, Boston, MA; et al)
Am J Cardiol 106:1770-1776, 2010

Progressive left ventricular (LV) dysfunction induces expression of the cytokine transforming growth factor-β1. Endoglin (CD105) is a transforming growth factor-β1 co-receptor that is released into the circulation as soluble endoglin (sEng). The objective of the present study was to assess the serum levels of sEng in patients with heart failure and to identify the predictive value of sEng for detecting elevated left ventricular end-diastolic pressures (LVEDPs). We measured the sEng levels in 82 consecutive patients with suspected LV dysfunction referred for determination of left heart filling pressures using cardiac catheterization. Among these subjects, the sEng levels correlated with the LVEDP (R = 0.689; p <0.0001), irrespective of the LV ejection fraction. Using a receiving operating characteristic curve, the sEng levels predicted an LVEDP of ≥16 mm Hg with an area under the curve of 0.85, exceeding the measured area under the curves for both atrial and brain natriuretic peptide, currently used biomarkers for heart failure diagnosis (atrial natriuretic peptide 0.68 and brain natriuretic peptide 0.65; p <0.01 vs sEng). In 10 subjects receiving medical therapy guided by invasive hemodynamic monitoring for heart failure, decreased a pulmonary capillary wedge pressure was associated with a reduced sEng level (R = 0.75, p = 0.008). Finally, compared to 25 healthy controls, the sEng levels were elevated in subjects with suspected LV dysfunction (3,589 ± 588 vs 4,257 ± 966 pg/ml, respectively, p <0.005) and correlated directly with the New York Heart Association class (R = 0.501, p <0.001). In conclusion, circulating levels of sEng are elevated in patients with increased LVEDP and New York Heart Association class, irrespective of the LV ejection fraction. sEng levels also decreased in association with a reduced cardiac filling pressure after diuresis. These findings have identified circulating sEng as a sensitive measure of elevated left heart filling pressures (Figs 1 and 3-5).

▶ This study for the first time describes a serum factor that correlates best with left ventricular filling pressure (LVFP) rather than with left ventricular (LV)

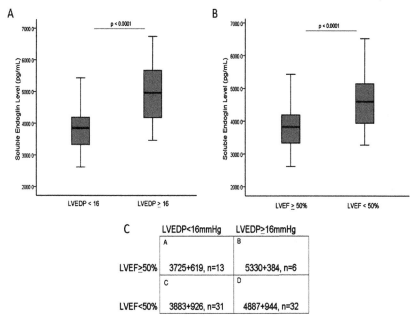

FIGURE 1.—sEng expression and LV filling pressure. *(A)* When grouped by LVEDP, sEng levels were significantly greater in patients with elevated LVEDP >16 mm Hg compared to low LVEDP <16 mm Hg (4,912 ± 922 vs 3,785 ± 724 pg/ml, respectively, p <0.0001). *(B)* When grouped by LVEF, those with low LVEF <50% had significantly increased sEng levels compared to controls (4,620 ± 980 vs 3,590 ± 588 pg/ml, respectively, p <0.001) or subjects with LVEF >50% (4,620 ± 980 vs 3,650 ± 550 pg/ml, p <0.001, respectively). *(C)* When grouped by both LVEF and LVEDP, sEng levels were significantly increased in subjects with elevated LVEDP, irrespective of LVEF (group A vs B or D, p <0.001; group A vs C, p = NS; group C vs B or D, p <0.001; group B vs D, p = NS). (Reprinted from the American Journal of Cardiology, Kapur NK, Heffernan KS, Yunis AA, et al. Usefulness of soluble endoglin as a noninvasive measure of left ventricular filling pressure in heart failure. *Am J Cardiol.* 2010;106:1770-1776. Copyright © 2010 with permission from Elsevier Inc.)

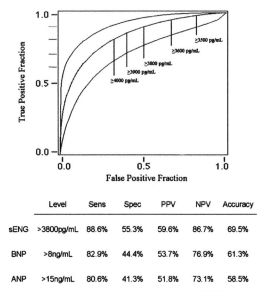

	Level	Sens	Spec	PPV	NPV	Accuracy
sENG	>3800pg/mL	88.6%	55.3%	59.6%	86.7%	69.5%
BNP	>8ng/mL	82.9%	44.4%	53.7%	76.9%	61.3%
ANP	>15ng/mL	80.6%	41.3%	51.8%	73.1%	58.5%

FIGURE 3.—Predictive value of sEng as determinant of elevated LVEDP. Receiver operating characteristic curve for sEng shown with specific cutpoints at various levels of sEng expression. AUC, area under curve; NPV, negative predictive value; PPV, positive predictive value; Sens, sensitivity; Spec, specificity. (Reprinted from the American Journal of Cardiology, Kapur NK, Heffernan KS, Yunis AA, et al. Usefulness of soluble endoglin as a noninvasive measure of left ventricular filling pressure in heart failure. *Am J Cardiol.* 2010;106:1770-1776. Copyright © 2010 with permission from Elsevier Inc.)

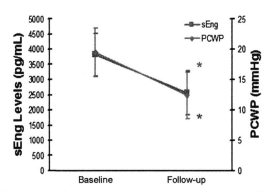

FIGURE 4.—Reduced sEng levels correlated with reduced pulmonary capillary wedge pressure (PCWP). Compared with baseline values, sEng levels were significantly reduced after 48 hours of diuretic therapy (3,830 ± 330 vs 2,540 ± 1,060 pg/ml, baseline vs follow-up, respectively, p<0.001) and corresponded with reduced PCWP (19.5 ± 3.1 vs 12.5 ± 4.5 mm Hg, baseline vs follow-up, respectively, p <0.001). Percentage of change in sEng strongly associated with percentage of change in LVEDP (R = 0.75, p = 0.008). In this group, ANP and BNP levels were also reduced after diuretic therapy (ANP, 10.5 ± 4.7 vs 5.2 ± 1.9 ng/mL, respectively, p = 0.02; BNP, 8.8 ± 2.5 vs 6.2 ± 1.7 ng/ml, respectively, p = 0.05). (Reprinted from Kapur NK, Heffernan KS, Yunis AA, et al. Usefulness of soluble endoglin as a noninvasive measure of left ventricular filling pressure in heart failure. *Am J Cardiol.* 2010;106:1770-1776. Copyright © 2010 with permission from Elsevier Inc.)

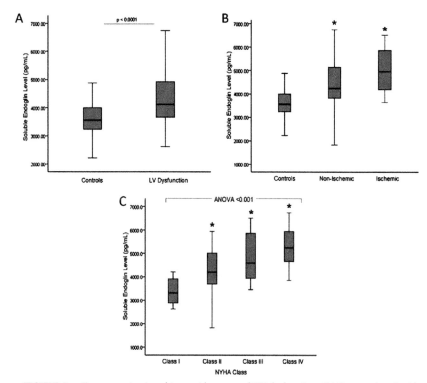

FIGURE 5.—sEng expression in subjects with suspected LV dysfunction. *(A)* Compared to healthy controls, sEng levels were significantly greater in total group of 82 study subjects (3,589 ± 588 vs 4,257 ± 966 pg/ml, respectively, p <0.005). *(B)* For study subjects with low LVEF <50%, sEng levels were increased regardless of whether underlying etiology was nonischemic or ischemic. sEng levels were greater in subjects with ischemic cardiomyopathy compared to patients with nonischemic heart failure (p = 0.06). *(C)* Among study subjects, worsening New York Heart Association (NYHA) class corresponded to increased sEng levels (NYHA class 1, 3,644.9 ± 579; class II, 4,307 ± 968; class III, 4,746 ± 947; and class IV, 5,089 ± 1,073 pg/ml; *p <0.01 vs class 1; analysis of variance [ANOVA], p <0.001). (Reprinted from the American Journal of Cardiology, Kapur NK, Heffernan KS, Yunis AA, et al. Usefulness of soluble endoglin as a noninvasive measure of left ventricular filling pressure in heart failure. *Am J Cardiol.* 2010;106:1770-1776. Copyright © 2010 with permission from Elsevier Inc.)

systolic function. Endoglin is a type III transforming growth factor-β1 coreceptor that promotes binding of transforming growth factors-β1 and -β3 to type II transforming growth factor-β1 in vascular tissue and regulates vascular tone.[1] In cardiac tissue, endoglin is expressed by endothelial cells, fibroblasts surrounding the muscle fibers, and in stromal cells of valve leaflets but not in muscle cells.[2] Soluble endoglin (sEng) is released from the extracellular domain of endoglin and has been associated with increased systemic vascular resistance observed in fibroproliferative conditions.[3,4] Since progressive heart failure (HF) is characterized by increased vascular resistance and transforming growth factor-β1 activity and increasing cardiac fibrosis,[5-7] the study was developed to test the hypothesis that sEng would increase in response to an increase in the LVFP and would therefore provide a sensitive noninvasive measure of cardiac overload. The sEng did correlate significantly with the LVFP and proved to be a more sensitive and specific predictor of cardiac pressure overload than the biomarkers atrial or brain natriuretic peptides. Furthermore, sEng strongly correlated with an elevated LV end-diastolic pressure regardless of the LV ejection fraction (LVEF), a reduced LVEF, and a worsening New York Heart Association class. With treatment and reduction of the LVFP, the sEng decreased proportionately. The implications of these findings are that sEng may have an important role in the pathophysiology of HF, that sEng may reduce the need for invasive measurement of LVFP, and that this biomarker of elevated LVFP might be useful in monitoring therapy of HF. Since sEng is expressed by endothelial cells and cardiac fibroblasts and not in myocytes, it may be of enhanced clinical utility because these cells are viable in the later stages of HF.

M. D. Cheitlin, MD

References

1. Lebrin F, Goumans MJ, Jonker L, et al. Endoglin promotes endothelial cell proliferation and TGF-beta/ALK1 signal transduction. *EMBO J*. 2004;23:4018-4028.
2. St-Jacques S, Cymerman U, Pece N, Letarte M. Molecular characterization and in situ localization of murine endoglin reveal that it is a transforming growth factor-beta binding protein of endothelial and stromal cells. *Endocrinology*. 1994;134: 2645-2657.
3. Leask A, Abraham DJ, Finlay DR, et al. Dysregulation of transforming growth factor beta signaling in scleroderma: overexpression of endoglin in cutaneous scleroderma fibroblasts. *Arthritis Rheum*. 2002;46:1857-1865.
4. Yagmur E, Rizk M, Stanzel S, et al. Elevation of endoglin (CD105) concentrations in serum of patients with liver cirrhosis and carcinoma. *Eur J Gastroenterol Hepatol*. 2007;19:755-761.
5. Zeisberg EM, Tarnavski O, Zeisberg M, et al. Endothelial-to-mesenchymal transition contributes to cardiac fibrosis. *Nat Med*. 2007;13:952-961.
6. Rosenkranz S. TGF-beta1 and angiotensin networking in cardiac remodeling. *Cardiovasc Res*. 2004;63:423-432.
7. Brutsaert DL. Role of endocardium in cardiac overloading and failure. *Eur Heart J*. 1990;11:G8-G16.

Myocarditis and Cardiomyopathy

Long-Acting Phosphodiesterase-5 Inhibitor Tadalafil Attenuates Doxorubicin-Induced Cardiomyopathy without Interfering with Chemotherapeutic Effect

Koka S, Das A, Zhu S-G, et al (Virginia Commonwealth Univ Med Ctr, Richmond)
J Pharmacol Exp Ther 334:1023-1030, 2010

Doxorubicin (DOX) is one of the most effective anticancer drugs. However, its cardiotoxicity remains a clinical concern that severely restricts its therapeutic usage. We designed this study to investigate whether tadalafil, a long-acting phosphodiesterase-5 (PDE-5) inhibitor, protects against DOX-induced cardiotoxicity. We also sought to delineate the cellular and molecular mechanisms underlying tadalafil-induced cardioprotection. Male CF-1 outbred mice were randomized into three groups ($n = 15–24$/group) to receive either saline (0.2 ml i.p.), DOX (15 mg/kg,

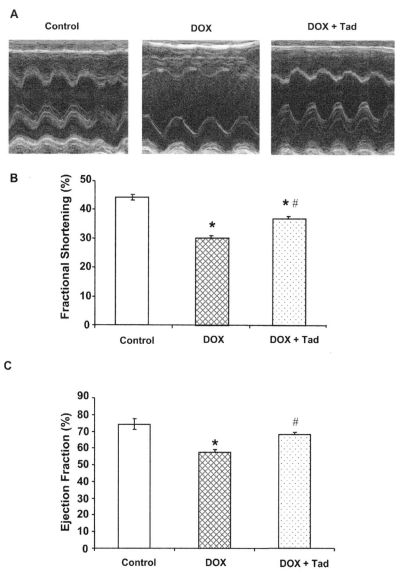

FIGURE 2.—Transthoracic echocardiography assessment of the effect of tadalafil on ventricular contractile dysfunction caused by DOX. A, representative echocardiographic tracings for each of the three experimental groups. B and C, the averaged data of fractional shortening (B) and ejection fraction (C) in the mice are presented as mean ± S.E. ($n = 6$ per group; *, $P < 0.05$ versus control; #, $P < 0.05$ versus DOX). (Reprinted from Koka S, Das A, Zhu S-G, et al. Long-acting phosphodiesterase-5 inhibitor tadalafil attenuates doxorubicin-induced cardiomyopathy without interfering with chemotherapeutic effect. *J Pharmacol Exp Ther.* 2010;334:1023-1030.)

given by a single intraperitoneal injection), or tadalafil (4 mg/kg p.o. daily for 9 days) plus DOX. Left ventricular function was subsequently assessed by transthoracic echocardiography and Millar conductance catheter.

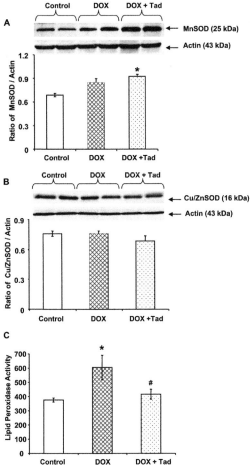

FIGURE 4.—Effect of tadalafil on superoxide dismutases and lipid peroxidation after DOX treatment. A and B, representative Western blots with specific bands of MnSOD (A) and Cu/ZnSOD (B) are shown. Bar graphs show densiometric quantification from four individual hearts per group, which was normalized against actin level for each sample. Data are expressed as mean ± S.E. *, $P < 0.05$ versus control. C, lipid peroxidation activity was quantified with a commercial kit. Data are represented as mean S.E. ($n = 8$/group). *, $P < 0.05$ versus control; #, $P < 0.05$ versus DOX. (Reprinted from Koka S, Das A, Zhu S-G, et al. Long-acting phosphodiesterase-5 inhibitor tadalafil attenuates doxorubicin-induced cardiomyopathy without interfering with chemotherapeutic effect. *J Pharmacol Exp Ther.* 2010;334:1023-1030.)

Cardiac contractile function was impaired by DOX, and it was significantly improved by cotreatment with tadalafil. Tadalafil attenuated DOX-induced apoptosis and depletion of prosurvival proteins, including Bcl-2 and GATA-4, in myocardium. Cardiac oxidative stress was attenuated and antioxidant capacity was enhanced by tadalafil possibly via upregulation of mitochondrial superoxide dismutase (MnSOD). Moreover,

Koka et al.

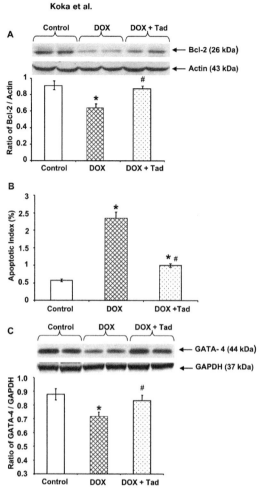

FIGURE 5.—Tadalafil attenuates apoptosis and down-regulation of GATA-4 in DOX-induced cardio-myopathy. A, representative Western blot and densitometric quantification showing Bcl-2 expression ($n = 6$/group). B, cardiac tissue apoptosis quantified by using TUNEL staining and expressed as apoptotic index for TUNEL-positive cells. Data are expressed as mean ± S.E. ($n = 6$/group). *, $P < 0.05$ versus control; #, $P < 0.05$ versus DOX group. C, cardiac protein expression of GATA-4 as measured by Western blot analysis. Bar graphs show densiometric quantification from four individual hearts per group, which is normalized against glyceraldehyde 3-phosphate dehydrogenase (GAPDH) level for each sample. *, $P < 0.05$ versus control; #, $P < 0.05$ versus DOX group. (Reprinted from Koka S, Das A, Zhu S-G, et al. Long-acting phosphodiesterase-5 inhibitor tadalafil attenuates doxorubicin-induced cardiomyopathy without interfering with chemotherapeutic effect. *J Pharmacol Exp Ther.* 2010;334:1023-1030.)

the tadalafil-treated group demonstrated increased cardiac cGMP level and protein kinase G (PKG) activity. Tadalafil did not interfere with the efficacy of DOX in killing human osteosarcoma cells in vitro or its anti-tumor effect in vivo in tumor xenograft model. We conclude that tadalafil improved left ventricular function and prevented cardiomyocyte apoptosis in DOX-induced cardiomyopathy through mechanisms involving up-regulation of cGMP, PKG activity, and MnSOD level without interfering with the chemotherapeutic benefits of DOX (Figs 2, 4, and 5).

▶ Doxorubicin (DOX) is one of the most effective antineoplastic agents in the treatment of certain malignant tumors including leukemias, lymphomas, and a variety of solid tumors.[1] Unfortunately, this anthracycline has a dose-dependent myocardial toxicity that is irreversible and results in heart failure (HF) and death.[2,3] Damage to the myocardium is characterized by myofibrillar disarray, mitochondrial injury, and cardiomyocyte apoptosis, leading to myofi-brillar loss and HF.[4] The mechanisms by which this myocardial damage occurs include free radical formation, lipid peroxidation, and inhibition of protein synthesis, in addition to mitochondrial edema, calcium overloading, and death of myocardial cells. A variety of approaches have been used to prevent or treat DOX toxicity in its early stages, including β-blockers, antioxidants, free radical scavengers, and renin-angiotensin inhibitors; however, in the late stages, cardiac transplantation is the only option available.[5] Sildenafil, a phos-phodiesterase type 5 (PDE-5) inhibitor, developed as an antianginal drug, was found by virtue of its inhibition of PDE-5, which antagonizes the hydrolysis of cyclic GMP (cGMP), thus prolonging smooth muscle relaxation. Sildenafil was first shown to prolong penile erection by increasing penile blood flow and so was useful in erectile dysfunction. Tadalafil is a long-acting PDE-5 inhibitor. Fisher et al[6] have shown that sildenafil attenuates cardiac dysfunction in DOX cardiomyopathy. The present mouse model study of DOX toxicity was designed first to demonstrate that tadalafil could attenuate DOX cardiomyocyte toxicity without diminishing the antineoplastic effects of the drug and second to elucidate the mechanism by which tadalafil diminishes DOX toxicity. They showed that tadalafil decreased DOX toxicity in mice without attenuating the antineoplastic effects on osteosarcoma cell lines. The mechanism of attenuation of toxicity appears to be by a variety of properties. These include increasing mitochondrial superoxide dismutase and inhibiting DOX-induced lipid peroxi-dation, thus reducing oxidative myocardial stress, preserving the antiapoptotic protein Bcl-2 and decreasing apoptosis, increasing cGMP and protein kinase G signaling pathways in the heart that play a role in protection against ischemia/reperfusion injury,[7,8] and increasing GATA-4 expression that plays an important role in nuclear events that modulate cell differentiation during cardiac development and stress responsiveness of the heart. So PDE-5 inhibi-tors have proved valuable first in erectile dysfunction, then in the treatment of pulmonary hypertension, and now possibly in the attenuation of DOX toxicity.

M. D. Cheitlin, MD

References

1. Hortobágyi GN. Anthracyclines in the treatment of cancer. An overview. *Drugs.* 1997;54:1-7.
2. Singal PK, Iliskovic N. Doxorubicin-induced cardiomyopathy. *N Engl J Med.* 1998;339:900-905.
3. Fu LX, Waagstein F, Hjalmarson A. A new insight into adriamycin-induced cardiotoxicity. *Int J Cardiol.* 1990;29:15-20.

4. Billingham ME, Mason JW, Bristow MR, Daniels JR. Anthracycline cardiomyopathy monitored by morphologic changes. *Cancer Treat Rep.* 1978;62:865-872.
5. Thomas X, Le QH, Fiere D. Anthracycline-related toxicity requiring cardiac transplantation in long-term disease-free survivors with acute promyelocytic leukemia. *Ann Hematol.* 2002;81:504-507.
6. Fisher PW, Salloum F, Das A, Hyder H, Kukreja RC. Phosphodiesterase-5 inhibition with sildenafil attenuates cardiomyocyte apoptosis and left ventricular dysfunction in a chronic model of doxorubicin cardiotoxicity. *Circulation.* 2005; 111:1601-1610.
7. Das A, Xi L, Kukreja RC. Protein kinase G-dependent cardioprotective mechanism of phosphodiesterase-5 inhibition involves phosphorylation of ERK and GSK3 beta. *J Biol Chem.* 2008;283:29572-29585.
8. Salloum FN, Chau VQ, Hoke NN, et al. Phosphodiesterase-5 inhibitor, tadalafil, protects against myocardial ischemia/reperfusion through protein kinase G-dependent generation of hydrogen sulfide. *Circulation.* 2009;120:S31-S36.

Iron Overload Cardiomyopathy: Better Understanding of an Increasing Disorder

Gujja P, Rosing DR, Tripodi DJ, et al (Univ of Cincinnati, OH; Natl Insts of Health, Bethesda, MD)
J Am Coll Cardiol 56:1001-1012, 2010

The prevalence of iron overload cardiomyopathy (IOC) is increasing. The spectrum of symptoms of IOC is varied. Early in the disease process, patients may be asymptomatic, whereas severely overloaded patients can have terminal heart failure complaints that are refractory to treatment. It has been shown that early recognition and intervention may alter outcomes. Biochemical markers and tissue biopsy, which have traditionally been used to diagnose and guide therapy, are not sensitive enough to detect early cardiac iron deposition. Newer diagnostic modalities such as magnetic resonance imaging are noninvasive and can assess quantitative cardiac iron load. Phlebotomy and chelating drugs are suboptimal means of treating IOC; hence, the roles of gene therapy, hepcidin, and calcium channel blockers are being actively investigated. There is a need for the development of clinical guidelines in order to improve the management of this emerging complex disease (Figs 1 and 3).

▶ Most patients with cardiomyopathy at the time of diagnosis cannot get it reversed and treatment is directed at the pathophysiology of heart failure, with drugs targeted to treat the fluid overload and block the excessive neurohormonal activation that results in symptoms and progressive left ventricular dysfunction and death. In those with alcoholic cardiomyopathy, if patients stop drinking alcohol, a large number of these patients will recover ventricular function. Iron overload cardiomyopathy is one of the other few treatable cardiomyopathies that, if discovered early, can be stopped in its progression. The key to early treatment is early recognition of the disease. Excess iron accumulates in the body as a result of increased gastrointestinal absorption (hemochromatosis), excess administration of exogenous iron by dietary sources, or, more commonly, red

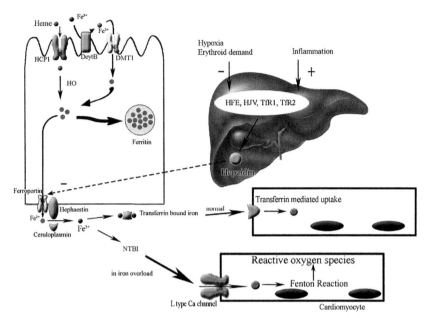

FIGURE 1.—Iron Kinetics. Heme is absorbed by Heme carrier protein (HCP)-1 and released from iron by hemoxygenase (HO)-1, but heme uptake overall still remains controversial. Non-heme iron is reduced by duodenal cytochrome b at the apical membrane of intestinal enterocytes (21), which is taken up by intestinal epithelium by the divalent metal transporter (DMT)-1 (22,23). Ferrous iron is then transported to the basolateral portion of the cell by iron carriers and later transported into the circulation by the duodenal iron exporter Ferroportin (regulated by hepcidin) when there is a need for iron. Ferrous iron is oxidized by ceruloplasmin in non-intestinal cells and also by a homolog of ceruloplasmin, Hephaestin, in intestinal cells to ferric iron and loaded on to transferrin. With the increase in intracellular concentrations of iron, ferritin synthesis also increases. Once the storage capacity is exceeded, metabolically active iron is released intracellularly in the form of hemosiderin and toxic nontransferrin-bound forms of iron (NTBI). *Editor's Note:* Please refer to original journal article for full references. (Reprinted from the Journal of the American College of Cardiology, Gujja P, Rosing DR, Tripodi DJ, et al. Iron overload cardiomyopathy: Better understanding of an increasing disorder. *J Am Coll Cardiol.* 2010;56:1001-1012. Copyright 2010, with permission from the American College of Cardiology Foundation.)

blood cell transfusions (hemosiderosis), the cornerstone of treatment for hereditary anemias such as thalassemia and sickle cell disease. The present paper is a very extensive review of the pathophysiology, diagnosis, and management of this disease. Described are the newer insights into iron homeostasis and a better understanding of how iron enters the body. Newer diagnostic techniques, including magnetic resonance imaging and diastolic function by tissue Doppler, are being developed to improve early diagnosis of iron overload, essential in treating early enough to halt progression to irreversible cardiomyopathy. To this end, a proposed clinical pathway algorithm is given to evaluate patients with idiopathic cardiomyopathy or those at risk of iron overload. New therapeutic options, other than repeated phlebotomy, include better chelating agents with fewer side effects, better efficacy, and absorption; calcium channel blocking agents; hepcidin, an amino acid that plays a major role in regulating iron homeostasis; genetic and stem cell therapy are being investigated. The incidence of iron overload cardiomyopathy is increasing worldwide, with patients with

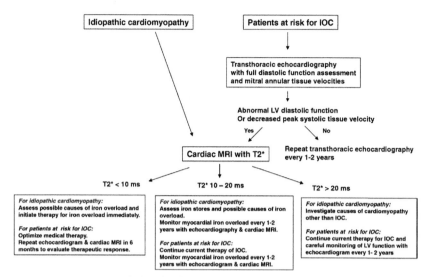

FIGURE 3.—Our Proposed Clinical Pathway to Evaluate Patients with Idiopathic Cardiomyopathy or Those at Risk for Iron Overload. IOC = iron overload cardiomyopathy; LV = left ventricle; MRI = magnetic resonance imaging. (Reprinted from the Journal of the American College of Cardiology, Gujja P, Rosing DR, Tripodi DJ, et al. Iron overload cardiomyopathy: Better understanding of an increasing disorder. *J Am Coll Cardiol.* 2010;56:1001-1012. Copyright 2010, with permission from the American College of Cardiology Foundation.)

thalassemia and sickle cell disease living longer, and in individuals with hematologic malignancies and increased treatment, especially with bone marrow transplants and stem cell therapy. Because cardiologists take care of most of these patients, an excellent review paper on this subject is a valuable resource.

M. D. Cheitlin, MD

Late benefits of dual-chamber pacing in obstructive hypertrophic cardiomyopathy: a 10-year follow-up study

Galve E, Sambola A, Saldaña G, et al (Hospital General Universitari Vall d'Hebron, Barcelona, Spain)
Heart 96:352-356, 2010

Objective.—To examine the mid-term and long-term outcomes in patients with obstructive hypertrophic cardiomyopathy (HCM) submitted to pacing.

Design.—Prospective, observational study.

Setting.—Single, non-referral centre.

Patients and Intervention.—Fifty patients (62 ± 11 years) with HCM refractory to medical treatment, all in New York Heart Association (NYHA) class III or IV, and with a rest gradient >50 mm Hg underwent a dual-chamber pacemaker implantation. Patients were followed-up for up to 10 years (mean 5.0 ± 2.9, range 0.6–10.1).

Results.—During the first year of follow-up, rest gradients decreased (baseline 86 ± 29 mm Hg; 3 months 55 ± 37; 1 year 41 ± 26; p=0.0001). NYHA class improved, as well as exercise tolerance (baseline 281 ± 112 m; 3 months 334 ± 106 m; 1 year 348 ± 78 m; p<0.0001). The physical and mental components of the quality of life instrument SF-36 also improved. Left ventricular wall thickness remained unchanged, while ejection fraction decreased (baseline $76 \pm 10\%$; 3 months $74 \pm 8\%$; 1 year $66 \pm 13\%$; p=0.002). During the long-term follow-up, an additional reduction in obstruction was found (final rest gradient 28 ± 24 mm Hg, p<0.02). Those patients who did not improve to NYHA class I or II and continued to have obstruction were given other treatments (six, alcohol ablation; three, surgical myectomy).

Conclusions.—Pacing in HCM results in a significant reduction in obstruction, improvement of symptoms and exercise capacity that is progressive and may be achieved after a long period of time. In this series, only 18% of cases needed a more aggressive treatment to relieve residual obstruction and obtain a satisfactory symptomatic status. In conclusion, these results emphasise the need for new controlled studies of pacing with a longer follow-up (Figs 1-4).

▶ Patients with hypertrophic obstructive cardiomyopathy (HOCM) who remain very symptomatic after medical management, including β blockers, verapamil, and disopyramide, are candidates for the more invasive procedures of septal ablation by surgery or by catheter-injected alcohol, each of which has a procedural mortality and complications such as complete heart block. Over 30 years ago, the observation that pacing the apex could reduce the outflow tract gradient in patients with HOCM was made by chance,[1] and since then there have been a number of studies on dual-chambered pacing in this disease, most of which showed a modest reduction in gradient and variable clinical improvement. Two small, randomized, crossover studies showed modest decrease in gradient with little or no improvement in functional capacity.[2,3]

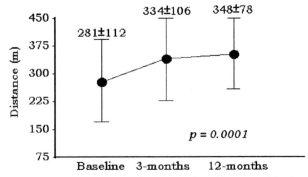

FIGURE 1.—6-Min walking test. Functional capacity evaluated by means of the distance covered in the 6-min corridor test. The baseline scale indicates before pacemaker implantation, and 3 months and 12 months after active pacing. (Reprinted from Galve E, Sambola A, Saldaña G, et al. Late benefits of dual-chamber pacing in obstructive hypertrophic cardiomyopathy: a 10-year follow-up study. *Heart.* 2010;96:352-356, with permission from the BMJ Publishing Group Ltd.)

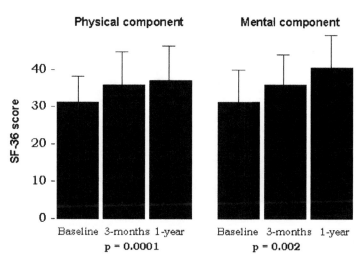

FIGURE 2.—SF-36 quality of life. Physical and mental components of the SF-36 quality-of-life instrument measured under basal conditions, and during the first year of follow-up after pacing. (Reprinted from Galve E, Sambola A, Saldaña G, et al. Late benefits of dual-chamber pacing in obstructive hypertrophic cardiomyopathy: a 10-year follow-up study. *Heart.* 2010;96:352-356, with permission from the BMJ Publishing Group Ltd.)

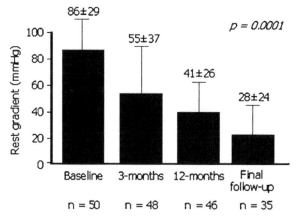

FIGURE 3.—Changes in outflow gradient. Evolution of peak left ventricular outflow tract gradient (mm Hg), before pacemaker implantation (baseline), and during early and late follow-up after pacing. (Reprinted from Galve E, Sambola A, Saldaña G, et al. Late benefits of dual-chamber pacing in obstructive hypertrophic cardiomyopathy: a 10-year follow-up study. *Heart.* 2010;96:352-356, with permission from the BMJ Publishing Group Ltd.)

Furthermore, the time of pacing was short, 2 to 3 months. This study is also small with only 50 patients, and all of them with New York Heart Association class III-IV on optimal medical management. However, the evaluation of systolic left ventricular function, degree of mitral regurgitation, functional capacity, and quality of life was comprehensive, and the follow-up period was a mean of 5 ± 2.9 years with a range from 0.6 to 10.1 years. The decrease in gradient

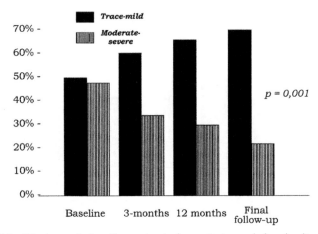

FIGURE 4.—Mitral regurgitation. Changes in mitral regurgitation grade from baseline before pacemaker implantation to 3 months and 12 months after pacing, and at final follow-up, expressed as percentages of the total number of patients. (Reprinted from Galve E, Sambola A, Saldaña G, et al. Late benefits of dual-chamber pacing in obstructive hypertrophic cardiomyopathy: a 10-year follow-up study. *Heart.* 2010;96:352-356, with permission from the BMJ Publishing Group Ltd.)

continued over the period of follow-up, and functional capacity also improved with time. The fact that apical pacing with short atrioventricular delay required a relatively long period to reduce gradient and improve the clinical symptoms suggests that the mechanism by which this is accomplished, although unknown, is more complicated than simply that pre-excitation of the right ventricular apex altering the dynamics and timing of contraction of the septal wall, reducing the projection of the basal septum into the outflow tract and thus decreasing obstruction. More likely, the dyssynchrony of contraction over time results in ventricular remodeling. Because many patients with HOCM have a cardioverter-defibrillator implanted to prevent sudden death, a study could be done randomizing patients to active/nonactive pacing as a therapeutic trial.

M. D. Cheitlin, MD

References

1. Hassenstein P, Storch HH, Schmitz W. [Results of electrical pacing in patients with hypertrophic obstruction cardiomyopathy (author's transl)]. *Thoraxchir Vask Chir.* 1975;23:496-498.
2. Kappenberger L, Linde C, Daubert C, et al. Pacing in hypertrophic obstructive cardiomyopathy. A randomized crossover study. PIC Study Group. *Eur Heart J.* 1997;18:1249-1256.
3. Maron BJ, Nishimura RA, McKenna WJ, Rakowski H, Josephson ME, Kieval RS. Assessment of permanent dual-chamber pacing as a treatment for drug-refractory symptomatic patients with obstructive hypertrophic cardiomyopathy. A randomized, double-blind, crossover study (M-PATHY). *Circulation.* 1999;99:2927-2933.

Myocardial Scar Visualized by Cardiovascular Magnetic Resonance Imaging Predicts Major Adverse Events in Patients With Hypertrophic Cardiomyopathy

Bruder O, Wagner A, Jensen CJ, et al (Elisabeth Hosp, Essen, Germany; Drexel College of Medicine, Philadelphia, PA; et al)
J Am Coll Cardiol 56:875-887, 2010

Objectives.—We sought to establish the prognostic value of a comprehensive cardiovascular magnetic resonance (CMR) examination in risk stratification of hypertrophic cardiomyopathy (HCM) patients.

Background.—With annual mortality rates ranging between 1% and 5%, depending on patient selection, a small but significant number of HCM patients are at risk for an adverse event. Therefore, the identification of and prophylactic therapy (i.e., defibrillator placement) in patients with HCM who are at risk of dying are imperative.

Methods.—Two-hundred forty-three consecutive patients with HCM were prospectively enrolled. All patients underwent initial CMR, and 220 were available for clinical follow-up. The mean follow-up time was 1,090 days after CMR. End points were all-cause and cardiac mortality.

Results.—During follow-up 20 of the 220 patients died, and 2 patients survived sudden cardiac death due to adequate implantable cardioverter-defibrillator discharge. Most events (n = 16) occurred for cardiac reasons; the remaining 6 events were related to cancer and accidents. Our data indicate that the presence of scar visualized by CMR yields an odds ratio of 5.47 for all-cause mortality and of 8.01 for cardiac mortality. This might be superior to classic clinical risk factors, because in our dataset the presence of 2 risk factors yields an odds ratio of 3.86 for all-cause and of 2.20 for cardiac mortality, respectively. Multivariable analysis also revealed the presence of late gadolinium enhancement as a good independent predictor of death in HCM patients.

Conclusions.—Among our population of largely low or asymptomatic HCM patients, the presence of scar indicated by CMR is a good independent predictor of all-cause and cardiac mortality (Figs 3-5).

► Hypertrophic cardiomyopathy (HC), the commonest genetic cardiovascular disease, has an annual mortality of 1% to 5% depending on patient selection.[1] Sudden death, frequently in a previously asymptomatic patient, is not unusual and a leading cause of sudden cardiac death in young people with HC.[2] The identification of those patients with HC at most risk of either deterioration of left ventricular function and heart failure or of sudden death would be extremely valuable. Clinical markers predictive of cardiac events in patients with HC, including a family history of sudden death, prior cardiac arrest, spontaneous ventricular tachycardia or syncope, extreme left ventricular wall thickness, and ventricular outflow tract obstruction, have been described, but all have a low positive predictive value.[3,4] Recently, myocardial scarring detected by late gadolinium enhancement (LGE) on cardiovascular MRI has been related to long-term clinical outcome and could be a better predictor of lethal adverse

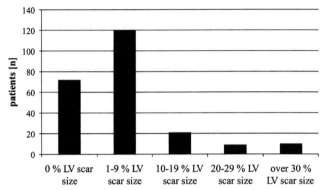

FIGURE 3.—Bar Graph Visualizing the Distribution of Scar Burden in Our Patient Cohort. Median scar percentage of left ventricular mass (%LV). It is important to note that, among most individuals in our largely low or asymptomatic hypertrophic cardiomyopathy population, scarring was present as indicated by late gadolinium enhancement. (Reprinted from Bruder O, Wagner A, Jensen CJ, et al. Myocardial scar visualized by cardiovascular magnetic resonance imaging predicts major adverse events in patients with hypertrophic cardiomyopathy. *J Am Coll Cardiol.* 2010;56:875-887, copyright 2010, with permission from the American College of Cardiology.)

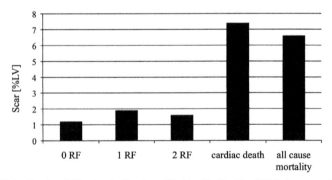

FIGURE 4.—Bar Graph Plotting the Number of Sudden Cardiac Death Risk Factors and All-Cause and Cardiac Mortality Versus the Amount of Scarring. Percentage of left ventricular mass (%LV). Note that patients who suffered an event during follow-up had the highest scar burden. Interestingly, patients without clinical risk factors (RF) also had scars. (Reprinted from Bruder O, Wagner A, Jensen CJ, et al. Myocardial scar visualized by cardiovascular magnetic resonance imaging predicts major adverse events in patients with hypertrophic cardiomyopathy. *J Am Coll Cardiol.* 2010;56:875-887, copyright 2010, with permission from the American College of Cardiology.)

events than the previously mentioned clinical markers.[5] Others have demonstrated that LGE is the substrate for ventricular arrhythmias in HC[5,6] and is associated with ventricular remodeling and heart failure. This study is a prospective 5-year follow-up of HC patients with cardiac MRI with gadolinium injection.

Hyperenhanced pixels have been shown to represent myocardial fibrosis/scarring in HC by autopsy comparison.[7] The 2 end points were all-cause death and cardiac death.

Most patients were only mildly symptomatic or without any symptoms; therefore, the finding that the presence of scar as visualized by LGE MRI was a good

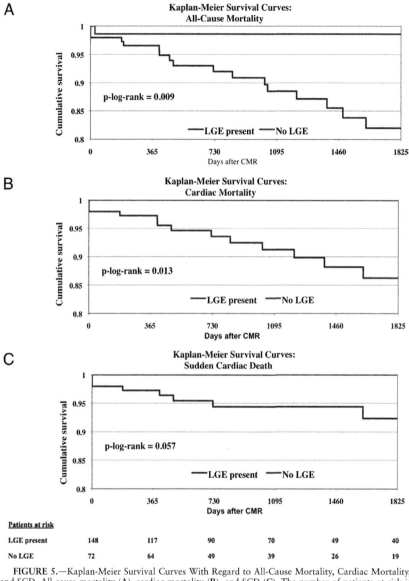

A

Kaplan-Meier Survival Curves:
All-Cause Mortality

p-log-rank = 0.009

—LGE present —No LGE

Days after CMR

B

Kaplan-Meier Survival Curves:
Cardiac Mortality

p-log-rank = 0.013

—LGE present —No LGE

Days after CMR

C

Kaplan-Meier Survival Curves:
Sudden Cardiac Death

p-log-rank = 0.057

—LGE present —No LGE

Days after CMR

Patients at risk

LGE present	148	117	90	70	49	40
No LGE	72	64	49	39	26	19

FIGURE 5.—Kaplan-Meier Survival Curves With Regard to All-Cause Mortality, Cardiac Mortality, and SCD. All-cause mortality (**A**), cardiac mortality (**B**), and SCD (**C**). The number of patients at risk is shown at the bottom of the figure. Note that in the group without any scar not a single patient suffered cardiac death (**B, C**) during the first 5 years of follow-up. Abbreviations as in Figure 1. (Reprinted from Bruder O, Wagner A, Jensen CJ, et al. Myocardial scar visualized by cardiovascular magnetic resonance imaging predicts major adverse events in patients with hypertrophic cardiomyopathy. *J Am Coll Cardiol.* 2010;56:875-887, copyright 2010, with permission from the American College of Cardiology.)

predictor for death in HC, with an odds ratio of 5.5 for all-cause mortality and 8.0 for cardiac mortality, suggests that this might be superior to the classical risk factors since sudden death in HC patients is not uncommon.[1,2] The fact that scar by LGE was the best independent predictor of all-cause and cardiac death supports the finding by Adabag and colleagues[5] that the presence of LGE was associated with a 7-fold risk of nonsustained ventricular tachycardia at follow-up. In this study, conventional risk factors were present in only 2 of the 22 patients who died on follow-up and not one patient without myocardial scar suffered cardiac death during the first 5 years of follow-up. Although 70% of patients had a small amount of scar (1%-9%) by LGE, only 16.4% had more than 10% of the left ventricle scarred. The patients with adverse events had the highest percent scarring, but there is no perfect association between the presence of a scar by LGE and cardiac death. A prospectively designed large study is still required to definitely establish LGE as causally related to the risk of death in patients with HC and evaluate the incremental value of additional cardiac MRI parameters, such as scar surface area.

M. D. Cheitlin, MD

References

1. Cannan CR, Reeder GS, Bailey KR, et al. Natural history of hypertrophic cardiomyopathy. A population-based study, 1976 through 1990. *Circulation.* 1995;92:2488-2495.
2. Maron BJ. Hypertrophic cardiomyopathy. *Lancet.* 1997;350:127-133.
3. Elliott PM, Poloniecki J, Dickie S, et al. Sudden death in hypertrophic cardiomyopathy: identification of high risk patients. *J Am Coll Cardiol.* 2000;36:2212-2218.
4. Spirito P, Seidman CE, McKenna WJ, Maron BJ. The management of hypertrophic cardiomyopathy. *N Engl J Med.* 1997;336:775-785.
5. Adabag AS, Maron BJ, Appelbaum E, et al. Occurrence and frequency of arrhythmias in hypertrophic cardiomyopathy in relation to delayed enhancement on cardiovascular magnetic resonance. *J Am Coll Cardiol.* 2008;51:1369-1374.
6. Leonardi S, Raineri C, De Ferrari GM, et al. Usefulness of cardiac magnetic resonance in assessing the risk of ventricular arrhythmias and sudden death in patients with hypertrophic cardiomyopathy. *Eur Heart J.* 2009;30:2003-2010.
7. Moon JC, Reed E, Sheppard MN, et al. The histologic basis of late gadolinium enhancement cardiovascular magnetic resonance in hypertrophic cardiomyopathy. *J Am Coll Cardiol.* 2004;43:2260-2264.

Risk of heart failure relapse in subsequent pregnancy among peripartum cardiomyopathy mothers

Fett JD, Fristoe KL, Welsh SN (Hôpital Albert Schweitzer, Deschapelles, Haiti; Peripartum Cardiomyopathy Support Network, Deschapelles, Haiti)
Int J Gynaecol Obstet 109:34-36, 2010

Objective.—To quantify the level of risk for heart failure relapse in a subsequent pregnancy in women who have had peripartum cardiomyopathy (PPCM), and to test the hypothesis that meeting additional criteria may help lower the risk.

Methods.—Prospectively-identified PPCM patients volunteering between 2003 and 2009 were identified from the PPCM Registry of Hôpital Albert Schweitzer, Deschapelles, Haiti, and an internet support group. Data were assessed for full adherence to monitoring and diagnostic criteria, clinical data, statistical analysis, and reporting.

Results.—Of 61 post-PPCM pregnancies identified, there were 18 relapses (29.5%) of heart failure. Of 26 pregnancies with a left ventricular ejection fraction (LVEF) of less than 0.55 prior to the pregnancy, relapse occurred in 12 (46.2%) pregnancies. Of 35 pregnancies with an LVEF of 0.55 or greater prior to the pregnancy, relapse occurred in 6 (17.1%) (*P* < 0.01). No relapses occurred in 9 women who also demonstrated adequate contractile reserve.

Conclusion.—The most important criterion associated with reduced risk for heart failure relapse in a post-PPCM pregnancy is recovery defined by an LVEF 0.55 or greater before the subsequent pregnancy. Exercise stress echocardiography showing adequate contractile reserve may help to identify women at an even lower risk of relapse (Figs 1 and 2, Table 1).

▶ Women with postpartum cardiomyopathy (PPCM) are at significant risk of relapsing heart failure during a subsequent pregnancy. To date, data support the concept that the risk of relapse in a subsequent pregnancy depends on the degree of left ventricular (LV) systolic functional recovery before becoming pregnant again. However, the degree of such risk is not well defined in these limited studies,[1-4] and there are no factors identified that are associated with the lowest risk. This study is the largest prospectively identified group of patients with PPCM with subsequent pregnancies, 61 post-PPCM pregnancies in 56 women, who were assessed for relapse of heart failure. In subsequent pregnancy, 18 relapses (29.5%) of heart failure occurred and the chance of recurrence was inversely related to the LV ejection fraction (LVEF) before the subsequent pregnancy. One of the important findings by these authors is that when a subsequent pregnancy occurred before the patient had fully recovered a LVEF > 50%, relapse of heart failure in the subsequent pregnancy occurred

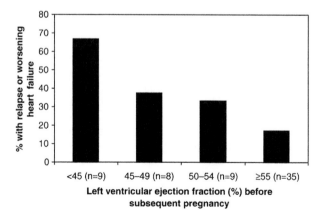

FIGURE 1.—Rate of relapse/worsening heart failure among 61 post-PPCM pregnancies, 2003–2009. (Reprinted from Fett JD, Fristoe KL, Welsh SN. Risk of heart failure relapse in subsequent pregnancy among peripartum cardiomyopathy mothers. *Int J Gynaecol Obstet.* 2010;109:34-36, with permission from Elsevier Ireland.)

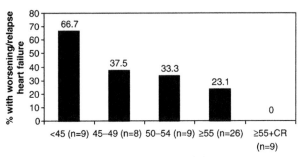

FIGURE 2.—Relapse or worsening of heart failure in 61 post-PPCM pregnancies, 2003–2009. (Reprinted from Fett JD, Fristoe KL, Welsh SN. Risk of heart failure relapse in subsequent pregnancy among peripartum cardiomyopathy mothers. *Int J Gynaecol Obstet.* 2010;109:34-36, with permission from Elsevier Ireland.)

TABLE 1.—Rate of Heart Failure Relapse Among 35 Post-PPCM Pregnancies in 30 Recovered (LVEF≥0.55) Patients From the USA, 2003–2009[a]

Criteria Met[b]	1 Only	1 and 2	1, 2, and 3	Total Relapses
Relapse of heart failure	3/11 (27.3)	3/15 (20.0)	0/9 (0)	6/35 (17.1)

[a]Values are given as number (percentage).
[b]Criterion 1: Recovered systolic heart function, with an LVEF of 0.55 or greater; Criterion 2: Maintained an LVEF of 0.55 or greater after phase-out of heart failure medications ("proof of recovery"); Criterion 3: Adequate contractile reserve demonstrated on exercise stress echocardiography (increase of LVEF at target exercise heart rate over resting heart rate by relative amount of at least 15%).

about 50% of the time.[1] Another unique observation in this study is that in patients with adequate contractile reserve before subsequent pregnancy, as defined by an increase of LVEF on exercise echocardiography at target exercise over resting heart rate ≥15%, there were no relapses of heart failure. Although the number of patients with exercise echocardiography was too small to reach significance, it is probable that this exercise test provides evidence that the heart can respond adequately to the stress of pregnancy, labor, and delivery.[5-7] It is never possible to say that in a patient who had PPCM, a subsequent pregnancy will not precipitate relapse of heart failure. However, it is true that a subsequent pregnancy in such a patient is at high risk of relapse until the patient's LV systolic function, as represented by LVEF, has returned to ≥50% or better ≥55%. If the patient has adequate contractile reserve on exercise echocardiography, the risk of relapse is even lower.

M. D. Cheitlin, MD

References

1. Fett JD, Christie LG, Murphy JG. Brief communication: Outcomes of subsequent pregnancy after peripartum cardiomyopathy: a case series from Haiti. *Ann Intern Med.* 2006;145:30-34.

2. Fett JD, Christie LG, Carraway RD, Murphy JG. Five-year prospective study of the incidence and prognosis of peripartum cardiomyopathy at a single institution. *Mayo Clin Proc.* 2005;80:1602-1606.
3. Elkayam U, Tummala PP, Rao K, et al. Maternal and fetal outcomes of subsequent pregnancies in women with peripartum cardiomyopathy. *N Engl J Med.* 2001;344: 1567-1571.
4. Habli M, O'Brien T, Nowack E, Khoury S, Barton JR, Sibai B. Peripartum cardiomyopathy: prognostic factors for long-term maternal outcome. *Am J Obstet Gynecol.* 2008;199:415.e1-415.e5.
5. Lampert MB, Weinert L, Hibbard J, Korcarz C, Lindheimer M, Lang RM. Contractile reserve in patients with peripartum cardiomyopathy and recovered left ventricular function. *Am J Obstet Gynecol.* 1997;176:189-195.
6. Moonen M, Senechal M, Cosyns B, et al. Impact of contractile reserve on acute response to cardiac resynchronization therapy. *Cardiovasc Ultrasound.* 2008;6:65.
7. Sicari R, Nihoyannopoulos P, Evangelista A, et al. Stress echocardiography expert consensus statement: European Association of Echocardiography (EAE) (a registered branch of the ESC). *Eur J Echocardiogr.* 2008;9:415-437.

Valvular Heart Disease and Infective Endocarditis

Aortic Valve Replacement With 17-mm Mechanical Prostheses: Is Patient–Prosthesis Mismatch a Relevant Phenomenon?

Garatti A, Mori F, Innocente F, et al (IRCCS Policlinico San Donato Hospital, San Donato Milanese, Milan, Italy; Casa Sollievo della Sofferenza, San Giovanni Rotondo, Foggia, Italy)
Ann Thorac Surg 91:71-78, 2011

Background.—We sought to evaluate the long-term performance of a consecutive cohort of patients implanted with a 17-mm bileaflet mechanical prosthesis.

Methods.—Between January 1995 and December 2005, 78 patients (74 women, mean age = 71 ± 12 years) underwent aortic valve replacement with a 17-mm mechanical bileaflet prosthesis (Sorin Bicarbon-Slim and St. Jude Medical-HP). Preoperative mean body surface area and New York Heart Association class were 1.6 ± 0.2 m^2 and 2.6 ± 0.8, respectively. Preoperative mean aortic annulus, indexed aortic valve area, and peak and mean gradients were 18 ± 1.6 mm, 0.42 cm^2/m^2, 89 ± 32 mm Hg, and 56 ± 21 mm Hg, respectively. Patients were divided into two groups, according to the presence (group A, 29 patients) or absence of patient–prosthesis mismatch (group B, 49 patients). Patient–prosthesis mismatch was defined by an indexed effective orifice area less than 0.85 cm^2/m^2.

Results.—Overall hospital mortality was 8.8%. Follow-up time averaged 86 ± 44 months. Actuarial 5-year and 10-year survival rates were 83.7% and 65.3%, respectively. The mean postoperative New York Heart Association class was 1.3 ± 0.6 ($p < 0.001$). Overall indexed left ventricular mass decreased from 163 ± 48 to 120 ± 42 g/m^2 ($p < 0.001$), whereas average peak and mean prosthesis gradients were 28 ± 9 mm Hg and 15 ± 6 mm Hg, respectively ($p < 0.001$). Early and long-term mortality were similar between the two groups as well as long-term hemodynamic performance (mean peak gradient was 28 mm Hg and 27 mm Hg in group A and

B, respectively, not significant); left ventricular mass regression occurred similarly in both groups (indexed left ventricular mass at follow-up was 136 ± 48 and 113 ± 40 in group A and B, respectively; not significant).

Conclusions.—Selected patients with aortic stenosis experience satisfactory clinical improvement after aortic valve replacement with modern small-diameter bileaflet prostheses (Figs 1-3).

▶ The problem of inserting a prosthetic valve into a small aortic annulus and creating a prosthesis-patient mismatch (PPM), defined as an indexed effective orifice area of <0.85 cm^2/m^2, is most common in elderly female patients and first described by Rahimtoola in 1978.[1] To avoid PPM in patients with small aortic roots, several strategies such as aortic root enlargement and stentless valve implantation have been developed and have shown good results.[2,3] Stentless 19- to 20-mm valves in patients with small aortic roots show hemodynamic improvement,[4] but there is little experience with 17-mm mechanical valves.[5,6] In the elderly, because of the necessity for anticoagulation in mechanical valves and better biologic valve survival, biologic valve prostheses are preferred. However, small stented biologic valves, especially in patients with a high body surface area, have high transprosthesis gradients, the PPM phenomenon. Root enlargement is more complicated, requires longer pump time, and is difficult or impossible in patients with heavily calcified aortic roots. Implanting a mechanical valve is quicker and simpler, but with 17-mm valves, the fear of PPM complicates the decision. This study of 78 patients with severe aortic stenosis, 34% of whom had coronary disease requiring bypass, had a 17-mm mechanical bileaflet valve implanted. Ninety-five percent of the patients were women with a body surface area (BSA) of 1.6 ± 0.2 m^2, and 90% were symptomatic. Almost 40% of the

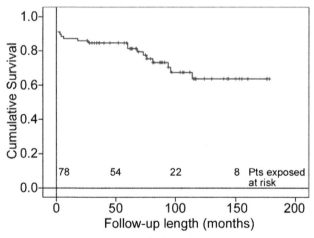

FIGURE 1.—Long-term postoperative survival. The Kaplan-Meier survival estimates were 83.7% at 5 years and 65.3% at 10 years. (Pts = patients.) (This article was published in The Annals of Thoracic Surgery, Garatti A, Mori F, Innocente F, et al. Aortic valve replacement with 17-mm mechanical prostheses: is patient–prosthesis mismatch a relevant phenomenon? *Ann Thorac Surg.* 2011;91:71-78, copyright The Society of Thoracic Surgeons 2011.)

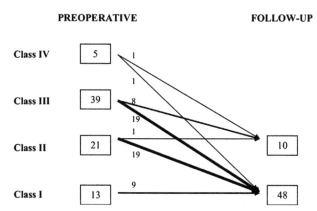

FIGURE 2.—Functional New York Heart Association class assessment before surgery and at follow-up. (This article was published in The Annals of Thoracic Surgery, Garatti A, Mori F, Innocente F, et al. Aortic valve replacement with 17-mm mechanical prostheses: is patient–prosthesis mismatch a relevant phenomenon? *Ann Thorac Surg.* 2011;91:71-78, copyright The Society of Thoracic Surgeons 2011.)

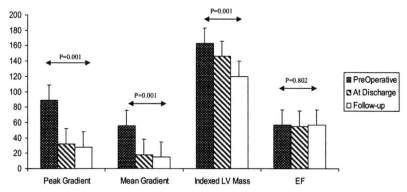

FIGURE 3.—Evolution of echocardiographic characteristics before surgery through discharge and follow-up. Probability value is calculated according to paired Student's t test between preoperative and follow-up results. (EF = ejection fraction; LV = left ventricle.) (This article was published in The Annals of Thoracic Surgery, Garatti A, Mori F, Innocente F, et al. Aortic valve replacement with 17-mm mechanical prostheses: is patient–prosthesis mismatch a relevant phenomenon? *Ann Thorac Surg.* 2011;91:71-78, copyright The Society of Thoracic Surgeons 2011.)

patients had PPM postoperatively, mainly because of a larger BSA. PPM did not affect early or long-term survival, postoperative functional capacity, and reduction in systolic gradient or regression of left ventricular mass. The major problem in this small study suggesting that PPM does not itself promise a poor prognosis is that there were only 6 patients with severe PPM (<0.65 cm²/m²). A larger study is necessary, but this study suggests that moderate PPM as presently defined does not adversely affect short- and long-term hemodynamic, functional, and survival results.

M. D. Cheitlin, MD

References

1. Rahimtoola SH. The problem of valve prosthesis-patient mismatch. *Circulation.* 1978;58:20-24.
2. Castro LJ, Arcidi JM Jr, Fisher AL, Gaudiani VA. Routine enlargement of the small aortic root: a preventive strategy to minimize mismatch. *Ann Thorac Surg.* 2002; 74:31-36.
3. Doss M, Martens S, Wood JP, et al. Performance of stentless versus stented aortic valve bioprostheses in the elderly patient: a prospective randomized trial. *Eur J Cardiothorac Surg.* 2003;23:299-304.
4. Vitale N, Caldarera I, Muneretto C, et al. Clinical evaluation of St Jude Medical Hemodynamic Plus versus standard aortic valve prostheses: The Italian multicenter, prospective, randomized study. *J Thorac Cardiovasc Surg.* 2001;122:691-698.
5. Okamura H, Yamaguchi A, Tanaka M, et al. The 17-mm St. Jude Medical Regent valve is a valid option for patients with a small aortic annulus. *Ann Thorac Surg.* 2009;87:90-94.
6. Casali G, Luzi G, Vicchio M, della Monica PL, Minardi G, Musumeci F. Echocardiographic follow-up after implanting 17-mm Regent mechanical prostheses. *Asian Cardiovasc Thorac Ann.* 2008;16:208-211.

Clinical course and predictors of death in prosthetic valve endocarditis over a 20-year period

Alonso-Valle H, Fariñas-Álvarez C, García-Palomo JD, et al (Universidad de Cantabria, Santander, Spain; Hosp Sierrallana, Torrelavega, Cantabria, Spain)
J Thorac Cardiovasc Surg 139:887-893, 2010

Objective.—To compare early and late outcome of patients with prosthetic valve endocarditis treated medically versus surgically and to determine predictors of in-hospital death. We retrospectively reviewed patient's clinical records, including laboratory findings, surgery, and pathologic files, in an acute-care, 1200-bed teaching hospital.

Methods.—One hundred thirty-three episodes of definite prosthetic valve endocarditis as defined by the Duke University diagnostic criteria occurred in 122 patients from January 1986 to December 2005. Logistic regression model was used to identify prognostic factors of in-hospital mortality. Long-term follow-up was made to assess late prognosis.

Results.—Bioprostheses were involved in 52% of cases and mechanical valves in 48%. The aortic valve was affected in 45% of patients. *Staphylococcus epidermidis* was isolated in 23% of cases, *Streptococcus* spp in 21%, *S aureus* in 13%, and *Enterococcus* in 8%. Cultures were negative in 18% of cases. Twenty-six patients were treated medically and 107 with combined antibiotics and valve replacement. The operative mortality was 6.5% and the in-hospital mortality, 29%. Presence of an abscess at echocardiography, urgent surgical treatment, heart failure, thrombocytopenia, and renal failure were significant predictors of in-hospital death. Kaplan-Meier survival at 12 months was 42% in patients treated medically and 71% in those treated surgically ($P = .0007$). Freedom from endocarditis was 91% at the end of follow-up.

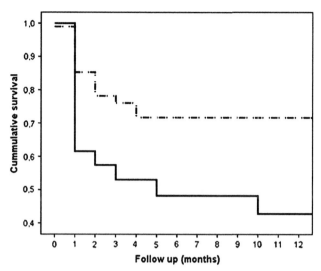

FIGURE 1.—Long-term survival of patients with prosthetic valve endocarditis after combined medical and surgical treatment (*upper line*) or medical treatment alone (*lower line*). (Reprinted from Alonso-Valle H, Fariñas-Álvarez C, García-Palomo JD, et al. Clinical course and predictors of death in prosthetic valve endocarditis over a 20-year period. *J Thorac Cardiovasc Surg.* 2010;139:887-893, with permission from The American Association for Thoracic Surgery.)

Conclusions.—Prosthetic valve endocarditis is a serious condition with high mortality. Patients with perivalvular abscess had a worse prognosis, and combined surgical and medical treatment could be the preferred approach to improve outcome (Fig 1).

▶ Prosthetic valve endocarditis is relatively uncommon but occurs in a cumulative incidence of 5% in a period of 10 years with a high case mortality varying from 25% to 59%.[1,2]

This study is the largest single-center study of patients with Duke criteria definite prosthetic valve endocarditis. Although it is a retrospective observational study with all the problems that implies, it supports the concept that the patients selected for surgery have a much better mid- to long-term prognosis than those treated medically.[3,4] Without randomization at a similar point in the course of their disease, it is impossible to definitely prove that surgery is better than medical management. The problems are that once the patient has undergone surgery, it is no longer possible to say how long he would have lived treated medically and those patients who died are included in the medically managed patients. This study provides further evidence that the presence of paravalvular abscesses is a bad prognostic sign. In this study, there was a worse prognosis with a low ejection fraction, an observation that is less often made in other studies.[5] Initial aggressive medical management is still essential in treating these patients, and the patients most likely to be handled by medical management alone are those with bioprosthetic valves where the infection is confined to the leaflets and the patient does not have severe valvular regurgitation. Even these patients are prone to progress and require surgery at a later time.

M. D. Cheitlin, MD

References

1. Rutledge R, Kim BJ, Applebaum RE. Actuarial analysis of the risk of prosthetic valve endocarditis in 1,598 patients with mechanical and bioprosthetic valves. *Arch Surg.* 1985;120:469-472.
2. Kuyvenhoven JP, van Rijk-Zwikker GL, Hermans J, Thompson J, Huysmans HA. Prosthetic valve endocarditis: analysis of risk factors for mortality. *Eur J Cardiothorac Surg.* 1994;8:420-424.
3. Fariñas MC, Pérez-Vázquez A, Fariñas-Álvarez C, et al. Risk factors of prosthetic valve endocarditis: a case-control study. *Ann Thorac Surg.* 2006;81:1284-1290.
4. Habib G, Tribouilloy C, Thuny F, et al. Prosthetic valve endocarditis: who needs surgery? A multicentre study of 104 cases. *Heart.* 2005;91:954-959.
5. Jassal DS, Neilan TG, Pradhan AD, et al. Surgical management of infective endocarditis: early predictors of short-term morbidity and mortality. *Ann Thorac Surg.* 2006;82:524-529.

Comparison Between Transcatheter and Surgical Prosthetic Valve Implantation in Patients With Severe Aortic Stenosis and Reduced Left Ventricular Ejection Fraction

Clavel MA, Webb JG, Rodés-Cabau J, et al (Laval Univ, Québec, Canada; Univ of British Columbia, Vancouver; et al)
Circulation 122:1928-1936, 2010

Background.—Patients with severe aortic stenosis and reduced left ventricular ejection fraction (LVEF) have a poor prognosis with conservative therapy but a high operative mortality when treated surgically. Recently, transcatheter aortic valve implantation (TAVI) has emerged as an alternative to surgical aortic valve replacement (SAVR) for patients considered at high or prohibitive operative risk. The objective of this study was to compare TAVI and SAVR with respect to postoperative recovery of LVEF in patients with severe aortic stenosis and reduced LV systolic function.

Methods and Results.—Echocardiographic data were prospectively collected before and after the procedure in 200 patients undergoing SAVR and 83 patients undergoing TAVI for severe aortic stenosis (aortic valve area ≤1 cm²) with reduced LV systolic function (LVEF ≤50%). TAVI patients were significantly older (81 ± 8 versus 70 ± 10 years; $P<0.0001$) and had more comorbidities compared with SAVR patients. Despite similar baseline LVEF ($34 \pm 11\%$ versus $34 \pm 10\%$), TAVI patients had better recovery of LVEF compared with SAVR patients (ΔLVEF, $14 \pm 15\%$ versus $7 \pm 11\%$; $P=0.005$). At the 1-year follow-up, 58% of TAVI patients had a normalization of LVEF ($>50\%$) as opposed to 20% in the SAVR group. On multivariable analysis, female gender ($P=0.004$), lower LVEF at baseline ($P=0.005$), absence of atrial fibrillation ($P=0.01$), TAVI ($P=0.007$), and larger increase in aortic valve area after the procedure (P=0.01) were independently associated with better recovery of LVEF.

Conclusion.—In patients with severe aortic stenosis and depressed LV systolic function, TAVI is associated with better LVEF recovery compared with SAVR. TAVI may provide an interesting alternative to SAVR in patients with depressed LV systolic function considered at high surgical risk.

▶ Patients with severe aortic stenosis (AS) and reduced left ventricular ejection fraction (LVEF) have a poor prognosis without valve replacement and an increased perioperative mortality compared with those with a normal LVEF.[1,2] In such patients, improvement after surgical prosthetic valve change in LVEF is variable, with improvement occurring because of a decrease in a pressure afterload and worsening because of ischemia, cardioplegia, oxidative stress, and inflammation-causing myocardial damage.[3,4] After prosthetic valve replacement, studies have shown that patients with depressed LVEF are very sensitive to the residual pressure afterload imposed by prosthesis-patient mismatch.[5] With the development of transcatheter aortic valve implantation (TAVI), there is now an alternative to surgical prosthetic valve replacement that avoids some of the serious negative consequences of bypass surgery and is being considered for patients at high or prohibitive surgical risk.[6,7] This retrospective observational study compared outcomes in patients with severe AS and reduced LVEF after surgical prosthetic valve replacement with those with TAVI and showed at 1 year postprocedure that the number of patients improving to an LVEF > 50% was significantly higher in the patients with thrombotic associated myocardial infarction. In another study by the same group, they reported that TAVI is associated with better hemodynamic performance and less incidence of prosthesis-patient mismatch compared with surgical valve replacement with either stented or stentless bioprostheses.[8] The duration of follow-up was short; the study was not a randomized study comparing surgical valve replacement with TAVI, but the results are extremely supportive in patients with severe AS and reduced LVEF or those considered inoperable of TAVI as an alternative therapy.

M. D. Cheitlin, MD

References

1. Powell DE, Tunick PA, Rosenzweig BP, et al. Aortic valve replacement in patients with aortic stenosis and severe left ventricular dysfunction. *Arch Intern Med.* 2000;160:1337-1341.
2. Pereira JJ, Lauer MS, Bashir M, et al. Survival after aortic valve replacement for severe aortic stenosis with low transvalvular gradients and severe left ventricular dysfunction. *J Am Coll Cardiol.* 2002;39:1356-1363.
3. Anselmi A, Abbate A, Girola F, et al. Myocardial ischemia, stunning, inflammation, and apoptosis during cardiac surgery: a review of evidence. *Eur J Cardiothorac Surg.* 2004;25:304-311.
4. Vähäsilta T, Saraste A, Kitö V, et al. Cardiomyocyte apoptosis after antegrade and retrograde cardioplegia. *Ann Thorac Surg.* 2005;80:2229-2234.
5. Ruel M, Al-Faleh H, Kulik A, Chan KL, Mesana TG, Burwash IG. Prosthesis-patient mismatch after aortic valve replacement predominantly affects patients

with pre-existing left ventricular dysfunction: effect on survival, freedom from heart failure, and left ventricular mass regression. *J Thorac Cardiovasc Surg.* 2006;131:1036-1044.

6. Webb JG, Pasupati S, Humphries K, et al. Percutaneous transarterial aortic valve replacement in selected high-risk patients with aortic stenosis. *Circulation.* 2007; 116:755-763.

7. Rodés-Cabau J, Webb JG, Cheung A, et al. Transcatheter aortic valve implantation for the treatment of severe symptomatic aortic stenosis in patients at very high or prohibitive surgical risk: acute and late outcomes of the multicenter Canadian experience. *J Am Coll Cardiol.* 2010;55:1080-1090.

8. Clavel MA, Webb JG, Pibarot P, et al. Comparison of the hemodynamic performance of percutaneous and surgical bioprostheses for the treatment of severe aortic stenosis. *J Am Coll Cardiol.* 2009;53:1883-1891.

Impact of Baseline Severity of Aortic Valve Stenosis on Effect of Intensive Lipid Lowering Therapy (from the SEAS Study)

Gerdts E, Rossebø AB, Pedersen TR, et al (Univ Hosp, Bergen, Norway; Aker Univ Hosp, Oslo, Norway; Oslo Univ Hosp Ulleval, Norway; et al)
Am J Cardiol 106:1634-1639, 2010

Retrospective studies have suggested a beneficial effect of lipid-lowering treatment on the progression of aortic stenosis (AS) in milder stages of the disease. In the randomized, placebo-controlled Simvastatin and Ezetimibe in Aortic Stenosis (SEAS) study, 4.3 years of combined treatment with simvastatin 40 mg and ezetimibe 10 mg did not reduce aortic valve events (AVEs), while ischemic cardiovascular events (ICEs) were significantly reduced in the overall study population. However, the impact of baseline AS severity on treatment effect has not been reported. Baseline and outcomes data in 1,763 SEAS patients (mean age 67 years, 39% women) were used. The study population was divided into tertiles of baseline peak aortic jet velocity (tertile 1: ≤2.8 m/s; tertile 2: >2.8 to 3.3 m/s; tertile 3: >3.3 m/s). Treatment effect and interaction were tested in Cox regression analyses. The rates of AVEs and ICEs increased with increasing baseline severity of AS. In Cox regression analyses, higher baseline peak aortic jet velocity predicted higher rates of AVEs and ICEs in all tertiles (all p values <0.05) and in the total study population (p <0.001). Simvastatin-ezetimibe treatment was not associated with a statistically significant reduction in AVEs in any individual tertile. A significant quantitative interaction between the severity of AS and simvastatin-ezetimibe treatment effect was demonstrated for ICEs (p <0.05) but not for AVEs (p = 0.10). In conclusion, the SEAS study results demonstrate a strong relation between baseline the severity of AS and the rate of cardiovascular events but no significant effect of lipid-lowering treatment on AVEs, even in the group with the mildest AS (Figs 1 and 2).

▶ Epidemiologic and experimental studies have implicated hypercholesterolemia as a risk factor in the development and progression of valvular aortic stenosis (AS), identifying cellular mechanisms similar to those involved in the

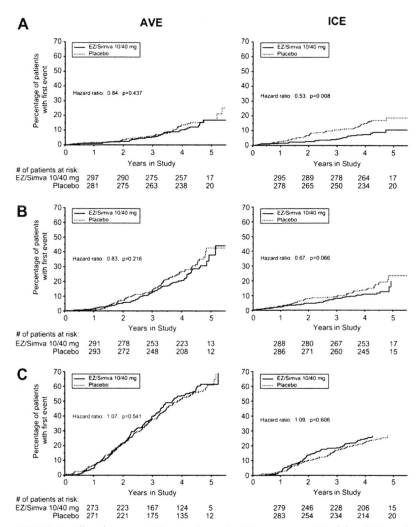

FIGURE 1.—Effect of simvastatin (Simva) and ezetimibe (EZ) treatment on AVEs *(left)* and ICEs *(right)*. Kaplan-Meier curve for intention-to-treat population in the lower tertile *(A)*, middle tertile *(B)*, and upper tertile *(C)* of baseline peak aortic jet velocity. (Reprinted from Gerdts E, Rossebø AB, Pedersen TR, et al. Impact of baseline severity of aortic valve stenosis on effect of intensive lipid lowering therapy (from the SEAS Study). *Am J Cardiol.* 2010;106:1634-1639, copyright © 2010 with permission from Elsevier.)

development of atherosclerosis. The possibility that statins (3-hydroxy-3-methyl-glutaryl-Coenzyme A reductase inhibitors) could slow or prevent the progression of AS has been proposed[1-3] and supported by a number of small, retrospective, observational studies.[4-6] However, in the 3 prospective treatment trials,[7-9] there was no evidence for statins decreasing the progression of or the adverse events from AS. Despite these disappointing results, retrospective analyses continue to suggest that statin therapy would be effective if it was started early enough in patients with the mildest degrees of AS.[10,11]

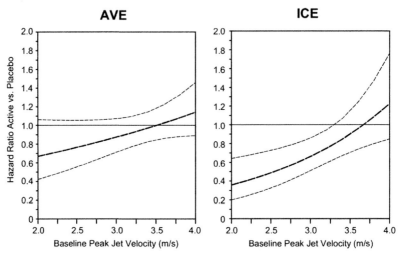

FIGURE 2.—Effect of simvastatin-ezetimibe treatment on AVEs *(left)* and ICEs *(right)* presented as hazard ratios and 95% confidence intervals as a function of baseline peak aortic jet velocity in the total study population. (Reprinted from Gerdts E, Rossebø AB, Pedersen TR, et al. Impact of baseline severity of aortic valve stenosis on effect of intensive lipid lowering therapy (from the SEAS Study). *Am J Cardiol.* 2010;106:1634-1639, copyright © 2010 with permission from Elsevier.)

This study is a substudy of the Simvastatin and Ezetimibe in Aortic Stenosis (SEAS) study, where 1763 patients with asymptomatic mild to moderate AS were randomized to placebo or to combination treatment with simvastatin 40 mg and ezetimibe 10 mg daily and followed up with an annual echocardiogram. The overall study found no effect of lipid-lowering drugs on progression or adverse events from AS. This study stratified the patients into tertiles (T) of baseline peak aortic jet velocity (T1: ≤ 2.8 m/sec, T2: > 2.8-3.3 m/sec, and T3: > 3.3 m/sec), and after a 4.3-year median follow-up duration, in the total study population, there was quantitative interaction between AS severity and simvastatin-ezetimibe treatment for ischemic cardiovascular events (ICEs) (cardiovascular death, nonfatal myocardial infarction, hospitalized unstable angina, coronary revascularization, and nonhemorrhagic stroke) but not for aortic valvular events (cardiovascular death, aortic valve replacement, and congestive heart failure because of progression of AS). The reduction in ICEs was significant only in the lowest tertile, borderline in the middle tertile, and absent in the highest tertile, possibly because in those with the highest gradient, the period of lipid-lowering drugs was too short before valve replacement became necessary. There was also no evidence for slowing annular progression of AS from the lowest to the highest tertile of aortic jet velocity.

These findings are consistent with the observation from the Cardiovascular Health Study that aortic valve sclerosis was associated with a 50% increased risk of myocardial infarction and is a marker for coronary artery disease, which is markedly benefited by lipid lowering. Although this study is evidence against statins reducing the progression of AS, it does not eliminate the possibility that the time of follow-up was too short or that patients with hypercholesterolemia, diabetes, or renal failure might not benefit because these patients were not included in the SEAS study. The negative results of these large randomized studies in patients with moderate AS must give caution to extrapolating results from retrospective, observational, or small studies suggesting otherwise.

M. D. Cheitlin, MD

References

1. Stewart BF, Siscovick D, Lind BK, et al. Clinical factors associated with calcific aortic valve disease. Cardiovascular Health Study. *J Am Coll Cardiol*. 1997;29:630-634.
2. Rajamannan NM, Subramaniam M, Springett M, et al. Atorvastatin inhibits hypercholesterolemia-induced cellular proliferation and bone matrix production in the rabbit aortic valve. *Circulation*. 2002;105:2660-2665.
3. Bossé Y, Mathieu P, Pibarot P. Genomics: the next step to elucidate the etiology of calcific aortic valve stenosis. *J Am Coll Cardiol*. 2008;51:1327-1336.
4. Novaro GM, Tiong IY, Pearce GL, Lauer MS, Sprecher DL, Griffin BP. Effect of hydroxymethylglutaryl coenzyme a reductase inhibitors on the progression of calcific aortic stenosis. *Circulation*. 2001;104:2205-2209.
5. Rosenhek R, Rader F, Loho N, et al. Statins but not angiotensin-converting enzyme inhibitors delay progression of aortic stenosis. *Circulation*. 2004;110: 1291-1295.
6. Moura LM, Ramos SF, Zamorano JL, et al. Rosuvastatin affecting aortic valve endothelium to slow the progression of aortic stenosis. *J Am Coll Cardiol*. 2007;49:554-561.
7. Cowell SJ, Newby DE, Prescott RJ, et al. Scottish Aortic Stenosis and Lipid Lowering Trial, Impact on Regression (SALTIRE) Investigators. A randomized trial of intensive lipid-lowering therapy in calcific aortic stenosis. *N Engl J Med*. 2005;352:2389-2397.
8. Rossebø AB, Pedersen TR, Boman K, et al. SEAS Investigators. Intensive lipid lowering with simvastatin and ezetimibe in aortic stenosis. *N Engl J Med*. 2008;359:1343-1356.
9. Chan KL, Teo K, Dumesnil JG, Ni A, Tam J, ASTRONOMER Investigators. Effect of lipid lowering with rosuvastatin on progression of aortic stenosis: results of the aortic stenosis progression observation: measuring effects of rosuvastatin (ASTRONOMER) trial. *Circulation*. 2010;121:306-314.
10. Antonini-Canterin F, Hîrşu M, Popescu BA, et al. Stage related effect of statin treatment on the progression of aortic valve sclerosis and stenosis. *Am J Cardiol*. 2008;102:738-742.
11. Antonini-Canterin F, Leiballi E, Enache R, et al. Hydroxymethylglutaryl coenzyme-a reductase inhibitors delay the progression of rheumatic aortic valve stenosis a long-term echocardiographic study. *J Am Coll Cardiol*. 2009;53:1874-1879.

Impact of Early Surgery on Embolic Events in Patients With Infective Endocarditis

Kim D-H, Kang D-H, Lee M-Z, et al (Univ of Ulsan, Seoul, Korea; et al)
Circulation 122:S17-S22, 2010

Background.—Surgical indications to prevent systemic embolism in infective endocarditis (IE) remain controversial. We sought to compare clinical outcomes of early surgery with conventional treatment in IE patients with embolic indications only.

Methods and Results.—From 1998 to 2006, we prospectively enrolled 132 consecutive patients (86 men; age, 49 ± 17 years) with definite IE.

Patients were included if they had a left-sided native valve endocarditis with vegetation. The choice of early surgery or conventional treatment was at the discretion of attending physician. Early surgery was performed on 64 patients (OP group) within 7 days of diagnosis, and conventional management was chosen for 68 patients (CONV group). The OP group had larger vegetations and a higher percentage of patients with severe valvular disease (88% versus 62%, $P = 0.001$). During initial hospitalization, there were no embolic events and 2 in-hospital deaths in the OP group and 14 embolic events and 2 in-hospital deaths in the CONV group. During a median follow-up of 1402 days, there were 2 cardiovascular deaths, 2 embolic events, and 1 recurrence of IE in the CONV group, and 1 cardiovascular death and 2 embolic events in the OP group. The 5-year event-free survival rate was significantly higher in the OP group ($93 \pm 3\%$) than in the CONV group ($73 + 5\%$, $P = 0.0016$). For 44 propensity score–matched pairs, the OP group had a lower event rate (hazard ratio, 0.18; $P = 0.007$).

Conclusions.—Compared with conventional treatment, an early surgery strategy is associated with improved clinical outcomes by effectively decreasing systemic embolism in patients with IE (Table 2).

▶ Infective endocarditis, in spite of the latest advances in diagnosis and therapy, continues to be the cause of increased mortality, the leading causes of which are congestive heart failure due to valvular regurgitation and stroke due to embolization.[1,2] The latest American College of Cardiology/American Heart Association guidelines for native valve endocarditis list surgery as class I indication for congestive heart failure, hemodynamic evidence of severe acute valvular regurgitation, fungal infection or persistent infection, refractory to treatment, and endocarditis complicated by heart block or other evidence of extravalvular destructive penetrating lesions, such as annular abscess or fistulae.[3] With vegetations, surgery is a class IIa indication if there are recurrent emboli and persistent vegetations in spite of appropriate antibiotic therapy. A class IIb recommendation for surgery is for patients with mobile vegetations in excess of 10 mm with or without emboli. Both recommendations concerning vegetations have a level of evidence: C, meaning that the recommendation is based on expert consensus, in other words, the opinion of the group writing

TABLE 2.—Comparison of In-Hospital and Follow-Up Events

	OP Group (n=64)	CONV Group (n=68)	P
In-hospital events			
Death, n	2	2	NS
Embolism, n	0	14	0.001
Follow-up events			
Death, n	1	2	NS
Thromboembolism, n	2	2	NS
Recurrence of IE, n	0	1	NS
5-year survival rate, %	95±3	94±3	NS
5-year event-free survival, %	93±3	73±5	0.002

the recommendations. There are studies that show that patients with large vegetations are at risk for embolization[4,5] and that the risk is especially high during the first 2 weeks of effective antibiotic therapy, but indication for surgery to prevent embolization is controversial[6,7] and must be balanced against the potential risks of perioperative mortality, prosthetic valve dysfunction, and infection.[8,9] With advances in surgical technique, the revised European Society of Cardiology guidelines recommend surgery as a class IIb indication for iso-lated very large vegetations (15 mm in diameter).[10] This study reports the clin-ical outcomes of early surgery within 1 week of diagnosis compared with those managed with a conventional treatment strategy based on present guidelines in infective native valve endocarditis with embolic indications only. The primary end point was a composite of embolic events occurring after the diagnosis of endocarditis, cardiovascular mortality, and recurrence of endocarditis during follow-up. In spite of the early operative group having larger and mobile vege-tations and a higher incidence of severe valvular disease, which should bias the study against early surgery, this study for the first time showed that early surgery within 1 week of diagnosis in patients with only vegetations as a possible surgical indication had an improved long-term clinical outcome with significant reduction in systemic embolic events and improved survival at about 4 years follow-up compared with conventional treatment strategy. These benefits were achieved without an increase in recurrent infective endocarditis relapse or prosthetic valve—related problems.

M. D. Cheitlin, MD

References

1. Sandre RM, Shafran SD. Infective endocarditis: review of 135 cases over 9 years. *Clin Infect Dis.* 1996;22:276-286.
2. Millaire A, Leroy O, Gaday V, et al. Incidence and prognosis of embolic events and metastatic infections in infective endocarditis. *Eur Heart J.* 1997;18: 677-684.
3. Bonow RO, Carabello BA, Chatterjee K, et al. 2008 focused update incorporated into the ACC/AHA 2006 guidelines for the management of patients with valvular heart disease: a report of the American College of Cardiology/American Heart Association Task Force on Practice Guidelines (Writing Committee to revise the 1998 guidelines for the management of patients with valvular heart disease): Endorsed by the Society of Cardiovascular Anesthesiologists, Society for Cardio-vascular Angiography and Interventions, and Society of Thoracic Surgeons. *J Am Coll Cardiol.* 2008;52:e1-e142.
4. Di Salvo G, Habib G, Pergola V, et al. Echocardiography predicts embolic events in infective endocarditis. *J Am Coll Cardiol.* 2001;37:1069-1076.
5. Thuny F, Di Salvo G, Belliard O, et al. Risk of embolism and death in infective endocarditis: prognostic value of echocardiography: a prospective multicenter study. *Circulation.* 2005;112:69-75.
6. Tleyjeh IM, Ghomrawi HM, Steckelberg JM, et al. The impact of valve surgery on 6-month mortality in left-sided infective endocarditis. *Circulation.* 2007;115: 1721-1728.
7. Cabell CH, Abrutyn E, Fowler VG Jr, et al. Use of surgery in patients with native valve infective endocarditis: results from the International Collaboration on Endocarditis Merged Database. *Am Heart J.* 2005;150:1092-1098.
8. Thuny F, Beurtheret S, Mancini J, et al. The timing of surgery influences mortality and morbidity in adults with severe complicated infective endocarditis: a propen-sity analysis. *Eur Heart J.* 2009 Mar 26 [Epub ahead of print].

9. Tleyjeh IM, Steckelberg JM, Georgescu G, et al. The association between the timing of valve surgery and 6-month mortality in left-sided infective endocarditis. *Heart.* 2008;94:892-896.

10. Habib G, Hoen B, Tornos P, et al. Guidelines on the prevention, diagnosis, and treatment of infective endocarditis (new version 2009): the Task Force on the Prevention, Diagnosis, and Treatment of Infective Endocarditis of the European Society of Cardiology (ESC). Endorsed by the European Society of Clinical Microbiology and Infectious Diseases (ESCMID) and the International Society of Chemotherapy (ISC) for Infection and Cancer. *Eur Heart J.* 2009;30:2369-2413.

Prognostic Implications of Mitral Regurgitation in Patients With Severe Aortic Regurgitation

Pai RG, Varadarajan P (Loma Linda Univ Med Ctr, CA)
Circulation 122:S43-S47, 2010

Background.—Mitral regurgitation (MR) is common in those with severe aortic regurgitation (AR) and can predispose to atrial fibrillation, heart failure, and a need for mitral valve surgery during aortic valve replacement (AVR). However, little data exist as to its clinical and prognostic implications.

Methods and Results.—Search of our echocardiographic data base between 1993 and 2007 yielded 756 patients with severe AR, with comprehensive clinical data from chart review and mortality data from National Death Index. Mortality was analyzed as a function of MR severity. Effect of AVR and concomitant mitral valve repair were investigated. Patient characteristics were age, 61 ± 17 years; female sex, 41%; and ejection fraction, 54 ± 19%. MR grade ≥2+ was present in 343 (45%) patients: 2+ in 152 (20%), 3+ in 93 (12%), and 4+ in 98 (13%). There was a progressive decrease in survival with each grade of MR ($P<0.0001$). Performance of AVR was associated with a better survival in those with 3 or 4+ MR ($P=0.02$). In addition, concomitant mitral valve repair in these patients resulted in a better survival (hazard ratio, 0.29; $P=0.02$).

Conclusions.—MR is common in patients with severe AR, with 3 or 4+ MR occurring in a quarter of these patients. It is an independent predictor of reduced survival. Performance of AVR and concomitant mitral valve repair is associated with a better survival. Development of MR should serve as an indication for AVR even in asymptomatic patients.

▶ The presence of mitral regurgitation (MR) in patients with severe aortic regurgitation (AR) can predispose to the development of atrial fibrillation, heart failure, and a need for mitral valve (MV) repair or replacement at the time of aortic valve replacement (AVR). This retrospective observational study from a single institution reports on a final cohort of 756 patients with severe AR with a follow-up of between 4 and 5 years. Twenty percent had 2 + MR, and 25% had 3 + or 4 + MR. Logistic regression analysis identified a lower left ventricular (LV) ejection fraction, thinner LV wall, female gender, atrial fibrillation, coronary artery disease, and renal insufficiency to be independent risk factors for 3+ or 4+ MR. Only 65 (34%) of the patients with 3+ or 4+ MR had AVR, and of these 39 (60%) had either MV replacement or MV repair. The study showed that 3+ to 4+ MR in patients with severe AR increases mortality and AVR improves survival. In a propensity score analysis, AVR was associated with a mortality hazard of 0.46 in patients with severe AR and 3+ or 4+ MR. Because 3+ or 4+ MR has deleterious consequences, asymptomatic patients with severe AR with still excellent systolic function should be watched closely for the development of progressive MR because severe MR represents an increased mortality risk. Even lesser degrees of MR increased mortality in patients with severe AR, and AVR in these patients also improved survival although to a lesser degree than with 3+ or 4+ MR. Although the latest American College of Cardiology/American Heart Association guidelines do not mention concomitant MR in patients with severe AR as an indication for AVR,[1] it might be prudent to consider surgery if progressive MR occurs.

M. D. Cheitlin, MD

Reference

1. Bonow RO, Carabello BA, Chatterjee K, et al. 2008 Focused update incorporated into the ACC/AHA 2006 guidelines for the management of patients with valvular heart disease: a report of the American College of Cardiology/American Heart Association Task Force on Practice Guidelines (Writing Committee to Revise the 1998 Guidelines for the Management of Patients With Valvular Heart Disease): endorsed by the Society of Cardiovascular Anesthesiologists, Society for Cardiovascular Angiography and Interventions, and Society of Thoracic Surgeons. *Circulation.* 2008;118:e523-e661.

Age-Dependent Profile of Left-Sided Infective Endocarditis: A 3-Center Experience

López J, Revilla A, Vilacosta I, et al (Hospital Clínico Universitario, Valladolid, Spain; Hospital Clínico San Carlos, Madrid, Spain; et al)
Circulation 121:892-897, 2010

Background.—The influence of age on the main epidemiological, clinical, echocardiographic, microbiological, and prognostic features of patients with infective endocarditis remains unknown. We present the series with the largest numbers and range of ages of subjects to date that analyzes the influence of age on the main characteristics of patients with isolated left-sided infective endocarditis. Furthermore, this series is the first one in which patients have been distributed according to age quartile.

Methods and Results.—A total of 600 episodes of left-sided endocarditis consecutively diagnosed in 3 tertiary centers were stratified into age-specific quartiles and 107 variables compared between the different groups. With increasing age, the percentage of women, previous heart disease, predisposing disease (diabetes mellitus and cancer), and infection by enterococci and *Streptococcus bovis* also increased. Valvular insufficiency and perforation and *Staphylococcus aureus* infection were more common in younger patients. The therapeutic approach differed depending on patient age because of the growing proportion of older patients who only received medical treatment. Clinical course and hospital prognosis were worse in the older patients because of increased surgical mortality among them.

Conclusions.—Increasing age is associated with less valvular impairment (insufficiency and perforation), a more favorable microbiological profile, and increased surgical mortality among adults with left-sided infective endocarditis.

▶ Infective endocarditis (IE), especially left-sided IE, in spite of advances in diagnosis and therapy, is still a disease with a poor prognosis. How age affects the clinical picture and the prognosis has become more important as the population ages and the expected numbers of cases of IE increase in the elderly. Although there have been reports of the influence of age in IE, the studies were limited in that many had small numbers of elderly patients,[1-3] reflected different demographics, focused on variable outcomes,[1-4] and used arbitrary age-specific cutoff points that were determined a posteriori.[1-4] This study examined the influence of patient age at the time of diagnosis on the epidemiological, clinical, echocardiographic, microbiological, and prognostic profile of patients with left-sided IE by distributing patients homogeneously by age in quartiles. The study included 600 patients with prospective recording of 107 variables for each episode analyzed. Although many of the findings were expected, this study found an age-related increase in the proportion of women, nosocomial IE, patients with previous heart disease, and conditions that increase the risk of IE, such as cancer and diabetes mellitus,[5] the proportion of patients with prosthetic valve IE, and a lower percentage of intravenous drug use and human immunodeficiency virus infection. With increasing age, there was a higher percentage of native mitral valve IE and a lower percentage of aortic valve involvement. Among the clinical and prognostic differences, as expected, as age increased there was an increased incidence of cardiac and renal failure. There was a lower incidence of valvular rupture in the elderly, and surgical intervention decreased as the patients aged but surgical mortality increased. The number of patients with surgical indications rejected for surgery increased significantly with increasing age. This study is unique in that it presents the largest number and age range of patients with prespecified data collected where arbitrary age limits were not set and the analysis limited only to those with left-sided IE.

M. D. Cheitlin, MD

References

1. Peled N, Pitlik S, Livni G, Ashkenazi S, Bishara J. Impact of age on clinical features and outcome of infective endocarditis. *Eur J Clin Microbiol Infect Dis.* 2006;25:473-475.
2. Di Salvo G, Thuny F, Rosenberg V, et al. Endocarditis in the elderly: clinical, echocardiographic, and prognostic features. *Eur Heart J.* 2003;24:1576-1583.
3. Cruz JM, Martínez R, García M, Zarzalejos JM, de la Peña F. Infective endocarditis in the elderly [in Spanish]. *An Med Interna.* 2003;20:569-574.
4. Durante-Mangoni E, Bradley S, Selton-Suty C, et al. International Collaboration on Endocarditis Prospective Cohort Study Group. Current features of infective

endocarditis in elderly patients: results of the International Collaboration on Endocarditis Prospective Cohort Study. *Arch Intern Med.* 2008;168:2095-2103.
5. Movahed MR, Hashemzadeh M, Jamal MM. Increased prevalence of infectious endocarditis in patients with type II diabetes mellitus. *J Diabetes Complications.* 2007;21:403-406.

Comprehensive Diagnostic Strategy for Blood Culture–Negative Endocarditis: A Prospective Study of 819 New Cases

Fournier P-E, Thuny F, Richet H, et al (Université de la Méditerranée, France; Centre Hospitalo-Universitaire de Grenoble, France; et al)
Clin Infect Dis 51:131-140, 2010

Background.—Blood culture–negative endocarditis (BCNE) may account for up to 31% of all cases of endocarditis.

Methods.—We used a prospective, multimodal strategy incorporating serological, molecular, and histopathological assays to investigate specimens from 819 patients suspected of having BCNE.

Results.—Diagnosis of endocarditis was first ruled out for 60 patients. Among 759 patients with BCNE, a causative microorganism was identified in 62.7%, and a noninfective etiology in 2.5%. Blood was the most useful specimen, providing a diagnosis for 47.7% of patients by serological analysis (mainly Q fever and *Bartonella* infections). Broad-range polymerase chain reaction (PCR) of blood and *Bartonella*–specific Western blot methods diagnosed 7 additional cases. PCR of valvular biopsies identified 109 more etiologies, mostly streptococci, *Tropheryma whipplei*, *Bartonella* species, and fungi. Primer extension enrichment reaction and autoimmunohistochemistry identified a microorganism in 5 additional patients. No virus or *Chlamydia* species were detected. A noninfective cause of endocarditis, particularly neoplasic or autoimmune disease, was determined by histological analysis or by searching for antinuclear antibodies in 19 (2.5%) of the patients. Our diagnostic strategy proved useful and sensitive for BCNE workup.

Conclusions.—We highlight the major role of zoonotic agents and the underestimated role of noninfective diseases in BCNE. We propose serological analysis for *Coxiella burnetii* and *Bartonella* species, detection of antinuclear antibodies and rheumatoid factor as first-line tests, followed by specific PCR assays for *T. whipplei*, *Bartonella* species, and fungi in blood. Broad-spectrum 16S and 18S ribosomal RNA PCR may be performed on valvular biopsies, when available (Figs 1 and 2, Table 5).

▶ Blood culture-negative endocarditis (BCNE), where no microorganism can be grown using the usual blood culture methods, occurs in 2.5% to 31% of infective endocarditis cases.[1] The reasons for the variation in the incidence of negative blood cultures in different series may be differences in diagnostic criteria used, fastidious zoonotic agents, early use of antibiotics prior to drawing blood cultures, differences in timing of serologic testing,[2] or involvement of

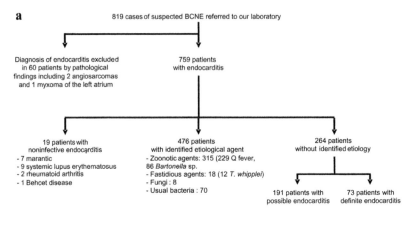

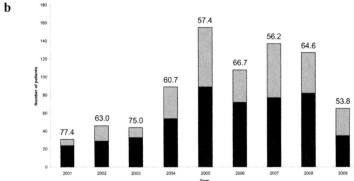

FIGURE 1.—Distribution of the 819 patients with suspected blood culture−negative endocarditis (BCNE) studied from 1 June 2001 to 1 September 2009, according to the etiological diagnosis *(a)* and the year *(b)*. *Black columns,* Number of patients per year for whom we obtained an etiological diagnosis (infectious or not). *Gray columns,* Number of patients without any etiological diagnosis. Values above each column represent percentages of etiological diagnoses obtained each year. Agents include *Tropheryma whipplei.* (Reprinted from Fournier P-E, Thuny F, Richet H, et al. Comprehensive diagnostic strategy for blood culture−negative endocarditis: a prospective study of 819 new cases. *Clin Infect Dis.* 2010;51:131-140, with permission from the Infectious Diseases Society of America and the University of Chicago.)

unknown organisms. This study is from an institution to which cases of BCNE are referred. The authors demonstrate the value of systematic serologic testing for not only various fastidious organisms such as *Coxiella burnetii* and *Bartonella* species but also *Brucella* species, *Legionella pneumophila*, and *Mycoplasma* species. Other methods that proved of value were histologic examination and molecular detection methods such as broad-range polymerase chain reaction, particularly when applied to excised valve tissue. Another useful tool in identifying the noninfectious cause of endocarditis was the detection of autoantibodies including rheumatoid factor, where 2.5% of the patients with BCNE were found to have marantic endocarditis, Libman-Sacks endocarditis, rheumatoid arthritis, and Behçet disease. Using this multimodal diagnostic strategy, they identified a causative microbial agent in 62.7% of 759 patients

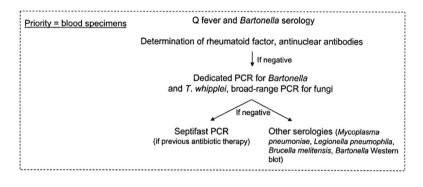

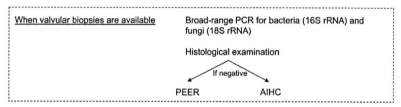

FIGURE 2.—Diagnostic tests applied to clinical specimens for identification of causative agents of blood culture−negative endocarditis. Agents include *Tropheryma whipplei*. AIHC, autoimmunohisto-chemistry; PCR, polymerase chain reaction; PEER, primer extension enrichment reaction; rRNA, ribosomal RNA. (Reprinted from Fournier P-E, Thuny F, Richet H, et al. Comprehensive diagnostic strategy for blood culture−negative endocarditis: a prospective study of 819 new cases. *Clin Infect Dis.* 2010;51:131-140, with permission from the Infectious Diseases Society of America and the University of Chicago.)

TABLE 5.—Comparison of Microorganisms Identified in Published Series of Blood Culture−Negative Endocarditis

Microorganism	Present Study[a] (n = 740)	France [3] (n = 348)	France [29] (n = 88)	Great Britain [30] (n = 63)	Algeria [31] (n = 62)
Bartonella species	12.4	28.4	0	9.5	22.6
Brucella melitensis	0	0	0	0	1.6
Chlamydia species	0	0	2.2	1.6	0
Corynebacterium species	0.5	0	1.1	0	1.6
Coxiella burnetii	37.0	48	7.9	12.7	3.2
Enterobacteriaceae	0.5	0	0	0	0
HACEK bacteria	0.5	0	0	0	3.2
Staphylococcus species	2.0	0	3.4	11.1	6.4
Streptococcus species	4.4	0	1.1	6.3	3.2
Tropheryma whipplei	2.6	0.3	0	0	0
Other bacteria	3.0	1.1	1.1	1.6	1.6
Fungi	1.0	0	0	6.3	1.6
No etiology	36.5	22.1	82.9	50.8	54.8

Note. Data are percentages. HACEK, Haemophilus, Actinobacillus, Cardiobacterium, Eikenella, Kingella.
Editor's Note: Please refer to original journal article for full references.
[a]Patients classified as excluded were not included in this analysis.

with BCNE and noninfective endocarditis in 2.5%. In hospitals where infective endocarditis is a relatively frequent problem, the physicians managing these patients should consult with their laboratory microbiologists whenever they have a case of BCNE and make certain that the patient has had the benefit of these latest techniques to make an etiologic diagnosis.

M. D. Cheitlin, MD

References

1. Brouqui P, Raoult D. Endocarditis due to rare and fastidious bacteria. *Clin Microbiol Rev.* 2001;14:177-207.
2. Raoult D, Casalta JP, Richet H, et al. Contribution of systematic serological testing in diagnosis of infective endocarditis. *J Clin Microbiol.* 2005;43:5238-5242.

Conclusion about the association between valve surgery and mortality in an infective endocarditis cohort changed after adjusting for survivor bias
Tleyjeh IM, Ghomrawi HMK, Steckelberg JM, et al (King Fahd Med City, Riyadh, Saudi Arabia; Cornell Univ, NY; Mayo Clinic College of Medicine, Rochester, MN; et al)
J Clin Epidemiol 63:130-135, 2010

Objective.—Survivor bias commonly weakens observational studies, even those published in premier journals. It occurs because patients who live longer are more likely to receive treatment than those who die early. We sought to quantify the effect of survivor bias on the association between valve surgery and mortality in infective endocarditis (IE).

Study Design and Setting.—The study cohort included 546 IE patients. We compared the hazard ratios (HR) resulting from two propensity score analysis approaches that adjusted for survivor bias (time-dependent variable and matching on follow-up time) with those achieved using the same models but without that adjustment (time-fixed variable).

Results.—In the total cohort, the HR of surgery in the time-dependent model was 1.9 (95% confidence interval [CI] = 1.1–3.2; $P = 0.03$) vs. 0.9 (95% CI = 0.5–1.4; $P = 0.53$) in the time-fixed model. In the propensity score–matched subset, the HR of surgery was 1.3 (95% CI = 0.5–3.1; $P = 0.56$) and 0.8 (95% CI = 0.4–1.7; $P = 0.57$) in the subset with and without matching on follow-up time, respectively.

Conclusion.—Adjusting for survivor bias changed the conclusion about the association between valve surgery and mortality in IE. Researchers should be aware of this bias when evaluating observational studies of treatment efficacy (Fig 1).

▶ This article addresses the problem of survivor bias in observational studies by reanalyzing 4 observational studies involving the effect of surgery in a group of 546 patients with left-sided infective endocarditis. Three of these studies had a propensity score analysis and found survival benefit for surgery, at least in a subset of patients. None had accounted for survivor bias, and when the

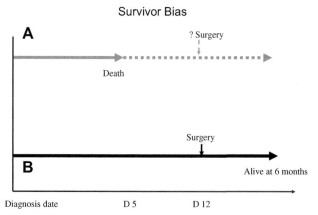

FIGURE 1.—An example of survivor treatment selection bias in a study that examines the association between valve surgery and 6-month mortality in patients with left-sided infective endocarditis. Patients who live longer (group B) have more opportunity to be selected for treatment (surgery) than those who die earlier (group A). A correlation between survival and treatment may mistakenly be interpreted as showing evidence that treatment improves survival. (Reprinted from Tleyjeh IM, Ghomrawi HMK, Steckelberg JM, et al. Conclusion about the association between valve surgery and mortality in an infective endocarditis cohort changed after adjusting for survivor bias. *J Clin Epidemiol.* 2010;63:130-135, with permission from Elsevier.)

data were recalculated to include a time-dependent variable and matching on follow-up time, the conclusion that surgery improved survival was changed. Fourteen years ago, Glesby and Hoover,[1] in an analysis of articles concerning survival effect of treatment of patients with human immunodeficiency virus infection, emphasized the importance of accounting for survivor bias in evaluating treatment, stating that any observational study that did not include this should not be published. In a more recent article, van Walraven and colleagues[2] reviewed 9 of the most widely read journals that included *Circulation, The New England Journal of Medicine,* and *Journal of the American Medical Association* for studies with time-dependent factors as susceptible to survivor bias if a time-dependent covariate analysis was not used and found that 18.6% contained a time-dependent factor, and of these, 41% were susceptible to survivor bias. Correction of the bias could have qualitatively changed the studies' conclusion in over half the studies. Whenever reading reports of surgery or other types of intervention, survivor bias should be taken into account. Reader, beware!

M. D. Cheitlin, MD

References

1. Glesby MJ, Hoover DR. Survivor treatment selection bias in observational studies: examples from the AIDS literature. *Ann Intern Med.* 1996;124:999-1005.
2. van Walraven C, Davis D, Forster AJ, Wells GA. Time-dependent bias was common in survival analyses published in leading clinical journals. *J Clin Epidemiol.* 2004;57:672-682.

Relation of Level of B-Type Natriuretic Peptide With Outcomes in Patients With Infective Endocarditis

Shiue AB, Stancoven AB, Purcell JB, et al (Univ of Texas Southwestern Med Ctr, Dallas; Univ of Chicago Med Ctr, IL; et al)
Am J Cardiol 106:1011-1015, 2010

Elevated B-type natriuretic peptide (BNP) is a marker of poor outcomes in heart failure, acute coronary syndromes, and sepsis. Elevated cardiac troponin I (cTnI) is associated with adverse outcomes in infective endocarditis. It was hypothesized that elevated BNP would be associated with increased rates of morbidity and mortality in patients with infective endocarditis, particularly when combined with elevated cTnI. Consecutively enrolled patients in the International Collaboration on Endocarditis Prospective Cohort Study (ICE-PCS) were evaluated at a single center. The association between elevated BNP and a composite outcome of death, intracardiac abscess, and central nervous system event and the individual components of the composite was determined. Similar analyses were performed in patients who had BNP and cTnI measured. Of 103 patients, 45 had BNP measured for clinical indications. The median BNP level was higher in patients with the composite outcome (1,498 vs 433 pg/ml, p = 0.03) and in those who died (2,150 vs 628 pg/ml, p = 0.04). Elevated BNP was significantly associated with the composite outcome (p <0.01) and intracardiac abscess (p = 0.02). Patients with elevation of BNP and cTnI had a significantly higher probability of the composite outcome (69%) than patients with either BNP or cTnI elevated (29%) or neither BNP nor troponin elevated (0%) (p for trend <0.01). In conclusion, these data demonstrate a significant association between elevated BNP alone and in combination with cTnI for serious outcomes in infective endocarditis and warrant prospective evaluation (Figs 1-4).

▶ Despite advances in diagnosis and treatment, infective endocarditis (IE) is still a disease with major morbidity and mortality.[1,2] Risk stratification that would identify those patients at an increased risk of complications, including mortality, would be valuable in deciding on more vigorous management of such patients. For this purpose, biomarkers have been useful in other diseases such as acute coronary syndromes,[3] and several studies have demonstrated that elevated cardiac troponins are associated with an increased morbidity and mortality in IE.[4,5] Circulating levels of B-type natriuretic peptide (BNP) appear to serve as an integrated marker of multiple pathologic insults.[6] Only 1 small study has shown that combined elevated BNP and troponin I (TnI) have prognostic value in IE,[7] and the end point was surgical intervention or death. The present observational retrospective study with an elevated BNP prespecified as > 400 pg/mL and TnI prespecified as 0.1 ng/mL showed that an elevated TnI and BNP predicted a higher incidence of composite outcome (death, intracardiac abscess, or central nervous system event), with the highest incidence when both

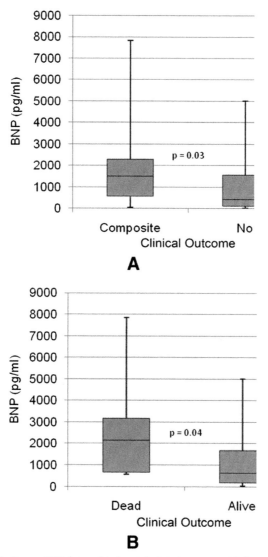

FIGURE 1.—Continuous BNP data and in-hospital clinical outcomes. Medians and IQRs of BNP levels of patients with and without composite outcomes *(A)* and those who were dead versus alive at hospital discharge *(B)*. (Reprinted from Shiue AB, Stancoven AB, Purcell JB, et al. Relation of level of B-type natriuretic peptide with outcomes in patients with infective endocarditis. *Am J Cardiol.* 2010;106:1011-1015, copyright 2010, with permission from Elsevier.)

TnI and BNP were elevated. An elevated BNP was associated with a 4.1-fold increase in the composite outcome. The fact that the poorest outcome was seen when both TnI and BNP were elevated emphasizes the point that these 2 biomarkers reflect different pathologic factors. TnI is released with cardiomyocyte necrosis and so reflects increasing loss of cardiomyocytes and increasingly poor

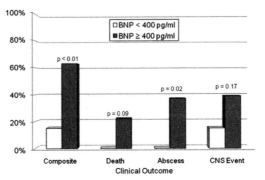

FIGURE 2.—Rate of composite and individual clinical outcomes stratified by BNP level. (Reprinted from Shiue AB, Stancoven AB, Purcell JB, et al. Relation of level of B-type natriuretic peptide with outcomes in patients with infective endocarditis. *Am J Cardiol.* 2010;106:1011-1015, copyright 2010, with permission from Elsevier.)

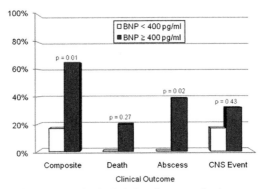

FIGURE 3.—Rate of composite and individual clinical outcomes by the presence of BNP elevation, restricted to patients with normal left ventricular systolic function. (Reprinted from Shiue AB, Stancoven AB, Purcell JB, et al. Relation of level of B-type natriuretic peptide with outcomes in patients with infective endocarditis. *Am J Cardiol.* 2010;106:1011-1015, copyright 2010, with permission from Elsevier.)

left ventricular function. Because BNP is released from ventricular cardiomyocytes in response to myocardial stretch and volume overload,[8] the development of severe valvular regurgitation could be the cause of BNP elevation and poorer outcome. However, the association of increased BNP and composite outcome was maintained when the analysis included only patients without severe aortic or mitral regurgitation and normal ventricular function. It is not clear what causes the elevated BNP, whether it is due to myocardial depression from sepsis or an inflammatory response similar to sepsis. The limitations to this study are such that it must be considered a pilot study and therefore must generate other larger prospective trials. Still, this is the first study to demonstrate the significant association of BNP elevation and poor outcomes in IE.

M. D. Cheitlin, MD

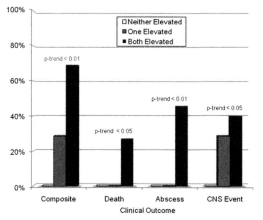

FIGURE 4.—Rate of composite and individual clinical outcomes by BNP and cTnI elevation in patients with BNP and cTnI drawn. (Reprinted from Shiue AB, Stancoven AB, Purcell JB, et al. Relation of level of B-type natriuretic peptide with outcomes in patients with infective endocarditis. *Am J Cardiol.* 2010;106:1011-1015, copyright 2010, with permission from Elsevier.)

References

1. Murdoch DR, Corey GR, Hoen B, et al. International Collaboration on Endocarditis-Prospective Cohort Study (ICE-PCS) Investigators. Clinical presentation, etiology, and outcome of infective endocarditis in the 21st century: the International Collaboration on Endocarditis-Prospective Cohort Study. *Arch Intern Med.* 2009;169:463-473.
2. Cabell CH, Jollis JG, Peterson GE, et al. Changing patient characteristics and the effect on mortality in endocarditis. *Arch Intern Med.* 2002;162:90-94.
3. de Lemos JA, Morrow DA, Bentley JH, et al. The prognostic value of B-type natriuretic peptide in patients with acute coronary syndromes. *N Engl J Med.* 2001; 345:1014-1021.
4. Purcell JB, Patel M, Khera A, et al. Relation of troponin elevation to outcome in patients with infective endocarditis. *Am J Cardiol.* 2008;101:1479-1481.
5. Tsenovoy P, Aronow WS, Joseph J, Kopacz MS. Patients with infective endocarditis and increased cardiac troponin I levels have a higher incidence of in-hospital mortality and valve replacement than those with normal cardiac troponin I levels. *Cardiology.* 2009;112:202-204.
6. Drazner MH, de Lemos JA. Unexpected BNP levels in patients with advanced heart failure: a tale of caution and promise. *Am Heart J.* 2005;149:187-189.
7. Kahveci G, Bayrak F, Mutlu B, et al. Prognostic value of N-terminal pro-B-type natriuretic peptide in patients with active infective endocarditis. *Am J Cardiol.* 2007;99:1429-1433.
8. Yasue H, Yoshimura M, Sumida H, et al. Localization and mechanism of secretion of B-type natriuretic peptide in comparison with those of A-type natriuretic peptide in normal subjects and patients with heart failure. *Circulation.* 1994;90: 195-203.

Natural History of Very Severe Aortic Stenosis

Rosenhek R, Zilberszac R, Schemper M, et al (Med Univ of Vienna, Austria)
Circulation 121:151-156, 2010

Background.—We sought to assess the outcome of asymptomatic patients with very severe aortic stenosis.

Methods and Results.—We prospectively followed 116 consecutive asymptomatic patients (57 women; age, 67 ± 16 years) with very severe isolated aortic stenosis defined by a peak aortic jet velocity (AV-Vel) ≥ 5.0 m/s (average AV-Vel, 5.37 ± 0.35 m/s; valve area, 0.63 ± 0.12 cm^2). During a median follow-up of 41 months (interquartile range, 26 to 63 months), 96 events occurred (indication for aortic valve replacement, 90; cardiac deaths, 6). Event-free survival was 64%, 36%, 25%, 12%, and 3% at 1, 2, 3, 4, and 6 years, respectively. AV-Vel but not aortic valve area was shown to independently affect event-free survival. Patients with an AV-Vel ≥ 5.5 m/s had an event-free survival of 44%, 25%, 11%, and 4% at 1, 2, 3, and 4 years, respectively, compared with 76%, 43%, 33%, and 17% for patients with an AV-Vel between 5.0 and 5.5 m/s ($P<0.0001$). Six cardiac deaths occurred in previously asymptomatic patients (sudden death, 1; congestive heart failure, 4; myocardial infarction, 1). Patients with an initial AV-Vel ≥ 5.5 m/s had a higher likelihood (52%) of severe symptom onset (New York Heart Association or Canadian Cardiovascular Society class >II) than those with an AV-Vel between 5.0 and 5.5 m/s (27%; $P=0.03$).

Conclusions.—Despite being asymptomatic, patients with very severe aortic stenosis have a poor prognosis with a high event rate and a risk of rapid functional deterioration. Early elective valve replacement surgery should therefore be considered in these patients.

► Severe calcific aortic stenosis (AS) in symptomatic patients has a poor prognosis without surgery,[1] so there is universal agreement that valve replacement is indicated. Asymptomatic patients with AS, even if severe, have a very low incidence of sudden death as the first symptom, lower than the operative mortality during valve replacement.[2,3] For this reason, the current guidelines of the European Society of Cardiology make no recommendation for surgery for those asymptomatic patients with very severe AS.[4] The American College of Cardiology/American Heart Association recommendation for surgery in asymptomatic patients with very severe AS (peak aortic jet velocity of 5.0 m/sec, a mean gradient of 60 mm Hg, and a valve area of 0.6 cm^2) is a Class IIb indication for surgery if the expected operative mortality is 1%.[5] The strategy of watchful waiting relies on performing regular follow-up examinations to detect the first evidence of developing symptoms before referring the patient for surgery. There is growing evidence that some asymptomatic patients with very severe AS will benefit from early elective surgery.[6]

Arguments in favor of early surgery include a higher operative risk for more symptomatic patients,[7] the development of symptoms unreported by the patient,[8] deaths while on the waiting list for surgery, and irreversible myocardial damage. These risks are balanced against the operative mortality, the long-term morbidity and mortality related to the prosthetic valve, and the potential need for reoperation.[9] This study assesses for the first time the outcome of the asymptomatic patient with very severe AS defined by a peak aortic jet velocity of 5 m/sec. The end points were defined as cardiac death or indication for valve replacement according to accepted guidelines, and the study showed that these patients have a very poor event-free survival rate. Other studies have shown that the peak aortic jet velocity is a marker of disease severity and a predictor of incrementally higher event rates in asymptomatic patients with mild, moderate, and severe AS.[2,3,10] The patients with a peak jet velocity of 5.5 m/sec had an even worse event-free survival and more severe symptom presentation than those with peak aortic jet velocities between 5.0 and 5.5 m/sec. Interestingly, the aortic valve area did not affect the outcome in patients with very severe AS (as defined by a peak velocity over 5 m/sec) possibly because of the technical limitations of measuring the aortic valve area by the continuity equation or, more likely, in the setting of an aortic valve area of 1 cm^2, the hemodynamic burden on the left ventricle is reflected more accurately by the peak transaortic velocity and gradient. With such a poor event-free survival in patients with a peak aortic jet velocity of ≥5.0 m/sec, this study supports the concept of elective surgery, even when asymptomatic, in such patients.

M. D. Cheitlin, MD

References

1. Horstkotte D, Loogen F. The natural history of aortic valve stenosis. *Eur Heart J.* 1988;9:57-64.
2. Otto CM, Burwash IG, Legget ME, et al. Prospective study of asymptomatic valvular aortic stenosis: clinical, echocardiographic, and exercise predictors of outcome. *Circulation.* 1997;95:2262-2270.
3. Rosenhek R, Binder T, Porenta G, et al. Predictors of outcome in severe, asymptomatic aortic stenosis. *N Engl J Med.* 2000;343:611-617.
4. Vahanian A, Baumgartner H, Bax J, et al. Guidelines on the management of valvular heart disease: the Task Force on the Management of Valvular Heart Disease of the European Society of Cardiology. *Eur Heart J.* 2007;28:230-268.
5. Bonow RO, Carabello BA, Chatterjee K, et al. ACC/AHA 2006 guidelines for the management of patients with valvular heart disease: a report of the American College of Cardiology/American Heart Association Task Force on Practice Guidelines (writing Committee to Revise the 1998 guidelines for the management of patients with valvular heart disease) developed in collaboration with the Society of Cardiovascular Anesthesiologists endorsed by the Society for Cardiovascular Angiography and Interventions and the Society of Thoracic Surgeons. *J Am Coll Cardiol.* 2006;48:e1-e148.
6. Rosenhek R, Maurer G, Baumgartner H. Should early elective surgery be performed in patients with severe but asymptomatic aortic stenosis? *Eur Heart J.* 2002;23:1417-1421.
7. Society of Thoracic Surgeons. STS National Database: STS U.S. cardiac surgery database: 1997 aortic valve replacement patients: preoperative risk variables, http://www.ctsnet.org/doc/3031. Accessed March 20, 2008.
8. Gjertsson P, Caidahl K, Odén A, Bech-Hanssen O. Diagnostic and referral delay in patients with aortic stenosis is common and negatively affects outcome. *Scand Cardiovasc J.* 2007;41:12-18.
9. Hammermeister K, Sethi GK, Henderson WG, Grover FL, Oprian C, Rahimtoola SH. Outcomes 15 years after valve replacement with a mechanical

versus a bioprosthetic valve: final report of the Veterans Affairs randomized trial. *J Am Coll Cardiol.* 2000;36:1152-1158.
10. Rosenhek R, Klaar U, Schemper M, et al. Mild and moderate aortic stenosis: natural history and risk stratification by echocardiography. *Eur Heart J.* 2004; 25:199-205.

Miscellaneous

Anti-heart and anti-intercalated disk autoantibodies: evidence for autoimmunity in idiopathic recurrent acute pericarditis

Caforio ALP, Brucato A, Doria A, et al (Univ of Padua, Italy; Ospedali Riuniti, Bergamo, Italy; et al)

Heart 96:779-784, 2010

Background.—Idiopathic recurrent acute pericarditis (IRAP) is a rare disease of suspected, yet unproved, immune-mediated origin. The finding of serum heart-specific autoantibodies in IRAP would strengthen the autoimmune hypothesis and provide aetiology-specific non-invasive biomarkers.

Objective.—To assess frequency of serum anti-heart (AHA), anti-intercalated-disk (AIDA) and non-cardiac-specific autoantibodies and their clinical and instrumental correlates in patients with IRAP.

Patients.—40 consecutive patients with IRAP, 25 male, aged 37 ± 16 years, representing a large single-centre cohort collected at a referral centre over a long time period (median 5 years, range 1—22 years). Control groups included patients with non-inflammatory cardiac disease (NICD) (n=160), ischaemic heart failure (n=141) and normal subjects (n=270).

Methods.—AHA (organ-specific, cross-reactive 1 and 2 types) and AIDA were detected in serum samples from patients, at last follow-up, and control subjects by indirect immunofluorescence (IIF) on human myocardium and skeletal muscle. Non-cardiac-specific autoantibodies were detected by IIF, and anti-Ro/SSA, anti-La/SSB by ELISA.

Results.—The frequencies of cross-reactive 1 AHA and of AIDA were higher (50%; 25%) in IRAP than in NICD (4%; 4%), ischaemic (1%; 2%) or normal subjects (3%; 0%) (p=0.0001). AHA and/or AIDA were found in 67.5% patients with IRAP. Of the non-cardiac-specific antibodies, only antinuclear autoantibodies at titre $\geq 1/160$ were more common in IRAP (5%) versus normal (0.5%, p<0.04). AIDA in IRAP were associated with a higher number of recurrences (p=0.01) and hospitalisations (p=0.0001), high titre (1/80 or higher) AHA with a higher number of recurrences (p=0.02).

Conclusions.—The detection of AHA and of AIDA supports the involvement of autoimmunity in the majority of patients with IRAP (Table 7).

▶ Idiopathic acute pericarditis is a relatively common disease with recurrences frequently distressing to both patient and physician occurring in up to 15% to 32% of patients.[1-3] The pathogenesis of acute pericarditis is generally suspected

TABLE 7.—Sensitivities, Specificities, Positive (PPV) and Negative Predictive Values (NPV) of Anti-Heart Autoantibody (AHA) and Anti-Intercalated-Disk AIDA Autoantibody Patterns in Idiopathic Recurrent Acute Pericarditis (IRAP)

	IRAP	Normal Subjects	p Value	Sensitivity (%)	Specificity (%)	PPV (%)	NPV (%)
AHA (any pattern): Positive/negative	25/15	23/247	0.0001	62	91	52	94
AHA (organ-specific or cross-reactive 1): Positive/negative	22/18	15/255	0.0001	55	94	59	93
AIDA: Positive/negative	10/30	0/270	0.0001	25	100	100	90
AHA (any pattern) and/or AIDA positive: Positive/negative	27/13	23/247	0.0001	54	95	67.5	91.5
AHA (organ-specific or cross-reactive 1) and/or AIDA: Positive/negative	22/18	15/255	0.0001	59	93	55	94

to be immune mediated, but this is not yet certain.[4,5] Patients with autoimmune disease have a high frequency of circulating autoantibodies to the target organ and other noninvolved tissues.[6] In patients with myocarditis and dilated cardiomyopathy, serum antiheart autoantibodies (AHA), and anti-intercalated disc autoantibodies (AIDA) have been detected by indirect immunofluorescence. In this study, a large group of patients with idiopathic recurrent acute pericarditis (IRAP) was found for the first time to have AHA and AIDA in significantly greater frequency than in serum from control patients, thus supporting the immune-mediated pathogenesis of this disease. Because the finding of increased serum AHA and AIDA is seen in myocarditis, a possible explanation is that patients with IRAP have epicardial involvement. This should not be surprising because the development of ST elevation in pericarditis is evidence for at least superficial epicardial inflammation. Whether an elevation in AHA and AIDA in patients with the first episode of acute pericarditis is more likely to have a recurrence is not yet known.

M. D. Cheitlin, MD

References

1. Spodick DH. Acute pericarditis: current concepts and practice. *JAMA.* 2003;289:1150-1153.
2. Shabetai R. Recurrent pericarditis: recent advances and remaining questions. *Circulation.* 2005;112:1921-1923.
3. Soler-Soler J, Sagristà-Sauleda J, Permanyer-Miralda G. Relapsing pericarditis. *Heart.* 2004;90:1364-1368.
4. Brucato A, Brambilla G, Adler Y, Spodick DH, Canesi B. Therapy of recurrent acute pericarditis: a rheumatological solution? *Clin Exp Rheumatol.* 2006;24:45-50.
5. Marcolongo R, Russo R, Laveder F, Noventa F, Agostini C. Immunosuppressive therapy prevents recurrent pericarditis. *J Am Coll Cardiol.* 1995;26:1276-1279.
6. Rose NR, Bona C. Defining criteria for autoimmune diseases (Witebsky's postulates revisited). *Immunol Today.* 1993;14:426-430.

COlchicine for the Prevention of the Post-pericardiotomy Syndrome (COPPS): a multicentre, randomized, double-blind, placebo-controlled trial

Imazio M, on behalf of the COPPS Investigators (Maria Vittoria Hosp, Torino, Italy; et al)

Eur Heart J 31:2749-2754, 2010

Aims.—No drug has been proven efficacious to prevent the post-pericardiotomy syndrome (PPS), but colchicine seems safe and effective for the treatment and prevention of pericarditis. The aim of the COlchicine for the Prevention of the Post-pericardiotomy Syndrome (COPPS) trial is to test the efficacy and safety of colchicine for the primary prevention of the PPS.

Methods and Results.—The COPPS study is a multicentre, double-blind, randomized trial. On the third post-operative day, 360 patients (mean age 65.7 ± 12.3 years, 66% males), 180 in each treatment arm, were randomized to receive placebo or colchicine (1.0 mg twice daily for the first day followed by a maintenance dose of 0.5 mg twice daily for 1 month in patients ≥70 kg, and halved doses for patients <70 kg or intolerant to the highest dose). The primary efficacy endpoint was the incidence of PPS at 12 months. Secondary endpoint was the combined rate of disease-related hospitalization, cardiac tamponade, constrictive pericarditis, and relapses. Baseline characteristics were well balanced between the study groups. Colchicine significantly reduced the incidence of the PPS at 12 months compared with placebo (respectively, 8.9 vs. 21.1%; $P = 0.002$; number needed to treat = 8). Colchicine also reduced the secondary endpoint (respectively, 0.6 vs. 5.0%; $P = 0.024$). The rate of side effects (mainly related to gastrointestinal intolerance) was similar in the colchicine and placebo groups (respectively, 8.9 vs. 5.0%; $P = 0.212$).

Conclusion.—Colchicine is safe and efficacious in the prevention of the PPS and its related complications and may halve the risk of developing the syndrome following cardiac surgery.

ClinicalTrials.gov number, NCT00128427 (Figs 2 and 3, Table 1).

▶ Postpericardiotomy syndrome (PPS) is a common complication after cardiac surgery, occurring several days to several weeks after the surgery in 10% to 40% of the patients.[1,2] The treatment is empirical, consisting of aspirin or nonsteroidal anti-inflammatory drugs or steroids if these drugs fail to control the symptoms. None of these drugs have been proven to prevent PPS when used prophylactically.[3,4] Colchicine has been shown to be effective in treating patients with recurrent PPS and in preventing recurrences.[5-7]

The Colchicine for the Prevention of the Postpericardiotomy Syndrome trial is the first large, double-blind, randomized, placebo-controlled trial to test the hypothesis that colchicine used prophylactically can be effective in the primary prevention of PPS following cardiac surgery. Although the diagnosis is made clinically, the criteria for the diagnosis of PPS were prospectively defined.[8] The study for the first time showed that colchicine was definitely effective in preventing PPS postsurgically and also in decreasing the rate of the combined

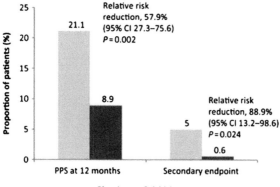

FIGURE 2.—Proportion of patients developing the primary endpoint (post-pericardiotomy syndrome at 12 months; relative risk reduction 57.9%, 95% confidence interval 27.3–75.6; $P = 0.002$) and the secondary endpoint (recurrence, cardiac tamponade, constrictive pericarditis, and post-pericardiotomy syndrome-related hospitalization; relative risk reduction 88.9%, 95% confidence interval 13.2–98.6; $P = 0.024$). (Reprinted from Imazio M, on behalf of the COPPS Investigators. COlchicine for the Prevention of the Post-pericardiotomy Syndrome (COPPS): a multicentre, randomized, double-blind, placebo-controlled trial. *Eur Heart J* 2010;31:2749-2754, with permission of The European Society of Cardiology.)

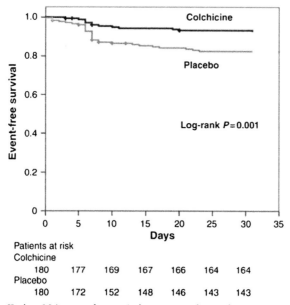

FIGURE 3.—Kaplan–Meier event-free survival curves according to the treatment groups in the first 30 days (85% of all postpericardiotomy syndrome events). Curves remained parallel after the first month. (Reprinted from Imazio M, on behalf of the COPPS Investigators. COlchicine for the Prevention of the Post-pericardiotomy Syndrome (COPPS): a multicentre, randomized, double-blind, placebo-controlled trial. *Eur Heart J* 2010;31:2749-2754, with permission of The European Society of Cardiology.)

TABLE 1.—Criteria for the Diagnosis of the Post-Pericardiotomy Syndrome

1. Fever lasting beyond the first post-operative week without evidence of systemic or focal infection
2. Pleuritic chest pain
3. Friction rub
4. Evidence of pleural effusion
5. Evidence of new or worsening pericardial effusion

The diagnosis of post-pericardiotomy syndrome was based on the presence of at least two criteria.

end point of disease-related hospitalization, cardiac tamponade, constrictive pericarditis, and recurrent pericarditis. The mechanism by which this happens is unknown, but the major action of colchicine is to disrupt microtubules[9] that can inhibit various leukocyte functions and interfere with the inflammatory response. PPS can vary from being simply an annoying painful complication postsurgically to a life-threatening problem with cardiac tamponade or rarely, pericardial constriction. Showing that colchicine can effectively prevent this postoperative complication is a significant advance.

M. D. Cheitlin, MD

References

1. Prince SE, Cunha BA. Postpericardiotomy syndrome. *Heart Lung.* 1997;26: 165-168.
2. Hoit BD. Pericardial and postpericardial injury syndromes. In: Rose BD, ed. *Upto-Date.* Wellesley, MA: Uptodate Online; 2010.
3. Gill PJ, Forbes K, Coe JY. The effect of short-term prophylactic acetylsalicylic acid on the incidence of postpericardiotomy syndrome after surgical closure of atrial septal defects. *Pediatr Cardiol.* 2009;30:1061-1067.
4. Mott AR, Fraser CD Jr, Kusnoor AV, et al. The effect of short-term prophylactic methylprednisolone on the incidence and severity of postpericardiotomy syndrome in children undergoing cardiac surgery with cardiopulmonary bypass. *J Am Coll Cardiol.* 2001;37:1700-1706.
5. Adler Y, Finkelstein Y, Guindo J, et al. Colchicine treatment for recurrent pericarditis: a decade of experience. *Circulation.* 1998;97:2183-2185.
6. Artom G, Koren-Morag N, Spodick DH, et al. Pretreatment with corticosteroids attenuates the efficacy of colchicine in preventing recurrent pericarditis: a multi-centre all-case analysis. *Eur Heart J.* 2005;26:723-727.
7. Imazio M, Spodick DH, Brucato A, Trinchero R, Adler Y. Controversial issues in the management of pericardial diseases. *Circulation.* 2010;121:916-928.
8. Finkelstein Y, Shemesh J, Mahlab K, et al. Colchicine for the prevention of post-pericardiotomy syndrome. *Herz.* 2002;27:791-794.
9. Imazio M, Brucato A, Trinchero R, Spodick D, Adler Y. Colchicine for pericarditis: hype or hope? *Eur Heart J.* 2009;30:532-539.

Atrial septal defects versus ventricular septal defects in BREATHE-5, a placebo-controlled study of pulmonary arterial hypertension related to Eisenmenger's syndrome: A subgroup analysis

Berger RMF, Beghetti M, Galiè N, et al (Univ of Groningen, The Netherlands; Children's Hosp, Geneva, Switzerland; Univ of Bologna, Italy; et al)
Int J Cardiol 144:373-378, 2010

Background.—Eisenmenger's syndrome (ES) is the most advanced form of pulmonary arterial hypertension related to congenital heart disease. Evolution of pulmonary vascular disease differs markedly between patients with atrial septal defects (ASD) versus ventricular septal defects (VSD), potentially affecting response to treatment. We compared the effects of bosentan and placebo in patients with isolated ASD (ASD subgroup) versus patients with isolated VSD or both defects (VSD subgroup).

Methods.—Post-hoc analysis of a 16-week, multicenter, randomized, double-blind, placebo-controlled trial was performed. Fifty-four patients (13: ASDs, 36: VSDs, 5: VSD + ASD) were randomized to bosentan 62.5-mg bid for four weeks (uptitrated to 125-mg bid thereafter) or placebo. Main outcome measures were: indexed pulmonary vascular resistance (PVRi), exercise capacity, mean pulmonary artery pressure (mPAP), pulmonary blood flow index (Qpi), and changes in oxygen saturation (SpO_2).

Results.—Placebo-corrected median (95% CI) treatment effects on PVRi were $-544.0 \text{ dyn·s·cm}^{-5}$ (-1593.8, 344.7) and $-436.4 \text{ dyn·s·cm}^{-5}$ (-960.0, 167.0) in the ASD and VSD subgroups, respectively. Effects of bosentan on exercise capacity and mPAP were similar in both subgroups. No changes in SpO_2 or Qpi were observed in either bosentan or placebo subgroups.

Conclusions.—Improvements in exercise capacity and cardiopulmonary hemodynamics, without desaturation, were observed in ES patients with both ASDs and VSDs. Although not reaching statistical significance, improvements were similar to those in the BREATHE-5 analyses, suggesting that the location of septal defects is not a key determinant of treatment response. These data further support the use of bosentan for the treatment of ES, independent of shunt location (Figs 1-3).

▶ Patients with ventricular septal defect (VSD) and atrial septal defect (ASD) with Eisenmenger syndrome in the past have had no definitive therapy to lower pulmonary vascular resistance (PVR) and consequently have a poor prognosis.[1-3] With the introduction of prostacyclin vasodilators and endothelin antagonists, patients with idiopathic pulmonary hypertension have been shown to increase exercise capacity and prolong survival. The Bosentan Randomized Trial of Endothelin Antagonist Therapy-5 (BREATH-5)[4] was the first placebo-controlled trial of bosentan in patients with Eisenmenger syndrome that showed improved exercise capacity and hemodynamics without a decrease in arterial oxygen saturation. Bosentan is an antagonist to both the A

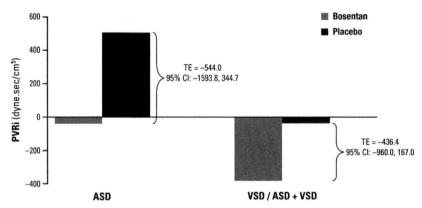

FIGURE 1.—Indexed pulmonary vascular resistance (PVRi): median change from baseline to week 16. (TE: treatment effect; CI: confidence interval). (Reprinted from Berger RMF, Beghetti M, Galiè N, et al. Atrial septal defects versus ventricular septal defects in BREATHE-5, a placebo-controlled study of pulmonary arterial hypertension related to Eisenmenger's syndrome: a subgroup analysis. *Int J Cardiol.* 2010;144:373-378, with permission from Elsevier Ireland.)

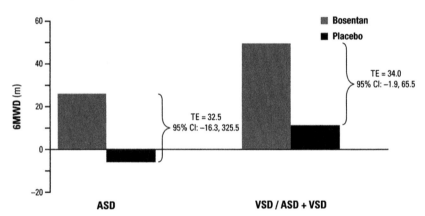

FIGURE 2.—6-minute walk distance (6MWD): median change from baseline to week 16. (TE: treatment effect; CI: confidence interval). (Reprinted from Berger RMF, Beghetti M, Galiè N, et al. Atrial septal defects versus ventricular septal defects in BREATHE-5, a placebo-controlled study of pulmonary arterial hypertension related to Eisenmenger's syndrome: a subgroup analysis. *Int J Cardiol.* 2010;144:373-378, with permission from Elsevier Ireland.)

and B subtypes of endothelin receptor[5] and blocks the deleterious effects of endothelin-1, including inflammation, vascular hypertrophy, fibrosis, and vasoconstriction.[5] The 2 congenital shunt lesions included in this study were ASD and VSD. In these defects, there is initially a left-to-right shunt with increased pulmonary to systemic blood flow ratio. With large defects, eventually in some patients, the increased pulmonary blood flow exposes the pulmonary vasculature to increased shear stress and circumferential stretch that leads to vascular remodeling and elevated PVR.[6,7] There is a fundamental difference between the 2 types of lesions. In the ASD, the damage to the pulmonary arteries and

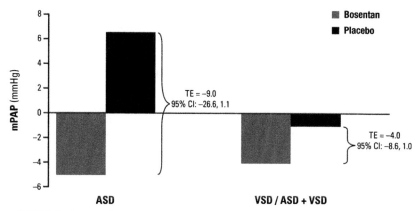

FIGURE 3.—Mean pulmonary artery pressure (mPAP): median change from baseline to week 16, (TE: treatment effect; CI: confidence interval). (Reprinted from Berger RMF, Beghetti M, Galiè N, et al. Atrial septal defects versus ventricular septal defects in BREATHE-5, a placebo-controlled study of pulmonary arterial hypertension related to Eisenmenger's syndrome: a subgroup analysis. *Int J Cardiol.* 2010;144:373-378, with permission from Elsevier Ireland.)

arterioles is related solely to the increased blood flow, whereas in the nonrestrictive VSD, because the pressures in both ventricles are equal from an early age, the shear stress is high due to both increased blood flow and pulmonary artery pressure. In the patient with ASD, the shunt reversal through the ASD occurs when the right ventricle fails and the resistance to diastolic filling of the right ventricle exceeds that of the left ventricle. In the patient with VSD, when the PVR becomes greater than the systemic vascular resistance (SVR), the shunt becomes right to left and the patient becomes desaturated and cyanotic. With vasodilatation affecting both the pulmonary and systemic vascular beds, the problem that could arise is that the effect could be greater on the systemic than the pulmonary vascular bed and the right-to-left shunt could increase, increasing the systemic arterial desaturation and worsening the exercise capacity. The present paper is a subgroup analysis of the BREATH-5 study and compares the effect of bosentan on exercise capacity, PVR/SVR, and arterial oxygen saturation in patients with ASD and VSD. It was found that there was an improvement in exercise capacity, a decrease in mean pulmonary artery pressure, and a significant decrease in PVR, all with no change in arterial saturation. The limitations of the small number of patients with ASD, the nature of a post hoc analysis, and the short 16-week follow-up must be recognized. However, the results of this analysis suggest that patients with Eisenmenger syndrome due to ASD or VSD can receive bosentan with similar clinical and hemodynamic benefits.

M. D. Cheitlin, MD

References

1. Daliento L, Somerville J, Presbitero P, et al. Eisenmenger syndrome: factors relating to deterioration and death. *Eur Heart J.* 1998;19:1845-1855.

2. Diller GP, Dimopoulos K, Okonko D, et al. Exercise intolerance in adult congenital heart disease: comparative severity, correlates, and prognostic implication. *Circulation.* 2005;112:828-835.
3. Oya H, Nagaya N, Uematsu M, et al. Poor prognosis and related factors in adults with Eisenmenger syndrome. *Am Heart J.* 2002;143:739-744.
4. Galiè N, Beghetti M, Gatzoulis MA, et al. Bosentan therapy in patients with Eisenmenger syndrome: a multicenter, double-blind, randomized, placebo-controlled study. *Circulation.* 2006;114:48-54.
5. Galiè N, Torbicki A, Barst R, et al. Guidelines on diagnosis and treatment of pulmonary arterial hypertension. The Task Force on Diagnosis and Treatment of Pulmonary Arterial Hypertension of the European Society of Cardiology. *Eur Heart J.* 2004;25:2243-2278.
6. Hoffman JI, Rudolph AM, Heymann MA. Pulmonary vascular disease with congenital heart lesions: pathologic features and causes. *Circulation.* 1981;64: 873-877.
7. Rabinovitch M. It all begins with EVE (endogenous vascular elastase). *Isr J Med Sci.* 1996;32:803-810.

Dabigatran versus Warfarin in Patients with Atrial Fibrillation

Connolly SJ, the RE-LY Steering Committee and Investigators (McMaster Univ and Hamilton Health Sciences, Ontario, Canada; et al)
N Engl J Med 361:1139-1151, 2009

Background.—Warfarin reduces the risk of stroke in patients with atrial fibrillation but increases the risk of hemorrhage and is difficult to use. Dabigatran is a new oral direct thrombin inhibitor.

Methods.—In this noninferiority trial, we randomly assigned 18,113 patients who had atrial fibrillation and a risk of stroke to receive, in a blinded fashion, fixed doses of dabigatran — 110 mg or 150 mg twice daily — or, in an unblinded fashion, adjusted-dose warfarin. The median duration of the follow-up period was 2.0 years. The primary outcome was stroke or systemic embolism.

Results.—Rates of the primary outcome were 1.69% per year in the warfarin group, as compared with 1.53% per year in the group that received 110 mg of dabigatran (relative risk with dabigatran, 0.91; 95% confidence interval [CI], 0.74 to 1.11; P<0.001 for noninferiority) and 1.11% per year in the group that received 150 mg of dabigatran (relative risk, 0.66; 95% CI, 0.53 to 0.82; P<0.001 for superiority). The rate of major bleeding was 3.36% per year in the warfarin group, as compared with 2.71% per year in the group receiving 110 mg of dabigatran (P=0.003) and 3.11% per year in the group receiving 150 mg of dabigatran (P=0.31). The rate of hemorrhagic stroke was 0.38% per year in the warfarin group, as compared with 0.12% per year with 110 mg of dabigatran (P<0.001) and 0.10% per year with 150 mg of dabigatran (P<0.001). The mortality rate was 4.13% per year in the warfarin group, as compared with 3.75% per year with 110 mg of dabigatran (P=0.13) and 3.64% per year with 150 mg of dabigatran (P=0.051).

Conclusions.—In patients with atrial fibrillation, dabigatran given at a dose of 110 mg was associated with rates of stroke and systemic embolism that were similar to those associated with warfarin, as well as lower rates of major hemorrhage. Dabigatran administered at a dose of 150 mg, as compared with warfarin, was associated with lower rates of stroke and systemic embolism but similar rates of major hemorrhage. (ClinicalTrials.gov number, NCT00262600.)

▶ For 60 years warfarin has been the only effective oral anticoagulant for use in venous and selected arterial thrombotic disorders and as a preventive medicine for systemic embolization and stroke in patients with atrial fibrillation. Problems with warfarin include a requirement for laboratory monitoring by prothrombin times, a narrow therapeutic index, a long half-life resulting in a slow onset of therapeutic effect, and a need for parenteral anticoagulation until warfarin becomes effective. In addition, there are numerous interactions with other drugs and foods, such as leafy green vegetables containing vitamin K. Dabigatran etexilate is an oral prodrug that is converted by a serum esterase to dabigatran, a potent competitive thrombin inhibitor. This is the first study establishing dabigatran etexilate as equally or, with the 150-mg dose twice a day (BID), more effective in preventing stroke or systemic emboli in patients with atrial fibrillation without increasing major bleeding and less likely than warfarin to cause hemorrhagic stroke. The first oral direct thrombin inhibitor, ximelagatran, almost a decade ago was effective in arterial and venous thrombotic disorders including atrial fibrillation but with long-term use was found to have hepatotoxicity.

Dabigatran has many advantages over warfarin in that it has a relatively short half-life, obviating the need for parenteral anticoagulation before the drug takes effect, little drug or dietary interactions, and especially no laboratory monitoring. In the 2-year follow-up, there has been no hepatotoxicity beyond that seen with warfarin. Subsequent substudies of this study have shown that the benefits of the 150 mg BID dose at reducing stroke, the 110-mg BID dose at reducing bleeding, and both doses at reducing intracranial bleeding versus warfarin were consistent regardless of the individual center's quality of international normalized ratio control[1] and that both doses were equally effective in those with and without previous stroke or transient ischemic attack.[2]

There are a number of other thrombin inhibitors and other drugs effective at the terminus of the coagulation cascade, such as direct factor Xa inhibitors, the most advanced ones being rivaroxaban and apixaban. Zikria and Ansell have published a very good review of the oral direct thrombin and factor Xa inhibitors.[3] If these initial reports are confirmed by other studies and no important adverse effects are noted on long-term follow-up, these novel oral anticoagulants will be a marked advance in the treatment of arterial and venous thrombotic disorders.

M. D. Cheitlin, MD

References

1. Wallentin L, Yusuf S, Ezekowitz MD, et al. Efficacy and safety of dabigatran compared with warfarin at different levels of international normalised ratio control for stroke prevention in atrial fibrillation: an analysis of the RE-LY trial. *Lancet.* 2010;376:975-983.

2. Diener HC, Connolly SJ, Ezekowitz MD, et al. Dabigatran compared with warfarin in patients with atrial fibrillation and previous transient ischaemic attack or stroke: a subgroup analysis of the RE-LY trial. *Lancet Neurol.* 2010;9: 1157-1163.
3. Zikria J, Ansell J. Oral anticoagulation with Factor Xa and thrombin inhibitors: Is there an alternative to warfarin? *Discov Med.* 2009;8:196-203.

Comparison of Prognostic Value of Echographic Risk Score With the Thrombolysis In Myocardial Infarction (TIMI) and Global Registry In Acute Coronary Events (GRACE) Risk Scores in Acute Coronary Syndrome

Bedetti G, Gargani L, Sicari R, et al ("S. Maria della Scaletta" Hosp, Imola, Italy; Natl Res Council, Pisa, Italy; et al)
Am J Cardiol 106:1709-1716, 2010

Risk stratification in patients with acute coronary syndromes (ACS) is achieved today by clinical models, "blind" to the prognostic support of imaging methods. To assess the value of simple at rest cardiac chest sonography in predicting the intra- and extrahospital risk of death or myocardial infarction, we enrolled 470 consecutive in-patients (312 men, age 71 ± 12 years) who had been admitted for ACS. On admission, all had received a clinical score using the Global Registry in Acute Coronary Events and Thrombolysis in Myocardial Infarction systems and, within 1 to 12 hours, a comprehensive cardiac-chest ultrasound scan. Each of the 16 echocardiographic parameters evaluating left and right, systolic and diastolic, ventricular function and structure, was scored from 0 (normal) to 3 (severely abnormal). The median follow-up was 5 months (interquartile range 1 to 10). Patients with hard events (n = 102) could be separated from patients without events (n = 368) using the Global Registry in Acute Coronary Events score, Thrombolysis in Myocardial Infarction score, and several echocardiographic parameters. On multivariate Cox analysis, ejection fraction (hazard ratio 1.45, 95% confidence interval 1.02 to 2.08, p = 0.040), tricuspid annular plane systolic excursion (hazard ratio 1.66, 95% confidence interval 1.13 to 2.45, p = 0.010) and ultrasound lung comets (hazard ratio 1.69, 95% confidence interval 1.25 to 2.27, p = 0.001) were independent predictors of cardiac events. The 3-variable echocardiographic score (from 0, normal to 9, severe abnormalities in ejection fraction, ultrasound lung comets, and tricuspid annular plane systolic excursion) effectively stratified patients and added value (hazard ratio 2.52, 95% confidence interval 1.89 to 3.37, p <0.0001) to the Global Registry in Acute Coronary Events score (hazard ratio 1.60, 95% confidence interval 1.07 to 2.39, p = 0.003). In conclusion, for patients with ACS, effective risk stratification can be achieved with cardiac and chest ultrasound imaging parameters, adding prognostic value to the clinical risk scores (Figs 1-4).

▶ Acute coronary syndromes (ACS) resulting from an abrupt change in the coronary circulation include ST-segment elevation myocardial infarction

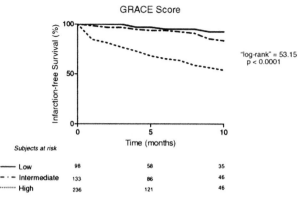

FIGURE 1.—Kaplan-Meier estimates of event-free survival (end point, intra-and extrahospital death or myocardial infarction), according to GRACE risk score categorization of patients in tertiles of risk: low, intermediate, high (GRACE risk score for non—ST-segment elevation ACS, low [1 to 108], intermediate [109 to 140], and high [141 to 372]; GRACE risk score for ST-segment elevation ACS, low [49 to 125], intermediate [126 to 154], and high [155 to 319]). (Reprinted from Bedetti G, Gargani L, Sicari R, et al. Comparison of prognostic value of echographic risk score with the Thrombolysis in Myocardial Infarction (TIMI) and Global Registry in Acute Coronary Events (GRACE) risk scores in acute coronary syndrome. *Am J Cardiol.* 2010;106:1709-1716, copyright © 2010 with permission from Elsevier.)

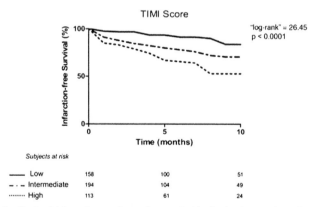

FIGURE 2.—Kaplan-Meier estimates of event-free survival (end point, intra-and extrahospital death or myocardial infarction), according to TIMI risk score categorization of patients in tertiles of risk: low, intermediate, high (TIMI risk score for unstable angina/NSTEMI, low [0 to 2], intermediate [3 to 4], and high [5 to 7]; TIMI risk score for STEMI, low [0 to 3], intermediate [4 to 6], and high [≥7]). (Reprinted from Bedetti G, Gargani L, Sicari R, et al. Comparison of prognostic value of echographic risk score with the Thrombolysis in Myocardial Infarction (TIMI) and Global Registry in Acute Coronary Events (GRACE) risk scores in acute coronary syndrome. *Am J Cardiol.* 2010;106:1709-1716, copyright © 2010 with permission from Elsevier.)

(STEMI), non-STEMI, and unstable angina. Although all ACS share similar pathophysiologic mechanisms, patients with resting ischemic discomfort have a wide spectrum of treatment options and prognosis.[1] Risk stratification is important in evaluating such patients, in deciding the urgency and type of treatment, and in estimating the prognosis. There are a number of risk scores

Echo score

Score	0	1	2	3
EF	≥50%	49-40%	39-30%	<30%
TAPSE	>20 mm	20-15 mm	14-10 mm	<10 mm
ULCs	≤ 5	6-15	16-30	>30

FIGURE 3.—Echocardiographic score obtained by selection of 3 most significant echocardiographic parameters in predicting hard events (ejection fraction, tricuspid annular plane systolic excursion, and ultrasound lung comets). (Reprinted from Bedetti G, Gargani L, Sicari R, et al. Comparison of prognostic value of echographic risk score with the Thrombolysis in Myocardial Infarction (TIMI) and Global Registry in Acute Coronary Events (GRACE) risk scores in acute coronary syndrome. *Am J Cardiol.* 2010;106:1709-1716, copyright © 2010 with permission from Elsevier.)

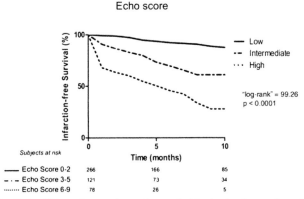

FIGURE 4.—Kaplan-Meier estimates of event-free survival (end point, intra-and extrahospital death or myocardial infarction), according to echocardiographic score categorization of patients in tertiles of risk: low, intermediate, and high. (Reprinted from Bedetti G, Gargani L, Sicari R, et al. Comparison of prognostic value of echographic risk score with the Thrombolysis in Myocardial Infarction (TIMI) and Global Registry in Acute Coronary Events (GRACE) risk scores in acute coronary syndrome. *Am J Cardiol.* 2010;106:1709-1716, copyright © 2010 with permission from Elsevier.)

available, including the Global Registry in Acute Coronary Events (GRACE) and the Thrombolysis in Myocardial Infarction (TIMI) scores, all of which have a high predictive value for in-hospital and 1- and 12-month mortality,[2-5] and all of which use clinical and electrocardiographic findings, but not echocardiographic imaging. This study compares the predictive value for the hard events of in-hospital and 6-month postdischarge mortality and recurrent myocardial infarction, of cardiac and chest ultrasound parameters with those of the GRACE and TIMI risk scores and finds that the cardiac chest ultrasound findings were independent predictors of these hard events. Unique to this prognostic imaging is the lung ultrasound examination for lung comets, an ultrasound index of extravascular lung water.[6] Of all the cardiac and chest ultrasound measurements, the 3 that were most helpful in determining the risk score were tricuspid annular plane excursion, left ventricular ejection fraction, and the number of lung comets. The chest ultrasound is done with the usual echocardiographic equipment, is simple to perform along the anterior and lateral right and left chest walls, and takes about 3 minutes.[6] The comets are hyperechogenic coherent bundles with a narrow base, spreading from the transducer to the further border of the screen, and arising only from the pleural line. The total number of comets found at each scanning site yields a score reflecting the extent of the extravascular fluid in the lung. The Kaplan-Meier survival estimates showed better outcome for patients with a low-risk echocardiographic score than for patients with an intermediate- or high-risk echocardiographic score. When the echocardiographic score was entered into the clinical model, it was accurate in predicting the outcome in patients with ACS and added value to the GRACE risk score. Because the cardiac and chest ultrasound adds information concerning right ventricular function and the degree of pulmonary congestion in addition to left ventricular function, the incorporation of these imaging findings to the traditional clinical and electrocardiographic-derived scores should improve the prognostic value of the presently used risk scores.

M. D. Cheitlin, MD

References

1. Kushner FG, Hand M, Smith SC Jr, et al. 2009 Focused Updates: ACC/AHA Guidelines for the Management of Patients With ST-Elevation Myocardial Infarction (updating the 2004 Guideline and 2007 Focused Update) and ACC/AHA/SCAI Guidelines on Percutaneous Coronary Intervention (updating the 2005 Guideline and 2007 Focused Update): a report of the American College of Cardiology Foundation/American Heart Association Task Force on Practice Guidelines. *Circulation.* 2009;120:2271-2306.
2. Antman EM, Cohen M, Bernink PJ, et al. The TIMI risk score for unstable angina/non-ST elevation MI: a method for prognostication and therapeutic decision making. *JAMA.* 2000;284:835-842.
3. Morrow DA, Antman EM, Charlesworth A, et al. TIMI risk score for ST-elevation myocardial infarction: a convenient, bedside, clinical score for risk assessment at presentation: an intravenous nPA for treatment of infarcting myocardium II trial substudy. *Circulation.* 2000;102:2031-2037.
4. Fox KA, Dabbous OH, Goldberg RJ, et al. GRACE Investigators. Prediction of risk of death and myocardial infarction in the six months after presentation with acute coronary syndrome: prospective multinational observational study (GRACE). *BMJ.* 2006;333:1091.
5. Ramsay G, Podogrodzka M, McClure C, Fox KA. Risk prediction in patients presenting with suspected cardiac pain: the GRACE and TIMI risk scores versus clinical evaluation. *QJM.* 2007;100:11-18.
6. Picano E, Frassi F, Agricola E, Gligorova S, Gargani L, Mottola G. Ultrasound lung comets: a clinically useful sign of extravascular lung water. *J Am Soc Echocardiogr.* 2006;19:356-363.

Combinations of prognostic tools for identification of high-risk normotensive patients with acute symptomatic pulmonary embolism

Jiménez D, Aujesky D, Moores L, et al (Ramón y Cajal Hospital, Madrid, Spain; Univ of Lausanne, Switzerland; Uniformed Services Univ, Bethesda, MD; et al)
Thorax 66:75-81, 2011

Background.—In haemodynamically stable patients with acute symptomatic pulmonary embolism (PE), studies have not evaluated the usefulness of combining the measurement of cardiac troponin, transthoracic echocardiogram (TTE), and lower extremity complete compression ultrasound (CCUS) testing for predicting the risk of PE-related death.

Methods.—The study assessed the ability of three diagnostic tests (cardiac troponin I (cTnI), echocardiogram, and CCUS) to prognosticate the primary outcome of PE-related mortality during 30 days of follow-up after a diagnosis of PE by objective testing.

Results.—Of 591 normotensive patients diagnosed with PE, the primary outcome occurred in 37 patients (6.3%; 95% CI 4.3% to 8.2%). Patients with right ventricular dysfunction (RVD) by TTE and concomitant deep vein thrombosis (DVT) by CCUS had a PE-related mortality of 19.6%, compared with 17.1% of patients with elevated cTnI and concomitant DVT and 15.2% of patients with elevated cTnI and RVD. The use of any two-test strategy had a higher specificity and positive predictive value compared with the use of any test by itself. A combined three-test strategy did not further improve prognostication. For a subgroup analysis of high-risk patients, according to the pulmonary embolism severity index (classes IV and V), positive predictive values of the two-test strategies for PE-related mortality were 25.0%, 24.4% and 20.7%, respectively.

Conclusions.—In haemodynamically stable patients with acute symptomatic PE, a combination of echocardiography (or troponin testing) and CCUS improved prognostication compared with the use of any test by itself for the identification of those at high risk of PE-related death (Fig 2, Table 5).

▶ The patient with an acute pulmonary embolism (PE) with hemodynamic instability, shock, or cardiac arrest has a high mortality and is a candidate for fibrinolysis or emergency thrombectomy. Recent guidelines of European Society of Cardiology[1] and American College of Chest Physician[2] recognize high-risk patients with PE as those having clinically evident right ventricular failure with refractory arterial hypotension and shock and recommend the use of thrombolysis. There is no agreement about identifying high-risk patients in patients with acute PE who remain normotensive and without overt right ventricular failure. This report is a prospective study of a large number of patients with acute PE, all of whom had bilateral proximal and lower extremity complete compression ultrasound study (CCUS) for deep vein thrombosis (DVT) within 48 hours, a transthoracic echocardiogram (TTE) within 24 hours, and a troponin I (TnI) within 12 hours of diagnosis. Criteria for a positive study of CCUS, for right ventricular dysfunction on TTE, and for

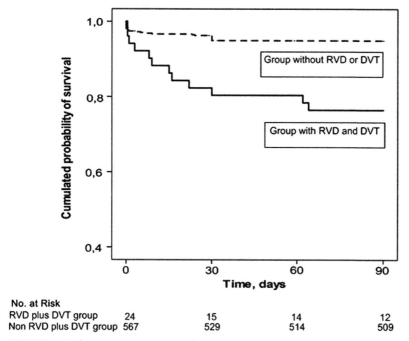

No. at Risk

RVD plus DVT group	24	15	14	12
Non RVD plus DVT group	567	529	514	509

FIGURE 2.—Kaplan—Meier survival curves of normotensive patients with acute symptomatic pulmonary embolism, stratified by the presence or absence of right ventricular dysfunction (RVD, by echocardiogram) and concomitant deep vein thrombosis (DVT, by lower extremity complete compression ultrasound) at the time of pulmonary embolism diagnosis. Log rank p<0.001. (Reprinted from Jiménez D, Aujesky D, Moores L, et al. Combinations of prognostic tools for identification of high-risk normotensive patients with acute symptomatic pulmonary embolism. *Thorax.* 2011;66:75-81, and reproduced/amended with permission from the BMJ Publishing Group.)

TABLE 5.—Prediction Rule Test Characteristics for 30-Day PE-Related Mortality in 228 Patients Deemed High Risk by the PESI

	Troponin Plus TTE Parameter (95% CI)	Troponin Plus CCUS Parameter (95% CI)	TTE Plus CCUS Parameter (95% CI)
Positive test N, %	29 (12.7%)	41 (18.0%)	51 (10.5%)
Sensitivity, %	27.3 (8.7 to 45.9)	45.4 (24.6 to 66.3)	27.3 (8.7 to 45.9)
Specificity, %	88.8 (84.5 to 93.1)	84.9 (80.1 to 89.8)	91.3 (87.4 to 95.1)
Positive predictive value, %	20.7 (5.9 to 35.4)	24.4 (11.2 to 37.5)	25.0 (7.7 to 42.3)
Negative predictive value, %	92.0 (88.2 to 95.7)	93.6 (90.1 to 97.1)	92.2 (88.5 to 95.8)
Positive likelihood ratio	2.44 (1.12 to 5.35)	3.02 (1.72 to 5.29)	3.12 (1.38 to 7.03)
Negative likelihood ratio	0.82 (0.63 to 1.06)	0.64 (0.44 to 0.94)	0.80 (0.61 to 1.03)

CCUS, lower extremity complete compression ultrasound; PE, pulmonary embolism; PESI, pulmonary embolism severity index; TTE, transthoracic echocardiography.

abnormality of TnI were defined a priori. Right ventricular dysfunction and an abnormal TnI are evidence for damage to the right ventricle because of the severe afterload caused by sudden obstruction to right ventricular ejection, and the finding of DVT by CCUS shows the presence of remaining thrombus and is predictive of the risk of recurrent episodes of PE that could destabilize a previously normotensive patient. Although there have been studies demonstrating that TTE evidence of right ventricular dysfunction has a low positive predictive value for PE-related death[3,4] and others investigating the prognostic power of combining a biomarker for injury and TTE,[5-7] the studies were all either small or included a limited number of hemodynamically stable patients.

This study identified high-risk normotensive patients with PE as those with 2 of the 3 noninvasive tests positive. A single positive test was of limited usefulness, whereas the positive likelihood of PE-related mortality doubled with the addition of a second positive test. All 3 of the tests were positive and did not appreciably improve the predictability of the 2-test strategy. If the patient was high-risk by the Pulmonary Embolism Severity Index,[8] a score based on 11 simple patient characteristics that stratified 30-day mortality rates into 5 severity classes, the 2-test strategy in these high-risk patients had the highest positive predictive value for PE-associated 30-day mortality. The finding of high-risk mortality in normotensive patients with acute PE suggests that such patients might benefit from more aggressive therapy than simply anticoagulation. The next step is to investigate the impact of risk stratification on the management of acute PE by a prospective randomized study.

M. D. Cheitlin, MD

References

1. Torbicki A, Perrier A, Konstantinides S, et al. Task Force for the Diagnosis and Management of Acute Pulmonary Embolism of the European Society of Cardiology. Guidelines on the diagnosis and management of acute pulmonary embolism: the Task Force for the Diagnosis and Management of Acute Pulmonary Embolism of European Society of Cardiology (ESC). *Eur Heart J.* 2008;29: 2276-2315.
2. Kearon C, Kahn SR, Agnelli G, et al. American College of Chest Physicians. Antithrombotic therapy for venous thromboembolic disease: American College of Chest Physicians Evidence-Based Clinical Practice Guidelines (8th Edition). *Chest.* 2008;133:454S-545S.
3. Ten Wolde M, Söhne M, Quak E, Mac Gillavry MR, Büller HR. Prognostic value of echocardiographically assessed right ventricular dysfunction in patients with pulmonary embolism. *Arch Intern Med.* 2004;164:1685-1689.
4. Sanchez O, Trinquart L, Colombet I, et al. Prognostic value of right ventricular dysfunction in patients with haemodynamically stable pulmonary embolism: a systematic review. *Eur Heart J.* 2008;29:1569-1577.
5. Binder L, Pieske B, Olschewski M, et al. N-terminal pro-brain natriuretic peptide or troponin testing followed by echocardiography for risk stratification of acute pulmonary embolism. *Circulation.* 2005;112:1573-1579.
6. Kucher N, Wallmann D, Carone A, Windecker S, Meier B, Hess OM. Incremental prognostic value of troponin I and echocardiography in patients with acute pulmonary embolism. *Eur Heart J.* 2003;24:1651-1656.
7. Scridon T, Scridon C, Skali H, Alvarez A, Goldhaber SZ, Solomon SD. Prognostic significance of troponin elevation and right ventricular enlargement in acute pulmonary embolism. *Am J Cardiol.* 2005;96:303-305.
8. Aujesky D, Obrosky DS, Stone RA, et al. Derivation and validation of a prognostic model for pulmonary embolism. *Am J Respir Crit Care Med.* 2005;172: 1041-1046.

Analysis of the Impact of Early Surgery on In-Hospital Mortality of Native Valve Endocarditis: Use of Propensity Score and Instrumental Variable Methods to Adjust for Treatment-Selection Bias

Lalani T, for the International Collaboration on Endocarditis—Prospective Cohort Study (ICE-PCS) Investigators (Duke Univ Med Ctr, Durham, NC; et al)
Circulation 121:1005-1013, 2010

Background.—The impact of early surgery on mortality in patients with native valve endocarditis (NVE) is unresolved. This study sought to evaluate valve surgery compared with medical therapy for NVE and to identify characteristics of patients who are most likely to benefit from early surgery.

Methods and Results.—Using a prospective, multinational cohort of patients with definite NVE, the effect of early surgery on in-hospital mortality was assessed by propensity-based matching adjustment for survivor bias and by instrumental variable analysis. Patients were stratified by propensity quintile, paravalvular complications, valve perforation, systemic embolization, stroke, *Staphylococcus aureus* infection, and congestive heart failure. Of the 1552 patients with NVE, 720 (46%) underwent early surgery and 832 (54%) were treated with medical therapy. Compared with medical therapy, early surgery was associated with a significant reduction in mortality in the overall cohort (12.1% [87/720] versus 20.7% [172/832]) and after propensity-based matching and adjustment for survivor bias (absolute risk reduction [ARR] −5.9%, *P*<0.001). With a combined instrument, the instrumental-variable—adjusted ARR in mortality associated with early surgery was −11.2% (*P*<0.001). In subgroup analysis, surgery was found to confer a survival benefit compared with medical therapy among patients with a higher propensity for surgery (ARR −10.9% for quintiles 4 and 5, *P*=0.002) and those with paravalvular complications (ARR −17.3%, *P*<0.001), systemic embolization (ARR −12.9%, *P*=0.002), *S aureus* NVE (ARR −20.1%, *P*<0.001), and stroke (ARR −13%, *P*=0.02) but not those with valve perforation or congestive heart failure.

Conclusions.—Early surgery for NVE is associated with an in-hospital mortality benefit compared with medical therapy alone (Fig 1).

► The indications for surgery in patients with native valve endocarditis are still debatable. Practice guidelines conclude that surgery is indicated in patients with infective endocarditis in those developing heart failure, repeated embolization, infection resistance to appropriate antibiotics, and paravalvular abscesses or intracardiac damage, but the evidence for these recommendations rests on consensus rather than on randomized studies.[1] In fact, because endocarditis is relatively uncommon, there are no large randomized studies of surgery versus medical management available. Almost all studies attempting to answer this question have been observational, with a small number of subjects and without accounting for the various biases that can influence the result. Such biases are referral bias, overt treatment bias relating to covariates measured in the study,

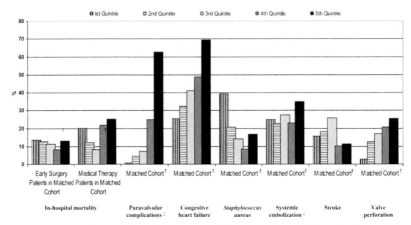

FIGURE 1.—Distribution of key characteristics of the propensity-matched, survivor-bias–adjusted cohort of patients with NVE by surgical propensity-score quintiles. *Propensity-matched, survivor-bias–adjusted cohort (n=1238 or 169 matched pairs); quintiles based on propensity scores. †Frequency based on the propensity-matched, survivor-bias–adjusted surgery and medical therapy patients within each quintile. Percentages calculated as fraction of patients with outcome (eg, paravalvular complication) out of total number of patients in the quintile. ‡Transesophageal or transthoracic echocardiographic evidence of paravalvular abscess or fistula formation. (Reprinted from Lalani T, for the International Collaboration on Endocarditis–Prospective Cohort Study (ICE-PCS) Investigators. Analysis of the impact of early surgery on in-hospital mortality of native valve endocarditis: use of propensity score and instrumental variable methods to adjust for treatment-selection bias. *Circulation.* 2010;121:1005-1013, with permission from the American Heart Association.)

survivor bias indicating that patients who live longer are more likely to have surgery than those who die early in the course of the disease, and hidden bias meaning those unmeasured patient characteristics that affect both the decision to treat and the outcome. This study from the International Collaboration on Endocarditis-Prospective Cohort Study database is the largest observational study that used powerful statistical instruments, such as propensity analysis to attempt to account for overt treatment bias, survivor bias by matching surgical patients to medical patients who lived at least as long, and hidden bias by a statistical method known as instrumental variable analysis. In this study, which comes as close to a randomized study as it is possible to do by accounting for these confounding biases, the authors concluded that there is an in-hospital mortality risk ratio in favor of early surgery in those patients with native valve infective endocarditis and paravalvular complications, systemic embolization, stroke, or *Staphylococcus aureus* infection. Peculiarly, there was no mortality benefit of early surgery in those with heart failure or perforated valve.

The problem with this referral center study is that patients with endocarditis who were intravenous drug users, had prosthetic valve endocarditis, had surgery before admission to the study hospital, and had a variety of missing data were excluded, so that only 44% of the entire cohort of patients with Duke criteria–proved endocarditis are included in the study. Also, those with heart failure are not graded by severity, and the follow-up was only for the in-hospital period, so the benefit of early surgery might be seen in those with more severe heart failure and in those with valve perforation. A very good editorial accompanies this article and is well worth reading.[2]

M. D. Cheitlin, MD

References

1. Bonow RO, Carabello BA, Chatterjee K, et al. ACC/AHA 2006 guidelines for the management of patients with valvular heart disease: a report of the American College of Cardiology/American Heart Association Task Force on Practice Guidelines (writing Committee to Revise the 1998 guidelines for the management of patients with valvular heart disease) developed in collaboration with the Society of Cardiovascular Anesthesiologists endorsed by the Society for Cardiovascular Angiography and Interventions and the Society of Thoracic Surgeons. *J Am Coll Cardiol.* 2006;48:e1-e148.
2. Farzaneh-Far R, Bolger AF. Surgical timing in infectious endocarditis: wrestling with the unrandomized. *Circulation.* 2010;121:960-962.

High prevalence of intramural coronary infection in patients with drug-resistant cardiac syndrome X: comparison with chronic stable angina and normal controls

Chimenti C, Sale P, Verardo R, et al (La Sapienza Univ, Rome Italy; IRCCS "Lazzaro Spallanzani", Rome, Italy; et al)
Heart 96:1926-1931, 2010

Background.—Coronary microvascular dysfunction has been reported along with myocardial viral infection. Whether intramural coronary vessels infection plays a role in patients with cardiac syndrome X (CSX) is unknown.

Methods.—Thirteen consecutive patients (four men, nine women, mean age 51 ± 10.5 years) with drug-resistant CSX underwent left ventricular endomyocardial biopsy. Myocardial tissue was examined for histology, immunohistochemistry and for the presence of cardiotropic viruses by PCR analysis. In the presence of a viral infection on the whole tissue, laser microdissection was performed to analyse the viral genome selectively in intramural vessels and cardiomyocytes. Controls were surgical cardiac biopsies from patients with chronic stable angina and from patients with mitral stenosis and normal cardiac function (normal controls).

Results.—Histology showed hypertrophy and degeneration of cardiomyocytes with interstitial and replacement fibrosis in all CSX, while focal lymphocytic myocarditis was additionally recognised in three patients. No vasculitis was observed. Viral genomes were detected in nine of 13 CSX (Epstein—Barr virus in four, adenovirus in three, human herpes virus (HHV) 6 in one, Epstein—Barr adenovirus co-infection in one). Laser microdissection showed that Epstein—Barr and adenovirus localised both in cardiomyocytes and intramural vessels, while HHV-6 infection was confined to the vessel wall.

Conclusions.—Viral genomes can be detected in intramural vessels of up to 69% of drug-resistant CSX. Coronary small vessels infection represents an alternative pathophysiological mechanism of this syndrome and can explain the poor response to anti-ischaemic drugs (Table 2).

▶ Cardiac syndrome X (CSX), defined as exertional typical angina pectoris with electrocardiographic and/or metabolic evidence of myocardial ischemia and angiographically normal epicardial coronary arteries,[1] is caused by dysfunction of small intramural coronary arteries affected by either structural or functional abnormalities of vascular smooth muscle and/or endothelial cells.[2] The causes of the microvascular dysfunction are not known, but mechanisms such as the usual coronary risk factors,[3] estrogen deficiency in females,[4] and low-grade inflammation[5] have been suggested. Also, there is the possibility that myocardial ischemia is not the cause of the clinical syndrome. Multiple studies have demonstrated coronary microvascular dysfunction in these patients, manifested by reversible perfusion defects on stress myocardial perfusion studies,[2] impaired endothelium-dependent coronary flow reserve,[4] and increased vasoconstrictor reactivity of small coronary artery vessels.[5] Multiple mechanisms that could influence this microvascular dysfunction have been suggested, among them altered autonomic tone, enhanced ion transport across cell membranes,[6] and increased endothelin-1 release.[7] The observation that myocardial viral infection

TABLE 2.—Comparison of Baseline, Histological and Molecular Characteristics Among CSX Patients, CSA Patients and Normal Controls

Variables	CSX Patients (n=13)	CSA Patients (n=15)	Normal Controls (n=20)	p Value
Age, years, (mean±SD)	51.0±10.5	53.3±6.8	52.6±7.3	0.750
Sex				0.638
Male, N (%)	4 (31%)	6 (40%)	5 (25%)	
CAD risk factors, N (%)				
Family history				0.060
Yes	4 (31)	10 (67)	6 (30)	
Hypertension				>0.001
Yes	0 (0)	13 (87)	6 (30)	
Diabetes				0.020
Yes	0 (0)	7 (47)	6 (30)	
Hypercholesterolaemia (>200 mg/dl)				0.112
Yes	2 (15)	8 (53)	7 (35)	
Cigarette smoking				0.077
Yes	4 (31)	11 (73)	10 (50)	
Echocardiography, mean±SD				
EDD (mm)	48.0±2.3	49.0±4.0	47.5±6.3	0.659
EF (%)	58±4.4	59±5.2	59±4.1	0.796
Histology				
Fibrosis, %, mean±SD	6.1±1.2	2.9±0.9	2.0±0.7	<0.001*
Myocyte degeneration, N (%)				<0.001*
Yes	13 (100)	3 (23)	0 (0)	
Focal myocarditis, N (%)				<0.001*
Yes	3 (23)	0 (0)	0 (0)	
Viral agent (PCR), N (%)				<0.001*
Yes	9 (69)	0 (0)	0 (0)	

CSA, chronic stable angina; CSX, cardiac syndrome X;
EDD, left ventricular end-diastolic diameter; EF, left ventricular ejection fraction.
*p<0.001 A versus B and A versus C.

can be associated with coronary microvascular dysfunction[8] initiated this study that carefully defined patients with CSX resistance to medication, and performed myocardial biopsies to study the presence of viral genomes in the cardiomyocytes and coronary intramural vessels with appropriate controls. The finding of virus in 69% of the CSX patients, without serologic evidence of an active infection or the presence of a viral genome in the blood, ruling out contamination from circulating cells, and none of the controls is intriguing, suggesting an explanation for the resistance to antianginal drugs in this population. Sixty-seven percent of the viruses detected were herpes viruses (Ebstein-Barr virus [EBV] and human herpes virus-6) that have preferential tropism for endothelial cells. Interestingly, a high prevalence of myocardial EBV infection has been reported in patients with myocarditis that mimics acute myocardial infarction.[9] For the first time, this study has shown that myocardial viral infection, localized in the coronary microvasculature, can be found in patients with CSX refractory to antianginal medication and may be implicated in the microcirculatory dysfunction seen in this disease.

M. D. Cheitlin, MD

References

1. Kemp HG Jr. Left ventricular function in patients with the anginal syndrome and normal coronary arteriograms. *Am J Cardiol.* 1973;32:375-376.
2. Mosseri M, Yarom R, Gotsman MS, Hasin Y. Histologic evidence for small-vessel coronary artery disease in patients with angina pectoris and patent large coronary arteries. *Circulation.* 1986;74:964-972.
3. Botker HE, Moller N, Schmitz O, Bagger JP, Nielsen TT. Myocardial insulin resistance in patients with syndrome X. *J Clin Invest.* 1997;100:1919-1927.
4. Rosano GM, Collins P, Kaski JC, et al. Syndrome X in women is associated with oestrogen deficiency. *Eur Heart J.* 1995;16:610-614.
5. Lanza GA, Sestito A, Cammarota G, et al. Assessment of systemic inflammation and infective pathogen burden in patients with cardiac syndrome X. *Am J Cardiol.* 2004;94:40-44.
6. Gaspardone A, Ferri C, Crea F, et al. Enhanced activity of sodium-lithium countertransport in patients with cardiac syndrome X: a potential link between cardiac and metabolic syndrome X. *J Am Coll Cardiol.* 1998;32:2031-2034.
7. Lanza GA, Lüscher TF, Pasceri V, et al. Effects of atrial pacing on arterial and coronary sinus endothelin-1 levels in syndrome X. *Am J Cardiol.* 1999;84:1187-1191.
8. Vallbracht KB, Schwimmbeck PL, Kühl U, Rauch U, Seeberg B, Schultheiss HP. Differential aspects of endothelial function of the coronary microcirculation considering myocardial virus persistence, endothelial activation, and myocardial leukocyte infiltrates. *Circulation.* 2005;111:1784-1791.
9. Angelini A, Calzolari V, Calabrese F, et al. Myocarditis mimicking acute myocardial infarction: role of endomyocardial biopsy in the differential diagnosis. *Heart.* 2000;84:245-250.

6 Cardiac Arrhythmias, Conduction Disturbances, and Electrophysiology

Atrial Fibrillation

Age as a Risk Factor for Stroke in Atrial Fibrillation Patients: Implications for Thromboprophylaxis

Marinigh R, Lip GYH, Fiotti N, et al (Univ of Birmingham Centre for Cardiovascular Sciences, UK; Univ of Trieste, Italy)
J Am Coll Cardiol 56:827-837, 2010

The prevalence of atrial fibrillation (AF) is related to age and is projected to rise exponentially as the population ages and the prevalence of cardiovascular risk factors increases. The risk of ischemic stroke is significantly increased in AF patients, and there is evidence of a graded increased risk of stroke associated with advancing age. Oral anticoagulation (OAC) is far more effective than antiplatelet agents at reducing stroke risk in patients with AF. Therefore, increasing numbers of elderly patients are candidates for, and could benefit from, the use of anticoagulants. However, elderly people with AF are less likely to receive OAC therapy. This is mainly due to concerns about a higher risk of OAC-associated hemorrhage in the elderly population. Until recently, older patients were underrepresented in randomized controlled trials of OAC versus placebo or antiplatelet therapy, and therefore the evidence base for the value of OAC in the elderly population was not known. However, analyses of the available trial data indicate that the expected net clinical benefit of warfarin therapy is highest among patients with the highest untreated risk for stroke, which includes the oldest age category. An important caveat with warfarin treatment is maintenance of a therapeutic international normalized ratio, regardless of the age of the patient, where time in therapeutic range should be ≥65%. Therefore, age alone should not prevent prescription of OAC in elderly patients, given an appropriate stroke and bleeding risk stratification (Tables 3 and 4).

▶ Thromboembolic complications of atrial fibrillation (AF) are associated with significant morbidity and mortality. Both risk of stroke and prevalence of AF increase with age, and older age has consistently been identified as an independent risk for thromboembolic complications of AF. However, reluctance persists to treat older patients with oral anticoagulants (OACs) because of a perceived prohibitive bleeding risk in this population. In this context, Marinigh et al performed a systematic review of published studies evaluating the relationship between age, thromboembolism, and bleeding risk in AF. Twelve of 17 identified studies evaluating the relationship between age and stroke in AF found age to be an independent risk factor for stroke, and a pooled analysis of 5 randomized controlled trials resulted in a relative risk of 1.4 (95% confidence interval [CI], 1.1-1.8) for stroke by increasing decade. This risk was evident in most studies whether patients were dichotomized by a threshold age (eg, > 75 years) or stratified by decade. The newer CHA_2DS_2-VASc schema also includes age of 65 to 74 years as a risk factor and > 75 years as a high-risk feature, consistent with data that age is a continuous variable for risk (Table 3). Elderly patients also appear to benefit from anticoagulation; a meta-analysis of 11 trials demonstrated a hazard ratio (HR) of 0.36 (95% CI, 0.29-0.45) for warfarin compared with aspirin that was not attenuated with increasing age. However, age has also consistently been shown to be a risk factor for bleeding; 1 recent meta-analysis reporting an HR of 1.6 (95% CI, 1.47-1.77) for major bleeding. Interestingly, the bleeding risk was similar for patients taking warfarin or aspirin. Further stratification of bleeding risk in elderly patients has been demonstrated with several risk prediction models, such as HAS-BLED (Table 4). Importantly, stroke and bleeding risks are affected by time in therapeutic range (TTR) with warfarin. TTR, in turn, has been shown to be affected by a variety of patient-specific factors, many of which are more common in the elderly. Despite this risk, the

TABLE 3.—Stroke Risk Assessment in AF: CHA_2DS_2-VASc*

Stroke Risk Factors	Score
Congestive heart failure/LV dysfunction	1
Hypertension	1
Age ≥75 yrs	2
Diabetes mellitus	1
Stroke/TIA/TE	2
Vascular disease (prior MI, PAD, or aortic plaque)	1
Age 65−74 years	1
Sex category (i.e., female sex)	1

The CHA_2DS_2-VASc schema assesses stroke risk in patients with nonvalvular atrial fibrillation (51).
TE = thromboembolic event; TIA = transient ischemic attack.
*For a CHA_2DS_2-VASc score >1, such patients are high risk and should have oral anticoagulation (e.g., warfarin); for a CHA_2DS_2-VASc score = 1, antithrombotic therapy is recommended, either as oral anticoagulation or aspirin 75 to 325 mg daily, but oral anticoagulation is preferred rather than aspirin; for a CHA_2DS_2-VASc score = 0 ("truly low risk"), either aspirin 75 to 325 mg daily or no antithrombotic therapy can be used, but no antithrombotic therapy may be preferred. Maximum score is 9 (51).

TABLE 4.—Bleeding Risk Assessment in AF: HAS-BLED Bleeding Risk Score

Letter	Clinical Characteristic*	Points Awarded
H	Hypertension	1
A	Abnormal renal and liver function (1 point each)	1 or 2
S	Stroke	1
B	Bleeding	1
L	Labile INRs	1
E	Elderly	1
D	Drugs or alcohol (1 point each)	1 or 2
		Maximum 9 points

*Hypertension is defined as systolic blood pressure >160 mm Hg. Abnormal kidney function is defined as the presence of chronic dialysis or renal transplantation or serum creatinine ≥200 μmol/l. Abnormal liver function is defined as chronic hepatic disease (e.g., cirrhosis) or biochemical evidence of significant hepatic derangement (e.g., bilirubin >2× upper limit of normal, in association with AST/ALT/ALP (aspartate aminotransferase/alanine aminotransferase/alkaline phosphatase) >3× upper limit normal, and so on). Bleeding refers to previous bleeding history and/or predisposition to bleeding (e.g., bleeding diathesis, anemia). LabileINRs (international normalized ratios) refers to unstable/high INRs or poor time in therapeutic range (e.g., <60%). Drugs/alcohol use refers to concomitant use of drugs, such as antiplatelet agents, nonsteroidal anti-inflammatory drugs (65).

authors identified 2 analyses evaluating the net clinical benefit (rate of thrombo-embolic complications minus bleeding complications) of OAC in older patients, and both suggested a significant benefit in this population over antiplatelet therapy. Based on their review, the authors conclude that while elderly patients are at higher risk for bleeding, OAC should be considered given the greater net clinical benefit of stroke prevention in a high-risk population. Although this systematic review reinforces the need for careful consideration of risks of using and avoiding OACs in elderly patients with AF, with an aging population and the recent development of alternative OACs, such as dabigitran and rivaroxaban, this will become an even more frequent and complex issue in clinical practice.

W. W. Brabham, MD

Association Between Familial Atrial Fibrillation and Risk of New-Onset Atrial Fibrillation

Lubitz SA, Yin X, Fontes JD, et al (Massachusetts General Hosp, Charlestown; Framingham Heart Study, MA; Boston Univ, MA)
JAMA 304:2263-2269, 2010

Context.—Although the heritability of atrial fibrillation (AF) is established, the contribution of familial AF to predicting new-onset AF remains unknown.

Objective.—To determine whether familial occurrence of AF is associated with new-onset AF beyond established risk factors.

Design, Setting, and Participants.—The Framingham Heart Study, a prospective community-based cohort study started in 1948. Original and Offspring Cohort participants were aged at least 30 years, were free of AF at the baseline examination, and had at least 1 parent or sibling enrolled in the study. The 4421 participants in this analysis (mean age,

54 [SD, 13] years; 54% women) were followed up through December 31, 2007.

Main Outcome Measures.—Incremental predictive value of incorporating different features of familial AF (any familial AF, premature familial AF [onset ≤65 years old], number of affected relatives, and youngest age of onset in a relative) into a risk model for new-onset AF.

Results.—Across 11 971 examinations during the period 1968-2007, 440 participants developed AF. Familial AF occurred among 1185 participants (26.8%) and premature familial AF occurred among 351 participants (7.9%). Atrial fibrillation occurred more frequently among participants with familial AF than without familial AF (unadjusted absolute event rates of 5.8% and 3.1%, respectively). The association was not attenuated by adjustment for AF risk factors (multivariable-adjusted hazard ratio, 1.40; 95% confidence interval [CI], 1.13-1.74) or reported AF-related genetic variants. Among the different features of familial AF examined, premature familial AF was associated with improved discrimination beyond traditional risk factors to the greatest extent (traditional risk factors, C statistic, 0.842 [95% CI, 0.826-0.858]; premature familial AF, C statistic, 0.846 [95% CI, 0.831-0.862]; $P = .004$). Modest changes in integrated discrimination improvement were observed with premature familial AF (2.1%). Net reclassification improvement (assessed using 8-year risk thresholds of <5%, 5%-10%, and >10%) did not change significantly with premature familial AF (index statistic, 0.011; 95% CI, −0.021 to 0.042; $P = .51$), although categoryless net reclassification was improved (index statistic, 0.127; 95% CI, 0.064-0.189; $P = .009$).

Conclusions.—In this cohort, familial AF was associated with an increased risk of AF that was not attenuated by adjustment for AF risk factors including genetic variants. Assessment of premature familial AF was associated with a very slight increase in predictive accuracy compared with traditional risk factors.

▶ The association between familial atrial fibrillation (AF) and the risk of new onset of AF was evaluated by an analysis of the Framingham Heart Study. Participants in this cohort had at least 1 parent or sibling enrolled in the study and were free of AF at the baseline evaluation. A total of 4421 participants were included. The study showed that a family history of AF was associated with an increased risk of AF and that this was not attenuated by adjustment of other risk factors or genetic variance. While there was an association of familial AF with new-onset AF, only 2% of the patient population had more than 2 affected relatives. There is direct association with increasing numbers of first-degree relatives with AF, but the small number of participants with multiple relatives is limiting. Premature onset of AF was defined as AF at age less than 65 years. This study did show an increased hazard ratio for the onset of AF and a linear increase in AF risk as the age of the youngest affected relative decreased. Patients with premature AF had an event rate of 4.3%, whereas it was only 1.2% without premature AF. Unfortunately, the genetic AF susceptibility loci were not seen in this study. There may be, as the authors stated, a "missing heritability" factor not seen or documented, and the population size may be too small to gather enough generic data.

While this study clearly shows the relationship between familial AF and new-onset AF, it also opens up many questions about genetics, genetic penetrance, environmental factors, and novel genetic variants.

R. B. Leman, MD

Effect of Combined Spironolactone–β-Blocker ± Enalapril Treatment on Occurrence of Symptomatic Atrial Fibrillation Episodes in Patients With a History of Paroxysmal Atrial Fibrillation (SPIR-AF Study)

Dabrowski R, Borowiec A, Smolis-Bak E, et al (Inst of Cardiology, Warsaw, Poland; et al)

Am J Cardiol 106:1609-1614, 2010

Angiotensin II and aldosterone are key factors responsible for the structural and neurohormonal remodeling of the atria and ventricles in patients with atrial fibrillation (AF). The aim of the present study was to evaluate the antiarrhythmic effects of spironolactone compared to angiotensin-converting enzyme inhibitors in patients with recurrent AF. A cohort of 164 consecutive patients (mean age 66 years, 87 men), with an average 4-year history of recurrent AF episodes, was enrolled in a prospective, randomized, 12-month trial with 4 treatment arms: group A, spironolactone, enalapril, and a β blocker; group B, spironolactone and a β blocker; group C, enalapril plus a β blocker; and group D, a β blocker alone. The primary end point of the trial was the presence of symptomatic AF episodes documented on the electrocardiogram. At 3-, 6-, 9-, and 12 months, a significant (p < 0.001) reduction had occurred in the incidence of AF episodes in both spironolactone-treated groups (group A, spironolactone, enalapril, and a β blocker; and group B, spironolactone plus a β blocker) compared to the incidence in patients treated with enalapril and a β blocker (group C) or a β blocker alone (group D). No significant difference was seen in AF recurrences between patients taking spironolactone and a β blocker with (group A) and without (group B) enalapril. No significant differences were found in the systolic or diastolic blood pressure or heart rate among the groups before and after 1 year of follow-up. In conclusion, combined spironolactone plus β-blocker treatment might be a simple and valuable option in preventing AF episodes in patients with normal left ventricular function and a history of refractory paroxysmal AF (Fig 2).

▶ Angiotensin II and aldosterone have been shown to be significant factors in structural, neurohormonal, and electrical remodeling of the atrium. In addition to stimulation of aldosterone production, actions of angiotensin II include reduction in β-adrenergic receptor density. Inflammatory processes, oxidative stress, collagen formation, and cardiomyocyte necrosis are all associated with aldosterone formation. This study by Dabrowski et al evaluated the effect of aldosterone versus angiotensin-converting enzyme inhibitor use for the

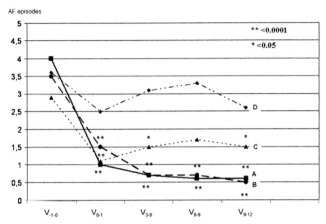

FIGURE 2.—Comparison of AF incidence among group A (spironoloctone, enalapril, and β blocker), group B spironolactone and β blocker), group C (enalapril and β blocker), and group D (β blocker) during 12 months of follow-up. (Reprinted from the American Journal of Cardiology, Dabrowski R, Borowiec A, Smolis-Bak E, et al. Effect of combined spironolactone−β-blocker ± enalapril treatment on occurrence of symptomatic atrial fibrillation episodes in patients with a history of paroxysmal atrial fibrillation (SPIR-AF Study). *Am J Cardiol.* 2010;106:1609-1614. Copyright © 2010 with permission from Elsevier Inc.)

reduction of symptomatic atrial fibrillation (AF) episodes in patients with recurrent AF. All patients were treated with a β-blocker, and 4 patient groups were studied in a prospective randomized fashion: group A, spironolactone and enalapril; group B, spironolactone; group C, enalapril; and group D, β-blocker only. After follow-up visits at 3, 6, 9, and 12 months, patients in both spironolactone-treated groups (A and B) had a significant reduction in the number of AF episodes compared with patients who did not receive spironolactone (group A: 4.0 vs 0.6 episodes, $P < .0001$; group B: 3.5 vs 0.5 episodes, $P < .0001$). Patients treated with enalapril and a β-blocker (group C) had a reduction in the number of episodes at 3- and 6-month visits but less pronounced results at 9- and 12-month visits (Fig 2). This small, pilot, randomized trial of spironolactone use in patients with recurrent AF suggests decreased burden of AF in patients treated with spironolactone. The mechanism of this result may be because of treatment of AF risk factors, including hypertension and congestive heart failure. Alternatively, spironolactone may have independent effects on fibrosis and atrial remodeling. This study requires further confirmation with a larger clinical trial, and use of atrial arrhythmia detection systems would provide further strength in assessing the efficacy of aldosterone blockade to decrease the number of AF episodes.

R. N. Vest III, MD

Efficacy and Safety of Prescription Omega-3 Fatty Acids for the Prevention of Recurrent Symptomatic Atrial Fibrillation: A Randomized Controlled Trial

Kowey PR, Reiffel JA, Ellenbogen KA, et al (Jefferson Med College, Philadelphia, PA; Columbia Univ Med Ctr, NY; Virginia Commonwealth Univ Med Ctr, Richmond, VA; et al)
JAMA 304:2363-2372, 2010

Context.—Atrial fibrillation (AF) is common, yet there remains an unmet medical need for additional treatment options. Current pharmacological treatments have limited efficacy and significant adverse events. Limited data from small trials suggest omega-3 polyunsaturated fatty acids may provide a safe, effective treatment option for AF patients.

Objective.—To evaluate the safety and efficacy of prescription omega-3 fatty acids (prescription omega-3) for the prevention of recurrent symptomatic AF.

Design, Setting, and Participants.—Prospective, randomized, double-blind, placebo-controlled, parallel-group multicenter trial involving 663 US outpatient participants with confirmed symptomatic paroxysmal (n = 542) or persistent (n = 121) AF, with no substantial structural heart disease, and in normal sinus rhythm at baseline were recruited from November 2006 to July 2009 (final follow-up was January 2010).

Interventions.—Prescription omega-3 (8 g/d) or placebo for the first 7 days; prescription omega-3 (4 g/d) or placebo thereafter through week 24.

Main Outcome Measures.—The primary end point was symptomatic recurrence of AF (first recurrence) in participants with paroxysmal AF. Secondary analyses included first recurrence in the persistent stratum and both strata combined. Participants were followed up for 6 months.

Results.—At 24 weeks, in the paroxysmal AF stratum, 129 of 269 participants (48%) in the placebo group and 135 of 258 participants (52%) in the prescription group had a recurrent symptomatic AF or flutter event. In the persistent AF stratum, 18 participants (33%) in the placebo group and 32 (50%) in the prescription group had documented symptomatic AF or flutter events. There was no difference between treatment groups for recurrence of symptomatic AF in the paroxysmal stratum (hazard ratio [HR], 1.15; 95% confidence interval [CI], 0.90-1.46; $P = .26$), in the persistent stratum (HR, 1.64; 95% CI, 0.92-2.92; $P = .09$), and both strata combined (HR, 1.22; 95% CI, 0.98-1.52; $P = .08$). Other, secondary end points were supportive of the primary result. A total of 5% of those receiving placebo and 4% of those receiving prescription omega-3 discontinued due to adverse events. Eicosapentaenoic and docosahexaenoic acid blood levels were significantly higher in the prescription group than in the placebo group at weeks 4 and 24.

Conclusion.—Among participants with paroxysmal AF, 24-week treatment with prescription omega-3 compared with placebo did not reduce recurrent AF over 6 months.

Trial Registration.—clinicaltrials.gov Identifier: NCT00402363.

▶ Atrial fibrillation (AF) is the most common arrhythmia resulting in hospitalization. The incidence of AF is growing as the population ages, which mandates better therapy. The results of the trial of antiarrhythmic drugs are largely disappointing with modest efficacy and frequent adverse effects often noted. This has led to alternative therapies, such as nontraditional pharmacologic therapy or catheter ablation. In this regard, a number of drugs have been reported to reduce AF incidence in small trials, such as angiotensin-converting enzyme (ACE) inhibitors, angiotensin receptor blockers (ARBs), statins, and omega-3 fatty acids. In this study, the effect of omega-3 fatty acids on the recurrence of symptomatic AF was evaluated in a well-designed and executed randomized, double blind, placebo-controlled trial. A relatively healthy cohort was studied who had either paroxysmal AF or persistent AF with no structural heart disease. There was no effect of omega-3 supplementation on symptomatic recurrences among patients with paroxysmal AF (Fig 2 in the original article) or any subgroup. These results are similar to other studies of adjunctive agents, such as ACE inhibitors or ARBs, that have failed to confirm an antiarrhythmic action in larger randomized studies. The present data indicate that although there may be beneficial effects of omega-3 fatty acids on cardiovascular health, these agents should not be used as treatment for paroxysmal AF. Although only symptomatic recurrences were assessed, it seems very unlikely that these agents will affect overall AF burden given the high incidence of symptomatic recurrences in both randomized groups.

M. R. Gold, MD, PhD

Efficacy and safety of dabigatran compared with warfarin at different levels of international normalised ratio control for stroke prevention in atrial fibrillation: an analysis of the RE-LY trial
Wallentin L, on behalf of the RE-LY investigators (Uppsala Univ, Sweden; et al)
Lancet 376:975-983, 2010

Background.—Effectiveness and safety of warfarin is associated with the time in therapeutic range (TTR) with an international normalised ratio (INR) of $2 \cdot 0 - 3 \cdot 0$. In the Randomised Evaluation of Long-term Anticoagulation Therapy (RE-LY) trial, dabigatran versus warfarin reduced both stroke and haemorrhage. We aimed to investigate the primary and secondary outcomes of the RE-LY trial in relation to each centre's mean TTR (cTTR) in the warfarin population.

Methods.—In the RE-LY trial, 18 113 patients at 951 sites were randomly assigned to 110 mg or 150 mg dabigatran twice daily versus warfarin dose adjusted to INR $2 \cdot 0 - 3 \cdot 0$. Median follow-up was $2 \cdot 0$ years. For 18 024 patients at 906 sites, the cTTR was estimated by averaging TTR for individual warfarin-treated patients calculated by the Rosendaal method. We compared the outcomes of RE-LY across the three treatment groups within four groups defined by the quartiles of cTTR. RE-LY is registered with ClinicalTrials.gov, number NCT00262600.

Findings.—The quartiles of cTTR for patients in the warfarin group were: less than $57 \cdot 1\%$, $57 \cdot 1-65 \cdot 5\%$, $65 \cdot 5-72 \cdot 6\%$, and greater than $72 \cdot 6\%$. There were no significant interactions between cTTR and prevention of stroke and systemic embolism with either 110 mg dabigatran (interaction p=$0 \cdot 89$) or 150 mg dabigatran (interaction p=$0 \cdot 20$) versus warfarin. Neither were any significant interactions recorded with cTTR with regards to intracranial bleeding with 110 mg dabigatran (interaction p=$0 \cdot 71$) or 150 mg dabigatran (interaction p=$0 \cdot 89$) versus warfarin. There was a significant interaction between cTTR and major bleeding when comparing 150 mg dabigatran with warfarin (interaction p=$0 \cdot 03$), with less bleeding events at lower cTTR but similar events at higher cTTR, whereas rates of major bleeding were lower with 110 mg dabigatran than with warfarin irrespective of cTTR. There were significant interactions between cTTR and effects of both 110 mg and 150 mg dabigatran versus warfarin on the composite of all cardiovascular events (interaction p=$0 \cdot 036$ and p=$0 \cdot 0006$, respectively) and total mortality (interaction p=$0 \cdot 066$ and p=$0 \cdot 052$, respectively) with reduced event rates at low cTTR, and similar rates at high cTTR.

Interpretation.—The benefits of 150 mg dabigatran at reducing stroke, 110 mg dabigatran at reducing bleeding, and both doses at reducing intracranial bleeding versus warfarin were consistent irrespective of centres' quality of INR control. For all vascular events, non-haemorrhagic events, and mortality, advantages of dabigatran were greater at sites with poor INR control than at those with good INR control. Overall, these results show that local standards of care affect the benefits of use of new treatment alternatives.

▶ Despite being the mainstay of anticoagulation for decades, warfarin remains a challenging drug to dose and to optimize efficacy. This substudy of the Randomized Evaluation of Long-term Anticoagulation Therapy trial examined the effects of optimal warfarin dosing (as measured by time in therapeutic range) on benefits and complications associated with using dabigatran versus warfarin. In this trial, the center's mean time in therapeutic range (cTTR) did not impact total strokes with dabigatran versus warfarin; therefore, dabigatran at 150 mg twice daily remains superior (while 110 mg is noninferior) to warfarin with regard to stroke reduction, regardless of the quality of a center's international normalized ratio (INR) control. As expected, better INR control was associated with fewer hemorrhagic strokes, while lower cTTR quartiles had less bleeding overall (likely because of subtherapeutic levels). The bleeding risk with dabigatran at 110 mg was lower regardless of cTTR, while dabigatran at 150 mg was better at centers with poor INR control. The results of this trial are consistent with previous studies; that is, better INR control is associated with better outcomes. However, this can be very difficult to achieve outside of the clinical trial setting, and overall, using dabigatran is associated with better efficacy and safety. Additionally, the 110-mg dose of dabigatran may have some benefits over both Coumadin and dabigatran at 150 mg with regard to safety and may warrant its use if approved in certain patient populations.

F. A. Cuoco, Jr, MD, MBA

Effect of Home Testing of International Normalized Ratio on Clinical Events
Matchar DB, for the THINRS Executive Committee and Site Investigators (Duke Univ Med Ctr, Durham, NC; et al)
N Engl J Med 363:1608-1620, 2010

Background.—Warfarin anticoagulation reduces thromboembolic complications in patients with atrial fibrillation or mechanical heart valves, but effective management is complex, and the international normalized ratio (INR) is often outside the target range. As compared with venous plasma testing, point-of-care INR measuring devices allow greater testing frequency and patient involvement and may improve clinical outcomes.

Methods.—We randomly assigned 2922 patients who were taking warfarin because of mechanical heart valves or atrial fibrillation and who were competent in the use of point-of-care INR devices to either weekly self-testing at home or monthly high-quality testing in a clinic. The primary end point was the time to a first major event (stroke, major bleeding episode, or death).

Results.—The patients were followed for 2.0 to 4.75 years, for a total of 8730 patient-years of follow-up. The time to the first primary event was not significantly longer in the self-testing group than in the clinic-testing group (hazard ratio, 0.88; 95% confidence interval, 0.75 to 1.04; P = 0.14). The two groups had similar rates of clinical outcomes except that the self-testing group reported more minor bleeding episodes. Over the entire follow-up period, the self-testing group had a small but significant improvement in the percentage of time during which the INR was within the target range (absolute difference between groups, 3.8 percentage points; P<0.001). At 2 years of follow-up, the self-testing group also had a small but significant improvement in patient satisfaction with anticoagulation therapy (P = 0.002) and quality of life (P<0.001).

Conclusions.—As compared with monthly high-quality clinic testing, weekly self-testing did not delay the time to a first stroke, major bleeding episode, or death to the extent suggested by prior studies. These results do not support the superiority of self-testing over clinic testing in reducing the risk of stroke, major bleeding episode, and death among patients taking warfarin therapy. (Funded by the Department of Veterans Affairs Cooperative Studies Program; ClinicalTrials.gov number, NCT00032591.)

▶ Anticoagulation with warfarin has been the clinical standard for decades to prevent stroke and other thromboembolic events among patients with mechanical valves and high-risk patients with atrial fibrillation. However, warfarin is one of the more difficult drugs to manage, requiring frequent monitoring of prothrombin time. One potential strategy to simplify regulation of warfarin dosing is to develop point of care management with home international normalized ratio testing. In this prospective randomized study of 2922 patients, this approach was evaluated. Compared with the control group strategy of regular clinic-based monitoring, home monitoring did not reduce embolic events or the primary composite end point of stroke, major bleed, or death (Fig 2 in the original article). The time in the therapeutic range was slightly greater in the home monitoring group, but this was not clinically meaningful. These results reinforce the challenges of warfarin use and the enthusiasm for alternative anticoagulants, such as dabigitran, to simplify patient care and improve outcomes.

M. R. Gold, MD, PhD

Atrial fibrillation termination as a procedural endpoint during ablation in long-standing persistent atrial fibrillation

Elayi CS, Di Biase L, Barrett C, et al (Univ of Lexington, KY; Texas Cardiac Arrhythmia Inst at St David's Med Ctr, Austin; Massachusetts General Hosp and Harvard Med School, Boston; et al)
Heart Rhythm 7:1216-1223, 2010

Background.—Ablation of long-standing persistent atrial fibrillation (AF) remains challenging, with a lower success rate than paroxysmal AF. A reliable ablation endpoint has not been demonstrated yet, although AF termination during ablation may be associated with higher long-term maintenance of sinus rhythm (SR).

Objective.—The purpose of this study was to determine whether the method of AF termination during ablation predicts mode of recurrence or long-term outcome.

Methods.—Three hundred six patients with long-standing persistent AF, free of antiarrhythmic drugs (AADs), undergoing a first radiofrequency ablation (pulmonary vein [PV] antrum isolation and complex fractionated atrial electrograms) were prospectively included. Organized atrial tachyarrhythmias (AT) that occurred during AF ablation were targeted. AF termination mode during ablation was studied in relation to other variables (characteristics of arrhythmia recurrence, redo procedures, the use of adenosine/isoproterenol for redo, and comparison of focal versus macroreentrant ATs). Long-term maintenance of SR was assessed during the follow-up.

Results.—During AF ablation, six of 306 patients converted directly to SR, 172 patients organized into AT (with 38 of them converting in SR with further ablation), and 128 did not organize or terminate and were cardioverted. Two hundred eleven of 306 patients (69%) maintained in long-term SR without AADs after a mean follow-up of 25 ± 6.9 months, with no statistical difference between the various AF termination modes during ablation. Presence or absence of organization during ablation clearly predicted the predominant mode of recurrence, respectively, AT or AF ($P = .022$). Among the 74 redo ablation patients, 24 patients

(32%) had extra PV triggers revealed by adenosine/isoproterenol. Termination of focal ATs was correlated with higher long-term success rate (24/29, 83%) than termination of macroreentrant ATs (20/35, 57%; $P = .026$).

Conclusion.—AF termination during ablation (conversion to AT or SR) could predict the mode of arrhythmia recurrence (AT vs. AF) but did not impact the long-term SR maintenance after one or two procedures. AT termination with further ablation did not correlate with better long-term outcome, except with focal ATs, for which termination seems critical (Fig 1).

▶ Initial results from mostly small nonprospective studies suggested that atrial fibrillation (AF) termination may be an end point associated with favorable long-term outcomes in ablation of long-standing persistent AF. Additionally, 1 prospective study[1] also showed that after multiple stepwise ablation procedures, termination of AF, and/or organization to atrial tachyarrhythmias (AT) may be associated with lower recurrence rates. This study from Elayi et al was a larger prospective trial that showed AF termination was not associated with better long-term outcomes. As shown in Fig 1, recurrence rates were

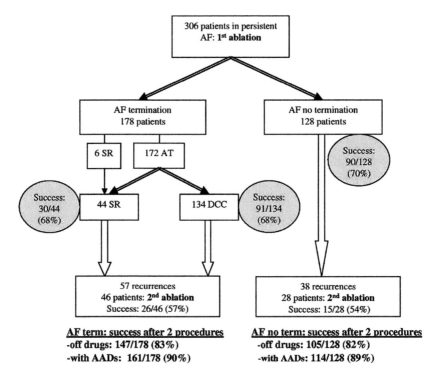

FIGURE 1.—Study design and results (AF termination mode and success rate after the first with ADDs and second procedure with and without AADs). (Reprinted from Elayi CS, Di Biase L, Barrett C, et al. Atrial fibrillation termination as a procedural endpoint during ablation in long-standing persistent atrial fibrillation. *Heart Rhythm*. 2010;7:1216-1223, with permission from Heart Rhythm Society.)

similar after ablation procedures regardless of AF organization and/or termination. Organization to atrial tachycardia did predict the mode of recurrence (ie, if AF organized to AT, AT would more likely be the recurrent arrhythmia). Of note, only a small minority of patients (14%) were actually converted to sinus rhythm during their initial ablation procedure. Over half of the patients were organized to AT with ablation, but a large percentage were macroreentrant or of undetermined mechanism, and these were difficult to terminate with ablation. The investigators in this study did not use empiric linear ablation sets as part of their strategy, and this may explain the difference between their results and those of previous studies. Nevertheless, this study reinforces the difficulties in identifying markers of successful ablation of AF.

F. A. Cuoco, Jr, MD, MBA

Reference

1. O'Neill MD, Wright M, Knecht S, et al. Long-term follow-up of persistent atrial fibrillation ablation using termination as a procedural endpoint. *Eur Heart J.* 2009;30:1105-1112.

Ablation of long-standing persistent atrial fibrillation with multielectrode ablation catheter

Miyazaki S, Wright M, Haïssaguerre M, et al (Hôpital Cardiologique du Haut-Lévêque and Université Victor Segalen Bordeaux II, France)
Heart Rhythm 7:1303-1305, 2010

A combination of pulmonary vein (PV) isolation, electrogram-based ablation, and linear lesions has been demonstrated to result in medium-term freedom from atrial fibrillation (AF) in the majority of patients with persistent AF. However, ablation using an irrigated-tip ablation catheter in these patients is a challenging and long procedure due to the number of potential targets requiring ablation. Next-generation catheters using different energy sources and multielectrode configurations have been developed to potentially simplify ablation. PV isolation can be reliably achieved with a circular multielectrode ring catheter (pulmonary vein ablation catheter [PVAC], Ablation Frontiers, Inc., Carlsbad, CA, USA) using duty-cycled bipolar and unipolar radiofrequency energy (GENius, Ablation Frontiers), and a successful outcome using multiple catheters has been demonstrated for patients with persistent AF. Recently, a novel linear multielectrode catheter (tip-versatile ablation catheter [T-VAC], Ablation Frontiers) has been developed to create linear lesions. We present the case of a patient with long-standing persistent AF who underwent stepwise ablation for the first time using a novel multielectrode linear catheter, which led to termination of AF in a procedure of relatively short duration.

▶ A combination of techniques for ablation of persistent atrial fibrillation (AF) is commonly used, including pulmonary vein isolation, wide-area pulmonary vein isolation, linear left atrial ablation, electrogram-guided ablation, and a step-wise approach using varying combinations of these techniques. Most operators currently use a 3.5-mm tip ablation catheter, but the procedural time required to perform appropriate ablation lines with this catheter is often extensive. Miyazaki et al reported the case of a 71-year-old patient who underwent AF ablation using a circular multielectrode ring catheter (pulmonary vein ablation catheter [PVAC], Ablation Frontiers) combined with a novel linear multielectrode catheter (tip-versatile ablation catheter [T-VAC], Ablation Frontiers). Pulmonary vein isolation was performed using PVAC followed by T-VAC electrogram-guided ablation. AF cycle length slowing was observed after each of these ablations. AF was terminated after right atrial electrogram-guided ablation, and the patient had no complications and no known atrial arrhythmias after 6 months of follow-up. This single-patient case report suggests potential feasibility of using multielectrode ablation technology, but study involving multiple patients is needed. Potential benefits of multielectrode ablation technology could include decreased fluoroscopy, ablation, and procedural time. Procedural efficacy and safety will need to be evaluated when multiple patients are studied.

R. N. Vest III, MD

Efficacy of catheter ablation and surgical *CryoMaze* procedure in patients with long-lasting persistent atrial fibrillation and rheumatic heart disease: a randomized trial
Liu X, Tan H-W, Wang X-H, et al (Shanghai Chest Hosp Affiliated to Shanghai Jiaotong Univ, China)
Eur Heart J 31:2633-2641, 2010

Aims.—Catheter ablation and surgical Maze procedure are effective in treating atrial fibrillation (AF) patients. However, there is no study that compares the effect of circumferential pulmonary vein isolation (CPVI) combined with substrate ablation after valvular surgery and the concomitant Maze procedure for the treatment of AF in patients with rheumatic heart disease (RHD). The aim of this study was to compare the effectiveness of CPVI combined with substrate modification and surgical Maze procedure using Saline-Irrigated Cooled-tip Radiofrequency Ablation (SICTRA) system for the treatment of long-lasting persistent AF in patients with RHD.

Methods and Results.—Between January 2006 and June 2008, 99 patients with long-lasting persistent AF and RHD were randomly assigned to undergo valvular operation and CPVI combined with substrate modification 6 months after the surgery (Group A, 49 patients) or valvular operation and concomitant Maze procedure (Group B, 50 patients). The mean follow-up periods were 15 ± 5 and 20 ± 8 months in Groups A and B, respectively. After one procedure, Group B had a significantly higher freedom from atrial arrhythmias compared with Group A (82% in Group B vs. 55.2% in Group A, $P < 0.001$). Fifteen patients in Group A underwent a redo procedure. Six patients in Group B underwent catheter

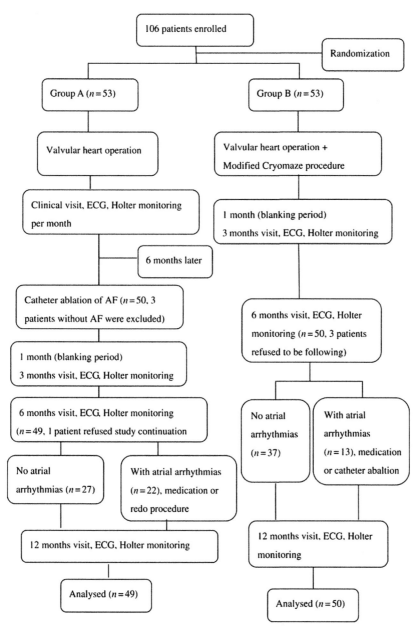

FIGURE 1.—Flowchart of the study protocol. (Reprinted from Liu X, Tan H-W, Wang X-H, et al. Efficacy of catheter ablation and surgical *CryoMaze* procedure in patients with long-lasting persistent atrial fibrillation and rheumatic heart disease: a randomized trial. *Eur Heart J* 2010;31:2633-2641, with permission of The European Society of Cardiology.)

ablation and four were treated successfully. The cumulative rates of sinus rhythm were 71% in Group A and 88% in Group B (*P* < 0.001).

Conclusion.—The concomitant Cox Maze procedure using SICTRA is more effective than subsequent CPVI combined with substrate modification in treating patients with long-lasting persistent AF and RHD (Fig 1).

▶ Catheter-based ablation and the surgical Maze procedure have both been used successfully to treat atrial fibrillation. Patients with rheumatic heart disease and coexisting atrial fibrillation suffer from reduced response rates with either of these procedures. Liu et al sought to compare 2 different strategies of atrial fibrillation ablation: (1) mitral valve replacement/repair followed by circumferential pulmonary vein isolation and substrate modification 6 months after valve surgery (group A) and (2) mitral valve replacement/repair with concomitant Cox Maze III procedure using a CryoMaze ablation energy source (group B). Ninety-nine patients were enrolled: 49 in group A and 50 in group B. Average follow-up was 15 ± 5 months for group A and 20 ± 8 months for group B. The groups were well matched with respect to age, sex, left atrial size, and duration of atrial fibrillation. After 1 procedure, group B had higher freedom from atrial arrhythmias compared with group A (82% in group B vs. 55.2% in group A). Fifteen patients in group A underwent repeat procedures as compared with 6 patients in group B who underwent catheter ablation upon postoperative recurrence of atrial fibrillation. At the conclusion of follow-up, cumulative rates of sinus rhythm were 71% in group A as compared with 88% in group B. This study shows that surgical Maze concomitant with mitral valve replacement/repair is superior to catheter-based ablation for patients with atrial fibrillation and rheumatic heart disease. Limitations of the study include small cohort size and routine amiodarone use in group B for 3 months during the postoperative period.

J. L. Sturdivant, MD

Prevention of Atrial Fibrillation Recurrence With Corticosteroids After Radiofrequency Catheter Ablation: A Randomized Controlled Trial
Koyama T, Tada H, Sekiguchi Y, et al (Univ of Tsukuba, Japan)
J Am Coll Cardiol 56:1463-1472, 2010

Objectives.—We sought to clarify the efficacy of corticosteroid therapy for preventing atrial fibrillation (AF) recurrence after pulmonary vein isolation (PVI).

Background.—The inflammatory process may cause acute AF recurrence after PVI. However, no studies have examined the relationship between corticosteroid administration and AF recurrence after PVI.

Methods.—A total of 125 patients with paroxysmal AF were randomized to receive either corticosteroids (corticosteroid group) or a placebo (placebo group). In the corticosteroid group, intravenous hydrocortisone (2 mg/kg) was given the day of the procedure, and oral prednisolone

(0.5 mg/kg/day) was administered for 3 days after the PVI. The body temperature and high-sensitivity C-reactive protein level were measured before and on each of the first 3 days after ablation.

Results.—The prevalence of immediate AF recurrence (≤3 days after the PVI) was significantly lower in the corticosteroid group (7%) than in the placebo group (31%). The maximum body temperature and C-reactive protein during the initial 3 days after ablation and the increase in the body temperature and C-reactive protein level from baseline were significantly lower in the corticosteroid group than in the placebo group. Corticosteroid treatment did not decrease AF recurrences between 4 and 30 days after ablation. The AF-free rate at 14 months post-ablation was greater in the corticosteroid group (85%) than in the placebo group (71%, p = 0.032 by the log-rank test).

Conclusions.—Transient use of small amounts of corticosteroids shortly after AF ablation may be effective and safe for preventing not only immediate AF recurrences but also AF recurrences during the mid-term follow-up period after PVI (Fig 1).

▶ Atrial fibrillation (AF) ablation with pulmonary vein isolation and often linear lesions is a rapidly growing procedure for the treatment of symptomatic AF. Recurrence rates remain high with this procedure, particularly in the early

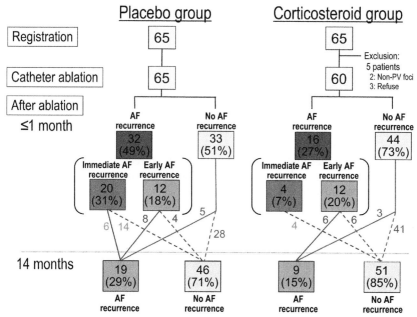

FIGURE 1.—Flow Diagram and Results of the Present Study. AF = atrial fibrillation; PV = pulmonary vein. (Reprinted from the Journal of the American College of Cardiology, Koyama T, Tada H, Sekiguchi Y, et al. Prevention of atrial fibrillation recurrence with corticosteroids after radiofrequency catheter ablation: a randomized controlled trial. *J Am Coll Cardiol.* 2010;56:1463-1472. Copyright 2010, with permission from the American College of Cardiology Foundation.)

postablation period. Clinically, recurrent arrhythmias in the first several months are not considered an ablation failure, and repeat procedures are performed only after more prolonged periods of arrhythmia recurrence. To test the hypothesis that inflammation is a cause of early recurrence of AF and possible overall success, this study was a randomized trial of corticosteroids during and immediately following AF ablation. The authors demonstrate that early recurrence was markedly reduced with corticosteroid administration, and the lack of early recurrence was associated with a smaller but still significant reduction in long-term AF (Fig 1). These provocative results suggest that postprocedural inflammation may be an important cause of early recurrence, and it may inhibit remodeling associated with long-term success. The small size of this study (n = 125) precludes advocating steroids routinely in all patients undergoing AF ablation; however, these provocative results warrant confirmation and further evaluation of other anti-inflammatory agents to improve success rates with this procedure.

M. R. Gold, MD, PhD

The CHADS Score Role in Managing Anticoagulation After Surgical Ablation for Atrial Fibrillation

Ad N, Henry L, Schlauch K, et al (Inova Heart and Vascular Inst, Falls Church, VA)
Ann Thorac Surg 90:1257-1262, 2010

Background.—Managing anticoagulation after surgical ablation is challenging, especially when sinus rhythm has been restored and the left atrial appendage has been surgically managed. The study purpose was to examine the applicability of the $CHADS_2$ in determining anticoagulation strategies after surgical ablation. $CHADS_2$ is a scoring system (0 to 6) used to indicate a patient's risk for a thromboembolic stroke and used for anticoagulation strategies. One point is given for any of the following conditions: C, congestive heart failure; H, hypertension; A, age 75 years old or greater; D, diabetes mellitus; and S, stroke which receives 2 points. A score of 2 or greater is an indication for a patient to be placed on warfarin unless otherwise contraindicated.

Methods.—A prospective, longitudinally designed study where $CHADS_2$ was calculated for all patients (n = 385). Clinical data on rhythm, anticoagulation medication, bleeding, and embolic stroke-transient ischemic attack (TIA) was obtained every 3 months. Logistic regression models were used to determine significant predictors of either event.

Results.—Of the 385 patients, 17% presented with a history of stroke-TIA. In a mean follow-up of 32.77 ± 16.33 months, embolic stroke-TIA events occurred in 4 patients (4.2 first events per 1,000 patient years) and bleeding events occurred in 69 patients (72.8 first events per 1,000 patient years). There was no significant difference in mean $CHADS_2$ between the stroke event and nonevent group (0.75 vs 1.46, respectively; $p = 0.21$), but there was a significant difference in $CHADS_2$ between the major bleed event group and the nonevent group (2.31 vs 1.41, respectively; $p < 0.003$). The logistic regression model was not predictive of stroke-TIA, but was significantly predictive of bleeding events ($\chi^2 = 10.30$, $p < 0.02$).

Conclusions.—The number of thromboembolic events after surgical ablation procedure is low and appears unrelated to the CHADS$_2$. This, together with the higher rate of bleeding, raises questions regarding the applicability of the CHADS$_2$ for patients after surgical ablation. A randomized study is required to define the risks and anticoagulation strategies for patients after surgical ablation.

▶ The congestive heart failure, hypertension, age > 75 years, diabetes, and previous stroke/transient ischemic attack (CHADS$_2$) scoring system is used to guide long-term anticoagulation strategies following catheter and surgical ablation for atrial fibrillation. A recent consensus statement suggests that warfarin be continued in patients who have a score ≥2 despite documentation of the absence of atrial fibrillation and/or flutter by continuous monitoring over a period of 2 years postablation, irrespective of the manner in which ablation is accomplished. Because surgical ablation typically involves surgical management of the left atrial appendage, Ad and colleagues sought to determine the usefulness of the CHADS$_2$ scoring system in patients who underwent surgical ablation in a prospective longitudinal fashion. A total of 385 patients were included in their investigation with a median CHADS$_2$ score of 1 (range, 0-5). All patients were discharged on warfarin for a period of 3 months unless otherwise contraindicated. Notable findings during a mean follow-up of 32.77 ± 16.33 months included (1) 7 thromboembolic events among 4 patients and (2) 120 bleeding events among 69 patients (22 major events and 98 minor events). Importantly, these investigators determined that for those patients undergoing surgical ablation with surgical management of the left atrial appendage, the CHADS$_2$ score did not reliably predict the occurrence of thromboembolic events postablation, irrespective of rhythm status. Moreover, they determined that the CHADS$_2$ score and administration of warfarin were the variables most associated with bleeding postablation and that patient age was the most significant predictor among the CHADS$_2$ variables. The authors appropriately acknowledged the fact that additional studies need to be performed to determine which patients would benefit most from anticoagulation postsurgical ablation. However, based upon their data, it seems reasonable to call into question the most recent consensus statement that advocates warfarin administration for those patients with a CHADS$_2$ score ≥2, at least within surgical populations. Perhaps anticoagulation should be used less frequently in those patients in whom the left atrial appendage is uniformly and completely excised and apposition of smooth endocardial surfaces is reliably achieved, particularly in the elderly.

W. M. Yarbrough, MD

Radiofrequency Catheter Ablation of Atrial Fibrillation: A Cause of Silent Thromboembolism?: Magnetic Resonance Imaging Assessment of Cerebral Thromboembolism in Patients Undergoing Ablation of Atrial Fibrillation

Gaita F, Caponi D, Pianelli M, et al (Univ of Turin, Asti, Italy; et al)
Circulation 122:1667-1673, 2010

Background.—Radiofrequency left atrial catheter ablation has become a routine procedure for treatment of atrial fibrillation. The aim of this study was to assess with preprocedural and postprocedural cerebral magnetic resonance imaging the thromboembolic risk, either silent or clinically manifest, in the context of atrial fibrillation ablation. The secondary end point was the identification of clinical or procedural parameters that correlate with cerebral embolism.

Methods and Results.—A total of 232 consecutive patients with paroxysmal or persistent atrial fibrillation who were candidates for radiofrequency left atrial catheter ablation were included in the study. Pulmonary vein isolation or pulmonary vein isolation plus linear lesions plus atrial defragmentation with the use of irrigated-tip ablation catheters was performed. All of the patients underwent preprocedural and postablation cerebral magnetic resonance imaging. A periprocedural symptomatic cerebrovascular accident occurred in 1 patient (0.4%). Postprocedural cerebral magnetic resonance imaging was positive for new embolic lesions in 33 patients (14%). No clinical parameters such as age, hypertension, diabetes mellitus, previous history of stroke, type of atrial fibrillation, and preablation antithrombotic treatment showed significant correlation with ischemic cerebral embolism. Procedural parameters such as activated clotting time value and, in particular, electric or pharmacological cardioversion to sinus rhythm correlated with an increased incidence of cerebral embolism. Cardioversion was also associated with an increased risk of 2.75 (95% confidence interval, 1.29 to 5.89; $P=0.009$).

Conclusions.—Radiofrequency left atrial catheter ablation carries a low risk of symptomatic cerebral ischemia but is associated with a substantial risk of silent cerebral ischemia detected on magnetic resonance imaging. Independent risk factors for cerebral thromboembolism are the level of activated clotting time and, in particular, the electric or pharmacological cardioversion to sinus rhythm during the procedure (Table 2).

▶ Radiofrequency catheter ablation is increasingly used for treatment of drug-refractory atrial fibrillation (AF). The 2011 American College of Cardiology Foundation/American Heart Association/Heart Rhythm Society updated guidelines for management of AF support its efficacy, assigning a class I recommendation for management of paroxysmal AF. It is not without complications, and symptomatic thromboembolic events, including cerebrovascular events, have been reported to occur in 0% to 7% of patients undergoing AF ablation. A few small studies reported silent cerebral ischemia in up to 11% of patients prior to ablation, although they were relatively small studies without baseline imaging

TABLE 2.—Clinical and Procedural Parameters Considered for Univariate Analysis

	Patients With Periprocedural Silent Cerebral Ischemic Lesion	Patients Without Periprocedural Cerebral Ischemic Lesion	OR	95% CI, Lower Limit of OR	95% CI, Upper Limit of OR	P
No. of patients	33	198				
Mean age, y	60±8	58±10	1.02	0.98	1.06	0.285
Male gender	24 (73)	156 (79)	0.74	0.32	1.72	0.495
Hypertension	17 (52)	95 (48)	1.08	0.52	2.24	0.828
Diabetes mellitus	0	10 (5)	0.00	0	Low	0.991
Structural heart disease	6 (18)	24 (12)	1.55	0.58	4.13	0.378
Dyslipidemia	8 (24)	49 (25)	0.93	0.39	2.20	0.879
Previous stroke or transient ischemic attack	2 (6)	13 (7)	1.37	0.37	5.11	0.633
Type of AF						
Paroxysmal	20 (61)	117(59)	0.89	0.42	1.88	0.77
Persistent	13 (39)	81 (41)				
Antithrombotic drugs						
Warfarin	23 (70)	154 (78)	0.68	0.30	1.54	0.361
Aspirin	10 (30)	44 (21)				
CHADS score						
0	15	92	Base	Base	Base	Base
1	16	83	1.18	0.55	2.53	0.668
2	0	16	0.38	0.04	3.10	0.369
>2	2	7	2.04	0.37	11.08	0.407
Spontaneous echo contrast	3	5	3.86	0.87	16.99	0.074
Mean ACT value during the procedure, s	269±28	282±32	0.98	0.97	0.99	0.014
Type of procedure		95 (48)	0.75	0.33	1.73	0.511
PV isolation	13 (39)	73 (37)				
PV+linear lesion	12 (37)	30 (15)	1.42	0.53	3.79	0.473
PV+linear lesion+atrial fragmented potential	8 (24)					
Transseptal approach	27 (79)	169 (85)	0.58	0.24	1.40	0.226
Patent foramen ovale	6 (21)	29 (15)	1.5	0.60	3.79	0.379
Procedure time, min	196±96	180±80	1.00	0.99	1.00	0.336
Radiofrequency time, min	50±20	47±20	1.00	0.99	1.00	0.336
Electric or pharmacological cardioversion during ablation	15 (45)	46 (23)	2.75	1.29	5.89	0.009

Values in parentheses are percentages. OR indicates odds ratio.

or control groups. Accordingly, Gaita et al performed a prospective multicenter cohort study of pre- and postprocedural cerebral MRI in 232 patients with paroxysmal or persistent AF undergoing ablation and 65 control patients undergoing elective electric cardioversion. The mean age of enrolled patients was 58 ± 10 years, with congestive heart failure, hypertension, age > 75 years, diabetes, and previous stroke/transient ischemic attack scores of 0 in 46%, 1 in 43%, 2 in 7%, and > 2 in 3%. The authors reported a single symptomatic cerebrovascular accident (0.4%), but postprocedure MRI demonstrated new asymptomatic ischemic lesions in 33 patients (14%). No differences were found in baseline clinical features between those with and without new ischemic lesions. However, significant differences were found for intraprocedure mean activated clotting time (ACT) (269 ± 28 seconds vs 282 ± 32 seconds; odds ratio [OR], 0.98; $P = .014$) and electrical or chemical cardioversion to sinus rhythm (45% vs 23%; OR, 2.75; $P = .009$) in those with and without new ischemic lesions, respectively (Table 2). Both parameters were independently associated with silent ischemic lesions on multivariable analysis. In the 65 patients undergoing elective cardioversion without ablation, no new ischemic lesions were detected on postprocedural MRI. Limitations of the study include the use of a procedural ACT target of 250 to 300 seconds, as many centers target an ACT of > 300 seconds. Additionally, the lack of long-term radiographic and clinical follow-ups makes the significance of these ischemic lesions uncertain. However, these results do raise concerns about the long-term safety of this approach and should encourage vigilance in catheter and anticoagulant management during AF ablation. Further data on long-term neurologic outcomes in these patients and possible alternative anticoagulant or cardioversion strategies are needed.

W. W. Brabham, MD

Clinical Significance of Early Recurrences of Atrial Tachycardia After Atrial Fibrillation Ablation
Choi J-I, Pak H-N, Park JS, et al (Korea Univ Med Ctr, Seoul, Republic of Korea; Yonsei Univ Health System, Seoul, Republic of Korea; et al)
J Cardiovasc Electrophysiol 21:1331-1337, 2010

Background.—Atrial tachycardia (AT) commonly recurs within 3 months after radiofrequency catheter ablation for atrial fibrillation (AF). However, it remains unclear whether early recurrence of atrial tachycardia (ERAT) predicts late recurrence of AF or AT.

Methods.—Of 352 consecutive patients who underwent circumferential pulmonary vein isolation with or without linear ablation(s) for AF, 56 patients (15.9%) with ERAT were identified by retrospective analysis. ERAT was defined as early relapse of AT within a 3-month blanking period after ablation.

Results.—During 21.7 ± 12.5 months, the rate of late recurrence was higher in patients with ERAT (41.1%) compared with those without ERAT (11.8%, P < 0.001). In a multivariable model, positive inducibility of AF or AT immediately after ablation (65.2% vs 36.4%, P = 0.046; odd ratio, 3.9; 95% confidence interval, 1.0–14.6) and the number of patients who underwent cavotricuspid isthmus (CTI) ablation (73.9% vs 42.4%, P = 0.042; odds ratio, 4.5; 95% confidence interval, 1.1–19.5) were significantly related to late recurrence in the ERAT group. The duration of ablation (174.3 ± 62.3 vs 114.7 ± 39.5 minutes, P = 0.046) and the procedure time (329.3 ± 83.4 vs 279.2 ± 79.7 minutes, P = 0.027) were significantly longer in patients with late recurrence than in those without late recurrence following ERAT.

Conclusions.—The late recurrence rate is higher in the patients with ERAT compared with those without ERAT following AF ablation, and is more often noted in the patients who underwent CTI ablation and had a prolonged procedure time. Furthermore, inducibility of AF or AT immediately after ablation independently predicts late recurrence in patients with ERAT (Fig 1, Tables 1 and 3).

▶ Early recurrence of atrial fibrillation (AF) is a known clinical predictor of late recurrence of AF; however, the significance of early recurrence of atrial tachycardia (ERAT) is not clear. This article describes a retrospective single-center review of 352 consecutive patients who underwent their first AF ablation between January 2004 and April 2008. All patients underwent circumferential antral ablation, and additional linear lesions (ie, cavotricuspid isthmus [CTI], left mitral isthmus [LMI], left atrium roofline) were performed if sinus rhythm was not restored during pulmonary vein isolation, with appropriate bidirectional block where indicated. Follow-up was performed at 1 week; 1, 3, 6, 9, and 12 months; and every 6 months (21.7 ± 12.5 months) after with a combination of Holter monitors, event recorders, and electrocardiographs.

Fig 1 shows the recorded outcomes; notably, ERAT was found in 56 patients, while it was absent in the other 296. Twenty-three of the 56 patients (41.1%) with ERAT went on to have a late recurrence after a 3-month blanking period, while only 35 of the 296 patients (11.8%) without ERAT had a late recurrence after the 3-month blanking period, a significant difference ($P < .001$).

At baseline (Table 1), ERAT patients were more likely to have persistent AF preablation, roofline ablations, and LMI ablation as well as procedure time and fluoroscopic time compared with those without ERAT. Importantly, more of the CTI ablations, roofline ablations, and LMI ablations were performed in the patients with persistent AF compared with paroxysmal AF. Additionally, 74% of the patients with ERAT and late recurrence had a CTI ablation, while only 42% of those without late recurrence had similar lesions made. Univariate analysis (Table 3) found the number of previously ineffective antiarrhythmic drugs, ablation number and length of time, procedure time, inducibility of AF or atrial tachycardia, and CTI ablation were significant predictors of late recurrence in the patients with ERAT.

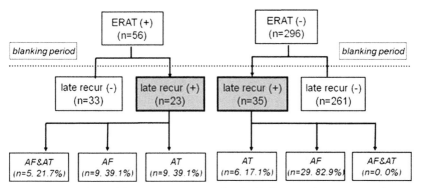

FIGURE 1.—Analysis of the recurrence patterns after the blanking periods in patients with ERAT. ERAT = early recurrence of atrial tachycardia; AF = atrial fibrillation; AT = atrial tachycardia. (Reprinted from Choi J-I, Pak H-N, Park JS, et al. Clinical significance of early recurrences of atrial tachycardia after atrial fibrillation ablation. *J Cardiovasc Electrophysiol.* 2010;21:1331-1337.)

TABLE 1.—Baseline Characteristics of Patients With and Without Early Recurrence of Atrial Tachycardia

	ERAT(+) (n = 56)	ERAT(−) (n = 296)	P-Value
Age (years)	57.2 ± 9.3	52.4 ± 11.0	0.002
Male	48 (85.7%)	237 (80.1%)	0.324
LVEF (%)	53.8 ± 7.3	54.9 ± 7.6	0.320
LA size (mm)	42.8 ± 5.5	40.5 ± 5.9	0.007
Persistent AF	31 (55.4%)	69 (23.3%)	<0.001
Prior AAD number	1.3 ± 0.7	1.1 ± 0.5	0.025
Structural heart disease	15 (26.8%)	36 (12.2%)	0.004
Hypertension	7 (12.5%)	36 (12.2%)	0.944
Procedure time (minutes)	299.8 ± 84.2	233.1 ± 75.1	<0.001
Fluoroscopic time (minutes)	83.5 ± 28.1	67.5 ± 30.5	<0.001
RF total duration (minutes)	129.1 ± 51.7	107.8 ± 53.9	0.500
CTI ablation	31 (55.4%)	171 (57.8%)	0.738
Roof line ablation	26 (46.4%)	69 (23.3%)	<0.001
LMI ablation	28 (50.9%)	81 (27.4%)	<0.001
Inducibility	27 (48.2%)	84 (28.4%)	0.003

Continuous variables are expressed as mean ± SD. ERAT = early recurrence of atrial tachycardia; LVEF = left ventricular ejection fraction; LA = left atrium; AF = atrial fibrillation; AAD = antiarrhythmic drug; RF = radiofrequency; CTI = cavotricuspid isthmus; LMI = left mitral isthmus.

TABLE 3.—Predictors of Late Recurrence Among Patients with ERAT in a Univariate Logistic Model

	Odds Ratio	95% CI	P-Value
Prior number of AADs	3.189	1.305−7.794	0.011
Ablation number	1.011	1.001−1.020	0.024
Ablation time (minutes)	1.025	1.004−1.047	0.019
Procedure time (minutes)	1.008	1.001−1.015	0.036
Inducibility (AT)	3.867	1.000−14.952	0.050
Inducibility (AF and AT)	3.281	1.078−9.989	0.036
CTI ablation	3.845	1.207−12.251	0.023

Continuous variables are expressed as mean ± SD. Abbreviations are same as in Table 1. CI = confidence interval.

This article demonstrates a statistically and possibly clinically significant increased risk of late recurrence of AF in patients with ERAT. Given the increased proportion of patients with persistent AF in the ERAT cohort, it is not clear if this was responsible for the higher recurrence rate or if this was because of the more extensive ablation performed in this group.

D. S. Sidney, MD

Characteristics of Complex Fractionated Electrograms in Nonpulmonary Vein Ectopy Initiating Atrial Fibrillation/Atrial Tachycardia

Lo L-W, Lin Y-J, Tsao H-M, et al (Taipei Veterans General Hosp, Taiwan; Natl Yang-Ming Univ, Taipei, Taiwan; et al)
J Cardiovasc Electrophysiol 20:1305-1312, 2009

Background.—Nonpulmonary vein (PV) ectopy initiating atrial fibrillation (AF)/atrial tachycardia (AT) is not uncommon in patients with AF. The relationship of complex fractionated atrial electrograms (CFAEs) and non-PV ectopy initiating AF/AT has not been assessed. We aimed to characterize the CFAEs in the non-PV ectopy initiating AF/AT.

Methods.—Twenty-three patients (age 53 ± 11 y/o, 19 males) who underwent a stepwise AF ablation with coexisting PV and non-PV ectopy initiating AF or AT were included. CFAE mapping was applied before and after the PV isolation in both atria by using a real-time NavX electroanatomic mapping system. A CFAE was defined as a fractionation interval (FI) of less than 120 ms over 8-second duration. A continuous CFAE (mostly, an FI < 50 ms) was defined as electrogram fractionation or repetitive rapid activity lasting for more than 8 seconds.

Results.—All patients (100%) with non-PV ectopy initiating AF or AT demonstrated corresponding continuous CFAEs at the firing foci. There was no significant difference in the FI among the PV ostial or non-PV atrial ectopy or other atrial CFAEs (54.1 ± 5.6, 58.3 ± 11.3, 52.8 ± 5.8 ms, $P = 0.12$). Ablation targeting those continuous CFAEs terminated the AF and AT and eliminated the non-PV ectopy in all patients (100%). During a follow-up of 7 months, 22% of the patients had an AF recurrence with PV reconnections. There was no recurrence of any ablated non-PV ectopy during the follow-up.

Conclusion.—The sites of the origin of the non-PV ectopies were at the same location as those of the atrial continuous CFAEs. Those non-PV foci were able to initiate and sustain AF/AT. By limited ablation targeting all atrial continuous CFAEs, the AF could be effectively eliminated (Fig 2).

▶ Mapping and ablation of nonpulmonary vein foci of atrial fibrillation (AF) initiation and regions of continuous fractionated atrial electrogram (CFAE) have both been shown potentially to improve the long-term results of AF ablation, particularly in persistent AF in which both of these phenomena occur more frequently. This study demonstrates that nonpulmonary vein foci usually arise in the same regions as nonpulmonary vein CFAE. If confirmed, this observation provides a much easier method for ablating potential nonpulmonary vein initiators. Mapping CFAE during AF is relatively quick and easy with 3-dimensional mapping systems, whereas mapping the first beat of AF initiation is technically difficult and time consuming. Thus, ablation of CFAE would provide a surrogate for nonpulmonary vein initiator ablation that would be quicker, easier, and potentially safer. These data also suggest that rapidly firing nonpulmonary vein foci contribute not only to AF initiation but also to AF maintenance. Why CFAE and nonpulmonary vein foci track to the same site is uncertain

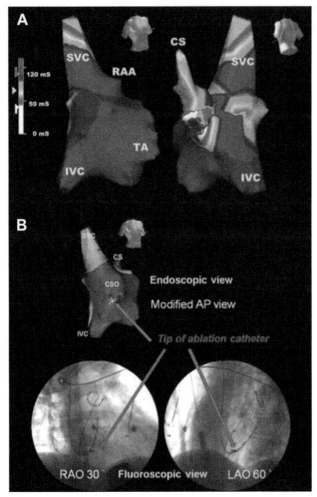

FIGURE 2.—Panel A, electroanatomic substrate mapping of the right atrium (the RAO and LAO of the right atrium). Panel B, endoscopic (upper) and fluoroscopic (lower) views showing the catheter location during radiofrequency ablation application. Panel A denotes CFAE mapping. The color annotation shows a range of colors with a fractionation interval of ≤50 ms shown in white, all the way through to an interval of >120 ms shown in purple. CS ostial ectopy initiating AF was found in this patient with the corresponding CFAE site around the coronary sinus ostium. Application of radiofrequency energy at this CFAE (brown spots in panel A and ablation catheter in panel B) terminated the AF. AP = anteroposterior; CS = coronary sinus; CSO = coronary sinus ostium; IVC = inferior vena cava; LAO = left anterior oblique; RAA = right atrial appendage; RAO = right anterior oblique; SVC = superior vena cava; TA = tricuspid annulus. For interpretation of the references to color in this figure legend, the reader is referred to web version of this article. (Reprinted from Lo L-W, Lin Y-J, Tsao H-M, et al. Characteristics of complex fractionated electrograms in nonpulmonary vein ectopy initiating atrial fibrillation/atrial tachycardia. *J Cardiovasc Electrophysiol*. 2009;20:1305-1312.)

but may reflect functional, anatomic, and autonomic milieu of the region. Regardless of the underlying cause, it provides a very clinically useful adjunctive ablation target to hopefully improve long-term results of AF ablation.

J. M. Wharton, MD

Atrial fibrillation following lung transplantation: double but not single lung transplant is associated with long-term freedom from paroxysmal atrial fibrillation

Lee G, Wu H, Kalman JM, et al (Univ of Melbourne, Australia; The Alfred Hosp, Melbourne, Australia)

Eur Heart J 31:2774-2782, 2010

Introduction.—The cornerstone of catheter ablation for atrial fibrillation (AF) is pulmonary vein electrical isolation (PVI). Recurrent AF post-PVI is a major limitation of the procedure with PV reconnection present in most patients. Single (SLT) and double (DLT) lung transplant surgery involves a 'cut and sew' PV antral isolation analogous to a catheter-based approach providing an opportunity to assess the efficacy of durable PVI.

Methods and Results.—A total of three hundred and twenty-seven consecutive lung transplant patients were compared with 201 control non-transplant thoracic surgery (THR) patients between 1998 and 2008. The primary analysis was the incidence of 'early' post-operative AF and 'late' AF (AF occurring following discharge from hospital after the index operation). Risk factors for the development of late AF were analysed using regression analysis. Acute post-operative AF was more common post-lung transplant (DLT 58/200 (29%) and SLT 36/127 (28%) vs. THR 28/201 (13.9%), $P < 0.001$) occurring at 4.7 ± 5.0 days in DLT, 3.4 ± 2.5 days after SLT, and 7.4 ± 11.2 days in the thoracic group ($P < 0.001$). At a mean follow-up of 5.4 ± 2.9 years late AF occurred in 1/200 (0.5%) in DLT vs. 16/127 (12.6%) in SLT and 23/201 (11.4%, $P < 0.001$) in THR groups. Kaplan—Meier survival analysis demonstrated the association of DLT with long-term freedom from AF. Significant variables [hazard ratio (HR) on univariate regression analysis of late AF were: DLT 0.06, age 1.09, LA diameter 1.2, hypertension 3.0, preoperative AF 12.2, early AF 8.8, rejection 3.2].

Conclusion.—Double but not SLT provides long-term freedom from AF despite a similar early post-operative incidence. This supports the critical role of the pulmonary veins in the pathogenesis of atrial fibrillation and the importance of durable electrical isolation of the pulmonary veins as the cornerstone in strategies for the long-term prevention of AF.

▶ Establishment of bilateral pulmonary vein electrical isolation, as is commonly attempted using percutaneous endocardial and/or minimally invasive epicardial techniques, remains a primary therapeutic goal in efforts to abolish atrial fibrillation (AF). However, whether and to what degree such abbreviated efforts provide long-term protection against recurrence of AF relative to the gold-standard albeit technically difficult Cox Maze surgical approach remains controversial. In their single-institution retrospective review, Lee and colleagues validated the concept that bilateral pulmonary vein isolation alone can be used to eliminate AF reliably. Specifically, these investigators compared the incidence of early and late AF in patients who underwent: (1) single lung transplantation (SLT) with unilateral vein isolation; (2) double lung transplantation

(DLT) with bilateral vein isolation; and (3) nontransplant unilateral thoracic surgery (thorSg) without vein isolation. Importantly, inclusion of patients who underwent DLT ensured beyond a shadow of a doubt that bilateral pulmonary vein electrical isolation was achieved analogous to the Cox Maze surgical procedure. Not surprisingly, the incidence of early AF was greater in the SLT (28%) and DLT (29%) groups relative to the thorSg group (14%, *P* < .05) and was presumably secondary to temporary left atrial irritation and manipulation from extensive hilar, left atrial, and pericardial dissection typically required for both SLT and DLT. Notably, the incidence of late AF was far less with DLT (0.5%) versus SLT and thorSg (12.4% and 11.4%, respectively, *P* < .05). While DLT tends to be a procedure carried out in younger more robust individuals who are perhaps less prone to developing AF than those who undergo SLT, it seems likely that bilateral pulmonary vein isolation confers added protection against AF occurrence. In fact, DLT was the only protective factor noted in the investigation. The findings reported in this study should not be used as evidence to promote DLT over SLT in patients with end-stage lung disease. Such decisions should continue to be made at the discretion of individual lung transplant centers based upon surgeon preference and institutional biases. However, these findings support the past findings of Haïssaguerra et al[1] and provide proof of the concept that the pulmonary veins are an initiation source for AF. Thus, these findings should be used to spearhead further efforts to achieve bilateral full-thickness and circumferential pulmonary vein electrical isolation via endocardial and/or epicardial techniques.

W. M. Yarbrough, MD

Reference

1. Haïssaguerre M, Jaïs P, Shah DC, et al. Spontaneous initiation of atrial fibrillation by ectopic beats originating in the pulmonary veins. *N Eng J Med.* 1998;339: 659-666.

Prophylactic ventral cardiac denervation: Does it reduce incidence of atrial fibrillation after coronary artery bypass grafting?
Omran AS, Karimi A, Ahmadi H, et al (Tehran Univ of Med Sciences, Iran)
J Thorac Cardiovasc Surg 140:1036-1039, 2010

Objective.—This study assessed the prophylactic effect of ventral cardiac denervation on reducing atrial fibrillation after coronary artery bypass grafting.

Methods.—This randomized prospective study recruited 220 adult patients (aged 42−79 years) who were scheduled to undergo coronary artery bypass grafting. Of these patients, 110 underwent ventral cardiac denervation in addition to coronary artery bypass grafting and 110 underwent only coronary artery bypass grafting. The demographic, intraoperative, and postoperative factors comprising atrial fibrillation were compared between the 2 groups. In addition, the predictive factors of atrial fibrillation in all 220 cases were assessed.

Results.—The mean age and the distribution of gender, body mass index, diabetes mellitus, chronic obstructive pulmonary disease, hypertension, hypercholesterolemia, and left main disease were not significantly different between the 2 groups. Atrial fibrillation incidence was significantly different between the groups ($P = .025$), with an incidence of 20.9% in the ventral cardiac denervation group and 10% in the control group. Atrial fibrillation occurred in 34 of the 220 patients, and ventral cardiac denervation was considered as a variable to evaluate its possible role in the prevention of postoperative atrial fibrillation. Our multivariate analysis showed age ($P = .002$; odds ratio, 1.098; confidence interval, 1.034–1.165) and ventral cardiac denervation ($P = .044$; odds ratio, 2.32; confidence interval, 1022–5.298) as the predictive factors of atrial fibrillation after coronary artery bypass grafting.

Conclusions.—Given the surprising results of the present study demonstrating that ventral cardiac denervation is a predictive factor of atrial fibrillation after coronary artery bypass grafting, ventral cardiac denervation should not be routinely considered for the prevention of atrial fibrillation after coronary artery bypass grafting (Table 2).

▶ Atrial fibrillation (AF) continues to plague both surgeons and patients following routine coronary artery bypass grafting (CABG) irrespective of whether these procedures are performed on- or off-pump. As pointed out by Omran and colleagues, the incidence of AF following CABG ranges widely among previously reported investigations and to date, no single pharmacologic or concomitant surgical intervention has proven superior in effectively

TABLE 2.—Univariate Analysis of Predictive Factors of Atrial Fibrillation After Coronary Artery Bypass Grafting*

Patient Characteristics	AF, n (%)	No AF, n (%)	P Value
Patient no.	34 (15.5%)	186 (84.5%)	
Age (y)	66.59 ± 6.69	62.14 ± 7.36	.001
Male	25 (79.4%)	150 (80.6%)	.868
Female	7 (20.6%)	36 (19.4%)	
COPD	1 (2.9%)	14 (7.5%)	.477
Diabetes mellitus	8 (23.5%)	55 (29.6%)	.474
Hypercholesterolemia	16 (47.1%)	94 (50.5%)	.709
Hypertension	21 (61.8%)	89 (47.8%)	.136
CCS grades III and IV	20 (60.6%)	79 (42.5%)	.054
K$^+$ (potassium)	4.49 ± 0.42	4.38 ± 0.40	.187
Left main disease	2 (6.5%)	14 (8%)	1
BMI	27.14 ± 4.66	26.66 ± 4.63	.588
CPB time (min)	66.32 ± 16.31	63.30 ± 14.94	.286
Crossclamp time (min)	38.26 ± 9.23	37.58 ± 14.33	.787
No. of grafts	3.67 ± 1	3.54 ± 0.79	.411
LITA graft as arterial conduit	34 (100%)	185 (99.5%)	1
SVG	2.67 ± 1	2.52 ± 0.79	.338
VCD	23 (67.6%)	87 (46.8%)	.025

AF, Atrial fibrillation; *COPD*, chronic obstructive pulmonary disease; *CCS*, Canadian Cardiovascular Society; *BMI*, body mass index; *CPB*, cardiopulmonary bypass; *LITA*, left internal thoracic artery; *SVG*, saphenous vein graft; *VCD*, ventral cardiac denervation.

*Data are presented as n (%) for categoric variables and mean ± standard deviation for numeric variables.

preventing AF. What is clear is that the occurrence of AF in the postoperative period can lead to lengthened postoperative hospital courses and a requirement for temporary anticoagulation in some instances. Surgical interventions short of creating prophylactic radiofrequency or cryoablation lesions include incising the posterior pericardium[1] and ventral cardiac denervation (VCD) as described by Omran et al as well as others.[2] Proponents for the former technique cite a decreased incidence of pericardial effusion as an inciting factor for the onset of AF, while proponents for the latter argue that VCD attenuates the effect of autonomic tone on the heart, thereby reducing the incidence of AF. In this randomized prospective study, a total of 220 patients undergoing routine on-pump CABG were subjected to CABG alone or CABG plus VCD by a single surgeon. VCD was carried out in a uniform fashion as described previously[2] and included removal of fat pads from around the great vessels at the base of the heart. Importantly, the authors observed no difference between groups with respect to the incidence for postoperative bleeding or requirement for reexploration, thereby demonstrating VCD to be a relatively safe intervention with respect to these parameters. However, they did observe a significant difference with respect to the incidence of postoperative AF. Specifically, and to the surprise of the authors, VCD was associated with a higher incidence of postoperative AF (20.9% vs 10%, $P = .025$). Only age and VCD predicted AF (Table 2). They suggested that their results may have differed from a past study[2] favoring VCD secondary to their rigorous monitoring of electrocardiographic events. In addition, they hypothesized that VCD may have damaged the blood supply to the sinoatrial node and that VCD may have altered the balance of the autonomic nervous system favoring preservation of sympathetic fibers relative to parasympathetic fibers. Irrespective of the cause, the authors concluded that routine VCD at the time of CABG could not be supported, and they appropriately acknowledged the fact that such an intervention could lead to excessive scarring around the base of the heart, maneuvers that inevitably render reoperative surgery more difficult for the operating surgeon.

W. M. Yarbrough, MD

References

1. Farsak B, Günaydin S, Tokmakoğlu H, Kandemir O, Yorgancioğlu C, Zorlutuna Y. Posterior pericardiotomy reduces the incidence of supra-ventricular arrhythmias and pericardial effusion after coronary artery bypass grafting. *Eur J Cardiothorac Surg.* 2002;22:278-281.
2. Melo J, Voigt P, Sonmez B, et al. Ventral cardiac denervation reduces the incidence of atrial fibrillation after coronary artery bypass grafting. *J Thorac Cardiovasc Surg.* 2004;127:511-516.

Gender Differences in the Clinical Characteristics and Atrioventricular Nodal Conduction Properties in Patients with Atrioventricular Nodal Reentrant Tachycardia

Suenari K, Hu Y-F, Tsao H-M, et al (Taipei Veterans General Hosp, Taiwan)
J Cardiovasc Electrophysiol 21:1114-1119, 2010

Introduction.—The detailed electrophysiological characteristics of the gender differences associated with atrioventricular nodal reentrant tachycardia (AVNRT) have not been clarified. This study investigated the gender-related electrophysiological differences in a large series of patients undergoing radiofrequency catheter ablation.

Methods and Results.—A total of 2,088 consecutive AVNRT patients (men/women 869/1,219) who underwent catheter ablation were enrolled in this study. We evaluated the gender differences in their electrophysiological characteristics. Women had a significantly younger age of onset, higher incidence of multiple jumps, shorter AH interval, atrial effective refractory period (ERP), anterograde fast pathway ERP, anterograde slow pathway ERP, and retrograde slow pathway ERP, and longer ventricular ERP than men. The incidence of baseline ventriculoatrial dissociation was lower in women than in men. Women needed less isoproterenol/atropine to induce AVNRT. No gender differences in the radiation exposure time, procedure time, complication rate, acute success rate, or second procedure rate were noted. Both typical and atypical AVNRT were more predominant in women. In the patients with atypical AVNRT, there was no significant gender difference in incidence of baseline ventriculoatrial dissociation; however, the retrograde slow pathway ERP was significantly shorter in women than in men. Women of premenopausal age (≤50 years old) had a significantly higher incidence of anterograde multiple jumps and a retrograde jump phenomenon, and a shorter anterograde slow pathway ERP and retrograde slow pathway ERP than those of women over 50 years old.

Conclusion.—Gender differences in the anterograde and retrograde AV nodal electrophysiology were noted in the patients with AVNRT.

▶ Cardiac arrhythmia gender differences are well described in this article, including higher prevalence of atrial tachycardias in women but higher prevalence of atrial fibrillation and Wolff-Parkinson-White syndrome in men. Atrioventricular nodal reentrant tachycardia (AVNRT) is much more common in women, and shorter slow pathway refractory periods, tachycardia cycle lengths, and atrioventricular block cycle lengths have been observed. Differences in AVNRT procedural success and complication rates have not been reported. This study by Suenari et al evaluated multiple aspects of gender differences in AVNRT ablation in a large series of patients. The patient population included 869 men and 1219 women who underwent AVNRT ablation. Women had a younger age at presentation compared with men, but no differences were observed with procedural success, radiation exposure, procedure time, or major complications. Compared with men, anterograde fast and slow pathway refractory periods were shorter as were retrograde slow pathway refractory periods in women. Comparisons of women older than 50 years with those younger than 50 years were performed to assess the effect of menopause. Women younger than 50 years had shorter refractory periods, while older women more frequently required use of isoproterenol for arrhythmia induction. In summary, this study evaluated a large cohort of patients undergoing AVNRT ablation and confirmed previously observed AVNRT gender differences. Further study is needed to assess the suggested role of gonadal hormones on multiple known arrhythmia differences between women and men.

R. N. Vest III, MD

Complication Rates Associated With Pacemaker or Implantable Cardioverter-Defibrillator Generator Replacements and Upgrade Procedures: Results From the REPLACE Registry
Poole JE, for the REPLACE Registry Investigators (Univ of Washington, Seattle; et al)
Circulation 122:1553-1561, 2010

Background.—Prospective studies defining the risk associated with pacemaker or implantable cardioverter-defibrillator replacement surgeries do not exist. These procedures are generally considered low risk despite results from recent retrospective series reporting higher rates.

Methods and Results.—We prospectively assessed predefined procedure-related complication rates associated with elective pacemaker or implantable cardioverter-defibrillator generator replacements over 6 months of follow-up. Two groups were studied: those without (cohort 1) and those with (cohort 2) a planned transvenous lead addition for replacement or upgrade to a device capable of additional therapies. Complications were adjudicated by an independent events committee. Seventy-two US academic and private practice centers participated. Major complications occurred in 4.0% (95% confidence interval, 2.9 to 5.4) of 1031 cohort 1 patients and 15.3% (95% confidence interval, 12.7 to 18.1) of 713 cohort 2 patients. In both cohorts, major complications were higher with implantable cardioverter-defibrillator compared with pacemaker generator replacements. Complications were highest in patients who had an upgrade to or a revised cardiac resynchronization therapy device (18.7%; 95% confidence interval, 15.1 to 22.6). No periprocedural deaths occurred in either cohort, although 8 later procedure-related deaths occurred in cohort 2. The 6-month infection rates were 1.4% (95% confidence interval, 0.7 to 2.3) and 1.1% (95% confidence interval, 0.5 to 2.2) for cohorts 1 and 2, respectively.

Conclusions.—Pacemaker and implantable cardioverter-defibrillator generator replacements are associated with a notable complication risk, particularly those with lead additions. These data support careful decision making before device replacement, when managing device advisories, and when considering upgrades to more complex systems.

▶ Pacemaker and implantable cardioverter-defibrillator (ICD) pulse generator replacement is typically considered a simple procedure. Anecdotal and retro- spective studies suggest a higher infection rate compared with new implants, but little is known of other complications. The Implantable Cardiac Pulse Generator Replacement Registry (REPLACE) was the first large prospective study of pulse generator replacements with or without lead replacements or upgrades. A major complication rate of 18.7% was noted, which was highest among those subjects receiving ICDs or cardiac resynchronization therapy upgrades. The longer follow-up (6 months) of this study illustrates the limita- tion of most device registries that assess in-hospital or 30-day events. REPLACE teaches us once again not to be cavalier about decisions regarding device implantation in populations with a high incidence of comorbidities.

M. R. Gold, MD, PhD

Atrioventricular nodal ablation predicts survival benefit in patients with atrial fibrillation receiving cardiac resynchronization therapy
Dong K, Shen W-K, Powell BD, et al (Zhejiang Univ School of Medicine, Hangzhou, China; Mayo Clinic, Rochester, MN; et al)
Heart Rhythm 7:1240-1245, 2010

Background.—Cardiac resynchronization therapy (CRT) benefits patients with advanced heart failure. The role of atrioventricular nodal (AVN) ablation in improving CRT outcomes, including survival benefit in CRT recipients with atrial fibrillation, is uncertain.

Objective.—The purpose of this study was to assess the impact of AVN ablation on clinical and survival outcomes in a large atrial fibrillation and heart failure population that met the current indication for CRT and to determine whether AVN ablation is an independent predictor of survival in CRT recipients.

Methods.—Of 154 patients with atrial fibrillation who received CRT-D, 45 (29%) underwent AVN ablation (+AVN-ABL group), whereas 109 (71%) received drug therapy for rate control during CRT (−AVN-ABL group). New York Heart Association (NYHA) class, electrocardiogram, and echocardiogram were assessed before and after CRT. Survival data were obtained from the national death and location database (Accurint).

Results.—CRT comparably improved left ventricular ejection fraction (8.1% ± 10.7% vs 6.8% ± 9.6%, $P = .49$) and left ventricular end- diastolic diameter (−2.1 ± 5.9 mm vs −2.1 ± 6.7 mm, $P = .74$) in both +AVN-ABL and −AVN-ABL groups. Improvement in NYHA class was significantly greater in the +AVN-ABL group than in −AVN-ABL group (−0.7 ± 0.8 vs −0.4 ± 0.8, $P = .04$). Survival estimates at 2 years were 96.0% (95% confidence interval [CI] 88.6%−100%) for +AVN-ABL group and 76.5% (95% CI 68.1%−85.8%) for−AVN-ABL group (*P* = .008). AVN ablation was independently associated with survival benefit from death (hazard ratio [HR] 0.13, 95% CI 0.03−0.58, *P* = .007) and from combined death, heart transplant, and left ventricular assist device (HR 0.19, 95% CI 0.06−0.62, *P* = .006) after CRT.

Conclusion.—Among patients with atrial fibrillation and heart failure receiving CRT, AVN ablation for definitive biventricular pacing provides greater improvement in NYHA class and survival benefit. Larger-scale randomized trials are needed to assess the clinical and survival outcomes of this therapy.

▶ Cardiac resynchronization therapy (CRT) has proven benefits in patients with reduced ejection fraction, interventricular conduction delay, and significant heart failure symptoms. Approximately one-third of patients with low ejection fraction also have atrial fibrillation. The benefit of CRT in indicated patients with atrial fibrillation has been largely unexplored. This study by Cha et al sought to define the benefit of CRT-defibrillator (CRT-D) therapy in patients with a high burden of atrial fibrillation who subsequently underwent atrioventricular node ablation (AVN-ABL). Of 154 patients with atrial fibrillation and standard indications for CRT therapy who also underwent implantation or upgrade to a CRT-D device, 45 patients (29%) also underwent AVN-ABL. About 71% of patients received medical therapy for ventricular rate control. Typical device settings were employed using a ventricular demand rate responsive mode, with a lower rate limit of 60 beats per minute and an upper rate limit of 120 to 130 beats per minute. Compared with the −AVN-ABL group, patients in the +AVN-ABL group were younger, had lower New York Heart Association (NYHA) class, had higher ejection fraction, and were not being treated with β-blockers. On average, all patients who underwent CRT-D implantation realized an improvement in left ventricular ejection fraction and left ventricular end-diastolic volume. Patients who also underwent AVN-ABL experienced greater improvement in NYHA class (−0.7 ± 0.8 for the +AVN-ABL group vs 0.4 ± 0.8 for the −AVN-ABL group, *P* = .04) and a significant survival benefit. Overall, biventricular pacing was seen in 99.0% in the +AVN-ABL group and 96% in the −AVN-ABL group (*P* = .05). Survival estimates at 2 years were 96.0% in the +AVN-ABL group as opposed to 76.5% in the −AVN-ABL group (*P* = .008). Severity of mitral regurgitation and AVN-ABL was the only univariate predictor of survival. This study suggests that AVN-ABL in patients with atrial fibrillation improves all-cause mortality and NYHA class. Limitations of the study include small study size, poorly matched study groups, potential variability in device programming, and poor heart rate control in the −AVN-ABL group. However, it suggests that a low threshold for AVN-ABL should be adopted in this cohort.

J. L. Sturdivant, MD

Devices

Effect of Cardiac Resynchronization Therapy on Reverse Remodeling and Relation to Outcome: Multicenter Automatic Defibrillator Implantation Trial: Cardiac Resynchronization Therapy

Solomon SD, for the MADIT-CRT Investigators (Brigham and Women's Hosp, Boston, MA; et al)
Circulation 122:985-992, 2010

Background.—Cardiac resynchronization therapy (CRT) plus implantation of an implantable cardioverter defibrillator (ICD) reduced the risk of death or heart failure event in patients with mildly symptomatic heart failure, left ventricular dysfunction, and wide QRS complex compared with an ICD only. We assessed echocardiographic changes in patients enrolled in the MADIT-CRT trial (Multicenter Automatic Defibrillator Implantation Trial: Cardiac Resynchronization Therapy) to evaluate whether the improvement in outcomes with CRT plus an ICD was associated with favorable alterations in cardiac size and function.

Methods and Results.—A total of 1820 patients were randomly assigned to CRT plus an ICD or to an ICD only in a 3:2 ratio. Echocardiographic studies were obtained at baseline and 12 months later in 1372 patients. We compared changes in cardiac size and performance between treatment groups and assessed the relationship between these changes over the first year, as well as subsequent outcomes. Compared with the ICD-only group, the CRT-plus-ICD group had greater improvement in left ventricular end-diastolic volume index (-26.2 versus -7.4 mL/m^2), left ventricular end-systolic volume index (-28.7 versus -9.1 mL/m^2), left ventricular ejection fraction (11% versus 3%), left atrial volume index (-11.9 versus -4.7 mL/m^2), and right ventricular fractional area change (8% versus 5%; $P<0.001$ for all). Improvement in end-diastolic volume at 1 year was predictive of subsequent death or heart failure, with adjustment for baseline covariates and treatment group; each 10% decrease in end-diastolic volume was associated with a 40% reduction in risk ($P<0.001$).

Conclusions.—CRT resulted in significant improvement in cardiac size and performance compared with an ICD-only strategy in patients with mildly symptomatic heart failure. Improvement in these measures accounted for the outcomes benefit.

Clinical Trial Registration Information.—URL: http://www.clinicaltrials. gov. Unique identifier: NCT00180271.

▶ Cardiac resynchronization therapy (CRT) has been shown to improve exercise capacity and quality of life, while reducing heart failure (HF) hospitalizations and mortality in selected populations. The early studies of CRT focused on patients with advanced HF. More recently, 3 studies were completed on CRT in mild HF (New York Heart Association class I or II): REsynchronization reVErses Remodeling in Systolic left vEntricular (REVERSE) dysfunction, Multicenter Automatic Defibrillator Implantation Trial: CRT (MADIT-CRT), and Resynchronization/Defibrillation for Ambulatory Heart Failure (RAFT). The results of these studies were largely concordant, with demonstration of improved functional status and reduced hospitalization. RAFT was the only study to show a reduced mortality with CRT-D devices, likely because of the longer follow-up. This study is an analysis of reverse remodeling from MADIT-CRT. Similar to other studies of CRT, a marked improvement of cardiac structure and function is noted with CRT. Specifically, left ventricular volumes decrease and ejection fraction increases with this treatment (Fig 1 in the original article). The important contribution of the present analysis is the demonstration of the correlation between reverse remodeling and clinical outcomes. Specifically, for every 10% decrease of left ventricular end-diastolic volume, there is a 40% reduction of HF event or death (Fig 3 in the original article). These data provide further confirmation of the similar response to CRT in mild and severe HF. Moreover, they provide support for the use of reverse remodeling as a surrogate end point for the response to CRT. Reverse remodeling is more pronounced in left bundle branch block versus right bundle branch block, with wider QRS duration and in women, all subgroups with a better clinical response to CRT.

M. R. Gold, MD, PhD

Cardiac Resynchronization Therapy in Asymptomatic or Mildly Symptomatic Heart Failure Patients in Relation to Etiology: Results From the REVERSE (REsynchronization reVErses Remodeling in Systolic Left vEntricular Dysfunction) Study
Linde C, on behalf of the REVERSE Study Group (Karolinska Univ Hosp, Stockholm, Sweden; et al)
J Am Coll Cardiol 56:1826-1831, 2010

Objectives.—The purpose of this study was to determine the effects of cardiac resynchronization therapy (CRT) with respect to heart failure etiology among patients in the REVERSE (REsynchronization reVErses Remodeling in Systolic Left vEntricular Dysfunction) study.

Background.—CRT improves outcomes in New York Heart Association functional class III/IV heart failure with wide QRS with a more pronounced effect on left ventricular (LV) reverse remodeling in nonischemic patients.

Methods.—A total of 277 patients with nonischemic heart disease (IHD) and 333 with IHD etiology in New York Heart Association functional class I or II with QRS ≥120 ms and left ventricular ejection fraction ≤40% received a CRT (± implantable cardioverter-defibrillator) and were randomized to CRT-ON or CRT-OFF for 12 months. The primary end point was the percentage of patients worsened by the HF clinical composite response, and multiple prespecified secondary end points were evaluated regarding etiology using univariable and multivariable analysis.

Results.—At baseline, IHD patients were significantly older and had more comorbidities and less dyssynchrony than non-IHD patients. In non-IHD patients, 10% worsened in CRT-ON compared with 19% in CRT-OFF (p = 0.01). In IHD patients, 20% worsened in the CRT-ON compared with 24% in the CRT-OFF group (p = 0.10). Non-IHD patients assigned to CRT-ON improved more in left ventricular end-systolic volume index than IHD patients. Randomization to CRT, left bundle branch block, and wider QRS duration independently predicted response to both end points, whereas non-IHD etiology was an independent predictor only for left ventricular end-systolic volume index.

Conclusions.—This substudy of REVERSE shows that CRT reverses left ventricular remodeling with a more extensive effect on nonischemic patients. Etiology was, however, not an independent predictor of clinical response. (REsynchronization reVErses Remodeling in Systolic Left vEntricular Dysfunction [REVERSE]; NCT00271154) (Figs 2 and 3).

▶ Controversy exists regarding the relative benefit of cardiac resynchronization therapy (CRT) among patients with ischemic cardiomyopathy (ICM) versus nonischemic cardiomyopathy. This substudy of the Resynchronization Reverses

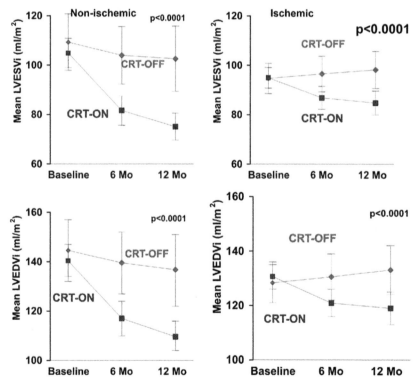

FIGURE 2.—Reverse Remodeling Left Ventricular End-Systolic and End-Diastolic Volume Index In Nonischemic and Ischemic Patients During CRT-ON and -OFF. The p values compare change from baseline to 12 months between cardiac resynchronization therapy (CRT)-ON and -OFF (2-sample *t* test). **Error bars** represent 95% confidence intervals. (Reprinted from the Journal of the American College of Cardiology, Linde C, on behalf of the REVERSE Study Group. Cardiac Resynchronization Therapy in Asymptomatic or Mildly Symptomatic Heart Failure Patients in Relation to Etiology: Results From the REVERSE (REsynchronization reVErses Remodeling in Systolic Left vEntricular Dysfunction) study. *J Am Coll Cardiol.* 2010;56:1826-1831. Copyright 2010, with permission from the American College of Cardiology.)

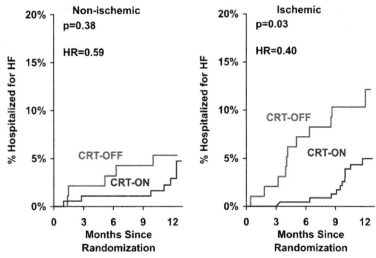

FIGURE 3.—Time to First Heart Failure–Related Hospitalization In Nonischemic and Ischemic Patients During CRT-ON and -OFF, Respectively. CRT = cardiac resynchronization therapy; HF = heart failure; HR = hazard ratio. (Reprinted from the Journal of the American College of Cardiology, Linde C, on behalf of the REVERSE Study Group. Cardiac Resynchronization Therapy in Asymptomatic or Mildly Symptomatic Heart Failure Patients in Relation to Etiology: results from the REVERSE (REsynchronization reVErses Remodeling in Systolic Left vEntricular Dysfunction) study. *J Am Coll Cardiol.* 2010;56:1826-1831. Copyright 2010, with permission from the American College of Cardiology.)

Remodeling in Systolic Left Ventricular Dysfunction trial examined the impact of etiology of cardiomyopathy on the clinical and mechanical benefits of CRT in patients with mild-moderate congestive heart failure (CHF). As depicted in Fig 2, patients with nonischemic heart disease (NIHD) had a larger benefit with respect to left ventricular (LV) remodeling (improved LV end-systolic volume index) compared with ICM; however, this did not correlate with improved clinical benefit, including decreased hospitalizations for CHF or death (Fig 3). The ischemic heart disease (IHD) group had statistically less dyssynchrony compared with the NIHD group, which may explain the lesser extent of reverse remodeling. The results of this study were consistent with those of prior CRT trials, and as noted previously, predictors of response included randomization to CRT-ON, as well as left bundle branch block (LBBB) morphology and QRS width. Etiology of cardiomyopathy (IHD vs NIHD) should not be a determinant in selecting patients for CRT; selecting patients with wide LBBB morphology QRS will likely result in greater remodeling and net clinical benefit.

F. A. Cuoco, Jr, MD, MBA

Bundle-Branch Block Morphology and Other Predictors of Outcome After Cardiac Resynchronization Therapy in Medicare Patients

Bilchick KC, Kamath S, DiMarco JP, et al (Univ of Virginia Health System, Charlottesville)
Circulation 122:2022-2030, 2010

Background.—Clinical trials of cardiac resynchronization therapy (CRT) have enrolled a select group of patients, with few patients in subgroups such as right bundle-branch block (RBBB). Analysis of population-based outcomes provides a method to identify real-world predictors of CRT outcomes.

Methods and Results.—Medicare Implantable Cardioverter-Defibrillator Registry (2005 to 2006) data were merged with patient outcomes data. Cox proportional-hazards models assessed death and death/heart failure hospitalization outcomes in patients with CRT and an implantable cardioverter-defibrillator (CRT-D). The 14 946 registry patients with CRT-D (median follow-up, 40 months) had 1-year, 3-year, and overall mortality rates of 12%, 32%, and 37%, respectively. New York Heart Association class IV heart failure status (1-year hazard ratio [HR], 2.23; 3-year HR, 1.98; *P*<0.001) and age ≥80 years (1-year HR, 1.74; 3-year HR, 1.75; *P*<0.001) were associated with increased mortality both early and late after CRT-D. RBBB (1-year HR, 1.44; 3-year HR, 1.37; *P*<0.001) and ischemic cardiomyopathy (1-year HR, 1.39; 3-year HR, 1.44; *P*<0.001) were the next strongest adjusted predictors of both early and late mortality. RBBB and ischemic cardiomyopathy together had twice the adjusted hazard for death (HR, 1.99; *P*<0.001) as left BBB and nonischemic cardiomyopathy. QRS duration of at least 150 ms predicted more favorable outcomes in left BBB but had no impact in RBBB. A secondary analysis showed lower hazards for CRT-D compared with standard implantable cardioverter-defibrillators in left BBB compared with RBBB.

Conclusions.—In Medicare patients, RBBB, ischemic cardiomyopathy, New York Heart Association class IV status, and advanced age were powerful adjusted predictors of poor outcome after CRT-D. Real-world mortality rates 3 to 4 years after CRT-D appear higher than previously recognized.

▶ Among patients with advanced heart failure (HF) symptoms, cardiac resynchronization therapy (CRT), with or without an implantable cardioverter-defibrillator (ICD), has been shown to prolong survival, decrease HF symptoms, increase exercise capacity, and result in beneficial reverse left ventricular remodeling in appropriately selected patients. There is evidence for CRT defibrillator (CRT-D) implantation in patients with left ventricular ejection fraction of ≤35%, QRS of ≥120 milliseconds, and New York Heart Association (NYHA) class II and worse; however, there remains uncertainty on which patients in the real world actually benefit most. In this study, these investigators analyzed 14 946 patients from the Medicare Implantable Cardioverter-Defibrillator Registry from

2005 to 2006 and merged this registry with outcome data. During the first 3 years of follow-up, this large retrospective study demonstrated that despite 80% of patients on optimal medical therapy with β-blockers and angiotensin-converting enzyme inhibitors or angiotensin receptor blockers and CRT-D device therapy, approximately one-third of patients died and about one-half died or were hospitalized for HF. Powerful predictors of outcome in this population included bundle branch block (BBB) morphology followed by NYHA class IV HF, age ≥80 years, ischemic cardiomyopathy (ICM), diabetes, and atrial fibrillation. Fig 3 in the original article demonstrates the mortality rates based on BBB morphology and cardiomyopathy type over time. The combination of right bundle branch block (RBBB) and ICM was associated with almost twice the unadjusted mortality rate at 1, 2, and 3 years compared with left bundle branch block (LBBB) and nonischemic cardiomyopathy (NICM) with combinations of RBBB and NICM and LBBB and ICM at intermediate risk. A major limitation of this study is the lack of a control group; therefore it is not clear whether these findings are because of the higher mortality rate of patients with ischemic heart disease or RBBB rather than a lower response rate to CRT. Further randomized controlled trials are needed to verify these findings.

P. Netzler, MD

The Value of Defibrillator Electrograms for Recognition of Clinical Ventricular Tachycardias and for Pace Mapping of Post-Infarction Ventricular Tachycardia
Yoshida K, Liu T-Y, Scott C, et al (Univ of Michigan, Ann Arbor)
J Am Coll Cardiol 56:969-979, 2010

Objectives.—The purpose of this study was to assess the value of implantable cardioverter-defibrillator (ICD) electrograms (EGMs) in identifying clinically documented ventricular tachycardias (VTs).

Background.—Twelve-lead electrocardiograms (ECG) of spontaneous VT often are not available in patients referred for catheter ablation of post-infarction VT. Many of these patients have ICDs, and the ability of ICD EGMs to identify a specific configuration of VT has not been described.

Methods.—In 21 consecutive patients referred for catheter ablation of post-infarction VT, 124 VTs (mean cycle length: 393 ± 103 ms) were induced, and ICD EGMs were recorded during VT. Clinical VT had been documented with 12-lead ECGs in 15 of 21 patients. The 12-lead ECGs of the clinical VTs were compared with 64 different inducible VTs (mean cycle length: 390 ± 91 ms) to assess how well the ICD EGMs differentiated the clinical VTs from the other induced VTs. The exit site of 62 VTs (mean cycle length: 408 ± 112 ms) was identified by pace mapping (10 to 12 of 12 matching leads). The spatial resolution of pace mapping to identify a VT exit site was determined for both the 12-lead ECGs and the ICD EGMs using a customized MATLAB program (version 7.5, The MathWorks, Inc., Natick, Massachusetts).

Results.—Analysis of stored EGMs by comparison of receiver-operating characteristic curve cutoff values accurately distinguished the clinical VTs from 98% of the other inducible VTs. The mean spatial resolution of a 12-lead ECG pace map for the VT exit site was $2.9 \pm 4.0 \, cm^2$ (range 0 to $17.5 \, cm^2$) compared with $8.9 \pm 9.0 \, cm^2$ (range 0 to $35 \, cm^2$) for ICD EGM pace maps. The spatial resolution of pace mapping varied greatly between patients and between VTs. The spatial resolution of ICD EGMs was $<1.0 \, cm^2$ for ≥ 1 of the target VTs in 12 of 21 patients and 19 of 62 VTs. By visual inspection of the ICD EGMs, 96% of the clinical VTs were accurately differentiated from previously undocumented VTs.

Conclusions.—Stored ICD EGMs usually are an accurate surrogate for 12-lead ECGs for differentiating clinical VTs from other VTs. Pace mapping based on ICD EGMs has variable resolution but may be useful for identifying a VT exit site.

▶ Many patients with implantable cardioverter-defibrillators (ICDs) who present with recurrent ventricular tachycardia (VT) have their arrhythmias terminated by antitachycardia pacing or shocks before a 12-lead electrocardiogram (ECG) can be obtained. Therefore, a method to distinguish clinical from nonclinical VTs induced at the time of electrophysiologic (EP) study and ablation would be valuable to facilitate targeting arrhythmias that are significant while avoiding unnecessary ablation and possibly limiting the time and risk of the procedure. The investigators in this study attempted to use ICD electrograms (EGMs) to distinguish clinical from nonclinical arrhythmias during the ablation of postinfarction VT. With a method that used receiver operating characteristic curves, the authors demonstrated that ICD EGMs can be useful in distinguishing clinical VTs from nonclinical VTs induced during EP study, independent of rate. Simple visual analysis of ICD EGM morphology was found to be as accurate as offline computer analysis, making this method clinically applicable. Additionally, the authors demonstrated that ICD EGMs may be useful in pace mapping VT exit sites; however, it is important to realize that these exit sites may not represent the ideal site (eg, critical isthmus) for ablation and termination of VT. Finally, the spatial resolution of ICD EGMs is inferior to that of traditional 12-lead ECG pace mapping. Nevertheless, these results indicate that there is useful information in the analysis of ICD therapy that can aid in the ablation of VT.

F. A. Cuoco, Jr, MD, MBA

Long-term outcomes and clinical predictors for pacemaker-requiring bradyarrhythmias after cardiac transplantation: Analysis of the UNOS/OPTN cardiac transplant database
Cantillon DJ, Tarakji KG, Hu T, et al (Heart and Vascular Inst, Cleveland, OH)
Heart Rhythm 7:1567-1571, 2010

Background.—Pacemaker-requiring bradyarrhythmias after cardiac transplantation are common, and rarely can lead to sudden cardiac death. Prior outcomes studies have been limited to single-center data.

Objective.—This study sought to define the long-term outcomes and clinical predictors for pacemaker-requiring bradyarrhythmias in the cardiac transplant population.

Methods.—This study used multivariable analysis of the United Network for Organ Sharing/Organ Procurement and Transplantation Network (UNOS/OPTN) database of sequential U.S. cardiac transplant recipients from 1997 to 2007 stratified by postoperative bradyarrhythmias requiring a pacemaker. The primary end point was all-cause mortality.

Results.—Among 35,987 cardiac transplant recipients (age 46.1 ± 18.3 years, 76% male, 22% bicaval technique) with a follow-up of 6.3 ± 4.7 years, pacemaker-requiring bradyarrhythmias occurred in 3,940 patients (10.9%). Pacemaker recipients demonstrated improved survival (median 8.0 years vs. 5.2 years, *P* < .001), decreased 5-year mortality (13.8% vs. 17.7%, *P* < .001), and overall crude mortality (42.9% vs. 45.9%, *P* < .001). Multivariable propensity-score-adjusted analysis demonstrated improved survival among pacemaker recipients (adjusted hazard ratio 0.84, 95% confidence interval [CI] 0.80 to 0.88, *P* < .001) after adjustment for donor/recipient age, UNOS listing status, donor heart ischemic time, surgical technique, graft rejection, and other common comorbidities. The bicaval surgical technique was strongly protective against a postoperative pacemaker requirement (odds ratio [OR] 0.33, 95% CI 0.29 to 0.36, *P* < .001) in multivariable analysis. Among the other variables studied, only increasing donor age (OR 1.04, 95% CI 1.00 to 1.09, *P* < .001) and recipient age (OR 1.09, 95% CI 1.0 to 1.12, *P* < .001) were associated with a permanent pacemaker requirement.

Conclusion.—Cardiac transplant recipients with pacemaker-requiring bradyarrhythmias have an excellent long-term prognosis. Increased mortality in the nonpacemaker group merits further investigation. Biatrial surgical technique and increasing donor/recipient age are associated with postoperative pacemaker requirement (Table 3).

▶ Cantillon and colleagues analyzed clinical outcomes in patients undergoing cardiac transplantation that required pacemaker insertion for postoperative bradyarrhythmias. They examined variables associated with bradyarrhythmias, such as donor heart ischemic time, surgical implant technique, allograft

TABLE 3.—Predictors for Pacemaker Requirement After Cardiac Transplant Surgery (n = 35,987)

	Odds Ratio (95% CI)	P Value
Age (yrs)		
Donor	1.04 (1.00−1.09)	<.001
Recipient	1.09 (1.00−1.12)	<.001
Bicaval anastomosis	0.33 (0.29−0.36)	<.001
Donor heart ischemic time (min)	1.03 (0.97−1.04)	.880
Transplant CAD, stenosis ≥50%	2.12 (0.92−2.33)	.409
Rejection requiring treatment	0.95 (0.84−1.07)	.367

CAD = coronary artery disease; CI = confidence interval.

coronary atherosclerosis, allograft rejection, and donor and recipient age. Their study was unique in that they assessed the United Network for Organ Sharing/Organ Procurement and Transplantation Network (UNOS/OPTN) database, and in this process, they eliminated bias frequently associated with single-center reviews. Pertinent findings included the following: (1) postoperative bradyarrhythmias requiring insertion of a permanent transvenous pacemaker occurred in approximately 11% of cardiac transplant recipients over a period of 10 years (ending 2007) and (2) the biatrial surgical technique and increasing donor and recipient age were identified as important associations with postoperative bradyarrhythmias and necessity for pacemaker insertion (Table 3). The importance of this investigation is not its findings, but rather the method in which it was conducted—specifically, its interrogation of the UNOS/OPTN database. While the biatrial implantation technique for cardiac transplantation is both tried and true, its association with postoperative rhythm disturbances relative to the bicaval technique is well known and has resulted in its abandonment in some transplant centers. The bicaval technique of cardiac transplantation preserves the sinus node artery and it can be performed in a straightforward fashion and without any significant increase in ischemic time. Moreover, a past study[1] demonstrated that transplantation using the bicaval technique was associated with a small but significant survival advantage compared with the biatrial technique. Accordingly, the bicaval technique for cardiac transplantation should supplant the biatrial technique if for no other reason than to minimize the risk for insertion of a permanent pacemaker in the postoperative setting.

W. M. Yarbrough, MD

Reference

1. Davies RR, Russo MJ, Morgan JA, Sorabella RA, Naka Y, Chen JM. Standard versus bicaval techniques for orthotopic heart transplantation: An analysis of the United Network for Organ Sharing database. *J Thorac Cardiovasc Surg.* 2010;140:700-708.

Sudden Cardiac Death

Effectiveness of prophylactic implantation of cardioverter-defibrillators without cardiac resynchronization therapy in patients with ischaemic or non-ischaemic heart disease: a systematic review and meta-analysis

Theuns DAMJ, Smith T, Hunink MGM, et al (Erasmus MC, Rotterdam, The Netherlands; et al)

Europace 12:1564-1570, 2010

Aims.—Much controversy exists concerning the efficacy of primary prophylactic implantable cardioverter-defibrillators (ICDs) in patients with low ejection fraction due to coronary artery disease (CAD) or dilated cardiomyopathy (DCM). This is also related to the bias created by function improving interventions added to ICD therapy, e.g. resynchronization therapy. The aim was to investigate the efficacy of ICD-only therapy in primary prevention in patients with CAD or DCM.

Methods and Results.—Public domain databases, MEDLINE, EMBASE, and Cochrane Central Register of Controlled Trials, were searched from 1980 to 2009 for randomized clinical trials of ICD vs. conventional therapy. Two investigators independently abstracted the data. Pooled estimates were calculated using both fixed-effects and random-effects models. Eight trials were included in the final analysis (5343 patients). Implantable cardioverter-defibrillators significantly reduced the arrhythmic mortality [relative risk (RR): 0.40; 95% confidence interval (CI): 0.27–0.67] and all-cause mortality (RR: 0.73; 95% CI: 0.64–0.82). Regardless of aetiology of heart disease, ICD benefit was similar for CAD (RR: 0.67; 95% CI: 0.51–0.88) vs. DCM (RR: 0.74; 95% CI: 0.59–0.93).

Conclusions.—The results of this meta-analysis provide strong evidence for the beneficial effect of ICD-only therapy on the survival of patients with ischaemic or non-ischaemic heart disease, with a left ventricular ejection fraction ≤35%, if they are 40 days from myocardial infarction and ≥3 months from a coronary revascularization procedure (Fig 2).

▶ The implantable cardioverter-defibrillator (ICD) has become important adjunctive therapy for high-risk patients. Although the ICD was approved for human implantation 25 years ago, it is more recently that it has been used for

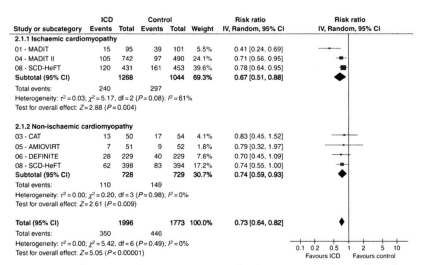

FIGURE 2.—All-cause mortality among patients with ischaemic or non-ischaemic heart disease randomized to implantable cardioverter-defibrillator (ICD) vs. conventional therapy in primary prevention. For each randomized trial, the number of deaths (Events) and the number assigned (Total) are shown. The point estimates of the relative risk (RR) for individual studies are represented by squares with 95% confidence intervals (CIs) shown as bars. The midpoint of the diamond represents the overall pooled estimate of the RR, and the 95% CI is represented by the horizontal tips of the diamond. AMIOVIRT, Amiodarone vs. Implantable Defibrillator Randomized Trial; CAT, Cardiomyopathy Trial; DEFINITE, Defibrillators in Non-Ischemic Cardiomyopathy Treatment Evaluation; MADIT, Multicenter Automatic Defibrillator Implantation Trial; SCD-HeFT, Sudden Cardiac Death in Heart Failure Trial. (Reprinted from Theuns DAMJ, Smith T, Hunink MGM, et al. Effectiveness of prophylactic implantation of cardioverter-defibrillators without cardiac resynchronization therapy in patients with ischaemic or non-ischaemic heart disease: a systematic review and meta-analysis. *Europace.* 2010;12:1564-1570.)

primary prevention. To help quantify the magnitude of benefit of the ICD, Theuns et al performed a meta-analysis of primary prevention ICD therapy among ischemic and nonischemic patients who did not receive cardiac resynchronization therapy. Their goal was to define the magnitude of ICD therapy alone on all-cause and arrhythmic mortality. Literature search and article selection identified 8 randomized clinical trials evaluating ICD-only therapy versus conventional medical therapy. All-cause mortality was reduced by 33% in ischemic cardiomyopathy patients and 26% in nonischemic cardiomyopathy patients (Fig 2). The reduction in all-cause and arrhythmic mortality for all patients was 27% and 60%, respectively. For studies that monitored delivery of ICD therapy, appropriate and inappropriate shocks occurred in 23% and 17% of patients, respectively. This meta-analysis demonstrates that ICD therapy provides a significant all-cause and arrhythmic mortality benefit and supports the present guidelines for primary prevention implantation.

M. L. Bernard, MD, PhD

Automated External Defibrillators and Survival After In-Hospital Cardiac Arrest

Chan PS, for the American Heart Association National Registry of Cardiopulmonary Resuscitation (NRCPR) Investigators (Saint Luke's Mid America Heart Inst, Kansas City, MO; et al)
JAMA 304:2129-2136, 2010

Context.—Automated external defibrillators (AEDs) improve survival from out-of-hospital cardiac arrests, but data on their effectiveness in hospitalized patients are limited.

Objective.—To evaluate the association between AED use and survival for in-hospital cardiac arrest.

Design, Setting, and Patients.—Cohort study of 11 695 hospitalized patients with cardiac arrests between January 1, 2000, and August 26, 2008, at 204 US hospitals following the introduction of AEDs on general hospital wards.

Main Outcome Measure.—Survival to hospital discharge by AED use, using multivariable hierarchical regression analyses to adjust for patient factors and hospital site.

Results.—Of 11 695 patients, 9616 (82.2%) had nonshockable rhythms (asystole and pulseless electrical activity) and 2079 (17.8%) had shockable rhythms (ventricular fibrillation and pulseless ventricular tachycardia). AEDs were used in 4515 patients (38.6%). Overall, 2117 patients (18.1%) survived to hospital discharge. Within the entire study population, AED use was associated with a lower rate of survival after in-hospital cardiac arrest compared with no AED use (16.3% vs 19.3%; adjusted rate ratio [RR], 0.85; 95% confidence interval [CI], 0.78-0.92; $P < .001$). Among cardiac arrests due to nonshockable rhythms, AED use was associated with lower survival (10.4% vs 15.4%; adjusted RR, 0.74; 95% CI, 0.65-0.83; $P < .001$). In contrast, for cardiac arrests due to shockable rhythms, AED use was not associated with survival (38.4% vs 39.8%; adjusted RR, 1.00; 95% CI, 0.88-1.13; $P = .99$). These patterns were consistently observed in both monitored and nonmonitored hospital units where AEDs were used, after matching patients to the individual units in each hospital where the cardiac arrest occurred, and with a propensity score analysis.

Conclusion.—Among hospitalized patients with cardiac arrest, use of AEDs was not associated with improved survival (Table 3).

▶ Strategies to improve survival associated with out-of-hospital cardiac arrest have developed over the past decade. Central in most approaches is the increased availability of automated external defibrillators (AEDs). This study evaluates the role of a similar strategy for in-hospital arrest. The cohort study was derived from 550 acute care hospitals with a total patient population of 110 132. The final study sample was 11 695 or 11% of the initial database and included only 204 hospitals (37%). The authors restricted their analysis to this smaller population to improve and ensure that the comparisons of AED use and survival were appropriate and contemporary. In the study population, there was a baseline difference in those with metastatic malignancy, baseline depression, and metabolic abnormality. These were all statistically higher in those with AED usage and may have some effect on survival.

Statistically, this study used multivariable hierarchy regression models to assess the relationship of AED use and survival. A propensity score was used to standardize the care of these patients and ensure balance. By doing this, the results showed a 16.3% decrease in the survival in those using AED versus 19.3% in those in whom it was not used ($P < .001$). In those with treatable arrhythmias, AED use showed a survival of 38.4% compared with 39% for no

TABLE 3.—Survival to Discharge[a]

	No. of Survivors/Total No. of Patients (%)		Unadjusted RR (95% CI)	Adjusted RR (95% CI)[b]	P Value
	AED Used	AED Not Used			
All units					
All arrests	734/4515 (16.3)	1383/7180 (19.3)	0.84 (0.78-0.92)	0.85 (0.78-0.92)	<.001
VF and pulseless VT	364/947 (38.4)	450/1132 (39.8)	0.97 (0.87-1.08)	1.00 (0.88-1.13)	.99
Asystole and PEA	370/3568 (10.4)	933/6048 (15.4)	0.67 (0.60-0.75)	0.74 (0.65-0.83)	<.001
Monitored units					
All arrests	488/2104 (23.2)	992/4156 (23.9)	0.97 (0.88-1.07)	0.87 (0.79-0.97)	.01
VF and pulseless VT	286/593 (48.2)	368/804 (45.8)	1.05 (0.94-1.18)	1.03 (0.89-1.18)	.71
Asystole and PEA	202/1511 (13.4)	624/3352 (18.6)	0.72 (0.62-0.83)	0.72 (0.62-0.85)	<.001
Nonmonitored units					
All arrests	246/2411 (10.2)	391/3024 (12.9)	0.79 (0.68-0.92)	0.82 (0.70-0.98)	.03
VF and pulseless VT	78/354 (22.0)	82/328 (25.0)	0.88 (0.67-1.16)	0.93 (0.63-1.36)	.71
Asystole and PEA	168/2057 (8.2)	309/2696 (11.5)	0.71 (0.60-0.85)	0.79 (0.65-0.96)	.02

Abbreviations: AED, automated external defibrillator; CI, confidence interval; PEA, pulseless electrical activity; RR, rate ratio; VF, ventricular fibrillation; VT, ventricular tachycardia.
[a]Crude and adjusted rates of survival to discharge by AED use are presented. Results for the entire cohort and stratified by monitoring status are depicted.
[b]Adjusted for hospital site and patient and hospital factors using hierarchical models.

AED use. Those in whom the AED would not expect to be helped (nontreatable arrhythmias), survival was worse with AED use 10.4% versus 15.5% (*P* < .001), suggesting that AEDs delayed treatment of the underlying cause of arrest.

The limitations of this study may be failure to implement AEDs efficiently from possibly poor training, which would attenuate the benefits. Smaller hospitals had a higher use of AEDs. Clearly, training to evaluate and treat an arrhythmia may have significant effects on survival. One of the most important items noted by the author is the huge increase in use of AEDs. Because 37% of hospitals now have AEDs, and more may be added annually, the effectiveness of their treatment should be established. These results indicate that a prospective randomized controlled study should be performed to evaluate the routine use of AEDs in hospitals.

R. B. Leman, MD

Chest Compression—Only CPR by Lay Rescuers and Survival From Out-of-Hospital Cardiac Arrest
Bobrow BJ, Spaite DW, Berg RA, et al (Arizona Dept of Health Services, Phoenix; Univ of Arizona, Tucson; Children's Hosp of Philadelphia, PA; et al)
JAMA 304:1447-1454, 2010

Context.—Chest compression—only bystander cardiopulmonary resuscitation (CPR) may be as effective as conventional CPR with rescue breathing for out-of-hospital cardiac arrest.

Objective.—To investigate the survival of patients with out-of-hospital cardiac arrest using compression-only CPR (COCPR) compared with conventional CPR.

Design, Setting, and Patients.—A 5-year prospective observational cohort study of survival in patients at least 18 years old with out-of-hospital cardiac arrest between January 1, 2005, and December 31, 2009, in Arizona. The relationship between layperson bystander CPR and survival to hospital discharge was evaluated using multivariable logistic regression.

Main Outcome Measure.—Survival to hospital discharge.

Results.—Among 5272 adults with out-of-hospital cardiac arrest of cardiac etiology not observed by responding emergency medical personnel, 779 were excluded because bystander CPR was provided by a health care professional or the arrest occurred in a medical facility. A total of 4415 met all inclusion criteria for analysis, including 2900 who received no bystander CPR, 666 who received conventional CPR, and 849 who received COCPR. Rates of survival to hospital discharge were 5.2% (95% confidence interval [CI], 4.4%-6.0%) for the no bystander CPR group, 7.8% (95% CI, 5.8%-9.8%) for conventional CPR, and 13.3% (95% CI, 11.0%-15.6%) for COCPR. The adjusted odds ratio (AOR) for survival for conventional CPR vs no CPR was 0.99 (95% CI, 0.69-1.43), for COCPR vs no CPR, 1.59 (95% CI, 1.18-2.13), and for COCPR vs conventional CPR, 1.60 (95% CI, 1.08-2.35). From 2005 to

2009, lay rescuer CPR increased from 28.2% (95% CI, 24.6%-31.8%) to 39.9% (95% CI, 36.8%-42.9%; *P* < .001); the proportion of CPR that was COCPR increased from 19.6% (95% CI, 13.6%-25.7%) to 75.9% (95% CI, 71.7%-80.1%; *P* < .001). Overall survival increased from 3.7% (95% CI, 2.2%-5.2%) to 9.8% (95% CI, 8.0%-11.6%; *P* < .001).

Conclusion.—Among patients with out-of-hospital cardiac arrest, layperson compression-only CPR was associated with increased survival compared with conventional CPR and no bystander CPR in this setting with public endorsement of chest compression-only CPR.

▶ Though survival of out-of-hospital cardiac arrest is improved with early and effective cardiopulmonary resuscitation (CPR), most patients suffering cardiac arrest do not receive bystander CPR; moreover, the optimal methods for CPR administration continue to evolve. As an alternative to conventional CPR with interruptions for ventilation, compression-only CPR (COCPR) has gained popularity for untrained medical personnel because of its simplicity and focus on effective chest compressions, a principle that has been emphasized as an important component of high-quality CPR.

The authors of this study sought to evaluate the effectiveness of a statewide public campaign to promote COCPR as compared with conventional bystander CPR and no bystander CPR. Following Arizona's statewide dissemination of information promoting COCPR, 5272 cardiac arrests between 2005 and 2009 were analyzed according to the type of CPR performed. During the study period, the number of bystanders performing any type of CPR increased from 28.2% in 2005 to 39.9% in 2009 (*P* < .001), while the proportion of bystanders performing COCPR increased from 19.6% to 75.9% during the same time period. The rate of survival to hospital discharge was 5.2% (95% confidence interval [CI], 4.4%-6.0%) for the no bystander CPR group, 7.8% (95% CI, 5.8-9.8%) for conventional CPR group, and 13.3% (95% CI, 11.0%-15.6%) for COCPR group. As shown in Table 3 in the original article, odds of survival were improved with COCPR compared with no bystander CPR (odds ratio, 1.59; 95% CI, 1.18-2.13) and conventional CPR (odds ratio, 1.60; 95% CI, 1.08-2.35). Overall survival increased from 3.7% (95% CI, 2.2%-5.2%) to 9.8% (95% CI, 9.0%-11.6%; *P* < .001).

There are several important findings in this study that have widespread implications for improvement in out-of-hospital cardiac arrest. First, it demonstrates the effectiveness of a public health campaign aimed at increasing awareness of the necessity for bystander CPR. Second, the results also suggest that COCPR is not only an alternative to traditional CPR but for the first time has been shown to be a superior method by increasing survival to hospital discharge and may be a preferable strategy for lay rescuers. Lastly, in addition to improved relative survival compared with conventional CPR, by increasing the number of bystanders performing CPR, this method also increases the absolute number of patients surviving out-of-hospital cardiac arrest. Despite these advances in provision and quality of bystander CPR, significant improvements are still required for patients with out-of-hospital cardiac arrest.

C. P. Rowley, MD

Long-Term Benefit of Primary Prevention With an Implantable Cardioverter-Defibrillator: An Extended 8-Year Follow-Up Study of the Multicenter Automatic Defibrillator Implantation Trial II

Goldenberg I, the Executive Committee of the Multicenter Automatic Defibrillator Implantation Trial II (Univ of Rochester Med Ctr, NY; et al)
Circulation 122:1265-1271, 2010

Background.—The Multicenter Automatic Defibrillator Implantation Trial II (MADIT-II) showed a significant 31% reduction in the risk of death with primary implantable cardioverter-defibrillator (ICD) therapy during a median follow-up of 1.5 years. However, currently there are no data on the long-term efficacy of primary defibrillator therapy.

Methods and Results.—MADIT-II enrolled 1232 patients with ischemic left ventricular dysfunction who were randomized to ICD and non-ICD medical therapy and were followed up through November 2001. For the present long-term study, we acquired posttrial mortality data through March 2009 for all study participants (median follow-up, 7.6 years). Multivariate Cox proportional hazards regression modeling was performed to calculate the hazard ratio for ICD versus non-ICD therapy during long-term follow-up. At 8 years of follow-up, the cumulative probability of all-cause mortality was 49% among patients treated with an ICD compared with 62% among non-ICD patients ($P<0.001$). Multivariate analysis demonstrated that ICD therapy was associated with a significant long-term survival benefit (hazard ratio for 0-through 8-year mortality = 0.66 [95% confidence interval, 0.56 to 0.78]; $P<0.001$). Treatment with an ICD was shown to be associated with a significant reduction in the risk of death during the early phase of the extended follow-up period (0 through 4 years: hazard ratio = 0.61 [95% confidence interval, 0.50 to 0.76]; $P<0.001$) and with continued life-saving benefit during the late phase of follow-up (5 through 8 years: hazard ratio = 0.74 [95% confidence interval, 0.57 to 0.96]; $P=0.02$).

Conclusions.—Our findings demonstrate a sustained 8-year survival benefit with primary ICD therapy in the MADIT-II population.

▶ Several large, landmark, multicenter trials led to the development of the implantable cardioverter-defibrillator (ICD) for primary prevention of sudden death. Multicenter Automatic Defibrillator Implantation Trial (MADIT) II and Sudden Cardiac Death in Heart Failure Trial are most responsible for the large increase in ICD implantation over the past 6 years. However, all of these studies had relatively short duration follow-up, which made cost-effectiveness questionable and potential applicability to real world patients. These factors have likely contributed to the underuse of ICD despite a class IA indication by guidelines. In this study, the MADIT II cohort was followed longitudinally for almost 8 years. The 31% mortality reduction at study completion was maintained at 8 years (34% reduction, Fig 1 in the original article) and provides strong evidence for the continued benefit of long-term ICD use among patients with ischemic cardiomyopathy. Patients with single-chamber devices had lower mortality than those with dual chambers, again calling into question the increased use of dual-chamber ICDs for primary prevention. While there was likely investigator bias in the crossover to ICD in the control arm that could have affected these results, the findings clearly show that ICD use is effective and that increased utilization is warranted according to evidence- and guideline-based recommendations.

M. R. Gold, MD, PhD

Long-Term Follow-Up of Idiopathic Ventricular Fibrillation Ablation: A Multicenter Study
Knecht S, Sacher F, Wright M, et al (Hôpital Cardiologique du Haut-Lévêque and the Université Victor Segalen Bordeaux II, France; et al)
J Am Coll Cardiol 54:522-528, 2009

Objectives.—This multicenter study sought to evaluate the long-term follow-up of patients ablated for idiopathic ventricular fibrillation (VF).

Background.—Catheter ablation of idiopathic VF that targets ventricular premature beat (VPB) triggers has been shown to prevent VF recurrences on short-term follow-up.

Methods.—From January 2000, 38 consecutive patients from 6 different centers underwent ablation of primary idiopathic VF initiated by short coupled VPB. All patients had experienced at least 1 documented VF, with 87% having experienced ≥2 VF episodes in the preceding year. Catheter ablation was guided by activation mapping of VPBs or pace mapping during sinus rhythm.

Results.—There were 38 patients (21 men) age 42 ± 13 years, refractory to a median of 2 antiarrhythmic drugs. Triggering VPBs originated from the right (n = 16), the left (n = 14), or both (n = 3) Purkinje systems and from the myocardium (n = 5). During a median post-procedural follow-up of 63 months, 7 (18%) of 38 patients experienced VF recurrence at a median of 4 months. Five of these 7 patients underwent repeat ablation without VF recurrence. Survival free of VF was predicted only by transient bundle-branch block in the originating ventricle during the electrophysiological study (p < 0.0001). The number of significant events (confirmed VF or aborted sudden death) was reduced from 4 (interquartile range 3 to 9) before to 0 (interquartile range 0 to 4) after ablation (p = 0.01).

Conclusions.—Ablation for idiopathic VF that targets short coupled VPB triggers is associated with a long-term freedom from VF recurrence.

▶ This study demonstrates the long-term efficacy of catheter ablation of focal premature ventricular contractions that initiate ventricular fibrillation (VF). While this study concentrates only on patients with idiopathic VF, other studies in limited numbers of patients with structural heart disease as well as genetic disorders such as long-QT and Brugada syndrome have shown similar efficacy. These studies represent the first attempts to cure VF with catheter ablation, which in the future will hopefully allow less dependence upon implantable cardiac defibrillators (ICDs). However, as the results of this study demonstrate, recurrence rates are still high (18%) and given the potential lethality of recurrences, ICDs are still recommended. Although the duration of follow-up in this study is impressive (median of 63 months), too little is known about idiopathic VF and its natural history to predict even long-term risk of developing further sites. In addition, acute success rates are high when there are spontaneously occurring premature ventricular contractions (PVCs) to map, but results are less impressive when PVCs are not occurring spontaneously since they are difficult to provoke with programmed stimulation and/or autonomic manipulation. This limits application at the present time to patients with frequent PVCs and requires timing the procedure to times when spontaneous ectopy is frequent. This obviously greatly limits application to the larger pool of patients at risk but confirms the use in this approach as a means of cure of VF.

J. M. Wharton, MD

Prophylactic Implantable Defibrillator in Patients With Arrhythmogenic Right Ventricular Cardiomyopathy/Dysplasia and No Prior Ventricular Fibrillation or Sustained Ventricular Tachycardia

Corrado D, Calkins H, Link MS, et al (Univ of Padua Med School, Italy; Johns Hopkins Hosp, Baltimore, MD; Tufts Med Ctr, Boston, MA; et al)
Circulation 122:1144-1152, 2010

Background.—The role of implantable cardioverter-defibrillator (ICD) in patients with arrhythmogenic right ventricular cardiomyopathy/dysplasia and no prior ventricular fibrillation (VF) or sustained ventricular tachycardia is an unsolved issue.

Methods and Results.—We studied 106 consecutive patients (62 men and 44 women; age, 35.6 ± 18 years) with arrhythmogenic right ventricular cardiomyopathy/dysplasia who received an ICD based on 1 or more arrhythmic risk factors such as syncope, nonsustained ventricular tachycardia, familial sudden death, and inducibility at programmed ventricular stimulation. During follow-up of 58 ± 35 months, 25 patients (24%) had appropriate ICD interventions and 17 (16%) had shocks for life-threatening VF or ventricular flutter. At 48 months, the actual survival rate was 100% compared with the VF/ventricular flutter—free survival rate of 77% (log-rank $P = 0.01$). Syncope significantly predicted any appropriate ICD interventions (hazard ratio, 2.94; 95% confidence interval, 1.83 to 4.67; $P = 0.013$) and shocks for VF/ventricular flutter (hazard ratio, 3.16; 95% confidence interval, 1.39 to 5.63; $P = 0.005$). The positive predictive value of programmed ventricular stimulation was 35% for any appropriate ICD intervention and 20% for shocks for VF/ventricular flutter, with a negative predictive value of 70% and 74%. None of the 27 asymptomatic patients with isolated familial sudden death had appropriate ICD therapy. Twenty patients (19%) had inappropriate ICD interventions, and 18 (17%) had device-related complications.

Conclusions.—One fourth of patients with arrhythmogenic right ventricular cardiomyopathy/dysplasia and no prior sustained ventricular tachycardia or VF had appropriate ICD interventions. Syncope was an important predictor of life-saving ICD intervention and is an indication for ICD. Prophylactic ICD may not be indicated in asymptomatic patients because of their low arrhythmic risk regardless of familial sudden death and programmed ventricular stimulation findings. Programmed ventricular stimulation had a low predictive accuracy for ICD therapy.

▶ Arrhythmogenic right ventricular dysplasia (ARVD) is an inherited disorder resulting in fibrofatty replacement of the right ventricular myocardium that places individuals at increased risk for lethal ventricular dysrhythmias. Patients with ARVD who have experienced sustained ventricular tachycardia (VT) or ventricular fibrillation (VF) are typically referred for placement of an internal cardioverter-defibrillator (ICD) for secondary prevention of sudden cardiac arrest. ICD implantation for patients who have ARVD without apparent clinical symptoms is reserved for those believed to have high-risk clinical features, including sudden death in a first-degree relative, syncope, nonsustained VT (NSVT), or inducible VT during programmed ventricular stimulation (PVS). However, the true arrhythmic risk in patients without previous VT/VF is not well established.

The authors of this study identified 106 patients with ARVD who received a primary prevention ICD based on one or more arrhythmic risk factors, including syncope, NSVT, familial sudden death, and inducibility at PVS. Patients were generally young (35.618 years) and were followed for an average of 58 ± 31 months during which time 25 (24%) had appropriate ICD interventions, including 17 who received defibrillation for VF/V flutter (Vfl). Patients receiving appropriate ICD interventions more often had syncope (72% vs 30%; $P < .001$) (Fig 3 in the original article), NSVT (72% vs 47%; $P = .04$), and left ventricular ejection fraction < 55% (44% vs 20%; $P = .03$). Only 26 (65%) of 40 patients who were inducible during PVS had appropriate ICD interventions. The positive predictive value of PVS was 35% for any appropriate ICD intervention and 20% for shock therapy of VF/Vfl, while the negative predictive value was 70% and 74%, resulting in an overall test accuracy of 49% and 42%. Of 27 patients who received ICDs because of a history of familial sudden death, none had appropriate ICD therapy. The predictive value of various factors for appropriate ICD shocks is summarized in Table 3 in the original article. Inappropriate ICD interventions and device-related complications occurred in 20 (19%) and 18 (17%) patients, respectively.

This study demonstrates the difficulty in identifying at-risk patients based on typical clinical factors and highlights the need for a refined understanding of the natural history of ARVD, including disease penetrance and its effect on arrhythmic risk. Importantly, the results suggest that patients who have ARVD with syncope are at high risk for lethal dysrhythmias and should receive prophylactic ICDs, whereas clinically asymptomatic patients whose only apparent risk factor for ICD is familial sudden death appear to have less benefit. Other clinical factors, including results of PVS, are insufficient to direct the care of patients with ARVD in isolation.

C. P. Rowley, MD

Role of Family History of Sudden Death in Risk Stratification and Prevention of Sudden Death With Implantable Defibrillators in Hypertrophic Cardiomyopathy
Bos JM, Maron BJ, Ackerman MJ, et al (Mayo Clinic, Rochester, MN; Minneapolis Heart Inst Foundation, MN)
Am J Cardiol 106:1481-1486, 2010

The selection of patients with hypertrophic cardiomyopathy (HC) for the primary prevention of sudden death (SD) with implantable cardioverter-defibrillators (ICDs) has been determined by the assessment of 5 risk factors. We examined one of these markers, the family history of HC-related SD in first-degree relatives, for which few data are available. The rate of appropriate ICD interventions was assessed in 177 consecutive patients with HC (63% men, age 45 ± 14 years) who had undergone prophylactic implantation at 2 tertiary centers, according to the identification of ≥1 risk markers. During a follow-up period of 4.6 ± 3 years, 25 patients (14%) had experienced appropriate ICD interventions for ventricular tachycardia/ fibrillation. The patients with a risk profile that included a family history of SD experienced interventions at a similar rate (3.7/100 person-years) as the patients without a family history of SD (3.1/100 person-years, p = 0.2). The rate and frequency of appropriate ICD interventions in 42 patients who had undergone implantation solely because of a family history of SD was 2.2/100 person-years (4/42, 10%), similar to that for patients with one risk factor other than SD family history (3.4%/100 person-years; 7/50, 14%; p = 0.2) and patients with multiple risk factors with (4.5/100 person-years; 9/49, 18%) and without (3.5/100 person-years; 5/36, 14%) a family history of SD (p = 0.8). In conclusion, a family history of SD is an important risk marker in patients with HC. Patients receiving ICDs for primary prevention because of a family history of HC-related SD, whether as an isolated risk factor or combined with other markers, experienced rates of appropriate ICD discharge comparable to that of other patient subsets with increased risk (Figs 1 and 4).

▶ This study attempted to identify the role of a family history of sudden death (SD) among patients with a history of hypertrophic cardiomyopathy (HM) who underwent implantable cardioverter-defibrillator (ICD) implantation for primary prevention of SD. In this cohort, appropriate ICD discharge was similar in groups who had a family history of SD as their sole risk factor compared with those with other risk factors. Fig 1 illustrates that rates of appropriate ICD discharges were similar in cohorts with and without a family history of SD,

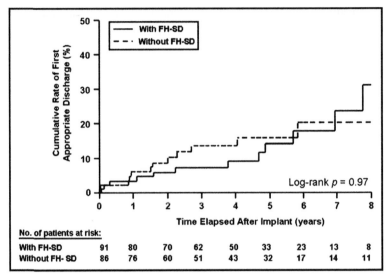

FIGURE 1.—Cumulative rates for first appropriate ICD intervention in patients with (With FH-SD) or without (Without FH-SD) a family history of SD. Kaplan-Meier curve showing cumulative rates for first appropriate ICD intervention in patients with or without family history of SD. (Reprinted from the American Journal of Cardiology, Bos JM, Maron BJ, Ackerman MJ, et al. Role of family history of sudden death in risk stratification and prevention of sudden death with implantable defibrillators in hypertrophic cardiomyopathy. *Am J Cardiol.* 2010;106:1481-1486. Copyright © 2010 with permission from Elsevier.)

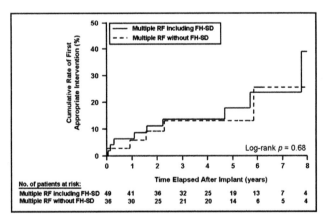

FIGURE 4.—Cumulative rates for first appropriate ICD intervention in patients with multiple risk factors. Kaplan-Meier curve showing cumulative rates for first appropriate ICD intervention in patients with multiple risk factors (RF), including family history of SD (multiple RF including FH-SD) or without family history of SD (multiple RF without FH-SD). (Reprinted from the American Journal of Cardiology, Bos JM, Maron BJ, Ackerman MJ, et al. Role of family history of sudden death in risk stratification and prevention of sudden death with implantable defibrillators in hypertrophic cardiomyopathy. *Am J Cardiol.* 2010;106:1481-1486. Copyright © 2010 with permission from Elsevier.)

while Fig 4 illustrates that these rates were similar between groups with and without a family history of SD when multiple risk factors were considered. The authors conclude that family history is an important and powerful predictor of events. In examining the results, it is clear that the group that did not have a family history of SD had a higher incidence and greater overall number of other classic risk factors for SD in HM (ie, nonsustained ventricular tachycardia, marked septal thickness, etc). Also, the numbers in this study were relatively small to draw meaningful conclusions to apply to the entire HM population. Finally, the rate of inappropriate ICD discharges in this cohort is quite high. Clinicians should carefully weight the overall risk for SD in individual patients with HM, taking into consideration family history but realizing that the presence or absence of other risk factors may be equally important when considering ICD implantation. Additionally, thoughtful programming of ICDs is necessary to avoid inappropriate therapy, which recently has been shown to have significant impact on morbidity and mortality in ICD patients.

F. A. Cuoco, Jr, MD, MBA

Light-to-moderate alcohol consumption and risk of sudden cardiac death in women
Chiuve SE, Rimm EB, Mukamal KJ, et al (Brigham and Women's Hosp and Harvard Med School, Boston, MA; Beth Israel Deaconess Med Ctr, Boston, MA)
Heart Rhythm 7:1374-1380, 2010

Background.—Moderate alcohol intake is associated with lower risk of coronary heart disease (CHD), but the association with sudden cardiac death (SCD) is less clear. In men, heavy alcohol consumption may increase risk of SCD, whereas light-to-moderate alcohol intake may lower risk. There are no parallel data among women.

Objective.—The purpose of this study was to assess the association between alcohol intake and risk of SCD among women and to investigate how this risk compared to other forms of CHD.

Methods.—We conducted a prospective cohort study among 85,067 women from the Nurses' Health Study who were free of chronic disease at baseline. Alcohol intake was assessed every 4 years through question-naires. Primary endpoints included SCD, fatal CHD, and nonfatal myocar-dial infarction.

Results.—We found a U-shaped association between alcohol intake and risk of SCD, with the lowest risk among women who drank 5.0−14.9 g/day of alcohol (P for quadratic trend $= 0.02$). Compared to abstainers, the multivariate relative risk (95% confidence interval) for SCD was 0.79 (0.55−1.14) for former drinkers, 0.77 (0.57-1.06) for 0.1−4.9 g/day, 0.64 (0.43−0.95) for 5.0−14.9 g/day, 0.68 (0.38−1.23) for 15.0−29.9 g/day, and 1.15 (0.7−01.87) for ≥30.0 g/day. In contrast, the relationship of alcohol intake and nonfatal and fatal CHD was more linear (P for linear trend <.001).

Conclusion.—In this cohort of women, the relationship between light-to-moderate alcohol intake and SCD is U-shaped, with a nadir at

5.0–14.9 g/day. Low levels of alcohol intake do not raise the risk of SCD and may lower risk in women (Fig 1).

▶ Alcohol consumption is associated with decreased all-cause mortality and cardiovascular disease in a J-shaped curve, with higher mortality observed in patients who do not consume alcohol or consume excessive amounts. Previous studies also demonstrated less sudden cardiac death (SCD) with moderate alcohol use, but these studies had limited inclusion of women. This study by Chiuve et al addresses the association of alcohol consumption and SCD in 121 700 women aged 30 to 55 years from the Nurses' Health Study. Extensive

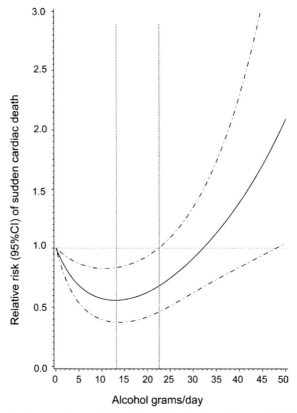

FIGURE 1.—Multivariate relative risk of sudden cardiac death as a function of alcohol intake. Data are fitted by a restricted cubic spline Cox proportional hazards model. The 95% confidence intervals (CI) are indicated by the *dashed lines*. Models adjusted for age, calories, smoking, body mass index, parental history of myocardial infarction, menopausal status, use of postmenopausal hormones, aspirin use, multivitamin and vitamin E supplements, physical activity, intake of omega-3 fatty acid, alpha-linolenic fatty acid, and trans-fatty acid, intake ratio of polyunsaturated to saturated fatty acids, diagnosis of coronary heart disease, stroke, diabetes, high blood pressure, and high cholesterol. The spline was based on 247 cases after the exclusion of former drinkers and women with intake >50 g/day. (Reprinted from Chiuve SE, Rimm EB, Mukamal KJ, et al. Light-to-moderate alcohol consumption and risk of sudden cardiac death in women. *Heart Rhythm*. 2010;7:1374-1380, with permission from Heart Rhythm Society.)

efforts were performed to increase the accuracy of SCD classification, and results were adjusted for age, diet, cardiovascular disease risk factors, and caloric intake. Women who consumed 5.0 to 14.9 g alcohol daily (approximately 0.5 to 1 drink/day) accounted for 50% of the study population and had the lowest risk of SCD in a U-shaped association ($P = .0003$) over 26 years of follow-up (Fig 1). There was no significant difference in risk of SCD between abstainers and women who had higher amounts of alcohol intake. Risk of SCD was unchanged when evaluated for type of alcohol intake (wine, beer, or liquor). A study of this size evaluating the association of alcohol consumption and SCD in women has not been performed previously, and the high number of study participants, significant number of SCD events, and extended period of follow-up time are notable. Despite the significant association demonstrated of decreased risk of SCD in women with moderate alcohol intake, clinicians must remember that current evidence demonstrates a strong association rather than cause.

R. N. Vest III, MD

Targeted Temperature Management for Comatose Survivors of Cardiac Arrest
Holzer M (Med Univ of Vienna, Austria)
N Engl J Med 363:1256-1264, 2010

A 62-year-old man collapses on the street, and emergency medical personnel who are called to the scene find that he is not breathing and that he has no pulse. The first recorded cardiac rhythm is ventricular fibrillation. Advanced cardiac life-support measures, including intubation, a total dose of 2 mg of epinephrine, and six defibrillation attempts, restore spontaneous circulation 22 minutes after the onset of the event. On admission to the emergency department, his condition is hemodynamically stable and he has adequate oxygenation and ventilation, but he is still comatose. A neurologic examination reveals reactive pupils and a positive cough reflex. The core body temperature is 35.5°C. A diagnosis of the post—cardiac arrest syndrome with coma is made. An intensive care specialist evaluates the patient and recommends the immediate initiation of targeted temperature management (Table 1).

▶ The case presented in this article illustrates an appropriate indication for use of targeted temperature management for a comatose survivor after successful restoration of spontaneous circulation status after a ventricular fibrillation arrest. There are about 350 000 to 450 000 out-of-hospital cardiac arrests yearly in the United States, and unfortunately only 40 000 survive to hospital admission. Many of these patients develop the post—cardiac arrest syndrome, including brain injury, myocardial dysfunction, systemic ischemia, and reperfusion responses, and less than half have a good neurologic recovery.

During cardiac arrest, oxygen stores are lost in seconds followed by loss of glucose and adenosine triphosphate (ATP) stores within 5 minutes. Ultimately,

TABLE 1.—Indications and Contraindications for Targeted Temperature Management in Comatose Patients after Cardiac Arrest

Patients for whom therapeutic hypothermia should be considered

Adult patients successfully resuscitated from a witnessed out-of-hospital cardiac arrest of presumed cardiac cause (patients after in-hospital cardiac arrest may also benefit)[28]

Patients who are comatose (i.e., patients with a score on the Glasgow Coma Scale of less than 8 or patients who do not obey any verbal command at any time after restoration of spontaneous circulation and before initiation of cooling)

Patients with an initial rhythm of ventricular fibrillation or nonperfusing ventricular tachycardia (patients presenting with other initial rhythms such as asystole or pulseless electrical activity may also benefit)[28]

Patients whose condition is hemodynamically stable (retrospective data suggest that patients in cardiogenic shock may also safely undergo hypothermia treatment)[29,30]

Patients for whom therapeutic hypothermia should not be considered

Patients with tympanic-membrane temperature below 30°C on admission

Patients who were comatose before the cardiac arrest

Pregnant patients

Patients who are terminally ill or for whom intensive care does not seem to be appropriate

Patients with inherited blood coagulation disorders

Editor's Note: Please refer to original journal article for full references.

excitotoxic cell death occurs. Reperfusion and reoxygenation cause reperfusion injury. Targeted temperature management (therapeutic hypothermia) limits neurologic injury by decreasing oxygen utilization and ATP consumption. Additionally, hypothermia decreases release of glutamate and dopamine as well as decreases apoptosis.

In 2002, 2 trials were published to support the use of therapeutic hypothermia. An Australian trial enrolled 77 comatose survivors of ventricular fibrillation or pulseless ventricular tachycardia. Half were cooled to 33°C for 12 hours. Forty-nine percent of the 43 patients treated with hypothermia had a favorable neurologic recovery at discharge compared with 26% of 34 normothermic patients (odds ratio, 5.25; 95% confidence interval [CI], 1.47-18.76; $P = .01$). A European multicenter trial enrolled 275 comatose survivors of a ventricular fibrillation or pulseless ventricular tachycardia arrest. Roughly half of these patients were cooled to 32°C to 34°C. Fifty-five percent of the 136 hypothermia-treated patients had a favorable neurologic outcome compared with 39% of the 137 normothermia-treated patients (risk ratio for a favorable outcome, 1.4; 95% CI, 1.08-1.81).

Based on the enrollment criteria of these studies, Table 1 describes indications and contraindications for targeted temperature management in comatose patients after cardiac arrest. Ideally, if chosen as a strategy, earlier cooling is better but should not be initiated if arrest was greater than 10 hours earlier. Fig 1 in the original article is an illustration demonstrating different methods of cooling, including precooled surface cooling pads, water-circulating surface cooling pads, and invasive catheter-based endovascular device for infusion of cold intravenous fluids. Sedation, analgesia, and paralysis should be initiated to prevent shivering, which may increase oxygen consumption via adrenergic response to hypothermia. Core body temperature is typically measured at central monitoring sites, such as the esophagus or Swan-Ganz catheter. Monitoring of metabolic disturbances (hypokalemia, hypomagnesemia, hypophosphatemia, and hyperglycemia) is necessary. Continuous electroencephalographic monitoring of seizures is prudent. After hypothermia is maintained for 24 hours, the patient should be rewarmed slowly (0.3°C-0.5°C per hour). Some patients may remain comatose for an extended period of time after resuscitation and rewarming; thus, it can be difficult to assess prognosis in the short term.

Adverse effects of targeted temperature management directly related to the cooling device or because of hypothermia occur in 1% (29 events of 3133 patients) and include bleeding, infection, deep-vein thrombosis, and pulmonary edema. There was no difference in adverse effects of targeted temperature management not related to cooling device compared with the patients treated without hypothermia (74% compared with 71%; $P = .31$).

In conclusion, therapeutic hypothermia is an important treatment strategy in patients who have return of spontaneous rhythm after cardiac arrest. The improvement in favorable outcome is worth the 1% event rate of adverse reactions. Furthermore, per the authors, this adds only $30 000 over the average cost for conventional care. There are still areas of uncertainty including the optimal sedation regimen and prognostic indicators once cooled, as hypothermia can confound traditional prognosticators. The 2003 and 2008 International Liaison Committee on Resuscitation, the 2005 European Resuscitation Council, and the American Heart Association all recommend that the core body temperature of unconscious adult patients with spontaneous circulation after an out-of-hospital ventricular fibrillation cardiac arrest should be lowered to 32°C to 34°C as soon as possible after the arrest and should be continued for at least 12 to 24 hours.

D. S. Sidney, MD

Vitamin D deficiency is associated with sudden cardiac death, combined cardiovascular events, and mortality in haemodialysis patients
Drechsler C, Pilz S, Obermayer-Pietsch B, et al (Univ of Würzburg, Germany; Med Univ of Graz, Austria; et al)
Eur Heart J 31:2253-2261, 2010

Aims.—Dialysis patients experience an excess mortality, predominantly of sudden cardiac death (SCD). Accumulating evidence suggests a role of vitamin D for myocardial and overall health. This study investigated the impact of vitamin D status on cardiovascular outcomes and fatal infections in haemodialysis patients.

Methods and Results.—25-hydroxyvitamin D [25(OH)D] was measured in 1108 diabetic haemodialysis patients who participated in the German Diabetes and Dialysis Study and were followed up for a median of 4 years. By Cox regression analyses, we determined hazard ratios (HR) for pre-specified, adjudicated endpoints according to baseline 25(OH)D levels: SCD ($n = 146$), myocardial infarction (MI, $n = 174$), stroke ($n = 89$), cardiovascular events (CVE, $n = 414$), death due to heart failure

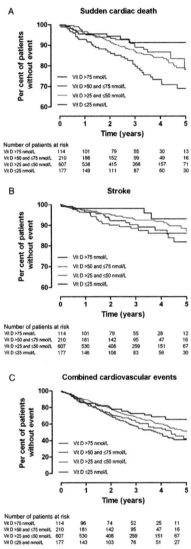

FIGURE 1.—Kaplan–Meier curves for the time to (A) sudden cardiac death, (B) stroke, (C) combined cardiovascular events in subgroups of patients according to 25-hydroxyvitamin D levels at baseline [severely vitamin D deficient (≤25 nmol/L), moderately vitamin D deficient (>25 and ≤50 nmol/L), vitamin D insufficient (>50 and ≤75 nmol/L), and vitamin D sufficient (>75 nmol/L)]. (Reprinted from Drechsler C, Pilz S, Obermayer-Pietsch B, et al. Vitamin D deficiency is associated with sudden cardiac death, combined cardiovascular events, and mortality in haemodialysis patients. *Eur Heart J.* 2010;31:2253-2261, with permission of The European Society of Cardiology.)

($n = 37$), fatal infection ($n = 111$), and all-cause mortality ($n = 545$). Patients had a mean age of 66 ± 8 years (54% male) and median 25(OH)D of 39 nmol/L (interquartile range: 28–55). Patients with severe vitamin D deficiency [25(OH)D of ≤ 25 nmol/L] had a 3-fold higher risk of SCD compared with those with sufficient 25(OH)D levels >75 nmol/L [HR: 2.99, 95% confidence interval (CI): 1.39—6.40]. Furthermore, CVE and all-cause mortality were strongly increased (HR: 1.78, 95% CI: 1.18—2.69, and HR: 1.74, 95% CI: 1.22—2.47, respectively), all persisting in multivariate models. There were borderline non-significant associations with stroke and fatal infection while MI and deaths due to heart failure were not meaningfully affected.

Conclusion.—Severe vitamin D deficiency was strongly associated with SCD, CVE, and mortality, and there were borderline associations with stroke and fatal infection. Whether vitamin D supplementation decreases adverse outcomes requires further evaluation (Fig 1).

▶ Hemodialysis patients experience high rates of cardiovascular events, including sudden cardiac death (SCD), myocardial infarction (MI), and stroke. Previous studies have demonstrated an association between cardiovascular events and low 25-hydroxyvitamin D [25(OH)D] levels that is often a clinical characteristic of patients with end-stage renal disease requiring dialysis. Therefore, the authors of this study aimed to characterize the association of vitamin D deficiency in hemodialysis patients with specific cardiac, vascular, and infection-related outcomes by analyzing the German Diabetes and Dialysis Study (4D study) population.

The 4D study comprises 1255 patients randomized to either low-dose atorvastatin 20 mg or placebo with a primary end point of death from cardiac causes, fatal or nonfatal stroke, and nonfatal MI over a median 4-year follow-up period. A total of 1108 patients in the 4D study had 25(OH)D levels measured at baseline and were included in this analysis. Patients were divided into 4 groups according to their baseline 25(OH)D levels and outcomes were evaluated. Hazard ratios for patients with the lowest quartile of 25(OH)D determined by Cox regression analysis were 2.99 (95% confidence interval [CI], 1.39-6.4) for SCD, 1.78 (95% CI, 1.18-2.69) for cardiovascular events (death from cardiac cause, fatal or nonfatal stroke, and nonfatal MI), and 1.74 (95%CI, 1.22-2.47) for all-cause mortality (Fig 1). Low 25(OH)D levels were not associated with an increase in death due to heart failure, MI, or infection.

While the authors suggest that these results implicate low 25(OH)D levels as a risk factor for SCD, cardiovascular events, and all-cause mortality, it is unclear if low vitamin D levels have a mechanistic role in these outcomes or if they are actually a risk marker for disease severity. This study is hypothesis generating and encourages further evaluation of the role of vitamin D in cardiovascular disease, including the possibility of risk modification through vitamin D supplementation in at-risk individuals.

C. P. Rowley, MD

Miscellaneous

Intracoronary ethanol ablation: A novel technique for ablation of ventricular fibrillation

Duncan E, Schilling RJ (Barts and the London NHS Trust, UK)
Heart Rhythm 7:1131-1134, 2010

Initiation of ventricular fibrillation (VF) by ventricular premature beats (VPBs) has been described in patients with heart disease and in those with structurally normal hearts. In both clinical scenarios, targeted endocardial

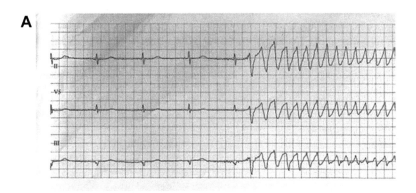

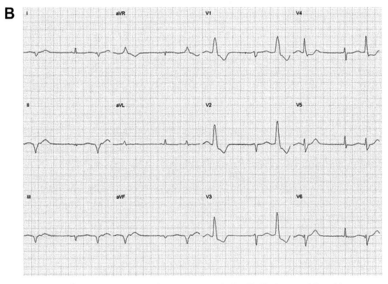

FIGURE 1.—A: The patient experienced recurrent ventricular fibrillation precipitated by a monomorphic ventricular ectopic. B: Twelve-lead ECG demonstrated frequent monomorphic ectopy. (Reprinted from Duncan E, Schilling RJ. Intracoronary ethanol ablation: a novel technique for ablation of ventricular fibrillation. *Heart Rhythm.* 2010;7:1131-1134, with permission from Heart Rhythm Society.)

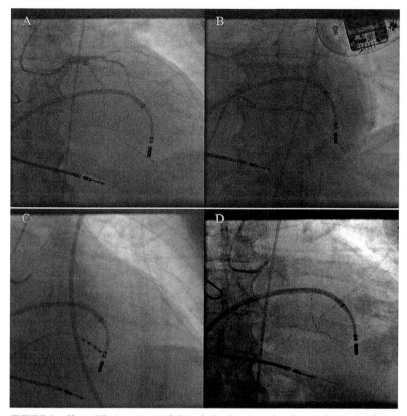

FIGURE 3.—Choice PT wire was passed through the chronic total occlusion of the circumflex coronary artery into the distal portion of an obtuse marginal branch. Fluoroscopy performed in the posteroanterior (**A**), left anterior oblique (**B**), and right anterior oblique (**C**) views confirmed that the vessel supplied the territory marked by the tip of the ablation catheter. **D:** A 1.0 × 14 over-the-wire balloon was inflated to occlude the midvessel, after which contrast was injected distal to the balloon. This technique confirmed that only the target vessel had been isolated, that the wire had remained intravascular, and that no extravasation had occurred. (Reprinted from Duncan E, Schilling RJ. Intracoronary ethanol ablation: a novel technique for ablation of ventricular fibrillation. *Heart Rhythm.* 2010;7:1131-1134, with permission from Heart Rhythm Society.)

catheter ablation of the site of origin of the VPB has resulted in long-term freedom from VF recurrence; however, acute procedural success is not always achieved. In this report, we describe intracoronary ethanol ablation of VF in a patient with ischemic cardiomyopathy who presented with electrical storm and in whom endocardial catheter ablation was unsuccessful (Figs 1A, B and 3).

▶ This article describes a 67-year-old man with multiple appropriate implantable cardioverter-defibrillator (ICD) shocks secondary to ventricular fibrillation triggered by a monomorphic ventricular premature beat (VPB). He initially underwent an endocardial ablation (both transseptal and retrograde approaches) after ruling out acute ischemia as a cause. Despite excellent pacemapping with

12/12 lead confirmation, and successful ablation, the patient returned in 72 hours after an additional 15 appropriate shocks, again initiated by a VPB (Fig 1A). A 12-lead electrocardiogram revealed frequent monomorphic VPB (Fig 1B) and so returned to the lab where VPB was again mapped to the inferior posterior wall of the ventricle. Pacemapping again demonstrated a 12/12 match to the clinical VPB and the map electrogram preceded the VPB surface electrogram by 82 milliseconds. The physician had extensively ablated this area 3 days earlier, so rather than reattempting to ablate the same region endocardially, the decision was made to proceed with ethanol ablation. Ninety-six percent absolute ethanol was injected into the distal circumflex, which had been chronically occluded and identified as the blood supply to the region of concern (Fig 3). Twelve months after the procedure, the patient has not received any therapy from his ICD, and VPBs did not recur.

The European Heart Rhythm Association/Heart Rhythm Society consensus on catheter ablation of ventricular arrhythmias reported that ethanol ablation should be considered only in unstable cases refractory to endocardial and epicardial ablation. This technique is currently used infrequently but may be useful in certain clinical scenarios such as this, in which endocardial ablation may not be successful. In this case, the target myocardium was low voltage, consistent with prior myocardial infarction, and was supplied by a chronically occluded vessel.

D. S. Sidney, MD

Impact of radiofrequency ablation of frequent post-infarction premature ventricular complexes on left ventricular ejection fraction

Sarrazin J-F, Labounty T, Kuhne M, et al (Univ of Michigan Health System, Ann Arbor)
Heart Rhythm 6:1543-1549, 2009

Background.—Frequent idiopathic premature ventricular complexes (PVC) are associated with a reversible form of cardiomyopathy. The effect of frequent PVCs on left ventricular function has not been evaluated in post-infarction patients.

Objective.—This study sought to evaluate the value of post-infarction PVC ablation and possible determinants of a reversible cardiomyopathy.

Methods.—Thirty consecutive patients (24 men, age 61 ± 12, left ventricular ejection fraction [LVEF] 0.36 ± 0.12) with remote myocardial infarction referred for implantable cardioverter-defibrillator (ICD) implantation for primary prevention of sudden death or for management of symptomatic ventricular tachycardia or PVCs were evaluated. Fifteen patients with a high PVC burden ($\geq 5\%$ of all QRS complexes on 24-h Holter monitor) underwent mapping and ablation of PVCs before ICD implantation. The remaining 15 patients served as a control group. LVEF was assessed by echocardiography, and scar burden was assessed by cardiac magnetic resonance imaging with delayed enhancement (DE-MRI) in both groups.

Results.—PVC ablation was successful in 15 of 15 patients and reduced the mean PVC burden from 22 ± 12% to 2.6 ± 5.0% (*P* <.001). After the procedure, LVEF increased significantly from 0.38 ± 0.11 to 0.51 ± 0.09 in the PVC ablation group (*P* =.0001). In the control group, LVEF remained unchanged within the same time frame (0.34 ± 0.14 vs. 0.33 ± 0.15; *P* =.6). Patients with frequent PVCs had a significantly smaller scar burden by DE-MRI compared with control patients. Five of the patients with frequent PVCs underwent ICD implantation.

Conclusion.—Post-infarction patients with frequent PVCs may have a reversible form of cardiomyopathy. DE-MRI may identify patients in whom the LVEF may improve after ablation of frequent PVCs (Fig 1).

▶ Frequent premature ventricular complexes (PVCs) have been shown to cause a potentially reversible tachycardia-induced cardiomyopathy similar to that observed with incessant supraventricular and ventricular tachycardias (VTs). This article extends this observation to patients with frequent PVCs in the setting of a previous myocardial infarction and ischemic cardiomyopathy with no significant ischemic areas. Successful endocardial ablation of PVCs resulted in significant improvement in left ventricular systolic function and functional class and decreased left ventricular diastolic dimension compared with their control group with ischemic cardiomyopathy and similar ejection fraction (EF) but infrequent PVCs. Of note, delayed enhancement MRI demonstrated less scarring in the ablation group compared with the control group (despite similar EFs), suggesting functional and thus potentially reversible dysfunction relative to the control group. PVCs were ablated in various sites but in most cases within the region of endocardial scar defined by MRI and voltage potential mapping similar to where sustained VTs are mapped.

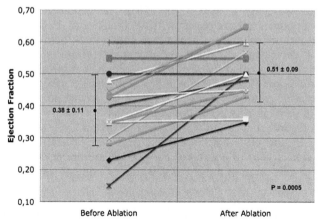

PVC Ablation Group

FIGURE 1.—Left ventricular ejection fractions before and after premature ventricular complex (PVC) ablation. (Reprinted from Sarrazin J-F, Labounty T, Kuhne M, et al. Impact of radiofrequency ablation of frequent post-infarction premature ventricular complexes on left ventricular ejection fraction. *Heart Rhythm.* 2009;6:1543-1549.)

Interestingly, 3 of the 4 patients in the ablation group with inducible sustained VT were no longer inducible after ablation of PVCs alone. In addition, most of the patients who were candidates for implantable cardioverter-defibrillators (ICDs) for secondary prevention of sudden cardiac death based upon an EF < 35% prior to ablation were no longer candidates after improvement in their EF after ablation. Thus, ablation of PVC foci is a useful clinical approach to improving systolic function in patients with ischemic cardiomyopathy and frequent ectopy. How much ventricular ectopy is needed to cause reversible dysfunction is not known, but delayed enhancement MRI demonstrating systolic dysfunction disproportionately decreased relative to fixed scar may suggest those most likely to benefit.

J. M. Wharton, MD

Cryoablation Versus Radiofrequency Energy for the Ablation of Atrioventricular Nodal Reentrant Tachycardia (the CYRANO Study): Results From a Large Multicenter Prospective Randomized Trial
Deisenhofer I, Zrenner B, Yin Y-H, et al (Technische Universität München, Munich, Germany; Krankenhaus Landshut-Achdorf, Germany; Chongqing Univ of Med Sciences, China; et al)
Circulation 122:2239-2245, 2010

Background.—Cryoablation has emerged as an alternative to radiofrequency catheter ablation (RFCA) for the treatment of atrioventricular (AV) nodal reentrant tachycardia (AVNRT). The purpose of this prospective randomized study was to test whether cryoablation is as effective as RFCA during both short-term and long-term follow-up with a lower risk of permanent AV block.

Methods and Results.—A total of 509 patients underwent slow pathway cryoablation (n=251) or RFCA (n=258). The primary end point was immediate ablation failure, permanent AV block, and AVNRT recurrence during a 6-month follow-up. Secondary end points included procedural parameters, device functionality, and pain perception. Significantly more patients in the cryoablation group than the RFCA group reached the primary end point (12.6% versus 6.3%; $P=0.018$). Whereas immediate ablation success (96.8% versus 98.4%) and occurrence of permanent AV block (0% versus 0.4%) did not differ, AVNRT recurrence was significantly more frequent in the cryoablation group (9.4% versus 4.4%; $P=0.029$). In the cryoablation group, procedure duration was longer (138 ± 54 versus 123 ± 48 minutes; $P=0.0012$) and more device problems occurred (13 versus 2 patients; $P=0.033$). Pain perception was lower in the cryoablation group ($P<0.001$).

Conclusions.—Cryoablation for AVNRT is as effective as RFCA over the short term but is associated with a higher recurrence rate at the 6-month follow-up. The risk of permanent AV block does not differ significantly between cryoablation and RFCA. The potential benefits of cryoenergy relative to ablation safety and pain perception are counterbalanced by longer procedure times, more device problems, and a high recurrence rate. *Clinical Trial Registration.*—URL: http://www.clinicaltrials.gov. Unique identifier: NCT00196222.

▶ The most common reentrant supraventricular tachycardia in clinical practice is atrioventricular nodal reentrant tachycardia (AVNRT). Ablation of this arrhythmia is common practice in symptomatic patients with high success rates and low recurrence rates. Slow pathway modification has emerged as the preferred ablation approach because of low rates of complete heart block. Although radiofrequency (RF) energy is most commonly used for ablation, other energy sources are used in selected cases. Cryoablation has the advantage of reversible freezing to test efficacy before permanent myocardial damage is achieved with more prolonged and lower temperature freezes. Cryoablation is commonly used in the pediatric population in attempts to minimize the risk of heart block in young patients with small hearts. The Cryoablation Versus Radiofrequency Energy for the Ablation of Atrioventricular Nodal Reentrant Tachycardia study was the first large randomized study comparing RF and Cryo for ablation of AVNRT in a typical adult population with this arrhythmia. Recurrence rates were higher with cryoablation, whereas there was no significant difference in heart block or clinical complications. These results indicate that Cryo has no advantage over RF for ablation of AVNRT in adults at experienced centers.

M. R. Gold, MD, PhD

Atrial Arrhythmias in Patients With Arrhythmogenic Right Ventricular Cardiomyopathy/Dysplasia and Ventricular Tachycardia

Chu AF, Zado E, Marchlinski FE (Hosp of the Univ of Pennsylvania, Philadelphia)

Am J Cardiol 106:720-722, 2010

Information on atrial arrhythmia associated with right ventricular cardiomyopathy/dysplasia (ARVC/D) is limited. In 36 patients with task force criteria for ARVC/D and history of ventricular tachycardia (VT), we confirmed the incidence and type of atrial arrhythmia, onset related to referral for VT ablation, fastest documented ventricular rate, management, and clinical and hemodynamic factors associated with their development. Thirty-six patients (28 men) had a mean age of 47 years (range 17 to 80) and mean follow-up of 56 ± 44 months. Thirty-five patients (97%) had implantable cardioverter—defibrillator (ICD) devices, 15 with atrial leads. Fifteen of 36 patients (42%) had documented atrial arrhythmias, with atrial flutter (aFL) in 11, atrial fibrillation (AF) in 11 patients, and aFL and AF in 7 patients. Maximum heart rate noted with atrial arrhythmia was 62 to 150 beats/min. In 9 patients, initial atrial arrhythmia preceded or was concurrent with presentation for VT ablation. In the remaining 6 patients, atrial arrhythmia (symptomatic in 4 patients) followed VT presentation. Three of these patients received ICD shock therapy for atrial arrhythmias. Seven of 11 patients with recurrent aFL required aFL ablation, 1 patient underwent His-bundle ablation for AF with rapid rate, and 8 patients required long-term drug therapy for AF control. Atrial arrhythmias were more common in patients with RV enlargement and moderate/severe tricuspid regurgitation. In conclusion, in patients with ARVC/D and VT, atrial arrhythmias are common, frequently necessitate ablative or pharmacologic treatment, and are more common in patients with moderate/severe tricuspid regurgitation and markedly enlarged right ventricle (Table 1).

▶ Little is known about the coexistence of atrial arrhythmias in patients with arrhythmogenic right ventricular dysplasia (ARVD). Chu et al performed an observational study of the incidence/type of atrial arrhythmias in sequential patients that met task force criteria for arrhythmogenic right ventricular cardiomyopathy/ARVD referred for ventricular tachycardia ablation. Analysis of surface electrocardiographs (as available) and stored implantable cardioverter-defibrillator (ICD) electrograms confirmed the incidence and type of arrhythmia. Atrial arrhythmias were also characterized with respect to timing of onset to presentation and fastest ventricular rate. Thirty-six patients met criteria for enrollment. Thirty-five patients (97%) had an ICD, of whom 15 (42%) had dual-chamber devices. Forty-two percent of patients had documented atrial arrhythmias, of whom 11 (31%) had typical cavotricuspid isthmus dependant flutter, 11 (31%) had atrial fibrillation, and 7 (19%) had both typical atrial flutter and atrial fibrillation. There were no incidences of atypical atrial flutter documented. This high incidence of atrial fibrillation and flutter was noted despite a relatively young age for this cohort (Table 1). The maximum heart rate noted with atrial arrhythmia was 62 to 150 beats per minute. Three patients received inappropriate ICD therapy because of atrial arrhythmias with rapidly conducted ventricular response. Patients with documented atrial arrhythmias were more likely to be older in age, have moderate to severe tricuspid regurgitation, and/or increased right ventricular volume (> 250 mL) as determined by endocardial mapping at the time of ablation. This study demonstrates the high prevalence of atrial arrhythmias in patients with ARVD. Furthermore, it may suggest implementation of dual chamber ICDs for

TABLE 1.—Clinical and Echocardiographic Imaging Characteristics of Patients With Versus Without Atrial Arrhythmias

| | AF/aFL | | |
Variable	Yes (n = 15)	No (n = 21)	p Value
Men (%)	12 (80%)	16 (76%)	NS
Age (years)	52 ± 16	43 ± 16	0.08
Moderate—severe tricuspid regurgitation	8/13* (62%)	4/19* (21%)	≤0.05
Moderate—severe right atrial dilatation	7/14* (50%)	5/19* (26%)	NS
Left ventricular ejection fraction (%)	43 ± 19	53 ± 11	NS
Right ventricular volume from electroanatomical map (ml)	313 ± 94	195 ± 53	≤0.01

*Not all transthoracic echocardiograms reported all values or were available for review.

documentation of atrial arrhythmias and attention to device programming in patients undergoing device implantation for ARVD.

J. L. Sturdivant, MD

A Novel Mutation in the *HCN4* Gene Causes Symptomatic Sinus Bradycardia in Moroccan Jews

Laish-Farkash A, Glikson M, Brass D, et al (Sheba Med Ctr, Tel Hashomer, Israel; Tel Aviv Univ, Israel; et al)
J Cardiovasc Electrophysiol 21:1365-1372, 2010

Objectives.—To conduct a clinical, genetic, and functional analysis of 3 unrelated families with familial sinus bradycardia (FSB).

Background.—Mutations in the hyperpolarization-activated nucleotide-gated channel (*HCN4*) are known to be associated with FSB.

Methods and Results.—Three males of Moroccan Jewish descent were hospitalized: 1 survived an out-of-hospital cardiac arrest and 2 presented with weakness and presyncopal events. All 3 had significant sinus bradycardia, also found in other first-degree relatives, with a segregation suggesting autosomal-dominant inheritance. All had normal response to exercise and normal heart structure. Sequencing of the *HCN4* gene in all patients revealed a C to T transition at nucleotide position 1,454, which resulted in an alanine to valine change (A485V) in the ion channel pore found in most of their bradycardiac relatives, but not in 150 controls. Functional expression of the mutated ion channel in *Xenopus* oocytes and in human embryonic kidney 293 cells revealed profoundly reduced function and synthesis of the mutant channel compared to wild-type.

Conclusions.—We describe a new mutation in the *HCN4* gene causing symptomatic FSB in 3 unrelated individuals of similar ethnic background that may indicate unexplained FSB in this ethnic group. This profound functional defect is consistent with the symptomatic phenotype.

▶ An increasing number of single-gene mutations that affect cardiac electrical activity have been recognized recently. These include mutations that cause channelopathies associated with long QT syndrome, Brugada syndrome, and short QT syndrome. Less frequently, inherited bradycardia syndromes have been recognized. In this study, Laish-Farakash et al report a novel inherited genetic mutation in the hyperpolarization-activated nucleotide-gated channel (*HCN4*) in members of 3 unrelated families in a community of Moroccan Jews, resulting in symptomatic familial sinus bradycardia. Genetic sequencing of affected and nonaffected individuals identified a new polymorphism in the affected group that results in an A485V mutation in the HCN4 protein. Patch clamp analysis using wild-type and mutant RNA–injected *Xenopus* oocytes demonstrated significantly reduced whole-cell currents using mutant RNA compared with wild type. Reduced whole-cell currents were also observed in A485V-transfected HEK 293 cells compared with wild type–transfected cells.

The A485V mutation results in alteration of the pore region of *HCN4*, which is the site of the G480R mutation, also associated with familial sinus bradycardia. A485V is the fifth reported *HCN4* mutation in humans, all of which result in sinus node dysfunction and/or arrhythmias. This report further implicates *HCN4* as an important regulator of sinus node function via its role as a modulator of the I$_f$ current.

M. L. Bernard, MD, PhD

Heart rate as a risk factor in chronic heart failure (SHIFT): the association between heart rate and outcomes in a randomised placebo-controlled trial
Böhm M, on behalf of the SHIFT Investigators (Universitätsklinikum des Saarlandes, Homburg/Saar, Germany; et al)
Lancet 376:886-894, 2010

Background.—Raised resting heart rate is a marker of cardiovascular risk. We postulated that heart rate is also a risk factor for cardiovascular events in heart failure. In the SHIFT trial, patients with chronic heart failure were treated with the selective heart-rate-lowering agent ivabradine. We aimed to test our hypothesis by investigating the association between heart rate and events in this patient population.

Methods.—We analysed cardiovascular outcomes in the placebo (n=3264) and ivabradine groups (n=3241) of this randomised trial, divided by quintiles of baseline heart rate in the placebo group. The primary composite endpoint was cardiovascular death or hospital admission for worsening heart failure. In the ivabradine group, heart rate achieved at 28 days was also analysed in relation to subsequent outcomes. Analysis adjusted to change in heart rate was used to study heart-rate reduction as mechanism for risk reduction by ivabradine directly.

Findings.—In the placebo group, patients with the highest heart rates (≥87 beats per min [bpm], n=682, 286 events) were at more than twofold higher risk for the primary composite endpoint than were patients with the lowest heart rates (70 to <72 bpm, n=461, 92 events; hazard ratio [HR] 2.34, 95% CI 1.84–2.98, p<0.0001). Risk of primary composite endpoint events increased by 3% with every beat increase from baseline heart rate and 16% for every 5-bpm increase. In the ivabradine group, there was a direct association between heart rate achieved at 28 days and subsequent cardiac outcomes. Patients with heart rates lower than 60 bpm at 28 days on treatment had fewer primary composite endpoint events during the study (n=1192; event rate 17.4%, 95% CI 15.3–19.6) than did patients with higher heart rates. The effect of ivabradine is accounted for by heart-rate reduction, as shown by the neutralisation of the treatment effect after adjustment for change of heart rate at 28 days (HR 0.95, 0.85–1.06, p=0.352).

Interpretation.—Our analysis confirms that high heart rate is a risk factor in heart failure. Selective lowering of heart rates with ivabradine

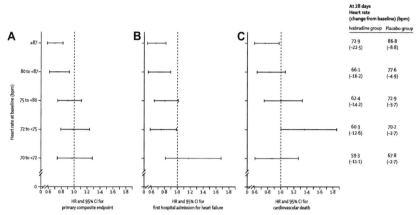

FIGURE 2.—Effect of ivabradine compared with placebo on (A) the primary composite endpoint, (B) first hospital admissions for worsening heart failure, and (C) cardiovascular deaths in the whole patient population, defined by quintiles of baseline heart-rate distribution. Primary composite endpoint includes cardiovascular deaths and hospital admissions for worsening heart failure. Adjusted for β-blocker intake at randomisation, New York Heart Association class, left-ventricular ejection fraction, ischaemic cause, age, systolic blood pressure, and creatinine clearance at baseline. HR=hazard ratio. bpm=beats per min. (Reprinted from Böhm M, on behalf of the SHIFT Investigators. Heart rate as a risk factor in chronic heart failure (SHIFT): The association between heart rate and outcomes in a randomised placebo-controlled trial. *Lancet*. 2010;376:886-894, with permission from Elsevier.)

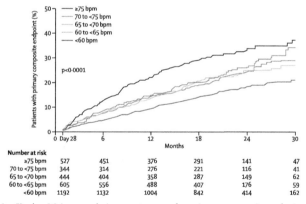

FIGURE 4.—Kaplan-Meier cumulative event curves for primary composite endpoint events in the ivabradine group, according to groups defined by heart rate achieved at 28 days. Data exclude patients reaching primary composite endpoint (cardiovascular death or hospital admission for worsening heart failure) during the first 28 days of follow-up. The log-rank p value is shown for the difference between the Kaplan-Meier curves. (Reprinted from Böhm M, on behalf of the SHIFT Investigators. Heart rate as a risk factor in chronic heart failure (SHIFT): The association between heart rate and outcomes in a randomised placebo-controlled trial. *Lancet*. 2010;376:886-894, with permission from Elsevier.)

improves cardiovascular outcomes. Heart rate is an important target for treatment of heart failure (Figs 2 and 4).

▶ Heart rate is a predictor of mortality in advanced heart failure (HF). β-Blockers have been shown to improve survival in this population, but it is not clear whether the mechanism is reducing heart rate or blocking other β-adrenergic functions. The Systolic Heart failure treatment with the I_f inhibitor ivabradine Trial (SHIFT) analyzed the effect of the I_f current antagonist, ivabradine, in a population with a chronic HF. A total of 6905 patients with New York Heart Association class II and higher symptoms, left-ventricular ejection fraction of < 35%, and sinus rhythm with rates above 70 beats per minute (bpm) were randomized to placebo or ivabradine and were assessed for cardiovascular death or hospitalization and worsening HF. As a selective bradycardic agent, ivabradine was studied to assess the effect of heart rate control alone on patients with HF. Baseline heart rate in the placebo group predicted a 2-fold difference in primary outcomes when comparing the highest (> 87 bpm) with the lowest (70-72 bpm) quintiles (Fig 2). Ivabradine-treated patients in the lowest on-treatment quintile (< 60 bpm) reached significantly fewer primary end points at 28 days compared with those in the highest quintile (> 75 bpm). As summarized in Fig 4, the SHIFT demonstrates that ivabradine can improve cardiovascular outcomes by providing rate control alone and baseline heart rate is a modifiable risk factor in population with a chronic HF.

M. L. Bernard, MD, PhD

Article Index

Chapter 1: Hypertension

Chapter 2: Pediatric Cardiovascular Disease Tetralogy of Fallot

Chapter 3: Cardiac Surgery Aortic Disease

Chapter 4: Coronary Heart DiseaseAcute ST-Segment Elevation Myocardial Infarction

Chapter 5: Non-Coronary Heart Disease in Adults

Chapter 6: Cardiac Arrhythmias, Conduction Disturbances, and ElectrophysiologyAtrial Fibrillation

Author Index

Printed and bound by CPI Group (UK) Ltd, Croydon, CR0 4YY

08/05/2025

01864677-0017